Nurse Practitioner
Certification
Examination and
Practice Preparation

Nurse Practitioner Certification Examination and Practice Preparation

SECOND EDITION

Margaret A. Fitzgerald

MS, APRN, BC, NP-C, FAANP, CSP
President, Fitzgerald Health Education Associates, Inc.
North Andover, Massachusetts
Family Nurse Practitioner
Adjunct Faculty, Family Practice Residency
Greater Lawrence Family Health Center
Lawrence, MA

F.A. DAVIS COMPANY • PHILADELPHIA

F. A. Davis Company
1915 Arch Street
Philadelphia, PA 19103
www.fadavis.com

Printed in the United States of America

Last digit indicates print number: 10 9 8 7 6

Acquisitions Editor: Joanne Patzek DaCunha, RN, MSN
Developmental Editor: Kristin L. Kern
Design & Illustration Manager: Joan Wendt

ISBN 10: 0-8036-1159-5   ISBN 13: 978-0-8036-1159-7

As new scientific information becomes available through basic and clinical research, recommended treatments and drug therapies undergo changes. The author(s) and publisher have done everything possible to make this book accurate, up to date, and in accord with accepted standards at the time of publication. The author(s), editors, and publisher are not responsible for errors or omissions or for consequences from application of the book, and make no warranty, expressed or implied, in regard to the contents of the book. Any practice described in this book should be applied by the reader in accordance with professional standards of care used in regard to the unique circumstances that may apply in each situation. The reader is advised always to check product information (package inserts) for changes and new information regarding dose and contraindications before administering any drug. Caution is especially urged when using new or infrequently ordered drugs.

To those who have contributed to the success of
Fitzgerald Health Education Associates, Inc..
My husband and business partner, Marc Comstock,
who believed in the company's potential
The FHEA, Inc. staff, whose dedication and hard work
have helped the company grow
Our family, who has supported and cheered us on
The NP community, whose commitment to their profession
and practice serve as a constant source of inspiration

Acknowledgments

This book represents a sum of the efforts of many people.

I thank Joanne Patzek DaCunha of F.A. Davis for her ongoing encouragement.

I thank my family, especially my husband and business partner Marc Comstock, for their good nature as they lived through this experience.

I thank the staff of Fitzgerald Health Education Associates, Inc., for sharing me with this project for many months.

I thank the patients and staff of the Greater Lawrence (MA) Family Health Center as they continue to serve as a source of inspiration as I developed this book.

Last but not least, I thank the thousands of nurse practitioners who, over the years, have attended the Fitzgerald Health Education Associates, Inc., Nurse Practitioner Certification and Practice Preparation courses. Your eagerness to learn, thirst for knowledge, and dedication to success continue to inspire me. It is indeed a privilege to be part of your professional development.

Introduction

This book represents a perspective on learning and practice that I have developed in my experience as a family nurse practitioner (NP) at the Greater Lawrence (MA) Family Health Center as well as an NP and family practice residency faculty member and professional speaker. In addition, my experience in the years of helping thousands of NPs achieve professional success through conducting NP Certification and Practice Preparation Courses influenced the development and presentation of the information within this book.

The scope of practice of the NP is wide, encompassing the care of the young, the old, the sick, and the well. This book has been developed to help the NP develop the knowledge and skills to successfully enter practice as well as achieve certification, an important landmark in professional achievement.

This book is not intended to be a comprehensive primary care text but rather a source to reinforce learning and a guide for the development of the information base needed for NP practice. The reader is encouraged to answer the questions given in each section and then check on the accuracy of his or her response. The discussion section is intended to enhance learning through highlighting the essentials of primary care NP practice. The numerous tables can serve as a quick-look resource not only as the NP prepares for entry to practice and certification but also in the delivery of ongoing care.

Margaret A. Fitzgerald, MS, APRN, BC, NP-C, FAANP, CSP
PRESIDENT
FITZGERALD HEALTH EDUCATION ASSOCIATES, INC.
NORTH ANDOVER, MA
FAMILY NURSE PRACTITIONER
ADJUNCT FACULTY, FAMILY PRACTICE RESIDENCY
GREATER LAWRENCE (MA) FAMILY HEALTH CENTER

Contents

1 Health Promotion and Disease Prevention — 1

2 Neurologic Disorders — 21

3 Skin Disorders — 39

4 Eye, Ear, Nose, and Throat Problems — 63

5 Chest Disorders — 87

6 Abdominal Disorders — 125

7 Male Genitourinary System — 153

8 Musculoskeletal Disorders — 169

9 Peripheral Vascular Disease — 199

10 Endocrine Disorders — 215

11 Hematologic and Immunologic Disorders — 241

12 Psychosocial Disorders — 261

13 Female Reproductive and Genitourinary Systems — 289

14 Pediatrics — 313

15 Childbearing — 359

Appendix: Answers to Your Most Common Test-Taking Questions — 383

Index — 393

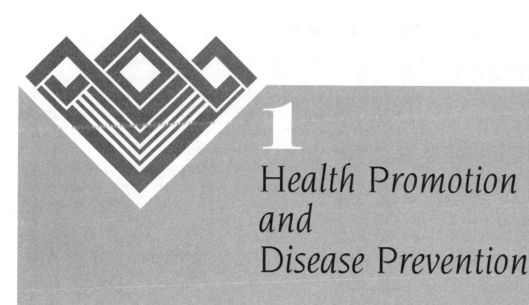

1
Health Promotion and Disease Prevention

1. An example of a primary prevention measure for a 78-year-old man with chronic obstructive pulmonary disease is:

    A. reviewing the use of prescribed medications.
    B. ensuring adequate illumination in the home.
    C. checking pulmonary function.
    D. performing a digital rectal examination and fecal occult blood test (FOBT).

2. Which of the following is an example of a primary prevention activity in a 76-year-old woman with osteoporosis?

    A. bisphosphonate therapy
    B. calcium supplementation
    C. home survey to identify fall hazards
    D. use of a back brace

3. Secondary prevention measures for a 78-year-old man with chronic obstructive pulmonary disease include:

    A. checking stool for occult blood.
    B. administering influenza vaccine.
    C. obtaining a serum theophylline level.

    D. advising about appropriate use of car passenger restraints.

4. Tertiary prevention measures for a 69-year-old woman with congestive heart failure include:

    A. administering antipneumococcal vaccine.
    B. adjusting therapy to minimize dyspnea.
    C. surveying skin for precancerous lesions.
    D. reviewing safe handling of food.

5. Which of the following provides passive immunity?

    A. hepatitis B immune globulin (HBIG)
    B. measles, mumps, and rubella (MMR) vaccine
    C. pneumococcal conjugate vaccine
    D. influenza vaccine

6. Active immunity is defined as:

    A. resistance developed in response to an antigen.
    B. immunity conferred by an antibody produced in another host.
    C. the resistance of a group to an infectious agent.
    D. defense against disease acquired naturally by the infant from the mother.

DISCUSSION

Primary prevention measures include activities provided to individuals to prevent the onset of a given disease. The goal of primary prevention measures is to spare individuals the suffering, burden, and cost associated with the clinical condition. Examples include health-protecting education and counseling, such as encouraging the use of car restraints and bicycle helmets and providing information on accident prevention.

Immunizations and chemoprophylaxis are also examples of primary prevention measures. Active immunization through the use of vaccines provides long-term protection from disease. The use of vaccines is preferred to passive immunization through the use of immune globulin (IG), because IG use provides only temporary protection. In herd immunity, a significant portion of a given population has immunity against an infectious agent; therefore the likelihood that the susceptible portion of the groups becomes infected is minimized (Table 1–1).

Secondary prevention measures include activities provided to identify and treat asymptomatic persons who have risk factors for a given disease or in preclinical disease. Examples include screening examinations for preclinical evidence of cancer, including mammography and cervical examination with Papanicolaou smear. Other examples of secondary prevention activities include screening for clinical conditions with a protracted asymptomatic period, such as blood pressure measurement to detect hypertension and lipid profile to detect hyperlipidemia.

Tertiary prevention measures are part of the management of a person with an established disease. The goal is to minimize disease-associated complications and the negative health effects of the conditions. Examples include medications and lifestyle modification to normalize blood glucose levels in individuals with diabetes mellitus and treatment of hyperlipidemia in patients who have coronary heart disease.

DISCUSSION SOURCE

U.S. Preventive Services Task Force (1996). Guide to Clinical Preventive Services (2nd ed.). Baltimore: Williams & Wilkins.

QUESTIONS

7. When advising a patient about injectable influenza immunization, the nurse practitioner (NP) considers the following about the vaccine:

    A. Its use is contraindicated during pregnancy.

    B. Its use is limited to children older than 6 years.

    C. It contains live virus.

    D. It is recommended for household members of high-risk patients.

8. A middle-aged man with chronic obstructive pulmonary disorder who is about to receive injectable influenza vaccine should be advised that:

    A. it is more than 90% effective in preventing influenza.

    B. its use is contraindicated in the presence of eczema.

    C. localized reactions from the immunization are fairly common.

    D. a short, intense flulike syndrome typically occurs after immunization.

9. A 44-year-old woman with asthma presents asking for influenza vaccine. She is currently taking ciprofloxacin for treatment of a urinary tract infection, does not have a fever, and is feeling better. You inform her that she:

    A. should return for the immunization after completing her antibiotic therapy.

TABLE 1–1

CLINICAL PREVENTIVE SERVICES FOR NORMAL-RISK ADULTS
RECOMMENDED BY THE U. S. PREVENTIVE SERVICES TASK FORCE

	Range of Recommended Ages											
Years of Age ►	**18**	**25**	**30**	**35**	**40**	**45**	**50**	**55**	**60**	**65**	**70**	**75**
▼ SCREENING												
Blood pressure, height, and weight	Periodically →											
Obesity	Periodically →											
Cholestrol*				Men: every 5 years →								
						Women: every 5 years →						
Pap smear	Women: every 1 to 3 years →											
Chlamydia	(18 only)											
Mammography					Every 1 to 2 years →							
Colorectal cancer*							Depends on test →					
Osteoporosis										Routinely →		
Alcohol use	Periodically →											
Vision, hearing										Periodically →		
▼ IMMUNIZATION												
Tetanus-diptheria (Td)	Every 10 years →											
Varicella (VZV)	Susceptibles only: two doses →											
Measles, mumps, rubella (MMR)**	Women of childbearing age: one dose →											
Pneumococcal										One dose →		
Influenza							Yearly →					
▼ CHEMOPREVENTION												
Assess cardiovascular disease (CVD) risk and discuss aspirin to prevent CVD events					Men: periodically →							
							Women: periodically →					
▼ COUNSELLING												
Calcium intake	Women: periodically →											
Folic acid	Women of childbearing age →											
Breastfeeding	Women after childbirth →											
Tobacco cessation, drug and alcohol use, STDs and HIV, nutrition, physical activity, sun exposure, oral health, injury prevention, and polypharmacy	Periodically →											

Upper age limits should be individualized for each patient.

*See www.preventiveservices.ahrq.gov for U.S. Preventive Services Task Force recommendations
on colorectal cancer screening and other clinical preventive services.

**If 2 MMR dose =>1 month apart not previously given or if demonstrated immunity to these diseases.

(continued)

TABLE 1–1

CLINICAL PREVENTIVE SERVICES FOR NORMAL-RISK ADULTS
RECOMMENDED BY THE U. S. PREVENTIVE SERVICES TASK FORCE *(continued)*

BY MEDICAL CONDITIONS

Medical Conditions	Vaccine						
	Tetanus-Diphtheria (Td)*,[1]	Influenza[2]	Pneumococcal (Polysaccharide) [3,4]	Hepatitis B*,[5]	Hepatitis A [6]	Measles, Mumps, Rubella (MMR)*,[7]	Varicella*,[8]
Pregnancy		A					
Diabetes, heart disease; chronic pulmonary disease; chronic liver disease; including chronic alcoholism		B	C		D		
Congenital immunodeficiency, leukemia, lymphoma, generalized malignancy, therapywith alkylating agents, antimetabolites, radiation, or large amounts of corticosteroids			E				F
Renal failure/end-stage renal disease, recipients of hemodialysis or clotting factor concentrates			E	G			
Asplenia, including elective splenectomy and terminal complement component deficiencies		H	E, I, J				
Human immunodeficiency virus (HIV) infection			E, K			L	

For all persons in this group	Catch-up on childhood vaccinations	For persons with medical/ exposure indications	Contraindicated

Special notes for medical conditions

A. For women without chronic diseases/conditions, vaccinate if pregnancy will be at second or third trimester during influenza season. For women with chronic diseases/conditions, vaccinate at any time during the pregnancy.

B. Although chronic liver disease and alcoholism are not indicator conditions for influenza vaccination, give 1 dose annually if the patient is age 50 years or older, has other indications for influenza vaccine, or requests vaccination.

C. Asthma is an indicator condition for influenza but not for pneumococcal vaccination.

D. For all persons with chronic liver disease.

E. For persons < 65 years, revaccinate once after 5 years or more have elapsed since initial vaccination.

F. Persons with impaired humoral immunity but intact cellular immunity may be vaccinated.
MMWR 1999; 48 (RR-06): 1–5.

G. Hemodialysis patients: Use special formulation of vaccine (40

μg/mL) or two 1.0-mL 20 μg doses given at one site. Vaccinate early in the course of renal disease. Assess antibody titers to hepatitis B surface antigen (anti-HBs) levels annually. Administer additional doses if anti-HBs levels decline to < 10 mlu/mL.

H. There are no data specifically on risk of severe or complicated influenza infections among persons with asplenia. However, influenza is a risk factor for secondary bacterial infections that may cause severe disease in asplenics.

I. Administer meningococcal vaccine and consider (Hib) vaccine.

J. Elective splenectomy: vaccinate at least 2 weeks before surgery.

K. Vaccinate as close to diagnosis as possible when CD4 cell counts are highest.

L. Withhold MMR or other measles containing vaccines from HIV-infected persons with evidence of severe immunosuppression.
MMWR 1998; 47 (RR-8):21–22;
MMWR 2002;51 (RR-02):22–24.

TABLE 1–1

(Footnote continued)

1. **Tetanus-diphtheria (Td)**—Adults, including pregnant women with uncertain histories of a complete primary vaccination series should receive a primary series of Td. A primary series for adults is 3 doses: the first 2 doses given at least 4 weeks apart and the 3rd dose, 6–12 months after the second. Administer 1 dose if the person had received the primary series and the last vaccination was 10 years ago or longer. Consult MMWR 1991; 40 (RR-10): 1–21 for administering Td as prophylaxis in wound management. The American College of Physicians (ACP) Task Force on Adult Immunization supports a second option for Td use in adults: a single Td booster at age 50 years for persons who have completed the full pediatric series, including the teenage/young adult booster.
ACP Task force on Adult Immunization
Guide for Adult Immunization. (3rd ed, 1994:20).

2. **Influenza vaccination**—Medical indications: chronic disorders of the cardiovascular or pulmonary system, including asthma; chronic metabolic diseases including diabetes mellitus, renal dysfunction, hemoglobinopathies, or immunosuppression (including immunosuppression caused by medications or by human immunodeficiency virus [HIV]), requiring regular medical follow-up or hospitalization during the preceding year; women who will be in the second or third trimester of pregnancy during the influenza season. Occupational indications: health care workers. Other indications: residents of nursing homes and other long-term care facilities; persons likely to transmit influenza to persons at high risk (in-home care givers to persons with medical indications, household contacts and out-of-home caregivers of children from birth to 23 months of age, or children with asthma or other indicator conditions for influenza vaccination, household members and caregivers of elderly and adults with high-risk conditions); and anyone who wishes to be vaccinated. For healthy persons aged 5–49 years without high-risk conditions, either the inactivated vaccine or the intranasally administered influenza vaccine (Flumist) may be given.
MMWR 2003; 52(RR-8): 1–36; *MMWR* 2003; 53(RR-13):1–8.

3. **Pneumococcal polysaccharide vaccination**—Medical indications: chronic disorders of the pulmonary system (excluding asthma); cardiovascular diseases, diabetes mellitus, chronic liver diseases, including liver disease as a result of alcohol abuse (e.g., cirrhosis); chronic renal failure or nephrotic syndrome; functional or anatomic asplenia (e.g., sickle cell disease or splenectomy); immunosuppressive conditions (e.g., congenital immunodeficiency, HIV infection, leukemia, lymphoma, multiple myeloma, Hodgkin disease, generalized malignancy, organ or bone marrow transplantation), chemotherapy with alkylating agents, antimetabolites; or long-term systemic corticosteroids. Geographic/other indications: Alaskan natives and certain American Indian populations. Other indications: residents of nursing homes and other long-term care facilities.
MMWR 1997; 46(RR-8): 1–24.

4. **Revaccination with pneumococcal polysaccharide vaccine**—One-time revaccination after 5 years for persons with chronic renal failure or nephrotic syndrome, functional or anatomic asplenia (e.g., sickle cell disease or splenectomy), immunosuppressive conditions (e.g., congenital immunodeficiency, HIV infection, leukemia, lymphoma, multiple myeloma, Hodgkin disease, generalized malignancy, organ or bone marrow transplantation), chemotherapy with alkylating agents, antimetabolites, or long-term systemic corticosteroids. For persons 65 years and older, one-time revaccination if they were vaccinated 5 or more years previously and were aged less than 65 years at the time of primary vaccination.
MMWR 1997; 46 (RR-8): 1–24.

5. **Hepatitis B vaccination**—Medical indications: hemodialysis patients, patients who receive clotting-factor concentrates. Occupational indications: health care workers and public safety workers who have exposure to blood in the workplace, persons in training in schools of medicine, dentistry, nursing, laboratory technology, and other allied health professions. Behavioral indications: injection drug users, persons with more than one sex partner in the previous 6 months, persons with a recently acquired sexually transmitted disease (STD), all clients in STD clinics, men who have sex with men. Other indications: household contacts and sex partners of persons with chronic HBV infection, clients and staff of institutions for the developmentally disabled, international travelers who will be in countries with high or intermediate prevalence of chronic HBV infection for more than 6 months, inmates of correctional facilities. *MMWR* 1991; 40(RR-13):1–19.
(www.cdc.gov/travel/diseases/hbv.htm).

6. **Hepatitis A vaccination**—For the combined hepatitis A–hepatitis B vaccine, use 3 doses at 0, 1, 6 months. Medical indications: persons with clotting factor disorders or chronic liver disease. Behavioral indications: men who have sex with men, users of injection and noninjection illegal drugs. Occupational indications: persons working with hepatitis A virus (HAV)–infected primates or with HAV in a research laboratory setting. Other indications: persons traveling to or working in countries that have high or intermediate endemicity of hepatitis A.
MMWR 1999; 48 (RR-12): 1–37. (www.cdc.gov/travel/diseases/hav.htm)

7. **Measles, mumps, rubella vaccination (MMR)**—Measles component: adults born before 1957 may be considered immune to measles. Adults born in or after 1957 should receive at least one dose of MMR unless they have a medical contraindication, documentation of at least 1 dose or other acceptable evidence of immunity. A 2nd dose of MMR is recommended for adults who:
   - are recently exposed to measles or in an outbreak setting.
   - were previously vaccinated with killed measles vaccine.
   - were vaccinated with an unknown vaccine between 1963 and 1967.
   - are students in postsecondary educational institutions.
   - work in health care facilities.
   - plan to travel internationally.

   Mumps component: 1 dose of MMR should be adequate for protection. Rubella component: give 1 dose of MMR to women whose rubella vaccination history is unreliable and counsel women to avoid becoming pregnant for 4 weeks after vaccination. For women of childbearing age, regardless of birth year, routinely determine rubella immunity and counsel women regarding congenital rubella syndrome. Do not vaccinate pregnant

(continued)

━━━ **TABLE 1–1** ━━━

CLINICAL PREVENTIVE SERVICES FOR NORMAL-RISK ADULTS
RECOMMENDED BY THE U. S. PREVENTIVE SERVICES TASK FORCE
(Footnote continued)

women or those planning to become pregnant in the next 4 weeks. If patient is pregnant and susceptible, vaccinate as early in postpartum period as possible.
MMWR 1998; 47(RR-8):1–57; *MMWR* 2001; 50:1117.

8. **Varicella vaccination**—Recommended for all persons who do not have reliable clinical history of varicella infection or serologic evidence of varicella-zoster virus (VZV) infection who may be at high risk for exposure or transmission. This includes health care workers and family contacts of immunocompromised persons, those who live or work in environments where transmission is likely (e.g., teachers of young children, day care employees, and residents and staff members in institutional settings), persons who live or work in environments where VZV transmission can occur (e.g., college students, inmates and staff members of correctional institutions, and military personnel), adolescents and adults living in households with children, women who are not pregnant but who may become pregnant in the future, international travelers who are not immune to infection. Note: Greater than 95% of U.S. born adults are immune to VZV. Do not vaccinate pregnant women or those planning to become pregnant in the next 4 weeks. If patient pregnant and susceptible, vaccinate as early in postpartum period as possible.

MMWR 1996; 45(RR-11):1–36; *MMWR* 1999; 48(RR-6): 1–5.

9. **Meningococcal vaccine (quadrivalent polysaccharide for serogroups A, C, Y, and W-135)**—Consider vaccination for persons with medical indications: adults with terminal complement component deficiencies, adults with anatomic or functional asplenia. Other indications: travelers to countries in which disease is hyperendemic or epidemic ("meningitis belt" of sub-Saharan Africa, Mecca, Saudi Arabia for Hajj). Revaccination at 3–5 years may be indicated for persons at high risk for infection (e.g., persons residing in areas in which disease is epidemic). Counsel college freshmen, especially those who live in dormitories, regarding meningococcal disease and the vaccine so that they can make an educated decision about receiving the vaccination.

Note: The AAFP recommends that colleges take the lead in providing education about meningococcal infection and vaccination and offer it to those who are interested. Physicians need not initiate discussion of the meningococcal quadrivalent polysaccharide vaccine as part of routine medical care.
MMWR 2000; 49 (RR-7): 1–20.

B. will likely develop a significant reaction if immunized today.

C. can receive the immunization today.

D. is not a candidate for influenza vaccine.

10. Which of the following best describes amantadine or rimantadine use in the care of patients with or at risk for influenza?

    A. Initiation of therapy early in acute influenza illness may minimize the severity of disease.

    B. The primary action of these therapies is in preventing influenza A during outbreaks.

    C. These therapies are active against influenza A and B.

    D. The use of these products is an acceptable alternative to influenza vaccine.

11. Which of the following best describes zanamivir (Relenza) or oseltamivir (Tamiflu) use in the care of patients with or at risk for influenza?

    A. Initiation of therapy early in acute influenza illness may minimize the severity of disease.

    B. Their primary action is in preventing influenza A during outbreaks.

    C. The drugs are active only against influenza B.

    D. Its use is an acceptable alternative to influenza vaccine.

12. When advising a patient about immunization with the nasal spray flu vaccine, the NP considers the following:

    A. Its use is acceptable during pregnancy.

    B. Its use is limited to children younger than 6 years.

    C. It contains live virus.

    D. It is recommended for household members of high-risk patients.

ANSWERS

7. D	**8.** C	**9.** C
10. B	**11.** A	**12.** C

DISCUSSION

Influenza is a viral illness that typically causes many days of incapacitation and suffering, as well as the risk of death. The influenza vaccine is about 70% to 80% effective in preventing influenza A or B or reducing the severity of the disease.

Mild to moderate illness or taking an antibiotic is not a contraindication to any immunization, including influenza immunization. Annual influenza vaccine is recommended for persons age 65 years and older, as well as for patients with some other disorders, including asthma. The injectable vaccine does not contain live virus and is not shed; therefore, there is no risk of transmitting an infectious agent to household contacts.

Injectable influenza vaccine may be used during pregnancy and is recommended for all pregnant women. The timing of flu shot administration is based largely on the vaccine's availability, as a formulation based on predicted influenza strains is produced annually. This vaccine may be given to infants as young as 6 months. Influenza vaccine is recommended for members of households with high-risk patients in order to avoid transmission of infection.

The nasal-spray flu vaccine, also known as attenuated influenza vaccine (LAIV) differs from the injectable influenza vaccine or "flu shot" because it contains weakened live influenza viruses instead of killed viruses and is administered by nasal spray instead of injection. The nasal-spray flu vaccine contains three different influenza viruses that are sufficiently weakened as to be incapable of causing disease but with sufficient strength to stimulate a protective immune response. The viruses in the LAIV are cold-adapted and temperature-sensitive. As a result, the viruses can grow in the nose and throat but not in the lower respiratory tract where the temperature is higher. LAIV is approved for use in healthy people between the ages of 5 and 49 years. Individuals who should not receive LAIV include patients younger than 5 years or older than 50 years of age with a medical condition that places them at high risk for complications from influenza, including those with chronic heart or lung disease, such as asthma or reactive airways disease, diabetes or kidney failure, and immunosuppression, and children or adolescents on chronic aspirin therapy, people with a history of Guillain-Barré syndrome, pregnant women, and people with a history of allergy to any of the components of LAIV or to eggs. In addition, there is a slight risk of transmission of the vaccine viruses and subsequent illness to close contacts. As a result, the use of inactivated influenza vaccine is the preferred method for vaccinating household members, health care workers, and others who have close contact with people who have weakened immune systems. LAIV's adverse effects include nasal irritation and discharge, muscle aches, sore throat, and fever. The optimal time to receive influenza vaccine is usually in October or November, about a month prior to the anticipated onset of the flu season. Children between the ages of 5 and 8 years who have never received influenza vaccine should receive the nasal spray flu vaccine for the first time in October or earlier because they need a second dose 6 to 10 weeks after the first dose.

If taken during the flu season, amantadine or rimantadine use is approximately 70% to 90% effective in preventing influenza A. These medications have a less favorable adverse reaction profile (nervousness, anxiety, difficulty concentrating, and lightheadedness, and gastrointestinal side effects) than does influenza vaccine, have a significantly higher cost, and have no activity against influenza B. As a result, active immunization against influenza A and B by administering the flu shot is the preferred method of disease prevention. Oseltamivir can also be used for prevention of influenza A and B by an at-risk person who comes in contact with a person with active influenza. Zanamivir and oseltamivir are used to treat influenza A and B infections, but treatment with any of these drugs can shorten the time a person infected with influenza feels ill by approximately 1 day, if treatment is started during the first 2 days of illness. Zanamivir is inhaled and can cause adverse effects such as bronchospasm, especially in patients with asthma or other chronic lung disease. Oseltamivir's adverse effects are largely gastrointestinal; the risk of nausea and vomiting is significantly reduced if the medication is taken with food. The use of all of these medications is significantly more expensive and less effective than influenza immunization.

DISCUSSION SOURCES

Recommendations for Using Antiviral Agents for Influenza (2004). Centers for Disease Control and Prevention. Available at http://www.CDC.GOV/flu/professionals/treatment/recommenda-tions.htm

National Immunization Program (2004). Atlanta, GA: Centers for Disease Control and Prevention. Available at www.cdc.gov/nip, accessed 9.12.04.

Center for Disease Control and Prevention, Q & A: The Nasal-Spray Flu Vaccine (Live Attenuated Influenza Vaccine [LAIV]), Available at http://www.cdc.gov/flu/about/qa/nasalspray.htm, accessed 7.20.04.

QUESTIONS

13. When considering an adult's risk for measles, mumps, and rubella (MMR), the NP considers the following:

    A. Patients born before 1957 are probably immune because of natural infection.
    B. Considerable mortality and morbidity occur with all three diseases.
    C. Most cases in the United States occur in infants.
    D. The use of the vaccine is often associated with protracted arthralgia.

14. Which of the following is true about the MMR vaccine?

    A. It contains inactivated virus.
    B. Its use is contraindicated in patients with a history of egg allergy.
    C. Revaccination of an immune person is associated with risk of allergic reaction.
    D. Two doses at least 1 month apart are recommended for young adults who have not been previously immunized.

15. A 22-year-old woman is starting a job in a college health center and needs proof of German measles and measles immunity. She received childhood immunizations and supplies documentation of MMR vaccination at age 1.5 years. Your best response is to:

    A. obtain rubella and rubeola titers.
    B. give MMR immunization now.
    C. advise her to obtain IG if she has been exposed to measles or rubella.
    D. advise her to avoid individuals with rashes.

ANSWERS

13. A   14. D   15. B

DISCUSSION

The MMR vaccine contains live but weakened (attenuated) virus. Two immunizations 1 month apart are recommended for adults born after 1957, because those born before then are considered immune as a result of having had these diseases (native or wild infection); vaccine against these three formerly common illnesses was not available until the 1960s. As with all vaccines, giving additional doses to patients with an unclear immunization history is safe (see Table 1–3).

Rubella typically causes a relatively mild, 3- to 5-day illness with little risk of complication to the person infected. However, when rubella is contracted during pregnancy, the effects on the fetus can be devastating. Immunizing the entire population against rubella protects unborn children from the risk of contracting congenital rubella syndrome. Measles can cause severe illness with serious sequelae, including encephalitis and pneumonia; sequelae of mumps include orchitis.

In the past, a history of egg allergy was considered a contraindication to receiving MMR vaccine. However, the vaccine now appears safe. Patients with a history of life-threatening allergic reaction to neomycin or gelatin should not receive MMR. The MMR vaccine is safe to use during lactation, but its use during pregnancy is discouraged because of the theoretical but unproven risk of congenital rubella syndrome from the live virus contained in the vaccine. MMR vaccine is well tolerated; there have been rare reports of mild, transient adverse reactions such as rash and sore throat.

DISCUSSION SOURCE

MMR vaccine. (2004). Atlanta, GA: Centers for Disease Control and Prevention. Available at www.cdc.gov/nip/vaccine/mmr/default.htm, accessed 9.12.04.

QUESTIONS

16. When advising a patient about antipneumococcal immunization, the NP considers the following about the vaccine:

    A. It contains inactivated bacteria.

    B. It is contraindicated after splenectomy.

    C. It protects against community-acquired pneumonia caused by atypical pathogens.

    D. It is generally well tolerated.

17. Of the following, who is at greatest risk for invasive pneumococcal infection?

    A. a 68-year-old man with chronic obstructive pulmonary disease

    B. a 34-year-old woman who underwent splenectomy after a motor vehicle accident

    C. a 50-year-old man with a 15-year history of type 2 diabetes

    D. a 75-year-old woman with decreased mobility caused by rheumatoid arthritis

18. All of the following patients received a dose of antipneumococcal vaccine 5 years ago. Who is not a candidate for receiving a second dose of antipneumococcal immunization?

    A. a 45-year-old man with chronic bronchitis

    B. a 72-year-old woman with hypertension

    C. a 25-year-old man with a history of surgical splenectomy

    D. a 58-year-old woman with immunosuppression

ANSWERS

16. D   **17.** B   **18.** B

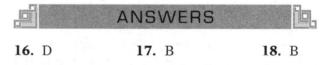

ANTIPNEUMOCOCCAL VACCINE ADVERSE REACTIONS	
Local reactions, including pain, redness	30%–50%
Fever, myalgia	Polysaccharide, < 1% Conjugate, 11%–64%
Severe, potentially life-threatening	Rare
Source: www.cdc.gov/nip/publications/pink/pneumon.pdf.	

DISCUSSION

Pneumococcal disease causes significant mortality and morbidity. The antipneumococcal vaccine contains purified polysaccharide from 23 of the most common strains of *Streptococcus pneumoniae*. These strains account for 90% of the bacteremic disease associated with this pathogen. The pneumococcal vaccine protects against pneumonia caused by *S. pneumoniae*, the leading cause of community-acquired pneumonia death in the United States. However, this immunization is ineffective against pneumonia caused by other infectious agents, including *Mycoplasma pneumoniae*, *Chlamydia pneumoniae*, *Legionella* species, and select gram-negative respiratory pathogens such as *Haemophilus influenzae* and *Moraxella catarrhalis*.

Antipneumococcal vaccine is recommended for persons age 65 years and older, for institutionalized individuals age 50 years and older, for persons younger than 65 years who have chronic cardiac or pulmonary conditions or diabetes mellitus, and for those who are asplenic. In particular, this vaccine is recommended for those with the greatest risk for invasive pneumococcal disease, including individuals with alcoholism, cirrhosis, chronic renal failure, nephrotic syndrome, congenital or acquired immunodeficiency, or malignancy, and those who are asplenic (see Tables 1–1 to 1–3).

Certain patients are candidates for antipneumococcal revaccination 5 years after the initial dose. These include everyone who was vaccinated before age 65, as well as people with functional or anatomic asplenia, immunosuppression, an organ transplant, chronic renal failure, and nephrotic syndrome. Reaction to pneumococcal vaccine is rare, but a mild local reaction may be seen, particularly with reimmunization.

DISCUSSION SOURCE

National Immunization Program (2004). Atlanta, GA: Centers for Disease Control and Prevention. Available at www.cdc.gov/nip, accessed 9.12.04.

QUESTIONS

19. Concerning hepatitis B virus (HBV) vaccine, which of the following is true?

    A. It contains live, whole HBV.
    B. All adults should have anti–hepatitis B surface antibody titers after three doses of vaccine.
    C. The vaccine should be offered during treatment for sexually transmitted diseases in unimmunized adults.
    D. Serologic testing for HBs antigen (HBsAg) should be done before hepatitis B vaccination is initiated in adults.

20. In which of the following groups is routine HBsAg screening recommended?

    A. hospital laboratory workers
    B. recipients of hepatitis B vaccine series
    C. pregnant women
    D. college students

21. You see a woman who has been sexually involved with a man newly diagnosed with acute hepatitis B. You advise her that she should:

    A. start a hepatitis B immunization series.
    B. limit the number of sexual partners.
    C. be tested for hepatitis B surface antibody (HBsAb).
    D. receive HBIG and hepatitis B immunization series

22. Hepatitis B vaccine should not be given to the person with a history of anaphylactic reaction to:

    A. egg.
    B. baker's yeast.
    C. neomycin.
    D. streptomycin.

23. Risks associated with chronic hepatitis B include all of the following except:

    A. hepatocellular carcinoma
    B. cirrhosis
    C. continued infectivity
    D. hypertension

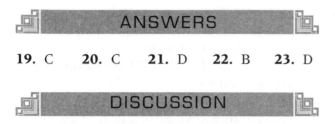

ANSWERS

19. C   **20.** C   **21.** D   **22.** B   **23.** D

DISCUSSION

Hepatitis B is caused by a small double-stranded DNA virus that contains an inner core protein of hepatitis B core antigen and an outer surface of HBsAg. The virus is transmitted through exchange of body fluids. Acute hepatitis B is a serious illness that can lead to hepatitic failure. Approximately 5% of those with acute hepatitis B develop chronic hepatitis B; chronic hepatitis B is a potent risk factor for hematoma or primary hepatocellular carcinoma and hepatic cirrhosis. The person with chronic hepatitis B continues to be able to transmit the virus.

Hepatitis B infection can be prevented by limiting exposure to blood and body fluids, as well as through immunization. Recombinant hepatitis B vaccine, which does not contain live virus, is well tolerated but is contraindicated in the person who has a history of anaphylactic reaction to baker's yeast (Table 1–3).

Infants who become infected perinatally with HBV have an estimated 25% lifetime chance of developing hepatocellular carcinoma or cirrhosis. As a result, all pregnant women should be screened for HBsAg at the first prenatal visit, regardless of HBV vaccine history. Because the HBV vaccine is not 100% effective, a woman may have carried HBsAg before becoming pregnant.

About 90% to 95% of those who receive the vaccine develop HBsAb (anti-HBs) after three doses, which implies protection from the virus. As a result, routine testing for the presence of HBsAb after immunization is not recommended. However, HBsAb testing should be considered to confirm the development of HBV protection in those with high risk for infection (e.g., select health care workers, injection drug users, sex workers) as well as those at risk for poor immune response (e.g., dialysis patients, immunosuppressed patients).

TABLE 1–2
IMMUNIZATION
CONTRAINDICATIONS

Anaphylaxis History	Immunization to Avoid
Neomycin	IPV, MMR, varicella
Streptomycin, polymyxin B, neomycin	IPV
Baker's yeast	Hepatitis B
Egg	Influenza vaccine

Source: www.cdc.gov/nip/recs/contraindications.htm guide, accessed 4/7/03.
IPV, inactivated poliovirus vaccine; MMR, measles, mumps, rubella vaccine.

Administration of HBIG after exposure, with a repeat dose in 1 month, is about 75% effective in protecting patients from hepatitis B after percutaneous, sexual, or mucosal exposure to HBV. HBV vaccine series should be started with postexposure HBIG.

DISCUSSION SOURCES

Friedman, L. (2003). Liver, biliary tract and pancreas. In Tierney, L., McPhee, S., and Papadakis, M. (eds.). Current Diagnosis and Treatment (38th ed., pp. 628–673). Norwalk, CT: Appleton & Lange.

Viral hepatitis (2004). National Center for Infectious Diseases. Available at www.CDC.GOV/NCIDOD/diseases/hepatitis, accessed 9.12.04.

QUESTIONS

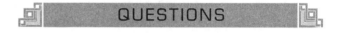

24. Which of the following best describes how smallpox is transmitted?

  A. direct deposit of infective droplets
  B. surface contact
  C. blood and body fluids
  D. vertical transmission

25. Smallpox disease includes which of the following characteristics?

  A. usually mild disease
  B. lesions that erupt over a number of days

C. loss of contagiousness once vesicles form

D. lesions all at the same stage

26. Smallpox vaccine contains:

A. live variola virus.

B. a virus fragment.

C. dead smallpox virus.

D. an antigenic protein.

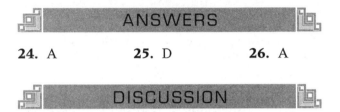

ANSWERS

24. A   **25.** D   **26.** A

DISCUSSION

Smallpox is a serious, contagious, and sometimes fatal infectious disease caused by the variola virus. There are a variety of clinical forms, of which variola major is the most common and severe form, carrying a fatality rate of around 30%. Smallpox in its naturally occurring form was globally eradicated after a successful worldwide vaccination program; the last U.S. case of smallpox was in 1949, and the last naturally occurring case in the world was in Somalia in 1977. As a result, routine vaccination for the general public was stopped in the United States in 1972. However, laboratory stockpiles of the variola virus do exist and could be used as a bioterrorism agent.

Smallpox is typically spread from person to person via direct deposit of infective droplets onto the nasal, oral, or pharyngeal mucosal membrane or in the alveoli of the lungs; direct and fairly prolonged face-to-face contact is required. Smallpox is sometimes contagious during the onset of fever (prodrome phase), but it becomes most contagious with the onset of rash. At this stage, the infected person is usually very sick and not able to move around in the community. The infected person is contagious until the last smallpox scab falls off. Less commonly, smallpox also can be spread through direct contact with infected bodily fluids or contaminated objects such as bedding or clothing. In rare cases, smallpox has been spread by virus carried in the air in enclosed settings such as buildings, buses, and trains. Smallpox cannot be transmitted to humans by insects or animals, nor can animals become ill with the disease.

Exposure to the virus is followed by an incubation period of about 7 to 17 days, during which the person does not have any symptoms and the disease is not contagious. The prodromal stage lasts 2 to 4 days, during which the person has a temperature of 101° to 104° F, malaise, headache, body aches, and sometimes vomiting. The person may be contagious at this time but is typically too sick to carry on normal activities. In the next stage, the rash appears first as small red spots on the tongue and in the mouth that develop into open sores that spread large amounts of the virus into the mouth and throat. At this time, the person becomes most contagious. The rash then appears on the skin, starting on the face and spreading first to the arms and legs and then to the hands and feet. Usually the rash spreads to all parts of the body within 24 hours, and the temperature typically falls. By day 3 of the rash, the skin lesions become raised, and by day 4 they fill with a thick, opaque fluid and become umbilicated. The temperature often rises again until the lesions crust over, in about 5 additional days. About 1 week later, the crusts begin to fall off, usually leaving a pitted scar. The person remains contagious until all of the crusts have fallen off.

Although both smallpox and varicella cause vesicular lesions, the clinical presentation of smallpox differs considerably from that of varicella (chickenpox). In varicella, the lesions typically erupt over days and are at various stages; some are vesicular, whereas some older lesions may be starting to crust over. In smallpox, all the skin lesions are usually at the same stage.

Smallpox treatment is largely supportive, inasmuch as there is no smallpox-specific therapy currently available. The person with suspect smallpox must be isolated swiftly. The NP should be aware of which local experts and governmental authorities need to be notified for a suspected case of smallpox.

In anticipation of possible exposure via bioterrorism, smallpox vaccination is being offered to or required of selected health and defense personnel such as first responders, emergency health care providers, and members of the military. Vaccination within 3 days of smallpox exposure prevents or significantly lessens the severity of smallpox symptoms in the vast majority of people, whereas vaccination 4 to 7 days after exposure likely offers some protection from disease or may modify the severity of disease.

Made from a live smallpox-related virus called vaccinia, the vaccine is given through a unique immunization method: A two-pronged needle is dipped into the vaccine solution. When removed, the needle retains a droplet of the vaccine. The needle is then used to prick the skin a number of times in a few seconds, producing a few drops of blood and some local discomfort. A red, itchy bump develops at the vaccine site in 3 to 4 days; this progresses to a large draining pustule over the next few days. During the second week, the blister begins to dry up, and a scab forms. The scab falls off in the third week, leaving a small scar. Until the scab falls off, the vaccine recipient can shed the vaccinia virus. This virus does not cause smallpox, but infection with this agent can result in serious cutaneous illnesses such as generalized vaccinia and eczema vaccinatum. As a result, the vaccination site must be cared for to prevent the vaccinia virus from spreading. The NP needs to be aware of current recommendations for smallpox vaccine candidates, as well as vaccine contraindications.

As with most vaccines, mild reactions include a few days of arm soreness and body aches. Fever may also be reported.

DISCUSSION SOURCE

Smallpox (2004). Atlanta, GA: Centers for Disease Control and Prevention. Available at www.bt.cdc.gov, accessed 9.12.04.

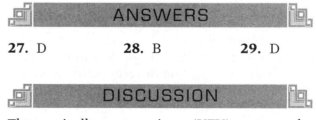

QUESTIONS

27. With the varicella vaccine, which of the following is correct?

   A. It contains killed varicella zoster virus.
   B. Its use is associated with an increase in reported cases of shingles.
   C. It should be offered to older adults who have a history of chickenpox.
   D. Although highly protective against invasive varicella disease, mild cases of chickenpox have been reported in immunized patients.

28. For which of the following patients should an NP order varicella antibody titers?

   A. a 14-year-old with an uncertain chickenpox history
   B. a health care worker who reports having had varicella as a child
   C. a 22-year-old woman who received two varicella immunizations 6 weeks apart
   D. a 72-year-old with shingles

29. A woman who has been advised to receive varicella-zoster IG asks about its risks. You respond that IG is a:

   A. synthetic product that is well tolerated.
   B. pooled blood product that often transmits infectious disease.
   C. blood product obtained from a single donor.
   D. pooled blood product with an excellent safety profile.

ANSWERS

27. D   28. B   29. D

DISCUSSION

The varicella-zoster virus (VZV) causes the highly contagious, systemic disease commonly known as chickenpox. Varicella infection usually confers lifetime immunity. However, reinfection may be seen in immunocompromised patients. More often, reexposure causes an increase in antibody titers without causing disease.

The VZV can lie dormant in sensory nerve ganglia. Later reactivation causes shingles, a painful, vesicular-form rash in a dermatomal pattern. About 15% of those who have had chickenpox develop shingles during their lifetimes. Shingles rates are markedly reduced in individuals who have received varicella vaccine compared with those who have had chickenpox.

A patient-reported history of varicella is considered a valid measure of immunity, with 97% to 99% having serologic evidence of immunity. Among adults with an unclear or negative varicella history, the majority are also seropositive. Confirming varicella immunity through varicella titers, even in the presence of a history of varicella infection, should be done in health care workers because of their risk of exposure and potential transmission of the disease.

Although the majority of cases are seen in children younger than 18 years, the greatest rate of mortality from varicella is in adults age 30 to 49 years.

The varicella vaccine, which contains attenuated virus, is administered in a single dose after the first birthday. Older children (13 years and older) and adults with no history of varicella infection or previous immunization should receive two immunizations 4 to 8 weeks apart. In particular, health care workers, family contacts of immunocompromised patients, and day care workers should be targeted for varicella vaccine, as should adults who are in environments with high risk of varicella transmission, such as college dormitories, military barracks, and long-term care facilities. The vaccine is highly protective against severe, invasive varicella. However, mild cases of chickenpox may be reported after immunization. (see Tables 1–1 and 1–3).

Varicella IG, as with all forms of IG, provides temporary, passive immunity to infection. IG is a pooled blood product with an excellent safety profile.

DISCUSSION SOURCE

Varicella (2004). Atlanta, GA: Centers for Disease Control and Prevention. Available at www.cdc. gov/nip/diseases/varicella, accessed 9.12.04.

QUESTIONS

30. An 18-year-old man has no primary tetanus immunization series documented. Which of the following represents the immunization needed?

   A. three doses of diphtheria, tetanus, and acellular pertussis (DTaP) vaccine 2 months apart
   B. tetanus IG now and two doses of tetanus-diphtheria (Td) vaccine 1 month apart
   C. Td vaccine now and repeated in 1 and 6 months
   D. Td vaccine as a single dose

31. Which wound presents the greatest risk for tetanus infection?

   A. a wound obtained while gardening
   B. a laceration obtained while trimming beef
   C. a human bite
   D. an abrasion obtained by falling on a sidewalk

ANSWERS

30. C   31. A

DISCUSSION

Tetanus infection is caused by *Clostridium tetani*, an anaerobic, gram-positive, spore-forming rod. This organism is found in soil, particularly if it contains manure. The organism enters the body through a contaminated wound, causing a life-threatening systemic disease characterized by painful muscle weakness and spasm ("lockjaw"). Diphtheria, caused by *Corynebacterium diphtheriae,* a gram-negative bacillus, is typically transmitted from person to person or through contaminated liquids such as milk. This organism causes severe respiratory tract infection, including the appearance of pseudomembranous pharyngitis.

Tetanus and diphtheria are uncommon infections because of widespread immunization. Because protective titers wane over time and adults are frequently lacking in up-to-date immunization, most cases of tetanus occur in persons older than 50 years.

A primary series of three Td vaccine injections sets the stage for long-term immunity. A booster Td dose every 10 years is recommended, but protection is probably present for 20 to 30 years after a primary series. Using Td vaccine rather than tetanus toxoid for primary series and booster doses in adulthood assists in keeping diphtheria immunity as well (see Tables 1–1 and 1–3).

At the time of wound-producing injury, tetanus IG affords temporary protection for persons who have not received tetanus immunization.

DISCUSSION SOURCE

Tetanus disease (2004). Atlanta, GA: Centers for Disease Control and Prevention. Available at www. cdc.gov/nip/diseases/tetanus, accessed 9.12.04.

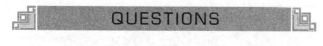

QUESTIONS

32. The most common source of hepatitis A infection is:

    A. needle sharing.
    B. raw shellfish.
    C. contaminated water supplies.
    D. intimate person-to-person contact.

33. When answering questions about hepatitis A vaccine, the NP considers that it:

    A. contains live virus.
    B. should be offered to those who frequently travel to developing countries.
    C. is required for all children.
    D. confers life-long protection after a single injection.

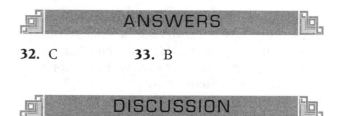

ANSWERS

32. C   **33.** B

DISCUSSION

Hepatitis A infection is caused by hepatitis A virus (HAV), a small RNA virus. Transmitted primarily by fecal-contaminated drinking water and food supplies, hepatitis A is typically a self-limiting infection with a very low mortality rate. Although eating raw shellfish that grew in contaminated water can be problematic, fecal-contaminated water supplies are the most common source of infection. In developing countries with limited pure water, the majority of the children contract this disease by age 5 years. In North America, adults age 20 to 39 years account for nearly 50% of the reported cases.

The hepatitis A vaccine, which contains inactivated virus, is given in two injections 6 to 12 months apart. Candidates include those who reside in or travel to areas where the disease is endemic, food handlers, sewage workers, animal handlers, day care attendees and workers, long-term care residents and workers, and military and laboratory personnel. Children who live in areas with a high incidence of hepatitis A should also be immunized. Injection drug users may also benefit from the vaccine. However, HAV is rarely transmitted sexually or from needle sharing; rather, injection drug users often live in conditions that facilitate the oral-fecal transmission of the hepatitis A virus. In addition, coinfection with hepatitis A and C, with hepatitis A and B, or acute hepatitis A in addition to a chronic liver disease may lead to a rapid deterioration in hepatic function. Therefore, persons with chronic hepatitis B and/or C or any chronic liver disease should be immunized against hepatitis A (see Tables 1–1 and 1–3).

DISCUSSION SOURCE

Friedman, L. (2003). Liver, biliary tract and pancreas. In Tierney, L., McPhee, S., and Papadakis, M. (eds.). Current Diagnosis and Treatment (42nd ed., pp 628–673). New York: Appleton Medical Books/McGraw-Hill.

Viral hepatitis (2004). National Center for Infectious Diseases. Available at www.CDC.GOV/NCIDOD/diseases/hepatitis, accessed 9.12.04.

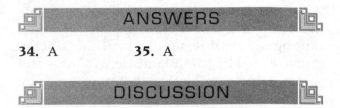

QUESTIONS

34. Which of the following is found in poliovirus infection?

    A. It is transmitted via the fecal-oral route.

    B. Rates of infection among household contacts are about 30%.

    C. Sporadic outbreaks continue to occur in North America.

    D. It is transmitted via aerosol and droplets.

35. A 30-year-old man with the human immunodeficiency virus (HIV) lives with his two preschool-aged children. Which of the following best represents advice you should give him about immunizing his children?

    A. Immunizations should take place without concern for his health status.

    B. The children should not receive influenza vaccine.

    C. MMR vaccine should not be given.

    D. The children should not receive poliovirus immunization.

ANSWERS

34. A   **35.** A

DISCUSSION

Polioviruses are highly contagious and capable of causing paralytic, life-threatening infections. Transmission is via the fecal-oral route, and rates of infection among household contacts can be as high as 96%.

For decades, North and South America have been free of indigenous poliomyelitis, largely because of the efficacy of the poliovirus vaccine and the safety of the drinking water supply. The use of inactivated poliovirus vaccine (IPV) is standard practice in the United States and Canada, whereas oral poliovirus vaccine (OPV) continues to be used in many developing nations. Oral poliovirus vaccine contains live virus, and its use is not recommended for people with immunosuppression, because of the small risk of the recipient's developing vaccine-associated paralytic poliomyelitis (VAPP). The recipient sheds attenuated virus in the stool for up to 3 months after receiving the dose. As a result, OPV use is not recommended if the vaccine recipient resides with a person with immunosuppression, including HIV, because this shedding places susceptible household members at risk for VAPP. Using IPV vaccine eliminates this risk (Table 1–3).

DISCUSSION SOURCE

Zimmerman, R., and Spann, S. (1999). Poliovirus vaccine options. American Family Physician 59(1):113–118.

QUESTIONS

36. When working with an obese middle-aged man on weight reduction, an NP considers that one of the first actions should be to:

    A. add an exercise program while minimizing the need for dietary changes.

TABLE 1–3

RECOMMENDED ADULT IMMUNIZATION SCHEDULE, UNITED STATES, 2003–2004 BY AGE GROUP

Vaccine	Age Group		
	19–49 Years	50–64 Years	65 Years and Older
Tetanus-diphtheria (Td)*	1 Dose booster every 10 years[1]		
Influenza	1 Dose annually[2]	1 Dose annually[2]	
Pneumococcal (polysaccharide)	1 Dose[3,4]		1 Dose[3,4]
Hepatitis B*	3 Doses (0, 1–2, 4–6 months)[5]		
Hepatitis A	2 Doses (0, 6–12 months)[6]		
Measles, mumps, rubella (MMR)*	1 Dose if measles, mumps, or rubella vaccination history is unreliable; 2 doses for persons with occupational or other indications[7]		
Varicella*	2 Doses (0, 4–8 weeks) for persons who are susceptible[8]		
Meningococcal (polysaccharide)	1 Dose[9]		

	For all persons in this group		Catch-up on childhood vaccinations		For persons with medical/ exposure indications

*Covered by the Vaccine Injury Compensation Program. For information on how to file a claim, call 800-338-2382. Please also visit www.hrsa.gov/osp/vicp. To file a claim for vaccine injury, contact U.S. Court of Federal Claims, 717 Madison Place, N.W., Washington D.C.20005, 202-219-9657.

This schedule indicates the recommended age groups for routine administration of currently licensed vaccines for persons 19 years of age and older. Licensed combination vaccines may be used whenever any components of the combination are indicated and the vaccine's other components are not contraindicated. Providers should consult the manufacturers' package inserts for detailed recommendations.

Report all clinically significant postvaccination reactions to the Vaccine Adverse Event Reporting System (VAERS). Reporting forms and instructions on filing a VAERS report are available by calling 800-822-7967 or from the VAERS website at www.vaers.org.

For additional information about the vaccines listed above and contraindications for immunization, visit the National Immunization Program Website at www.cdc.gov/nip/ or call the National Immunization Hotline at 800-232-2522 (English) or 800-232-0233 (Spanish).

Approved by the Advisory Committee on Immunization Practices (ACIP) and accepted by the American College of Obstetricians and Gynecologists (ACOG) and the American Academy of Family Physicians (AAFP).

    B. ask the patient about what he believes contributes to his weight problem.

    C. refer the patient to a nutritionist for diet counseling.

    D. ask for a commitment to lose weight.

37. A sedentary, obese 52-year-old woman is diagnosed with hypertension. What is the least helpful response to her statement "It is going to be too hard to diet, exercise, and take these pills"?

    A. "Try taking your medication when you brush your teeth."

B. "You really need to try to improve your health."

C. "Tell me what you feel will get in your way of improving your health."

D. "Could you start with reducing the amount of salt in your diet?"

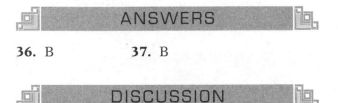

ANSWERS

36. B   **37.** B

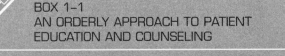

DISCUSSION

Possessing information about methods for preventing disease and maintaining health is an important part of patient education. However, knowledge alone does not ensure a change in behavior. NPs need to consider a number of factors in patient counseling and education (Box 1–1).

DISCUSSION SOURCE

U.S. Preventive Services Task Force (1996). Guide to Clinical Preventive Services (2nd ed.). Baltimore: Williams & Wilkins.

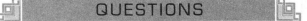

QUESTIONS

38. Which of the following is the most effective method of cancer screening?

   A. skin examination
   B. fecal occult blood test (FOBT)
   C. pelvic examination
   D. chest radiograph

39. Which of the following is a recommended method of annual colorectal cancer screening for a 62-year-old man?

   A. digital rectal examination
   B. in-office FOBT

BOX 1–1
AN ORDERLY APPROACH TO PATIENT EDUCATION AND COUNSELING

▼ Assess the patient's knowledge base about factors contributing to the problem.
▼ Evaluate the contribution of the patient's belief system to the problem.
▼ Ask the patient about perceived barriers to action as well as supporting factors.
▼ Match teaching to the patient's perception of the problem.
▼ Inform the patient about the purpose and benefit of an intervention.
▼ Give the patient an anticipated time of onset of effect of a therapy.
▼ Suggest small rather than large changes in behavior.
▼ Give accurate, specific information.
▼ Consider adding new positive behaviors rather than attempting to discontinue established behaviors.
▼ Link desired behavior with established behavior.
▼ Give a strong, personalized message about the seriousness of health risk.
▼ Ask for a commitment from the patient.
▼ Use a combination of teaching strategies, such as visual, oral, and written methods.
▼ Strive for an interdisciplinary approach to patient education and counseling, with all members of the team giving the same message.
▼ Maintain frequent contact with the patient to monitor progress.
▼ Expect gains and periodic setbacks.

Adapted from U.S. Preventive Services Task Force (1996). Guide to Clinical Preventive Services (2nd ed.). Baltimore: Williams & Wilkins.

C. at-home FOBT

D. sigmoidoscopy

40. According to the American Cancer Society recommendations, which of the following men should be screened for prostate cancer?

A. a 46-year-old African-American man

B. a 49-year-old man of Asian ancestry

C. a 86-year-old man with end-stage renal failure

D. a 38-year-old man with a recent history of acute prostatitis

41. Which of the following types of cancer screening is not routinely recommended in a 55-year-old woman?

A. breast

B. skin

C. endometrium

D. colorectal

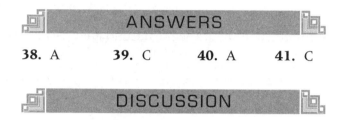

ANSWERS

38. A   **39.** C   **40.** A   **41.** C

DISCUSSION

Cancer screening is an important part of providing comprehensive health care. Adherence to current, nationally recognized guidelines is critical (Table 1–4).

TABLE 1–4

AMERICAN CANCER SOCIETY CANCER DETECTION GUIDELINES

BREAST

Breast self-examination monthly for women aged 20 and older

Breast clinical physical examination for women aged 20–40, every 3 years; older than 40, every year

- This examination should be done close to the time of the scheduled mammogram Ideally, the clinical breast examination should be done before the scheduled mammogram.

Mammography for women aged 40 and older, every year.

COLON AND RECTUM

Beginning at age 50, both men and women should follow one of these five testing schedules:

- Yearly fecal occult blood test (FOBT)
  - For FOBT, the take-home multiple sample method should be used.
- Flexible sigmoidoscopy every 5 years
- Yearly fecal occult blood test plus flexible sigmoidoscopy every 5 years
  - The combination of FOBT and flexible sigmoidoscopy is preferred over either of these two tests alone.
- Double-contrast barium enema study every 5 years
- Colonoscopy every 10 years
  - All positive test results should be followed up with colonoscopy

People should begin colorectal cancer screening earlier and/or undergo screening more often if they have any of the following colorectal cancer risk factors:

- Personal history of colorectal cancer or adenomatous polyps
- Strong family history of colorectal cancer or polyps (cancer or polyps in a first-degree relative younger than 60 or in two first-degree relatives of any age). Note: a first-degree relative is defined as a parent, sibling, or child.
- Personal history of chronic inflammatory bowel disease or a family history of hereditary colorectal cancer syndromes (familial adenomatous polyposis and hereditary nonpolyposis colon cancer).

Cervical

- Papanicolaou test and pelvic examination for women who are or have been sexually active or have reached age 18, every year; after three or more consecutive satisfactory normal annual examination results, the Papanicolaou test may be performed less frequently at the discretion of the health care provider.

(continued)

▬▬▬ **TABLE 1–4** ▬▬▬▬▬▬▬▬▬▬▬▬▬▬▬▬▬▬▬▬▬▬▬▬▬▬▬▬

AMERICAN CANCER SOCIETY CANCER DETECTION GUIDELINES *(continued)*

Prostate
- Guideline statement
  - Both the prostate-specific antigen (PSA) test and digital rectal examination (DRE) should be offered annually, beginning at age 50 years, to men who have at least a 10-year life expectancy. Men at high risk should begin testing at age 45 years.
- Information should be provided to men regarding potential risks and benefits of early detection and treatment of prostate cancer
  - Men who choose to undergo testing should begin at age 50 years. However, men in high-risk groups, such as African-Americans and men who have a first-degree relative in whom prostate cancer was diagnosed at a young age, should begin testing at 45 years. Note: a first-degree relative is defined as a father, brother, or son.
  - Men who ask their health care provider to make the decision on their behalf should be tested. Discouraging testing is not appropriate. Not offering testing is also not appropriate.
  - Testing for prostate cancer in asymptomatic men can detect tumors at a more favorable stage (anatomic extent of disease). There has been a reduction in mortality from prostate cancer, but it has not been established that this is a direct result of screening.
  - An abnormal PSA test result has been defined as a value of above 4.0 ng/mL. Some elevations in PSA may be due to benign conditions of the prostate.
  - Health care workers skilled in recognizing subtle prostate abnormalities, including those of symmetry and consistency, as well as the more classic findings of marked induration or nodules, should perform the DRE of the prostate. The DRE is less effective in detecting prostate carcinoma than is the PSA test.

Endometrium
  - All women should be informed about the risks and symptoms of endometrial cancer and strongly encouraged to report any unexpected bleeding or spotting. For women with or at high risk for hereditary nonpolyposis colon cancer (HNPCC), annual screening should be offered for endometrial cancer, with endometrial biopsy beginning at age 35.

Sources: American Cancer Society (2002). Cancer Facts and Figures 2002. Atlanta, GA: American Cancer Society; American Cancer Society Cancer Detection Guidelines (2002). Available at www.cancer.org, accessed 4/7/03.

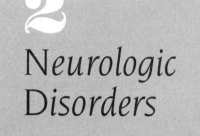

Neurologic Disorders

QUESTIONS

1. Assessing vision and visual fields involves testing cranial nerve (CN):

   A. I.
   B. II.
   C. III.
   D. IV.

2. You perform an extraocular movement test on a middle-aged patient. He is unable to move his eyes upward and inward. This indicates a possibility of paralysis of CN:

   A. II.
   B. III.
   C. V.
   D. VI.

3. Loss of corneal reflex is seen in dysfunction of CN:

   A. III.
   B. IV.
   C. V.
   D. VI.

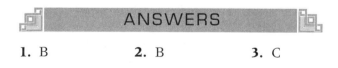

ANSWERS

1. B   2. B   3. C

DISCUSSION

Knowledge of the CNs is critical for performing an accurate neurologic assessment. Because these are paired nerves arising largely from the brainstem, a unilateral CN dysfunction is common, often reflecting a problem in the ipsilateral cerebral hemisphere.

CRANIAL NERVE MNEMONIC

A commonly used mnemonic for identifying and remembering the cranial nerves is: *On Old Olympus Towering Tops, A Finn And German Viewed Some Hops.* The details of the cranial nerves are as follows.

- CN I—Olfactory: You have one nose, where CN I resides. Its function contributes to the sense of smell.
- CN II—Optic: You have two eyes, where you will find CN II. Function of this cranial nerve is vital to vision and visual fields and, in conjunction with CN III, pupillary reaction.
- CN III—Occulomotor: CN III, the eye (*occulo-*) movement (motor) nerve works with CN III, IV, and VI (*abducens*, which helps the eyeball abduct or move). The actions of these CNs are largely responsible for the movement of the eyeball and eyelid.

- CN IV—Trochlear.
- CN V—Trigeminal: Three (*tri*) types of sensation (temperature, pain, and tactile) come from this three-branched nerve that covers three territories of the face. For normal corneal reflexes to be present, the afferent limb of the first division of CN V and the effect limb of CN VII need to be intact.
- CN VI—Abducens.
- CN VII—Facial: Dysfunction of this nerve gives the characteristic findings of Bell's palsy (facial asymmetry, droop of mouth, absent nasolabial fold, impaired eyelid movement).
- CN VIII—Auditory or vestibulocochlear: When this does not function properly, hearing (auditory) or balance is impaired (vestibulocochlear). The Rinne test is part of the evaluation of this cranial nerve.
- CN IX—Glossopharyngeal: The name of this CN provides a clue that its function affects the tongue (*glosso*) and throat (*pharynx*). Along with CN X, the function of this nerve is critical to swallowing, palate elevation, and gustation.
- CN X—Vagus.
- CN XI—Accessory or spinal root of the accessory: Function of this CN can be tested by evaluating shoulder shrug and lateral neck rotation.
- CN XII—Hypoglossal: Function of this CN is tested by noting movement and protrusion of the tongue.

DISCUSSION SOURCE

Devinsky, O., and Feldmann, E. (2000). Neurological Pearls. Philadelphia: F. A. Davis.

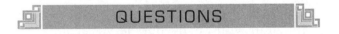

QUESTIONS

4. You examine a 29-year-old woman who has a sudden onset of right-sided facial asymmetry. She is unable to tightly close her right eyelid, frown, or smile on the affected side. Her examination is otherwise unremarkable. This may represent paralysis of CN:

    A. III.
    B. IV.
    C. VII.
    D. VIII.

5. Which represents the most appropriate diagnostic test for the patient in the previous question?

    A. complete blood cell count with white blood cell (WBC) differential
    B. Lyme disease antibody titer
    C. computed tomography (CT) scan of the head with contrast medium
    D. blood urea nitrogen and creatinine levels

6. In prescribing prednisone for the person with Bell palsy, the nurse practitioner (NP) considers that its use:

    A. helps in reversing facial paralysis even when given late in the course of illness.
    B. should be initiated at the onset of facial paralysis.
    C. will likely help minimize ocular symptoms.
    D. may prolong the course of the disease.

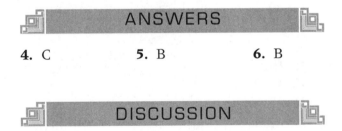

ANSWERS

4. C   5. B   6. B

DISCUSSION

Bell palsy is an acute paralysis of CN VII (in the absence of brain dysfunction) that is seen in the absence of other signs and symptoms. Because this condition can be a complication of Lyme disease, it is important to get the appropriate antibody titer. According to patient presentation and risk factors, rapid plasma reagin (RPR)/Venereal Disease Research Laboratory (VDRL) test and/or human immunodeficiency virus (HIV) screening should be obtained. However, neuroimaging is not needed, because a unilateral CN dysfunction is not consistent with the typical clinical presentation of an intracranial neoplasm. Corticosteroid therapy may help limit the length and severity of the paralysis. It is most effective when started early in the disease and is of no use if begun more than 10 days after the onset of symptoms. Acyclovir in patients with Bell palsy is controversial but is often given, inasmuch as herpes simplex virus is hypothesized to be a possible cause of the disease. Supportive care to help avoid ocular and oral injury, as well as counseling about the natural history of the disease, is critically important.

DISCUSSION SOURCE

Hedges, T. Bell Palsy. Available at http://www.emedicine.com/oph/topic508.htm, accessed 9.22.03.

QUESTIONS

7. A 40-year-old patient presents with a 5-week history of recurrent headaches that awaken him during the night. The pain is severe, lasts about 1 hour, and is located behind his left eye. Additional symptoms include lacrimation and nasal discharge. His physical examination is within normal limits. The most likely diagnosis is:

    A. common migraine.
    B. classic migraine.
    C. cluster headache.
    D. increased intracranial pressure (ICP).

8. Linda is a 22-year-old woman with a 3-year history of recurrent, unilateral, pulsating headaches with vomiting and photophobia. The headaches, which generally last 3 hours, can be aborted by resting in a dark room. She can usually tell that she is going to get a headache. She explains, "I see little 'squiggles' before my eyes for about 15 minutes." Her physical examination is unremarkable. This presentation is most consistent with:

    A. tension-type headache.
    B. migraine without aura.
    C. migraine with aura.
    D. cluster headache.

9. Prophylactic treatment for migraine headaches includes:

    A. propranolol.
    B. ergotamine.
    C. naproxen sodium.
    D. enalapril.

10. You are examining a 55-year-old woman who has a history of angina and migraine headache. Which of the following represents the best choice of acute headache treatment, called abortive migraine therapy, for this patient?

    A. verapamil
    B. ergotamine
    C. ibuprofen
    D. sumatriptan

11. With migraine headache, which of the following is true?

    A. Migraine with aura is the most common form.
    B. Most migraineurs are in ongoing health care for the condition.
    C. The condition is equally as common in men and women.
    D. The pain is typically described as pulsating.

12. In tension-type headache, which of the following is true?

    A. Photophobia is seldom reported.
    B. The pain is typically described as "pressing" in quality.
    C. The headache is usually unilateral.
    D. Activity makes the discomfort worse.

13. Treatment options in cluster headache include:

    A. nonsteroidal anti-inflammatory drugs (NSAIDs).
    B. oxygen.
    C. triptans.
    D. all of the above.

14. Which of the following affords the most rapid analgesic onset?

    A. naproxen
    B. liquid ibuprofen
    C. diclofenac
    D. celecoxib

15. Limitations of butalbital with acetaminophen and caffeine (Fioricet) use include its:

    A. energizing effect.
    B. gastrointestinal (GI) upset profile.
    C. high rate of rebound headache if used frequently.
    D. excessive cost.

16. The use of neuroleptics in migraine headache therapy should be limited to less than 3 times per week due to their:

    A. addictive potential.
    B. extrapyramidal movement risk.
    C. ability to cause rebound headache.
    D. sedative effect.

17. With appropriately prescribed headache prophylactic therapy, the patient should be informed to expect:

    A. virtual resolution of headaches.
    B. no fewer but less severe headaches.
    C. approximately 50% reduction in the number of headaches.
    D. that lifelong therapy is advised.

18. A 48-year-old woman presents with a monthly 4-day premenstrual migraine headache, poorly responsive to triptans and analgesics, and accompanied by hot flashes. The NP considers prescribing all of the following except:

    A. continuous monophasic oral contraceptive.
    B. phasic oral contraceptive with a 7-day-per-month withdrawal period.
    C. estrogen patch.
    D. triptan prophylaxis.

19. Prophylactic treatment options for the prevention of tension-type headaches include:

    A. desipramine.
    B. lisinopril.
    C. oxycodone.
    D. butalbital.

20. A 68-year-old man presents with new onset of headaches. He describes the pain as bilateral frontal to occipital and worst when he arises in the morning and when coughing. He feels much better by midafternoon. The history is most consistent with headache caused by:

    A. vascular compromise.
    B. increased ICP.
    C. brain tumor.
    D. tension-type with geriatric presentation.

ANSWERS

7. C	8. C	9. A
10. C	11. D	12. B
13. D	14. B	15. C
16. B	17. C	18. B
19. A	20. B	

DISCUSSION

The primary headaches, including migraine, tension-type, and cluster headache, are the most common chronic pain syndromes seen in primary care practice. The development of the appropriate diagnosis is critical to caring for the patients who have headaches (Table 2–1). In addition, headaches can be the presenting symptoms of a serious illness. The key points

TABLE 2–1

PRIMARY HEADACHE: CLINICAL PRESENTATION
AND DIAGNOSIS

Headache Type	Headache Characteristics
Tension-type headache	Lasts 30 mins to 7 d w/=>2 of the following characteristics: • Pressing, nonpulsatile pain • Mild to moderate in intensity • Usually bilateral location • Notation 0–1 of the following (>1 suggests migraine) • Nausea • Photophobia • Phonophobia
Headache w/o aura	Lasts 30 mins to 7 d w/=>2 of the following characteristics: • Usually unilateral location, although occasionally bilateral • Pulsating quality, moderate to severe in intensity • Aggravation by normal activity During headache, =>1 of the following: • Nausea and/or vomiting • Photophobia and phonophobia
Migraine with aura	Migraine-type headache occurs with or after aura • Focal dysfunction of cerebral cortex or brainstem causes =>1 aura symptom develops over 4 min, or =>2 sx occur in succession. • No aura symptom should last > 1 h. If this occurs, an alternate diagnosis should be considered.
Cluster headache	Tendency of headache to occur daily in groups or clusters: • Clusters usually last several weeks to months, then disappear for months to years. • Usually occur at characteristic times of year such as vernal and autumnal equinox, with 1–8 episodes/d, at the same time of day. Common time is ~ 1 h into sleep, hence the term "alarm clock" headache, as the pain awakens the person. • Headache location is often located behind one eye with a steady, intense, severe pain in a crescendo pattern lasting 15 mins to 3 h, with most in the range of 30–45 minutes. Pain intensity has helped earn the condition the term "suicide headache." Most often with ipsilateral autonomic signs such as lacrimation, conjunctival injection, ptosis, and nasal stuffiness.

to consider in assessing the person with headache are given in Box 2–1 and Table 2–2. The question of whether to obtain neuroimaging with head CT or magnetic resonance imaging (MRI) to evaluate for underlying disease often arises in the care of the person with nonacute primary headache. In the absence of a normal neurologic examination, the results of neuroimaging yield little additional information but add significantly to health care cost (Table 2–3).

Migraine without aura affects about 80% of persons with migraine. However, on careful questioning many patients report a migraine

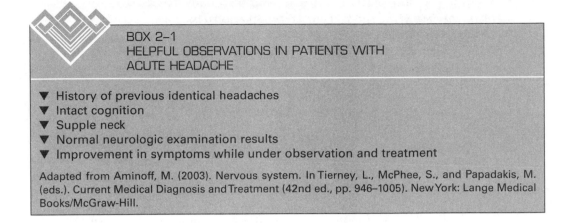

Adapted from Aminoff, M. (2003). Nervous system. In Tierney, L., McPhee, S., and Papadakis, M. (eds.). Current Medical Diagnosis and Treatment (42nd ed., pp. 946–1005). New York: Lange Medical Books/McGraw-Hill.

warning, such as agitation, jitteriness, disturbed sleep, or unusual dreams (see Table 2–1 for diagnostic criteria for headache). Migraine with aura is found in about 20% of those with migrainous disorders. The aura is a recurrent neurologic symptom that arises from the cerebral cortex or brainstem. Typically, the aura develops over 5 to 20 minutes, lasts less than 1 hour, and is accompanied or followed by migraine. Patients who have migraines with aura do not necessarily have more severe headaches than those without aura, but the former patients are more likely to be offered a fuller range of therapies. Patients without aura may be misdiagnosed as having tension-type headaches and therefore not offered headache therapies specifically suited for migraines, such as the triptans.

Although much of headache care is focused on the relief and prevention of migraine, tension-type headaches are a significant source of suffering and lost function (see Table 2–1 for diagnosis). Abortive treatment options include the use of acetaminophen; NSAIDs; and combination products such as butalbital with acetaminophen and acetaminophen, aspirin, and caffeine. Prophylactic therapies are highly effective at limiting the number and frequency of tension-type headache.

Cluster headaches, also known as migrainous neuralgia, are most common in middle-aged men, particularly those with heavy alcohol and tobacco use. Sometimes called the "suicide headache" because of the severity of the associated pain, cluster headache occurs periodically in clusters of several weeks, with associated lacrimation and rhinorrhea. Treatment includes reduction of triggers, such as tobacco and alcohol use, and initiation of prophylactic therapy, as well as appropriate abortive therapy (triptans, high-dose NSAIDs, and high-flow oxygen).

Headache treatment is aimed at identifying and reducing headache triggers. In addition,

---

■■■■ **TABLE 2–2** ■■■■
HEADACHE RED FLAGS:
"SNOOP" SIGNS

Systemic symptoms
- Fever, weight loss, or secondary headache risk factors (HIV, cancer)

Neurologic signs, symptoms
- Confusion, impaired alertness or consciousness

Onset
- Sudden, abrupt, or split-second

Older
- New onset and progressive headache, especially in adult ≥50

Previous headache history
- First headache
- Different headache
- Change in attack frequency, severity, or clinical features

Adapted from Silberstein, S. D., Lipton, R.B., and Dalessio, D.J. (eds.). Wolff's Headache and Other Head Pain (pp. 6–26). New York: Oxford University Press. HIV, human immunodeficiency virus.

TABLE 2-3

EVIDENCE-BASED GUIDELINES IN THE PRIMARY CARE
SETTING: NEUROIMAGING IN PATIENTS WITH NONACUTE
HEADACHE

- Significantly increased odds of finding abnormality on neuroimaging
  - Rapidly increasing headache frequency
  - History
    - Dizziness or lack of coordination
    - Subjective numbness or tingling
    - Headache causing awakening from sleep
    - Headache worse w/ Valsalva maneuver
    - Accelerating, new onset headache
  - Abnormal neurologic examination
  - Increasing age
    - More likely nonacute finding such as old infarct, atrophy
- Unlikely to correlate with abnormal neuroimaging
  - Neurologic examination within normal limits
  - Long-standing history of similar headache
  - "Worst headache of my life"
- Consensus-based principles
  - Testing should be avoided if it will not lead to a change in management
  - Not recommended if individual no more likely than general population to have significant abnormality
  - Testing not normally recommended as population policy may make sense at individual level
    - Patient or provider fear

U.S. Headache Consortium, available at www.aafp.org/clinical/migraine, accessed 9.12.04

---

abortive therapy should be offered. Prophylactic therapy, aimed at limiting the number and severity of future headaches, may also be indicated. Rescue therapy is used when abortive therapy is ineffective in providing headache relief.

When a migraine abortive agent is chosen, a number of considerations should be kept in mind. These medications are available in a number of forms (i.e., oral, parenteral, nasal spray, suppository). Migraine headaches are also present in a number of forms. A thoughtful match between the presentation of typical migraine and the form of medication is helpful. Here are some examples:

- Oral products generally take $1/2$ to 1 hour before there is significant relief of migraine pain. These products are best suited for patients with migraine who have a slowly developing headache with minimum GI distress. They should be used at the onset of symptoms. The use of oral products to manage migraine is the least expensive option and also facilitates patient self-care.

- Injectable products (e.g., sumatriptan and dihydroergotamine) have a rapid onset of action, usually within 15 to 30 minutes. These products are best suited for patients with rapidly progressing migraines accompanied by significant GI upset. Sumatriptan is available as a self-injector for patient administration. Dihydroergotamine is usually given intravenously in severe migrainosus along with parenteral hydration. Injectables are usually the most expensive treatment option, and using these products sometimes means that the patient with migraine requires a provider visit to facilitate the medication's use. Some triptans and dihydroergotamine are available as nasal sprays, have a similarly rapid onset of action, and are tolerable in the presence of GI upset. Suppositories have a slightly longer onset of action but may be used when nausea and vomiting are present.

- The triptans act as selective serotonin receptor agonists and work at the 5-HT1D serotonin receptor site, allowing an increase uptake of serotonin. Because of potential vasoconstrictor effect, their use is contraindicated in patients with Prinzmetal angina or coronary artery disease, in pregnant patients, and those who have recently used ergots. Because of the risk of serotonin syndrome, a condition of excessive availability of this neurotransmitter, the triptans should be used with caution with monamine oxidase inhibitor inhibitors (MAOIs) or high-dose selective serotonin reuptake inhibitors. Although the triptans are specifically labeled for use only in migraine, some patients with severe tension-type headache benefit from their use, which further supports the hypothesis there is a shared mechanism in migraine and tension-type headache.

- Ergotamines act as 5-HT1A and 5-HT1D receptor agonists and do not alter cerebral blood flow. Because of potential vasoconstrictor effect, their use should be avoided in the presence of coronary artery disease and pregnancy. Ergotamines are available in a variety of forms, including oral and sublingual tablets, suppositories, injectables, and nasal sprays. These products are helpful in the treatment of migraine but not tension-type headache.

- NSAIDs can be highly effective in both tension-type and migraine headache. These products inhibit prostaglandin and leukotriene synthesis and are most helpful when used at the first sign of headache, when GI upset is not a significant issue. The National Health Foundation Guidelines advise the use of rapid onset NSAIDs such as ibuprofen in high doses with booster doses. Acetaminophen and aspirin can also provide relief in migraine and tension-type headache but provide less analgesic effect.

- Fioricet is a combination of caffeine, butalbital, and acetaminophen. Whereas caffeine enhances the analgesic properties of acetaminophen, butalbital's barbiturate action enhances select neurotransmitter action, helping to relieve migraine and tension-type headache pain. With infrequent use, this product offers an inexpensive and generally well-tolerated headache treatment. Frequent or excessive Fioricet use should be discouraged because of the potential for barbiturate dependency from butalbital and analgesic rebound headache from acetaminophen.

- Midrin is a multidrug product that includes a vasoconstrictor (isometheptene mutate), analgesic (acetaminophen), and relaxant (65 mg of dichloralphenazone). It should be used in multiple doses at the beginning of a migraine headache or tension-type headache. Caution should be used when vasoconstriction is contraindicated.

- Excedrin Migraine is an aspirin, acetaminophen, and caffeine combination product. This is an over-the-counter product given Food and Drug Administration approval for migraine therapy and is also effective in tension-type headache. Its advantages include ease of patient access to the product, excellent side effect profile, and low cost. Excessive acetaminiphen use can lead to analgesic rebound headache.

- Neuroleptics may be used as adjuncts in migraine headache therapy because they help control nausea and vomiting. Because these drugs generally are highly sedating, using them in the clinician's office may make it difficult for patients to return home. Use should be limited to 3 days a week because of the risk of extrapyramidal movements (EPMs). Examples of neuroleptics are prochlorperazine (Compazine) and promethazine (Phenergan).

- Opioids such as hydrocodone, oxycodone, and codeine can provide analgesia and are often prescribed for migraine rescue. These products are sedating and potentially habituating, as well as being substances of abuse.

Use of prophylactic therapy of migraine, tension-type, or cluster headache should be considered if abortive headache therapy is used frequently or if inadequate symptom relief is obtained from appropriate use of these therapies. The goal of headache prophylactic therapy is a minimum of a 50% reduction in number of headaches in about two thirds of all patients, along with easier-to-control headaches. Most agents work through blockade of the 5HT2 receptor, and 1 to 2 months of use is needed before an effect is seen. Before headache prophylaxis is initiated, headache-inducing medications such as estrogen, progesterone, and vasodilators (Table 2–4) must first be eliminated or limited.

Secondary headaches are caused by an underlying disease process, often with increased ICP. The headache in increased ICP is usually reported as worst on awakening, which is when brain swelling is the worst. The pain is less intense as the day progresses and as the pressure lessens, in contrast to a tension-type headache, which usually worsens as the day goes on. Establishing the appropriate diagnosis is critical because treatment is guided by the reason for the increased ICP.

DISCUSSION SOURCES

Drew-Gastes, J., and Gross, R. (1999). Neurologic disorders. In Youngkin, E., Sawin, K., Kissinger, J., and Israel, D. (eds.). Pharmacotherapeutics: A Primary Care Clinical Guide (pp. 621–681). Norwalk, CT: Appleton & Lange.

Goadsby, P. J., Lipton, R. B., and Ferrari, M. D. (2002). Migraine—Current understanding and treatment. New England Journal of Medicine 346:257–270.

Solomon, S. (1997). Diagnosis of primary headache disorders: Validity of the International Headache Society criteria in clinical practice. Neurologic Clinics 15(1):107–114.

QUESTIONS

21. An 18-year-old college freshman is brought to the student health center with a chief complaint of headache and fever. On physical examination, he has positive Kernig and Brudzinski signs. The most likely diagnosis is:

A. encephalitis.

B. meningitis.

C. subarachnoid hemorrhage.

D. epidural hematoma.

TABLE 2–4
HEADACHE MEDICATIONS

Headache Therapy	Intervention	Comment
Lifestyle modification	Recognize and avoid triggers	Highly effective and infrequently uses
Analgesics	NSAIDs, acetaminophen, others	Risk of analgesic rebound headache, especially with excessive acetaminophen use
Migraine-specific medications	Ergots, triptans	Caution in pregnancy, CHD, uncontrolled IITN
Prophylactic medications	BB, CCB, TCA, AED (valproate, topiramate, others)	Goal — reduce headache frequency and severity

American Association for the Study of Headache Profiles. vol. 1, no. 2. Available at www.ahsnet.org/education/Prflsfall99.pdf, accessed 9.17.04.
AED, antiepileptic drug; BB, β blocker; CCB, calcium channel blocker; CHD, coronary heart disease; HTN, hypertension; NSAID, nonsteroidal anti-inflammatory drug; TCA, tricyclic antidepressant.

22. A 19-year-old college sophomore has meningococcal meningitis. You speak to the school health officers about the possible risk to other students. You inform them that:

    A. the patient does not have a contagious disease.
    B. all students need to receive antimicrobial prophylaxis, regardless of their degree of contact with the infected person.
    C. only intimate partners need prophylaxis.
    D. those with household-type contact with the patient should receive antimicrobial prophylaxis.

23. When evaluating the person who has bacterial meningitis, the NP expects to find cerebrospinal fluid (CSF) results of:

    A. low protein.
    B. predominance of lymphocytes.
    C. glucose at about 30% of serum levels.
    D. low opening pressure.

24. When evaluating the person who has aseptic or viral meningitis, the NP expects to find CSF results of:

    A. low protein.
    B. predominance of lymphocytes.
    C. glucose at about 30% of serum levels.
    D. low opening pressure.

25. Which of the following describes the Kernig sign?

    A. Neck pain with passive flexion of one hip and knee causes flexion of the contralateral leg.
    B. Passive neck flexion in a supine patient results in flexion of the knees and hips.
    C. Elicited with the patient lying supine and the hip flexed at 90 degrees, it is present when extension of the knee from this position elicits resistance or pain in the lower back or posterior thigh.
    D. The headache worsens when the patient is supine.

26. Physical examination findings in papilledema include:

    A. arteriovenous nicking.
    B. macular hyperpigmentation.
    C. optic disk bulging.
    D. pupillary constriction.

ANSWERS

21. B	**22.** D	**23.** C
24. B	**25.** C	**26.** C

DISCUSSION

Meningitis is an infection of the meninges, CSF, and ventricles. The disease is typically further defined by its cause, such as bacterial (pyogenic) or viral (aseptic).

In bacterial meningitis, the causative pathogens differ according to patient age and certain risk characteristics. Bacterial seeding usually occurs via hematogenous spread. Organisms can enter the meninges through the bloodstream from other parts of the body; the pathogen may have originally been asymptomatically carried in the nose and throat. Another mechanism of acquisition is local extension from another infection such as acute otitis media or bacterial rhinosinusitis. Congenital problems and trauma can provide a pathway via facial fractures or malformation (cleft lip or palate).

The presence of Kernig and Brudzinki signs along with headache and fever indicates a high probability of meningitis. Encephalitis is more likely viral in origin and usually presents with fewer meningeal signs. To eliminate or support the diagnosis of meningitis, lumbar puncture with cerebrospinal fluid (CSF) evaluation should be part of the evaluation of the febrile younger child who has altered findings of neurologic examination. Pleocytosis, defined as a WBC count of more than 5 cells/mm^3 of CSF, is an expected finding in meningitis caused by bacterial, viral, tubercular, fungal, or protozoan infection; an elevated CSF opening pressure is also a nearly universal finding. The typical CSF response in bacterial meningitis includes a WBC median count of 1200 cells/mm³ of CSF with 90% to 95% neutrophils; additional findings are a reduced CSF glucose amount below the normal level of about 60% of the plasma level and an elevated CSF protein level. In viral or aseptic meningitis, CSF results include normal glucose level, normal to slightly elevated protein levels, and lymphocytosis. Further testing to ascertain the causative organism is warranted. A head CT or MRI should be considered before lumbar puncture is performed.

Common pathogens in bacterial meningitis in the adult include *Streptococcus pneumoniae, Neisseria meningitidis, Staphylococcus* species, and *Haemophilus influenzae.* The clinical presentation of bacterial meningitis in the adult usually includes the classic triad of fever, headache, and nuchal rigidity, or stiff neck. The Brudzinski sign is elicited when passive neck flexion in a supine patient results in flexion of the knees and hips. The Kernig sign is elicited with the patient lying supine and the hip flexed at 90 degrees. A positive sign is present when extension of the knee from this position elicits resistance or pain in the lower back or posterior thigh. Papilledema or absence of venous pulsations upon funduscopic examination indicates increased ICP. Less common presenting symptoms include vomiting, seizures, and altered consciousness. In meningitis caused by *N. meningitidis,* rash is noted in about 50% of patients. The patient with viral meningitis usually has less severe symptoms that have a gradual onset.

The issue of meningitis contagion needs to be addressed. *N. meningitidis* is transmitted through droplets. Prophylaxis should be offered to persons with household-type or intimate contact with the infected patient, in particular if they have had more than 4 hours of exposure to the patient the week before the onset of illness. Antimicrobial options include rifampin, ciprofloxacin, and ceftriaxone. Meningitis caused by most other agents is a result of a patient rather than contagion factor;

that is, the meningitis is a result of extension of an existing illness such as bacterial sinusitis and otitis media.

Treatment of the person with meningitis includes supportive care and the use of the appropriate anti-infective agents. Ceftriaxone with vancomycin is usually the treatment of choice in suspected bacterial meningitis, pending bacterial sensitivity results. Acyclovir is an option in aseptic meningitis, pending identification of the offending virus.

DISCUSSION SOURCES

Centers for Disease Control and Prevention (2003). Meningococcal Disease. Available at http://www.cdc.gov/ncidod/dbmd/diseaseinfo/meningococcal_g.htm, accessed 9/22/03.

Gilbert, D., Moellering, R., and Sande, M. (2004). The Sanford Guide to Antimicrobial Therapy (34th ed.). Hyde Park, VT: Antimicrobial Therapy.

QUESTIONS

27. A 34-year-old woman has recently been diagnosed with multiple sclerosis (MS). When providing primary care for this patient, you consider that MS:

    A. has a predictable course of progressive decline in intellectual and motor function.
    B. presents with a classic pattern of myalgia, blurred vision, and ataxia.
    C. is often seen with a variable pattern of exacerbation and remissions.
    D. is accompanied by classic central nervous system lesions detectable on skull films.

28. Treatment options in MS to attenuate disease progression include:

    A. interferon β-1b.
    B. methylprednisolone.
    C. ribavirin.
    D. phenytoin.

29. Which of the following is most consistent with findings in patients with Parkinson disease?

   A. rigid posture with poor muscle tone
   B. masklike facies and continued cognitive function
   C. tremor at rest and bradykinesia
   D. excessive arm swinging with ambulation and flexed posture

30. Treatment options in Parkinson disease include all of the following except:

   A. levodopa.
   B. chlorpromazine.
   C. ropinirole.
   D. pramipexole.

31. Pallidotomy can be a helpful in the management of Parkinson disease–associated refractory _____ .

   A. dyskinesia
   B. anosmia
   C. seizure
   D. memory loss

ANSWERS

27. C	**28.** A	**29.** C
30. B	**31.** A	

DISCUSSION

MS is a disease characterized by episodes of focal neurologic dysfunction, with symptoms occurring acutely, worsening over a few days, and lasting weeks, followed by a period of partial to full resolution. Common symptoms include weakness or numbness of a limb, monocular visual loss, diplopia, vertigo, facial weakness or numbness, sphincter disturbances, ataxia, and nystagmus. MS is usually classified into two forms: (1) relapsing-remitting MS, in which episodes resolve with good neurologic function between exacerbations and minimal to no accumulative defects, and (2) chronic progressive MS, in which episodes do not fully resolve and there are accumulative defects. A person may have relapsing-remitting MS and later develop the chronic progressive form of the disease. The diagnosis of MS is often difficult to make because the signs of recurrent fatigue, muscle weakness, and other nonspecific signs and symptoms are often attributed to other diseases or to simply stress and fatigue. MRI can reveal demyelinating plaques, a typical finding in MS. Characteristic CSF findings include pleocytosis with predominance of monocytes and abnormal protein levels, including a modest increase in total protein, a markedly increased gammaglobulin fraction, a high immunoglobulin G index, presence of oligoclonal bands, and an increase in myelin basic protein.

MS is a disease characterized by exacerbation and remission. Triggers for exacerbations are varied but often include onset of common infectious disease such as urinary tract infection. Treatment of exacerbations includes treatment of the underlying precipitating illness, if present, and high-dose corticosteroids. Although discord exists as to the utility of this treatment, this therapy appears to shorten the course of the exacerbation but does not appear to have an impact on long-term disease progression. Maintenance immunomodulatory therapy with interferon β-1b (Betaseron) or interferon β-1a (Avonex) has been shown to significantly reduce frequency of exacerbations and long-term disability in relapsing-remitting MS. Immunosuppressive therapy with methotrexate or mitoxantrone is also used with some utility in reducing the rate of progression.

Parkinson disease is a slowly progressive movement disorder that is largely caused by an alteration in dopamine-containing neurons of the pars compacta of the substantia nigra. Age at onset is usually in the sixth decade and beyond, but the onset may occur in much younger adults.

The diagnosis of Parkinson disease is made by clinical evaluation and consists of a combination of six cardinal features: tremor at rest, rigidity, bradykinesia, flexed posture, loss of postural reflexes, and masklike facies. At least two of these, one being tremor at rest or bradykinesia, must be present. Typically, patients with Parkinson disease hold their arms rigidly at their sides with little movement during ambulation; forward falls are unfortunately common. The parkinsonian gait usually consists of a series of rapid small steps; to turn, patients must take several small steps, moving forward and backward.

Because Parkinson disease is characterized by an alteration in the dopaminergic pathway, dopamine agonists such as ropinirole (Requip) and pramipexole (Mirapex) are usually the early disease treatment of choice, in part because of a proposed neuroprotective effect, as well as having a better adverse effect profile than levodopa. Levodopa—a metabolic precursor of dopamine—continues to be used to minimize symptoms but tends to be less effective with more adverse effects as the disease progresses; the majority of patients who take levodopa for more than 5 to 10 years develop dyskinesia. Levodopa is often given with carbodopa in the fixed-dose combination know as Sinemet. Other medications used in the treatment of Parkinson disease include anticholinergics, such as benztropine, to help with tremor; however, this class of drugs is well known to cause dry mouth, urinary retention, and altered mentation, particularly in the older adult. Amantadine (Symmetrel) is an antiviral drug incidentally with time-limited (usually <1 year) antiparkinsonian benefits but can be used in later stages of the disease to help reduce dyskinesias. In view of the complexity of prescribing Parkinson disease medications, the prescriber should be well versed in these products and seek expert opinion as appropriate.

Surgical therapy, such as pallidotomy, can be helpful in the management of refractory dyskinesia, and brain stimulators can provide relief for refractory tremor.

DISCUSSION SOURCES

Martin, C. O. (2003). Multiple sclerosis. In Virtual Hospital: University of Iowa Family Practice Handbook, Fourth Edition: Neurology. Available at http://www.vh.org/adult/provider/family medicine/FPHandbook/Chapter09/11–9.html, accessed 9/22/03.

Martin, C. O. (2003). Parkinson disease, in Virtual Hospital: University of Iowa Family Practice Handbook, Fourth Edition: Neurology. Available at http://www.vh.org/adult/provider/family medicine/FPHandbook/Chapter09/05–9.html, accessed 9/22/03.

QUESTIONS

32. Which of the following best describes patient presentation during an absence (petit mal) seizure?

    A. blank staring lasting 3 to 50 seconds, accompanied by impaired level of consciousness

    B. awake state with abnormal motor behavior lasting seconds

    C. rigid extension of arms and legs, followed by sudden jerking movements with loss of consciousness

    D. abrupt muscle contraction with autonomic signs

33. Which of the following best describes patient presentation during a simple partial seizure?

    A. blank staring lasting 3 to 50 seconds, accompanied by impaired level of consciousness

    B. awake state with abnormal motor behavior lasting seconds

    C. rigid extension of arms and legs, followed by sudden jerking movements with loss of consciousness

    D. abrupt muscle contraction with autonomic signs

34. Which of the following best describes patient presentation during a tonic-clonic (grand mal) seizure?

    A. blank staring lasting 3 to 50 seconds, accompanied by impaired level of consciousness

B. awake state with abnormal motor behavior lasting seconds

C. rigid extension of arms and legs, followed by sudden jerking movements with loss of consciousness

D. abrupt muscle contraction with autonomic signs

35. Which of the following best describes patient presentation during a myoclonic seizure?

   A. blank staring lasting 3 to 50 seconds, accompanied by impaired level of consciousness

   B. awake state with abnormal motor behavior lasting seconds

   C. rigid extension of arms and legs, followed by sudden jerking movements with loss of consciousness

   D. brief, jerking contractions of arm(s), legs(s), and/or trunk.

36. Treatment options for the adult with seizures include all of the following except:

   A. carbamazepine.

   B. phenytoin.

   C. gabapentin.

   D. trandolapril.

37. A patient taking phenytoin may exhibit drug toxicity when concurrently taking:

   A. theophylline.

   B. famotidine.

   C. acetaminophen.

   D. aspirin.

ANSWERS

32. A	**33.** B	**34.** C
35. D	**36.** D	**37.** A

DISCUSSION

The type of seizure directs the treatment of the seizure disorder. Thus, knowledge of the presentation of the more common forms of seizures is critical (Table 2–5).

A number of standard seizure therapies, such as phenytoin, carbamazepine, clonazepam, ethosuximide, and valproic acid, and newer antiepileptic drugs (AEDs), such as gabapentin, lamotrigine, and topiramate, are now available. Expert knowledge of the indications and adverse reaction profiles of these medications is needed before AED therapy is initiated or continued.

Certain AEDs, including phenytoin and carbamazepine, are members of a group known as narrow therapeutic index drugs. A certain

TABLE 2–5
DESCRIPTION OF COMMON SEIZURE DISORDERS

Seizure Type	Description of Seizure	Comments
Absence (AKA petit mal)	Blank staring lasting 3–50 sec accompanied by impaired level of consciousness	Usual age of onset = 3–15 years
Myoclonic	Awake state or momentary loss of conciousness with abnormal motor behavior lasting seconds to minutes; one or more muscle groups causing brief jerking contractions of the limbs and trunk, occasionally flinging patient	Difficult to control; at least half also have tonic-clonic seizures. Usual age of onset = 2–7 years

Seizure Type	Description of Seizure	Comments
Tonic-clonic (grand mal)	Rigid extension of arms and legs followed by sudden jerking movements with loss of consciousness; bowel and bladder incontinence common with postictal confusion	Onset at any age; in adults, new onset may be found in brain tumor, post–head injury, alcohol withdrawal
Simple partial or focal seizure (jacksonian)	Awake state with abnormal motor, sensory, autonomic, or psychic behavior; movement can affect any part of body, localized or generalized	Typical age of onset 3–15 years
Complex partial	Aura characterized by unusual sense of smell or taste, visual or auditory hallucinations, image or sound, stomach upset; followed by vague stare and facial movements, muscle contraction and relaxation, and autonomic signs; can progress to loss of consciousness	Onset at any age

Adapted from Dunphy, LH (2004). Management Guidelines for Nurse Practitioners Working with Adults, Philadelphia: F.A. Davis, pp. 446–453; Aminoff, M. (2003). Nervous system. In Tierney, L, McPhee, S, and Papadakis, M: Current Medical Diagnosis and Treatment (42nd ed). New York: Lange Medical Books/McGraw-Hill, pp. 946–1005.

amount of such drugs is therapeutic, and just slightly more than this amount is potentially toxic. Other drugs in this category include warfarin, theophylline, and digoxin. Many of these drugs have high levels of protein binding, as well as significant utilization of hepatic enzymatic pathways for drug metabolism, such as cytochrome P-450. Phenytoin is highly (>90%) protein bound; when taken with other highly protein-bound drugs, it can be displaced from its protein-binding site, leading to increased free phenytoin and a risk of toxicity. Carbamazepine can increase the metabolic capacity of hepatic enzymes, which leads to more rapid metabolism of the drug and reduced levels of this and other drugs. The prescriber should be familiar with the drug interactions of all AEDs and monitor therapeutic levels as well as for adverse reactions.

DISCUSSION SOURCES

Aminoff, M. (2003). Nervous system. In Tierny, L., McPhee, S., and Papadakis, M. (eds.). Current Medical Diagnosis and Treatment (42nd ed., pp 946–1005). New York: Lange Medical Books/ McGraw-Hill.

Dunphy, L.H. (2004). Central and Peripheral Nervous Systems Disorders, In Dunphy's Management Guidelines for Nurse Practitioners Working with Adults, Philadelphia: F.A. Davis, pp 425–453.

QUESTIONS

38. Risk factors for transient ischemic attack (TIA) include all of the following except:

   A. atrial fibrillation.
   B. carotid artery disease.
   C. oral contraceptive use.
   D. pernicious anemia.

39. A TIA is characterized as an episode of reversible neurologic symptoms that may last up to:

  A. 1 hour.
  B. 6 hours.
  C. 12 hours.
  D. 24 hours.

40. When caring for a patient with a recent TIA, you consider that:

  A. long-term antiplatelet therapy is indicated.
  B. this person has a relatively low risk of future stroke.
  C. women present with this disorder more often than men.
  D. rehabilitation will be needed to minimize the effects of the resulting neurologic insult.

41 to 47. When considering the diagnosis of acute stroke, which of the following can be part of the presentation? (Answer yes or no.)

  41. partial loss of visual field
  42. unilateral hearing loss
  43. facial muscle paralysis
  44. vertigo
  45. diplopia
  46. headache
  47. ataxia

ANSWERS

38. D	**39.** D	**40.** A
41. Yes	**42.** Yes	**43.** Yes
44. Yes	**45.** Yes	
46. Yes	**47.** Yes	

DISCUSSION

A TIA is an acute neurologic event in which all signs and symptoms, including numbness, weakness, and flaccidity, as well as visual changes, ataxia, or dysarthria, resolve usually within minutes but certainly by 24 hours after onset. If changes persist beyond 24 hours, the diagnosis of stroke should be entertained. Indeed, TIA should be considered a "stroke warning." Risk factors include carotid artery atherosclerosis; structural cardiac problems, such as valvular problems that lead to increased risk of embolization; and hypercoagulable conditions, such as antiphospholipid antibody and oral contraceptive use. Intervention includes minimizing risk factors through lifestyle modification (e.g., smoking cessation, diet, exercise, and cardiovascular and cerebrovascular disease risk reduction such as aggressive treatment of dyslipidemia, hypertension, and diabetes mellitus) as well as long-term antiplatelet therapy.

Acute stroke is often thought of as presenting with a sudden-onset unilateral limb weakness and motor dysfunction. Although these findings are often part of the clinical presentation, other findings such as changes in hearing and vision, seizure, and head and neck pain are often noted (Table 2–6). Acute stroke should be thought of as a "brain attack," in which a portion of the brain is acutely ischemic, a potentially reversible condition if blood flow is reestablished. If blood flow is not restored, the ischemic tissue will be future compromised, and the ischemia evolves into a cerebral infarction, often with devastating long-term consequences. If acute stroke is suspected, the patient must undergo emergency neuroimaging (see Table 2–3) and be evaluated for thrombolytic and/or revascularization therapy in the appropriate health care setting.

DISCUSSION SOURCE

The Internet Stroke Center (2003). Emergency Stroke Evaluation & Diagnosis. Available at http://www.strokecenter.org/education/ais_evaluation/lt_rt_hemisphere.htm, accessed 5/26/03.

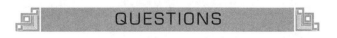

QUESTIONS

Identify the following as most likely associated with delirium or dementia:

TABLE 2–6
ACUTE STROKE PRESENTATION

Sign/Symptom	Clinical Presentation
Alteration in consciousness	Stupor Confusion Agitation Memory loss Delirium Seizures Coma
Headache	Intense or unusually severe Altered level of consciousness and/or neurologic deficit Unusual/severe neck or facial pain
Aphasia	Incoherent speech or difficulty understanding speech
Facial weakness or asymmetry	Paralysis of facial muscles (e.g., when patients speaks or smiles) May be on same side (ipsilateral) or opposite side contralateral to limb paralysis
Altered coordination	Incoordination, weakness, paralysis, or sensory loss of one or more limbs (usually one half of the body and in particular the hand) Ataxia (poor balance, clumsiness, or difficulty walking)
Visual loss	Monocular or binocular May be partial loss of the field
Miscellaneous	Vertigo Diplopia Unilateral hearing loss Nausea, vomiting Photophobia Phonophobia

Emergency Stroke Evaluation & Diagnosis, Internet Stroke Center, available at http://www.strokecenter.org/education/ais_evaluation/lt_rt_hemisphere. htm, accessed 5.26.03.

48. Insidious onset over months to years
49. Acute onset change in mental status
50. Associated with use of medications with anticholinergic effect
51. Treatment includes use of a NMDA-receptor antagonist
52. Mental status should return to baseline with recovery

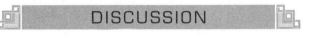

ANSWERS

48. Dementia	**49.** Delirium
50. Delirium	**51.** Dementia
52. Delirium	

DISCUSSION

Delirium is a condition in which the patient exhibits an acute onset, over hours to a few days, of reduced ability to maintain attention to external stimuli and appropriately shift attention to new stimuli. The result is disorganized thinking. The notation of =>2 of the following are usually noted: an altered level of consciousness from baseline; memory impairment; perceptual disturbance such as hallucinations; altered sleep; a change in psychomotor activity; and disorientation to time, place, and person. Delirium is not a diagnosis but rather a clinical state caused by an underlying health problem. Here is a helpful mnemonic as to the most common causes of delirium.

*D*rugs (anticholinergics, neuroleptics, long-acting benzodiazepines, others)
*E*motional (mood disorder, loss)
*L*ow PO$_2$ (hypoxemia from pneumonia, chronic obstructive pulmonary disorder, pulmonary embolus)
*I*nfection (urinary tract, respiratory tract, others)
*R*etention of urine or feces
*I*ctal or postictal state
*U*ndernutrition (protein/calorie malnutrition, vitamin B$_{12}$ or folate deficiency, dehydration)
*M*etabolic (thyroid, diabetes mellitus)
*S*ubdural hematoma

The evaluation of the person with delirium should be focused on defining its underlying cause. A thorough health history including social and home assessment and a physical examination should be conducted. A standardized evaluation of mental status, such as the Mini Mental Status Examination, must be included in the evaluation. At minimum, a hemogram with white blood cell count differential, urinalysis with urine culture and sensitivity, serum vitamin B$_{12}$ and folate, toxic screen, chemistry profile, thyroid stimulating hormone, and electrocardiogram should be obtained. Additional testing as indicated includes a rapid plasma reagent (RPR for syphilis testing), erythrocyte sedimentation rate, HIV antibody, hepatic profile, chest x-ray, and other images. Delirium treatment is aimed at assessing patients at greatest risk to help avoid its occurrence. When delirium occurs, treatment is focused on the condition's underlying cause. Mental status should return to baseline with recovery.

Dementia is defined by a chronic loss of intellectual or cognitive function of sufficient severity to interfere with social or occupational function; it is a symptom of an underlying diagnosis. In dementia, mental status changes can evolve insidiously over months or years with a gradually worsening course. The most common causes of dementia are Alzheimer disease and multi-infarct or vascular dementia. The evaluation of the person with suspected dementia is similar to assessment in delirium; the two conditions often overlap and can mimic each other. As indicated, additional dementia testing includes brain imaging and PET scan. In addition to behavior and supportive therapies, patients with dementia often benefit from the use of a cholinesterase inhibitor such as donepezil (Aricept), tacrine (Cognex), rivastigmine (Exelon), or a NMDA-receptor antagonist such as memantine (Namenda). These classes of medications have different mechanisms of action and can be given together.

DISCUSSION SOURCES

Devinsky, O., Feldmann, E. (2000). Neurological Pearls. Philadelphia: F. A. Davis.
Miller, C. (2004) Update on Dementia Medications, available at http://www.medscape.com/viewarticle/470704, accessed 7/24/04.

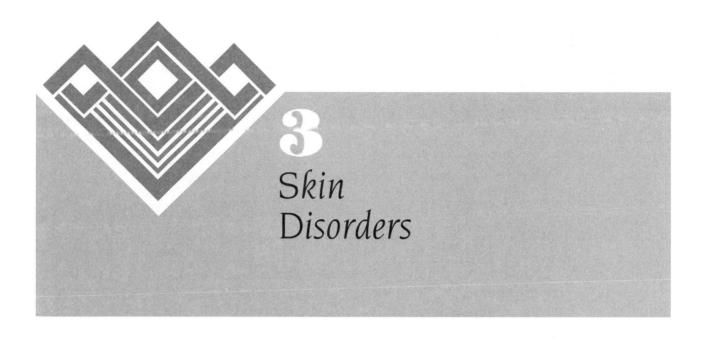

3

Skin Disorders

1 to 10. Match the following descriptions to the correct lesion or distribution name.

1. multiple lesions blending together
2. flat discoloration less than 1 cm in diameter
3. circumscribed area of skin edema
4. narrow linear crack into epidermis, exposing dermis
5. vesicle-like lesion with purulent content
6. flat discoloration greater than 1 cm in diameter
7. raised lesion, larger than 1 cm, may be same or different color from the surrounding skin
8. netlike cluster
9. loss of epidermis and dermis
10. loss of skin markings and full skin thickness

A. ulcer
B. atrophy
C. fissure
D. reticular
E. wheal
F. pustule
G. patch
H. plaque
I. macule
J. confluent

ANSWERS

J. **1.** coalescent or confluent
E. **3.** wheal
F. **5.** pustule
H. **7.** plaque
A. **9.** ulcer

I. **2.** macule
C. **4.** fissure
G. **6.** patch
D. **8.** reticular
B. **10.** atrophy

Identification of common dermatologic lesions is important to safe clinical practice (Table 3–1).

DISCUSSION SOURCE

Bickley, L. (2004) Bates' Guide to Physical Examination and History Taking (8th ed.) Philadelphia: Lippincott Williams and Wilkins.

TABLE 3-1

SKIN DISORDERS

Common Primary Skin Lesions

LESION	Description	Example
MACULE	Flat discoloration, usually < 1 cm in diameter	Freckle
PATCH	Flat area of skin discoloration, larger than a macule	Vitiligo
PAPULE	Raised lesion, < 1 cm, may be same or different color from the surrounding skin	Raised nevus
VESICLE	Fluid-filled, < 1 cm	Varicella
PLAQUE	Raised lesion, > 1 cm, may be same or different color from the surrounding skin	Psoriasis
PURPURA	Lesions caused by red blood cells leaving circulation and becoming trapped in skin	Petechiae, ecchymosis
PUSTULE	Vesicle-like lesion with purulent content	Impetigo, acne
WHEAL	Circumscribed area of skin edema	Hive
NODULE	Raised lesion, > 1 cm, usually mobile	Epidermal cyst
BULLAE	Fluid-filled, =>1 cm	Blister with 2nd-degree burn

Common Secondary Skin Lesions

EXCORIATION	Marks produced by scratching	Seen in areas of pruritic skin diseases
LICHENIFICA-TION	Skin thickening resembling callus formation	Seen in areas of recurrent scratching
FISSURE	Narrow linear crack into epidermis, exposing dermis	Split lip, athlete's foot
EROSION	Partial focal loss of epidermis; heals without scarring	Area exposed after bullous lesion opens
ULCER	Loss of epidermis and dermis; heals with scarring	Pressure sore
SCALE	Raised, flaking lesion	Dandruff, psoriasis
ATROPHY	Loss of skin markings and full skin thickness	Area treated excessively with higher potency corticosteroids

Terms Describing Patterns of Skin Lesions

ANNULAR	In a ring	Erythema migrans in Lyme disease
CONFLUENT OR COALESCENT	Multiple lesions blending together	Multiple skin conditions
RETICULAR	Netlike cluster	Multiple skin conditions
DERMATOMAL	Along a neurocutaneous dermatome	Herpes zoster
LINEAR	In streaks	Poison ivy

Grossman, D., and Guzzo, C. (2000). The skin. In Mangione, S. Physical Diagnosis Secrets. Philadelphia: Hanley & Belfus, Inc., pp. 35–68.

11. How many grams of a topical cream or ointment are needed for a single application to the hands?

    A. one
    B. two
    C. three
    D. four

12. How many grams of a topical cream or ointment are needed for a single application to an arm?

    A. one
    B. two
    C. three
    D. four

13. How many grams of a topical cream or ointment are needed for a single application to the entire body?

    A. 10 to 30
    B. 30 to 60
    C. 60 to 90
    D. 90 to 120

ANSWERS

11. B   12. C   13. B

DISCUSSION

Knowledge of the amount of a cream or ointment needed to treat a dermatologic condition is an important part of the prescriptive practice (Table 3–2). Prescribers often write prescriptions for an inadequate amount of a topical medication with insufficient numbers of refills, possibly creating a situation in which treatment fails because of an inadequate length of therapy.

DISCUSSION SOURCE

Arndt, K, and Bowers, K. (2001). Manual of Dermatologic Therapeutics (6th ed., pp. 120–121). Philadelphia: Lippincott Williams and Wilkins.

QUESTIONS

14. You write a prescription for a topical agent and anticipate the greatest rate of absorption when it is applied to the:

    A. palms of the hands.
    B. soles of the feet.
    C. face.
    D. abdomen.

TABLE 3–2
TOPICAL MEDICATION-DISPENSING FORMULA

	Amount Needed for One Application	Amount Needed in Twice-a-Day Application for 1 Week	Amount Needed in Twice-a-Day Application for 1 Month
Hands, head, face, anogenital region	2 g	28 g	120 g (4 oz)
One arm, anterior or posterior trunk	3 g	42 g	180 g (6 oz)
One leg			
Entire body	30–60 g	420–840 g (14–28 oz)	1.8–3.6 kg (60–120 oz or 3.75–7.5 lb)

Adapted from Arndt, K, and Bowers, K (2001). Manual of Dermatologic Therapeutics (6th ed., pp. 120–121). Philadelphia: Lippincott Williams and Wilkins.

15. You prescribe a topical medication and want it to have maximum absorption, so you choose the following vehicle:

A. gel
B. lotion
C. cream
D. ointment

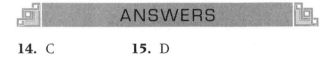

14. C   **15.** D

DISCUSSION

Safe prescription of a topical agent for patients with dermatologic disorders requires knowledge of the best vehicle for the medication. Certain parts of the body, notably the face, axillae, and genital area, are quite permeable, allowing greater absorption of medication than less permeable areas such as the extremities and trunk. In particular, the thickness of the palms of the hands and soles of the feet create a barrier so that relatively little topical medication is absorbed when applied to these sites. A general rule of cutaneous drug absorption is that it is inversely proportional to the thickness of the stratum corneum. For example, hydrocortisone absorption from the forearm is less than one third of the amount that is absorbed from the forehead.

In general, the less viscous the vehicle containing a topical medication, the less of the medication is absorbed. As a result, medication contained in a gel or lotion is absorbed in smaller amounts than that held in a cream or ointment. Besides enhancing absorption of the therapeutic agent, creams and ointments provide lubrication to the region, often a desirable effect in the presence of xerosis or lichenification.

DISCUSSION SOURCES

Woo, T. (2002). Drugs affecting the integumentary system. In Wynne, A., Woo, T., and Millard, M. (eds.). Pharmacotherapeutics for Nurse Practitioner Prescribers (pp. 565–618). Philadelphia: F. A. Davis.

QUESTIONS

16. One of the mechanisms of action of a topical corticosteroid preparation is as:

A. an antimitotic.
B. an exfoliant.
C. a vasoconstrictor.
D. a humectant.

17. To enhance the potency of a topical corticosteroid, the nurse practitioner (NP) recommends that the patient apply the preparation:

A. to dry skin by gentle rubbing.
B. and then apply an occlussive dressing.
C. before bathing.
D. with an emollient.

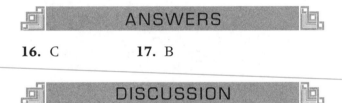

16. C   **17.** B

DISCUSSION

Corticosteroids are a class of drugs often used for treating inflammatory and allergic dermatologic disorders. Although corticosteroids reduce inflammatory and allergic reactions through a number of mechanisms (including immunosuppressive and inflammatory properties), their relative potency is based on vasoconstrictive activity; that is, the more potent topical steroids such as betametha-sone (class 1) have significantly greater vasoconstricting action than do the least potent agents such as hydrocortisone (class 7) (Table 3–3).

DISCUSSION SOURCES

Robertson, D., and Maibach, H. (2001). Dermatologic pharmacology. In Katzung, B. G. (ed.). Basic and Clinical Pharmacology (8th ed., pp. 1045–1063). New York: McGraw-Hill/Appleton & Lange.

Woo, T. (2002). Drugs affecting the integumentary system. In Wynne, A., Woo, T., and Millard, M. (eds.). Pharmacotherapeutics for Nurse Practitioner Prescribers (pp. 565–618). Philadelphia: F. A. Davis.

━━━ **TABLE 3–3** ━━━
EXAMPLES OF TOPICAL STEROID POTENCY

LOW POTENCY
Hydrocortisone (0.5%, 1%, 2.5%)
Fluocinolone acetonide 0.01% (Synalar)
Triamcinolone acetonide 0.025% (Aristocort)
Fluocinolone acetonide 0.025% (Synalar)
Hydrocortisone butyrate 0.1%
Hydrocortisone valerate 0.2% (Westcort)
Triamcinolone acetonide 0.1%

HIGH POTENCY
Fluocinolone acetonide 0.2% (Synalar-HP)
Desoximetasone 0.25% (Topicort)
Fluocinonide 0.05% (Lidex)
Betamethasone dipropionate, augmented, 0.05% (Diprolene AF cream)

SUPER-HIGH POTENCY
Betamethasone dipropionate, augmented, 0.05% (Diprolene gel, ointment)
Clobetasol propionate 0.05% (Temovate)
Halobetasol propionate 0.05% (Ultravate 0.05%)

Adapted from Arndt, K, and Bowers, K. (2001). Manual of Dermatologic Therapeutics (6th ed., pp. 120–121). Philadelphia: Lippincott Williams and Wilkins, and Woo, T. (2002). Drugs affecting the integumentary system. In Wynne, A., Woo, T., and Millard M. (eds.). Pharmacotherapeutics for Nurse Practitioner Prescribers (pp. 565–618). Philadelphia: F. A. Davis.

QUESTIONS

18. Antihistamines exhibit therapeutic effect by:

    A. inactivating circulating histamine.
    B. preventing the production of histamine.
    C. blocking activity at histamine receptor sites.
    D. acting as a procholenergic agent.

19. A possible adverse effect with the use of a first-generation antihistamine such as diphenhydramine in an 80-year-old man is:

    A. urinary retention.
    B. hypertension.
    C. tachycardia.
    D. urticaria.

ANSWERS

18. C   19. A

DISCUSSION

Antihistamines prevent action of formed histamine, a potent inflammatory mediator, and therefore can be used to control acute symptoms of itchiness and allergy. All antihistamines work by blocking histamine-1 (H_1) receptor sites, thus preventing the action of histamine.

Systemic antihistamines are usually divided into two groups: the standard or first-generation products such as diphenhydramine (Benadryl) or chlorpheniramine (Chlor-Trimeton) and the newer or second-generation products such as loratadine (Claritin), desloratadine (Clarinex), cetirizine (Zyrtec), and fexofenadine (Allegra). The first-generation antihistamines readily cross the blood-brain barrier, causing sedation. Their anticholinergic activity can result in drying of secretions, visual changes, and urinary retention, particularly in the older man with benign prostatic hyperplasia. The second-generation antihistamines do not easily cross the blood-brain barrier, which results in lower rates of sedation, and they have little anticholinergic effect.

DISCUSSION SOURCES

Arndt, K, and Bowers, K. (2001). Manual of Dermatologic Therapeutics (6th ed., pp. 120–121). Philadelphia: Lippincott Williams and Wilkins.

Woo, T. (2002). Drugs affecting the integumentary system. In Wynne, A., Woo, T., and Millard, M. (eds.). Pharmacotherapeutics for Nurse Practitioner Prescribers (pp. 565–618). Philadelphia: F. A. Davis.

QUESTIONS

20. Clinical features of impetigo include:

    A. intense itch.
    B. vcsiculopustular lesions.
    C. dermatomal pattern.
    D. being accompanied by fever and chills.

21. An oral antimicrobital option for the treatment of impetigo is to include all of the following except:

    A. amoxicillin.
    B. dicloxacillin.
    C. cephalexin.
    D. cefadroxil.

22. Mupirocin's (Bactroban's) spectrum of antimicrobial activity includes:

    A. primarily gram-negative organisms.
    B. select *Staphylococcus* and *Streptococcus* species.
    C. *Pseudomonas* species and anaerobic organisms.
    D. only organisms that do not produce beta-lactamase.

ANSWERS

20. B   **21.** A   **22.** B

DISCUSSION

Impetigo is a common, contagious skin condition usually caused by staphylococci or streptococci. Clinical features include groups of vesiculopulstular lesion with honey-colored crusts, often in a pattern reflecting autoinoculation. Treatment options include antibiotics effective against gram-positive organisms with stability in the presence of beta-lactamase. Dicloxacillin and first-generation cephalosporins such as cefadroxil or cephalexin are effective. For milder cases involving a small surface area, mupirocin (Bactroban), a topical antibacterial agent effective in eradicating select gram-positive organisms such as methicillin-resistant and methicillin-sensitive *Staphylococcus aureus* and streptococci, is an effective treatment option. Mupirocin is also prescribed for the temporary elimination of nasal carriage of *S. aureus*.

DISCUSSION SOURCES

Arndt, K, and Bowers, K. (2001). Manual of Dermatologic Therapeutics (6th ed., pp. 120–121). Philadelphia: Lippincott Williams and Wilkins.

Woo, T. (2002). Drugs affecting the integumentary system. In Wynne, A., Woo, T., and Millard, M. (eds.). Pharmacotherapeutics for Nurse Practitioner Prescribers (pp. 565–618). Philadelphia: F. A. Davis.

QUESTIONS

23. Which of the following medications contributes to the development of acne vulgaris?

    A. lithium
    B. propranolol
    C. tetracycline
    D. oral contraceptives

24. First-line therapy for acne vulgaris with closed comedones includes:

    A. oral antibiotics.
    B. isotretinoin.

C. benzoyl peroxide.

D. hydrocortisone cream.

25. When prescribing tretinoin (Retin-A), the NP advises the patient to:

   A. use it with benzoyl peroxide to minimize irritating effects.

   B. use a sunscreen because the drug is photosensitizing.

   C. add a sulfa-based cream to enhance antiacne effects.

   D. expect a significant improvement in acne lesions after approximately 1 week of use.

26. In the treatment of acne vulgaris, which type of lesions responds best to topical antibiotic therapy?

   A. open comedones

   B. cysts

   C. inflammatory lesions

   D. superficial lesions

27. Which of the following is indicated for the treatment of acne rosacea?

   A. metronidazole gel (MetroGel)

   B. clindamycin lotion (Cleocin)

   C. erythromycin 2% solution

   D. azelaic acid 20% (Azelex cream)

28. You have initiated therapy for an 18-year-old man with acne vulgaris and have prescribed tetracycline. He returns in 3 weeks, complaining that his skin is "no better." Your next action is to:

   A. counsel him that 6 to 8 weeks of treatment is often needed before significant improvement is achieved.

   B. discontinue the tetracycline and initiate minocyline therapy.

   C. advise him that antibiotics are likely not an effective treatment for him and should not be continued.

   D. add a second antimicrobial agent.

29. Of the following, who is the best candidate for isotretinoin (Accutane) therapy?

   A. a 17-year-old patient with pustular lesions and poor response to benzoyl peroxide

   B. a 20-year-old patient with cystic lesions who had tried a variety of therapies with minimal effect

   C. a 14-year-old patient with open and closed comedones and a family history of "ice pick" lesions

   D. an 18-year-old patient with inflammatory lesions and improvement with tretinoin (Retin-A)

30. In a 22-year-old woman using isotretinoin (Accutane) therapy, the NP ensures follow-up to monitor for all of the following tests except:

   A. aspartate aminotransferase (AST) measurement

   B. triglyceride measurements

   C. pregnancy test

   D. platelet count

ANSWERS

| 23. A | 24. C | 25. B | 26. C |
| 27. A | 28. A | 29. B | 30. D |

DISCUSSION

Acne vulgaris is a common pustular disorder caused by a combination of factors. An increase in sebaceous activity causes plugging of follicles and retention of sebum, allowing an overgrowth of *Propionibacterium acnes*. This allows an inflammatory reaction with the resulting wide variety of lesions, including open and closed comedones, cysts, and pustules.

Both topical and systemic antibiotics are used to treat acne and are particularly helpful as therapy for pustular lesions. However, the mechanism of action of antibiotics in acne therapy is probably not based solely on their antimicrobial action but may be caused in part by their anti-inflammatory activity. Additional acne vulgaris agents include topical vitamin A derivatives such as tretinoin (Retin-A), synthetic retinoid (Accutane), and comedolytics (benzoyl peroxide) (Table 3–4).

Nearly all adolescents develop acne vulgaris. Most discover that the skin clears considerably by early adulthood. Only 15% seek treatment for this problematic condition that affects teenagers at a time in their lives when body image and social acceptance are usually of greater influence than they are at any other

TABLE 3–4
ACNE MEDICATIONS

Acne medication	Mechanism of action and considerations for use
BENZOYL PEROXIDE CREAM, LOTION, VARIOUS CONCENTRATIONS	• Antimicrobial against *P. acnes* as well as comedolytic effects • Use lower strength formulation; may cause skin irritation • Often given with topical antibiotics
AZELAIC ACID (AZELEX) 20% CREAM	• Likely antimicrobial against *P. acnes*, keratolytic, possibly alters androgen metabolism • Expect ~6 weeks therapy prior to noting improvement • Mild skin irritation with redness and dryness common with initial use, improves over time • Less potent but less irritating than tretinoin preparations
TRETINOIN (RETINOIC ACID) GEL, CREAM, VARIOUS CONCENTRATIONS	• Decreases cohesion between epidermal cells, increases epidermal cell turnover, transforms closed to open comedones • Mild skin irritation with redness and dryness common with initial use, improves over time; expect ~6 weeks therapy prior to noting improvement • Photosensitizing; advise patient to use sunscreen
ORAL ANTIBIOTICS (CLINDAMYCIN, ERYTHROMYCIN, TETRACYCLINE, AZITHROMYCIN, OTHERS)	• Antimicrobial against *P. acnes*, anti-inflammatory • Indicated for the treatment of moderate papular inflammatory acne, usually when topical therapy has been inadequate • Once skin is clear, taper off slowly over a few months while adding topical antibiotic agents; rapid discontinuation results in return of acne • Long-term therapy is often needed
TOPICAL ANTIBIOTICS (CLINDAMYCIN, ERYTHROMYCIN, TETRACYCLINE, OTHERS)	• Antimicrobial against *P. acnes*, anti-inflammatory • Indicated in treatment of mild to moderate inflammatory acne vulgaris; less effective than oral antibiotics; often given in combination with benzoyl peroxide.
ORAL CONTRACEPTIVES	• Reduction in ovarian androgen production, decreased sebum production
ISOTRETINOIN (ACCUTANE) CAPSULES, VARIOUS STRENGTHS	• Likely inhibits sebaceous gland function • Indicated for treatment of cystic acne that does not respond to other therapies • Usual course of treatment is 4–6 months; discontinue when nodule count is reduced by 70%; repeat course only if needed after 2 months off drug • Prescriber must be properly trained in use of drug and fully aware of adverse reactions profile, including cheilitis, conjunctivitis, hypertriglyceridemia, xerosis, photosensitivity, and potent teratogenicity

Adapted from Woo, T. (2002). Drugs affecting the integumentary system. In Wynne, A., Woo, T., and Millard, M. (eds.): Pharmacotherapeutics for Nurse Practitioner Prescribers, pp. 565–618. Philadelphia: F. A. Davis. Gilbert, D., Moellering, R., and Sande, M. (2004). The Sanford Guide to Antimicrobial Therapy, 34th ed. Hyde Park, VT: Antimicrobial Therapy, Inc., p 34.

time of life. However, a number of effective treatment options are available.

Acne-inducing drugs should be avoided, if possible. However, certain medications such as lithium and phenytoin (Dilantin) may need to be used. These medications can also cause acne in adults. In any event, drug-induced acne can be treated with conventional therapy (see Table 3–4).

Isotretinoin (Accutane) is effective in cystic acne that does not respond to conventional therapy. Although most patients who take it have adverse effects related only to dry skin, the prescriber and patient need to be well aware of potentially serious problems associated with its use, including pseudotumor cerebri, birth defects, and depression.

DISCUSSION SOURCE

Berger, A. (2003). Skin, hair, and nails. In Tierney, L., McPhee, S., and Papadakis, M. (eds.). Current Medical Diagnosis and Treatment (pp. 80–145). New York: McGraw-Hill/Appleton & Lange.

QUESTIONS

31. A common infective agent in domestic pet cat bites is:

    A. rabies virus.
    B. *Pasteurella multocida.*
    C. *Bacteroides* species.
    D. *Haemophilus influenzae.*

32. Cat bite wound treatment should include prescribing:

    A. erythromycin.
    B. topical bacitracin.
    C. amoxicillin clavulanate.
    D. rifampin.

33. A 24-year-old man arrives at the walk-in center. He reports that he was bitten in the thigh by a raccoon while walking in the woods. The examination reveals a wound that is 1 cm deep on his right thigh. The wound is oozing bright red blood. Your next best action is to:

    A. administer high-dose parenteral penicillin.
    B. initiate antibacterial prophylaxis with amoxicillin.
    C. give rabies immune globulin and rabies vaccine.
    D. suture the wound after proper cleansing.

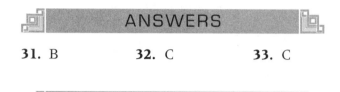

ANSWERS

31. B   **32.** C   **33.** C

DISCUSSION

Bite wounds should not be considered benign or inevitable. Intervention includes education to avoid further bites; therefore, a patient's history must include a complete documentation of events leading up to the bite.

All bites should be considered to carry significant infectious risk. This may vary from the relatively low rate of infection from dog bites (~5%) to the very high rate from cat bites (~80%). Initial therapy includes vigorous wound cleansing with antimicrobial agents as appropriate and débridement if necessary. Starting short-term prophylactic therapy within 12 hours of the injury should be considered, and tetanus immunization should be updated as needed (Table 3–5).

There has been an increase in domestic cases of rabies, primarily from bites by usually docile, often nocturnal wild animals that attack without provocation. These include bats, foxes, woodchucks, squirrels, and skunks. The NP should check with local authorities for information on rabies when a bite involves domestic pets, because the rabies risk in this situation is usually negligible and rabies prophylaxis is not indicated.

DISCUSSION SOURCES

Gilbert, D., Moellering, R., and Sande, M. (2004). The Sanford Guide to Antimicrobial Therapy

TABLE 3–5

INFECTIOUS AGENTS AND TREATMENT IN BITES

Type of Bite	Infective Agent	Prophylaxis or Treatment of Infection
Bat, raccoon, skunk	Uncertain; significant rabies risk	For bacterial infection Primary: amoxicillin with clavulanate, 875 mg/125 mg BID Alternative: doxycycline, 100 mg BID Animal should be considered rabid, and patients should be given rabies immune globulin and vaccine
Cat	*Pasteurella multocida, Staphylococcus aureus*	Primary: amoxicillin with clavulanate, 875 mg/125 mg BID Alternative: cefuroxime, 0.5 g BID; doxycycline, 100 mg orally BID Switch to penicillin if *P. multocida* is cultured from wound
Dog	Viridans spp., *P. multocida, S. aureus, Bacteroides* spp., others	Primary: amoxicillin with clavulanate, 875 mg/125 mg BID Alternative: clindamycin, 300 mg QID; a fluoroquinolone; or clindamycin with TMP-SMX (children)
Human	Viridans spp., *Staphylococcus epidermidis, S. corynebacterium, S. aureus, Bacteroides* spp., others	Early, not yet infected: amoxicillin with clavulanate, 875 mg/125 mg BID for 5 days Later (3–24 hr, signs of infections): parenteral therapy with ampicillin with sulbactam, cefoxitin, others
Rat	*Streptobacillus moniliformis, Spirillum minus*	Primary: amoxicillin with clavulanate, 875 mg/125 mg BID Alternative: doxycycline Rabies prophylaxis not indicated
Swine	Polymicrobial gram-positive cocci, gram-negative bacilli, anaerobes, Pasteurella spp.	Primary: amoxicillin with clavulanate, 875 mg/125 mg BID Alternative: parenteral third-generation cephalosporin, others
Nonhuman primate	Herpes virus simiae	Acyclovir

Adapted from Gilbert, D., Moellering, R., and Sande, M. (2004). The Sanford Guide to Antimicrobial Therapy (34th ed.). Hyde Park, VT: Antimicrobial therapy, p. 35.
BID, twice a day; QID, four times a day; TMP-SMX, trimethoprim-sulfamethoxazole.

(34th ed.). Hyde Park, VT: Antimicrobial Therapy.

Britton, I, and Hektor Dunphy, L. (2004). Skin disorders. In Hektor Dunphy: Management Guidelines for Nurse Practitioners Working with Adults. Philadelphia: F.A. Davis.

QUESTIONS

34. A patient presents with a painful blistering thermal burn involving the first, second, and third digits of his right hand. The most appropriate plan of care is to:

A. apply an anesthetic cream to the area and open the blisters.

B. apply silver sulfadiazine cream (Silvadene) to the area and then apply a bulky dressing.

C. refer the patient to burn specialty care.

D. loosely wrap the burn with a nonadherent dressing and prescribe an analgesic agent.

35. You examine a patient with a red, tender thermal burn that has excellent capillary refill involving the anterior right leg. The estimated involved body surface area is appropriately:

    A. 5%.
    B. 9%.
    C. 13%.
    D. 18%.

36. Which of the following best describes a second-degree burn?

    A. The affected skin blanches with ease.
    B. The surface is raw and moist.
    C. The affected area is white and leathery.
    D. The affected area is lichenified.

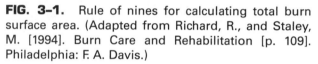

Anterior   **Posterior**

FIG. 3–1. Rule of nines for calculating total burn surface area. (Adapted from Richard, R., and Staley, M. [1994]. Burn Care and Rehabilitation [p. 109]. Philadelphia: F. A. Davis.)

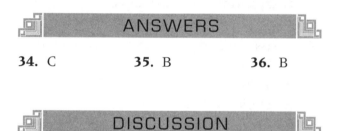

ANSWERS

34. C   **35.** B   **36.** B

DISCUSSION

As with bites, burn intervention includes asking for a complete history of the events leading up to the injury, to develop a plan for avoiding future events. In addition, education for burn avoidance for high-risk individuals for burn injury such as children, the elderly, and smokers should be a routine part of primary care.

In general, smaller (<10% of body surface area), minor (second-degree or lower) burns not involving a high-function area such as the hand or foot and of minimal cosmetic consequence can be treated in the outpatient setting. Treatment options include prevention of infection by the use of a topical antibiotic such as silver sulfadiazine. Patients with any burn involving areas of high function, such as the hands and feet, or of significant cosmetic consequence, such as the face, should be referred promptly to specialty care.

First- and second-degree burns are characterized by erythema, hyperemia, and pain. With first-degree burns, the skin blanches with ease; skin with second-degree burns has blisters and a raw, moist surface. In third-degree burns, pain may be minimal, but the burns are usually surrounded by areas of painful first- and second-degree burns. The surface of third-degree burns is usually white and leathery. It is important to estimate the surface area of the body affected by the burn (Fig. 3–1).

DISCUSSION SOURCES

Gilbert, D., Moellering, R., and Sande, M. (2004). The Sanford Guide to Antimicrobial Therapy (34th ed., pp. 36). Hyde Park, VT: Antimicrobial Therapy.

Britton, I, and Hektor Dunphy, L. (2004). Skin disorders. In Hektor Dunphy: Management Guidelines for Nurse Practitioners Working with Adults. Philadelphia: F.A. Davis.

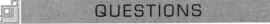

QUESTIONS

37. The most common causative organisms in cellulitis are:

   A. *Escherichia coli* and *Haemophilus influenzae.*

   B. *Bacteroides* species and other anaerobes.

   C. group A beta-hemolytic streptococci and *S. aureus.*

   D. pathogenic viruses.

38. Which of the following is the best treatment option for cellulitis?

   A. cephalexin

   B. doxycycline

   C. metronidazole

   D. trimethoprim-sulfamethoxazole

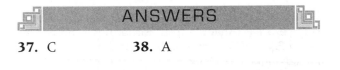

ANSWERS

37. C   **38.** A

DISCUSSION

Cellulitis is an acute infection of the subcutaneous tissue and skin. It usually spreads rapidly and is most commonly found in the extremities. The cause is usually a gram-positive organism such as group A beta-hemolytic streptococci and *S. aureus.* On occasion, particularly in immunocompromised individuals, select gram-negative organisms are the causative agent.

Treatment for cellulitis involves the choice of an antimicrobial agent with strong gram-positive coverage (in streptococcal and staphylococcal infection) and stability in the presence of beta-lactamase (in staphylococcal infection). The *Sanford Guide* recommends the following oral agents, all demonstrating the characteristics just described:

- erythromycin
- a cephalosporin
- amoxicillin with clavulanate (Augmentin)
- clarithromycin (Biaxin)
- azithromycin (Zithromax)
- dicloxacillin

DISCUSSION SOURCES

Gilbert, D., Moellering, R., and Sande, M. (2004). The Sanford Guide to Antimicrobial Therapy (34th ed., p. 36). Hyde Park, VT: Antimicrobial Therapy.

Britton, I, and Hektor Dunphy, L. (2004). Skin disorders. In Hektor Dunphy: Management Guidelines for Nurse Practitioners Working with Adults. Philadelphia: F.A. Davis.

QUESTIONS

39. The most important aspect of skin care for individuals with atopic dermatitis is:

   A. frequent bathing with antibacterial soap.

   B. consistent use of medium- to high-potency topical steroids.

   C. application of lubricants.

   D. treatment of dermatophytes.

40. A common trigger agent for contact dermatitis is:

   A. nickel.

   B. fabric softener.

   C. soaps.

   D. spicy foods.

41. One of the more common sites for atopic dermatitis in the adult is:

   A. the dorsum of the hand.

   B. the face.

   C. the neck.

   D. flexor surfaces.

42. One of the more common sites for atopic dermatitis in the infant is:

   A. the diaper area.

   B. the face.

   C. the neck.

   D. the posterior trunk.

43. The mechanism of action of tacrolimus in the treatment of atopic dermatis is as:

   A. an immunomodulator.

   B. an antimitotic.

   C. a mast cell activator.

   D. an exfoliant.

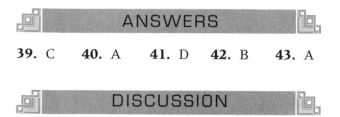

ANSWERS

39. C   **40.** A   **41.** D   **42.** B   **43.** A

DISCUSSION

Atopic dermatitis, or eczema, is one manifestation of a type I hypersensitivity reaction. This type of reaction is caused when immunoglobulin E (IgE) antibodies occupy receptor sites on mast cells. This causes a degradation of the mast cell and subsequent release of histamine, vasodilatation, mucous gland stimulation, and tissue swelling. Type I hypersensitivity reactions belong to two subgroups: atopy and anaphylaxis.

The atopy subgroup includes a number of common clinical conditions, such as allergic rhinitis, atopic dermatitis, allergic gastroenteropathy, and allergy-based asthma. Atopic diseases have a strong familial component and tend to cause localized rather than systemic reactions. Individuals with atopic disease are often able to identify allergy-inducing agents.

The diagnosis of atopic dermatitis includes the presence of itching and scratching, plus three or more of the following: red or inflamed rash, presence of excessive dryness/scaling, and location in skin folds of arms or legs. Additional findings include early age at initial onset (0 to 5 years) and elevated serum IgE and peripheral blood eosinophil levels. In infants, the face is often involved, whereas the diaper area, owing to the occlusive, damp enviroment, is usually spared.

Treatment for atopic dermatitis includes avoiding offending agents, minimizing skin dryness by limiting soap and water exposure, and the consistent use of lubricants. In general, the patient should be encouraged to treat the skin with care because it tends to be sensitive. When flares occur, the skin eruption is caused largely by histamine release. Antihistamines and/or topical and systemic corticosteroids are typically used to control flares. With an acute flare, an intermediate-potency topical corticosteroid is usually needed to control acute symptoms. After this is achieved, the topical corticosteroid of lowest potency that yields the desired effect should be used (see Table 3–3). Tacrolimus and pimecrolimus are immunomodulators that are helpful in the treatment of atopic dermatitis and offer a noncorticosteroid option for atopic dermatitis; these products block T cell stimulation by antigen-presenting cells and inhibit mast cell activation.

Itch (pruritus) is a very distressing symptom; many patients say it is more distressing than pain. It is a cardinal symptom of many forms of dermatitis. Histamine contributes to the development of itching; therefore, antihistamines can provide relief. Pruritus tends to be worst at night, often causing disturbance in sleep. In particular, providing the patient with a bedtime dose of antihistamine can yield tremendous relief from itch and improve sleep. Hydroxyzine (Atarax) appears to provide somewhat better relief of itch than do other antihistamines. Certirizine (Zyrtec) is a nonsedating antihistamine that is a metabolite of hydroxyzine.

DISCUSSION SOURCES

Berger, A. (2003). Skin, hair, and nails. In Tierney, L., McPhee, S., and Papadakis, M. (eds.). Current Medical Diagnosis and Treatment (pp. 80–145). Philadelphia: Lange Medical Books/McGraw-Hill.

Britton, I, and Hektor Dunphy, L. (2004). Skin disorders. In Hektor Dunphy: Management Guidelines for Nurse Practitioners Working with Adults. Philadelphia: F.A. Davis.

QUESTIONS

44. A 38-year-old woman with advanced human immunodeficiency virus (HIV) disease presents with a chief complaint of a painful, itchy rash over her trunk. Examination reveals linear vesicular lesions that do not cross the midline and are distributed over the posterior thorax. This is most consistent with:

    A. herpes zoster.
    B. dermatitis herpetiformis.
    C. molluscum contagiosum.
    D. impetigo.

45. A Tzanck smear that is positive for giant multinucleated cells was taken from a lesion caused by:

    A. herpesvirus.
    B. *S. aureus.*
    C. streptococci.
    D. allergic reaction.

46. When caring for an adult with an outbreak of shingles, you advise that:

    A. there is no known treatment for this condition.
    B. during outbreaks, the chickenpox virus is shed.
    C. although they are acutely painful, the lesions will heal well without scarring or lingering discomfort.
    D. this condition commonly strikes young and old alike.

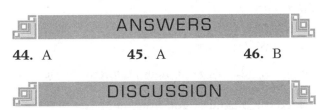

ANSWERS

44. A   **45.** A   **46.** B

DISCUSSION

Herpes zoster infection, commonly known as shingles, is an acutely painful condition caused by the varicella-zoster virus, the same agent that causes chickenpox. The virus lies dormant in the dorsal root ganglia of a dermatome. When activated, the characteristic blistering lesions occur along a dermatome, usually not crossing the midline. Any person who has had chickenpox is at risk for shingles, whereas recipients of varicella-zoster immunization have virtually no risk. Shingles is usually seen in persons of advanced age, those who are immunocompromised, and those with some other underlying health problem. When it is seen in younger adults, the possibility of HIV infection or other immunocompromise should be considered. During the acute attack, the chickenpox (varicella zoster) virus is shed;

therefore, patients may transmit this infection. Shingles, however, is not communicable from person to person.

Diagnosis of shingles is usually straightforward because of its characteristic lesions. If confirmation is needed, a Tzanck smear will reveal giant multinucleated cells, a finding in all herpetic infections.

Scarring and post-herpetic neuralgia are problematic sequelae of shingles. Initiating antiviral therapy with high-dose acyclovir (Zovirax), valacyclovir (Valtrex), or famciclovir (Famvir), preferably within the first 72 hours of herpes zoster outbreak, helps limit the severity of the lesions as well as minimize the risk of post-herpetic neuralgia and scarring.

Adequate analgesia should be offered to the person with shingles. Using a combination of topical agents such as Burow solution along with a high-potency nonsteroidal anti-inflammatory drug or opioid, or both, helps provide considerable relief. The patient should also be monitored for suprainfection of lesions. Because of the risk of complication and possible compromise of vision, expert consultation should be sought if herpes zoster involves a facial dermatome. Nonsteroidal anti-inflammatory drugs should not be prescribed during acute varicella infection because of the risk of necrotizing fasciitis.

DISCUSSION SOURCES

Berger, A. (2003). Skin, hair, and nails. In Tierney, L., McPhee, S., and Papadakis, M. (eds.). Current Medical Diagnosis and Treatment (pp. 80–145). Philadelphia: Lange Medical Books/McGraw-Hill.

Britton, I, and Hektor Dunphy, L. (2004). Skin disorders. In Hektor Dunphy: Management Guidelines for Nurse Practitioners Working with Adults. Philadelphia: F.A. Davis.

QUESTIONS

47. Characteristics of onychomycosis include all of the following except:

    A. it is readily diagnosed by clinical examination.
    B. nail hypertrophy.

C. brittle nails.

D. fingernails respond more readily to therapy than toenails.

18. When prescribing itraconazole (Sporanox), the NP considers that:

A. the drug is a cytochrome P-450 3A4 inhibitor.

B. one pulse cycle is recommended for fingernail treatment, and two cycles are needed for toenail therapy.

C. continuous therapy is preferred in the presence of hepatic disease.

D. taking the drug on an empty stomach enhances the efficacy of the product.

49. When prescribing pulse dosing with itraconazole (Sporanox) for the treatment of fingernail fungus, the NP realizes that:

A. a transient increase in AST levels may be seen.

B. drug-induced leukopenia is a common problem.

C. the patient needs to be warned about excessive bleeding because of the drug's antiplatelet effect.

D. its use is contraindicated in the presence of iron-deficiency anemia

50. In diagnosing onychomycosis, the NP considers that:

A. nails often have a single midline groove.

B. pitting is often seen.

C. microscopic examination reveals hyphae.

D. Beau's lines are present.

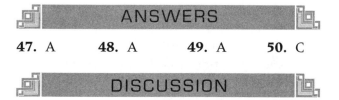

ANSWERS

47. A   **48.** A   **49.** A   **50.** C

DISCUSSION

Onychomycosis, or dermatophytosis of the nail, is a chronic disfiguring disorder. The nails are dull, thickened, and lusterless with a pithy consistency. Parts of the nail often break off. Because trauma and other conditions can cause a similar appearance, confirmation of the diagnosis with microscopic examination for hyphae of the nail scrapings mixed with potassium hydroxide (KOH) is important.

Until recently, therapeutic options were limited. Topical treatment proved to be of little value because the fungal agent is held within the nail matrix. Oral products such as griseofulvin required months of therapy because the drug was taken up by the developing nailbed and still yielded a high rate of relapse.

Antifungals such as itraconazole (Sporanox) and terbinafine (Lamisil) offer well-tolerated effective treatment for fingernail and toenail fungal infections. Both can be used in pulse cycles, with times of drug use alternating with abstinent periods. An example of pulse dosing is itraconazole, 400 mg daily for the first week of the month for 2 months, to treat the fingernails and for 3 months to treat the toenails. These products are held within the nail matrix for months after therapy; this produces effective treatment at a considerably reduced cost in comparison with constant therapy. In addition, all oral antifungals have hepatotoxic potential and may cause an increase in AST levels. However, pulse therapy lessens this risk considerably.

Caution is needed when itraconazole is prescribed because it inhibits by cytochrome P-450 3A4, a pathway also used by drugs such as diazepam, digoxin, anticoagulants, and certain HIV protease inhibitors. When these agents attempt to use this metabolic pathway, levels of both potentially increase, causing toxicity. Terbinafine has significantly fewer drug interactions.

DISCUSSION SOURCES

Berger, A. (2003). Skin, hair, and nails. In Tierney, L., McPhee, S., and Papadakis, M. (eds.). Current Medical Diagnosis and Treatment (pp. 80–145). Philadelphia: Lange Medical Books/McGraw-Hill.

Britton, I, and Hektor Dunphy, L. (2004). Skin disorders. In Hektor Dunphy: Management Guidelines for Nurse Practitioners Working with Adults. Philadelphia: F. A. Davis.

QUESTIONS

51. A 78-year-old resident of a long-term care facility complains of generalized itchiness at night that disturbs her sleep. Her examination is consistent with scabies. Which of the following do you expect to find on examination?

   A. excoriated papules on the interdigital area
   B. annular lesions over the buttocks
   C. vesicular lesions in a linear pattern
   D. honey-colored crusted lesions that began as vesicles

52. Which of the following represents the most accurate patient advice when using permethrin (Elimite) for treating scabies?

   A. To avoid systemic absorption, the medication should be applied over the body and rinsed off within 1 hour.
   B. The patient will notice a marked reduction in pruritus within 48 hours of using the product.
   C. Itch often persists for a few weeks after successful treatment.
   D. It is a second-line product in the treatment of scabies.

53. When advising the patient about scabies contagion, you inform her that:

   A. mites can live for a number of weeks away from the host.
   B. close personal contact with an infected person is usually needed to contract this disease.
   C. casual contact with an infected person is likely to result in infestation.
   D. bedding used by an infected person must be destroyed.

ANSWERS

51. A   **52.** C   **53.** B

DISCUSSION

Scabies is a communicable skin disease generally requiring close personal contact, such as sexual relations, to achieve contagion. However, contact with used, unwashed bedding and clothing from an infected person can result in infection. As a result, bedclothes and other items used by a person with scabies must be either washed in hot water or placed in a clothes dryer for a normal cycle. As an alternative, items can be placed in plastic storage bags for at least 1 week because mites do not survive for more than 3 to 4 days without contact with the host. Mites tend to burrow in areas of warmth, such as the finger webs, axillary folds, the belt line, areolae, the scrotum, and the penis, with lesions developing in these areas. The lesions may start with the characteristic burrows but usually progress to a vesicular or papular form, often with excoriation caused by scratching.

Permethrin (Elimite) lotion is the preferred method of treatment for scabies. The lotion must be left on for 8 to 14 hours to be effective. Despite effective therapy, individuals with scabies often have a significant problem with pruritus after permethrin treatment because of the presence of dead mites and their waste trapped in the skin, which causes an inflammatory reaction. This debris is eliminated from the body over a few weeks; therefore, the distress of itchiness passes at that time. Oral antihistamines, particularly for nighttime use, and low-to-medium-potency topical corticosteroids should be offered to help with this problem (Table 3–6). In the past, lindane (Kwell) was used, but this product presents potential problems with neurotoxicity and a resulting seizure risk, as well as lower efficacy. In particular, lindane should not be used by pregnant women, children, and elderly patients.

DISCUSSION SOURCE

Britton, I, and Hektor Dunphy, L. (2004). Skin disorders. In Hektor Dunphy: Management Guidelines for Nurse Practitioners Working with Adults. Philadelphia: F. A. Davis.

TABLE 3–6

MEDICATIONS USED IN THE TREATMENT OF ACUTE IgE–MEDIATED
HYPERSENSITIVITY REACTION

Medications	Mechanism of Action	Comments
Antihistamines	Antagonize H1-receptor sites. Prevent action of formed histamine so helpful in treatment of acute allergic reaction.	In acute reaction, give parenterally or in a quickly absorbed oral form such as chewable tablet or liquid. 1st generation products (diphenhydramine {Benadryl}, chlorpheniramine {Chlor-Trimeton}) • Cross blood-brain barrier causing sedation • Anticholinergic activity can cause blurred vision, dry mucous membranes. 2nd generation products (Loratadine {Claritin}, certirizine {Zyrtec}, fexofenadine {Allergra}) • Little transfer across blood-brain barrier. Low rates of sedation • Less anticholinergic effect
Epinephrine	Alpha-1, beta-1, beta-2 agonists. Potent vasoconstrictor, cardiac stimulant, bronchodilator	• Initial therapy for anaphylaxis due to its multiple modes of reversing airway and circulatory dysfunction • Anaphylaxis usually responds quickly to epinephrine given parenterally.
Oral corticosteroids	Inhibit eosinophilic action and other inflammatory mediators	• In higher dose and with longer therapy (>2 weeks), adrenal suppression may occur. • Taper usually not needed if use is short term (<10 days)and at lower dose (prednisone 40–60 mg/day) • Potential for causing gastropathy

www.anaphylaxis.org, accessed 9/17/04

QUESTIONS

54. You examine a patient with psoriasis vulgaris and expect to find the following lesions:

    A. lichenified areas in flexor areas
    B. red, well-demarcated plaques on the knees
    C. greasy lesions throughout the scalp
    D. vesicular lesions over the upper thorax

55. Psoriatic lesions are caused by:

    A. decreased exfoliation.
    B. rapid cell turnover, leading to decreased maturation and keratinization.
    C. inflammatory changes.
    D. lichenification.

56. Anthralin (Drithocreme) is helpful in treating psoriasis because it has what kind of activity?

    A. antimitotic
    B. exfoliative
    C. vasoconstrictor
    D. humectant

57. Treatment options in generalized psoriasis include all of the following except:

    A. psoralen with ultraviolet A light (PUVA) therapy.
    B. methotrexate.
    C. cyclosporine.
    D. systemic corticosteroids.

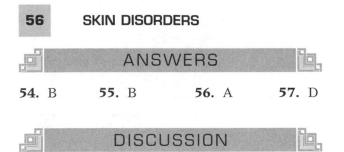

ANSWERS

54. B   **55.** B   **56.** A   **57.** D

DISCUSSION

Psoriasis vulgaris is a chronic skin disorder caused by accelerated mitosis and rapid cell turnover, which lead to decreased maturation and keratinization. This process prevents the dermal cells from "sticking" together, allowing for a shedding of cells in the form of characteristic silvery scales and leaving an underlying red plaque. Psoriasis is typically found in extensor surfaces; therefore, it is most often found in plaquelike lesions over the elbows and knees. The scalp and other surfaces are occasionally involved.

Topical corticosteroids have some antimitotic activity, which allows for regression of psoriatic plaques. It is often effective to use a medium- to high-potency drug for short periods of time until the plaques resolve and then to use a lower potency product three to four times a week to maintain remission. As with all dermatoses, consistent use of high-potency topical steroids is discouraged. Tar preparations can be very helpful, but they have a low level of patient acceptance because of their messiness and odor.

Additional treatment options include use of anthralin (Drithocreme), an antimitotic, and calciprotriene, a vitamin D_3 derivative. Although they do offer effective psoriasis therapy, these products are significantly more expensive than topical corticosteroids and tars. Use should be reserved for steroid-resistant cases.

If psoriasis is generalized, covering more than 30% of body surface area, treatment with topical products is difficult and expensive. Ultraviolet A light exposure three times weekly is highly effective. Light therapy is associated with an increase in skin cancer risk.

For severe, recalcitrant psoriasis, cyclosporine, methotrexate, and systemic retinoid are also used. Referral to a dermatologist or NP with expertise in prescribing these agents is indicated for these patients.

DISCUSSION SOURCES

Berger, A. (2003). Skin, hair, and nails. In Tierney, L., McPhee, S., and Papadakis, M. (eds.). Current Medical Diagnosis and Treatment (pp. 80–145). Philadelphia: Lange Medical Books/McGraw-Hill.

Britton, I, and Hektor Dunphy, L. (2004). Skin disorders. In Hektor Dunphy: Management Guidelines for Nurse Practitioners Working with Adults. Philadelphia: F. A. Davis.

QUESTIONS

58. Which of the following best describes seborrheic dermatitis lesions?

   A. flaking lesions in the antecubital and popliteal spaces
   B. greasy, scaling lesions on the scalp
   C. intensely itchy lesions in the groin folds
   D. silvery lesions on the elbows and knees

59. In counseling a patient with seborrheic dermatitis on the scalp about efforts to clear lesions, you advise her to:

   A. use an antifungal shampoo.
   B. apply petroleum jelly nightly to the affected area.
   C. coat the area with high-potency corticosteroid cream three times a week.
   D. periodically expose the lesions to sunlight.

ANSWERS

58. B   **59.** A

DISCUSSION

Seborrheic dermatitis is a chronic, recurrent skin condition found in areas with a high concentration of sebaceous glands, such as the scalp, eyelid margins, nasolabial folds, ears, and upper trunk. A number of theories are proposed for its cause. Because of the lesions' response to antifungal agents, the backbone of therapy, seborrheic dermatitis is most likely caused by an inflammatory reaction to *Pityrosporum ovale,* a yeast present on the scalp of all humans. Further supporting this hypothesis is the fact that seborrhea is often found in immunocompromised patients and in those who are chronically ill (e.g., the elderly population and those with Parkinson disease).

The use of lubricants such as petroleum jelly may help remove stubborn lesions so that the lesions can be exposed to antifungal therapy (e.g., selenium sulfide or ketaconazole shampoo), but this does not constitute first-line therapy. As with any skin condition, high-potency topical corticosteroid use is discouraged because of the risk of subcutaneous atrophy, telangiectatic vessels, and other problems. Although seborrhea usually worsens in the winter and improves in the summer, exposing lesions to sunlight is not recommended because of the potential increase in skin cancer risk.

DISCUSSION SOURCE

Britton, I, and Hektor Dunphy, L. (2004). Skin disorders. In Hektor Dunphy: Management Guidelines for Nurse Practitioners Working with Adults. Philadelphia: F. A. Davis.

QUESTIONS

60. A 49-year-old man presents with a lesion suspect for malignant melanoma. You describe it as having:

    A. deep black-brown coloring throughout.
    B. sharp borders.
    C. a diameter of 3 mm or less.
    D. variable pigmentation.

61. A 72-year-old woman presents with a newly formed, painless, pearly, ulcerated nodule with an overlying telangiectasis on the upper lip. This most likely represents:

    A. an actinic keratosis.
    B. a basal cell carcinoma.
    C. a squamous cell carcinoma.
    D. molluscum contagiosum.

62. Which of the following represents the most effective method of cancer screening?

    A. skin examination
    B. stool for occult blood
    C. pelvic examination
    D. chest radiography

63. Risk factors for malignant melanoma include:

    A. Asian ancestry.
    B. history of blistering sunburn.
    C. use of sunscreen in childhood.
    D. presence of atopic dermatitis.

64. Actinic keratoses can be described as:

    A. a slightly rough, pink or flesh-colored lesion in a sun-exposed area.
    B. a well-defined, slightly raised, red, scaly plaque in a skinfold.
    C. a blistering lesion along a dermatome.
    D. a crusting lesion along flexor aspects of the fingers.

65. Treatment options for actinic keratoses include topical:

    A. hydrocortisone.
    B. fluorouracil.
    C. acyclovir.
    D. doxepin.

ANSWERS

60. D	**61.** B	**62.** A
63. B	**64.** A	**65.** B

DISCUSSION

As with any area of dermatology, accurate diagnosis of a condition depends on knowledge of the description of the lesion as well as its most likely site of occurrence. The most potent risk factor for any skin cancer is sun exposure; instruct patients on sun avoidance. The consistent use of high–sun protection factor (SPF) sunscreen is critical and helps reduce but not eliminate the risk of squamous or basal cell carcinoma. Sunscreen use likely does little to minimize malignant melanoma risk.

Skin examination has the benefit of enabling the examiner to detect premalignant lesions (e.g., actinic keratoses and precursor lesions to squamous cell carcinoma) as well as malignant lesions. The American Cancer Society proposes the "ABCDE" mnemonic for assessing malignant melanoma:

A = asymmetric with nonmatching sides
B = borders are irregular
C = color is not uniform; brown, black, red, white, blue
D = diameter usually larger than 6 mm, or the size a pencil eraser
E = evolving lesions, either new or changing

Similar memory aids for squamous and basal cell carcinoma are as follows:
- For basal cell carcinoma ("PUT ON S'unscreen"):
P = pearly papule
U = ulcerating
T = telangiectasia
O = on the face, scalp, pinnae
N = nodule
S = slow growing
- Squamous cell carcinoma—early lesions ("NO SUN"):
N = nodular
O = opaque
S = sun-exposed areas
U = ulcerating
N = nondistinct borders

Later lesions may also include scale and firm margins.

Treatment of actinic keratoses, also known as solar keratoses, includes cryotherapy with liquid nitrogen. This causes the lesions to crust for about 2 weeks, revealing healed tissue, with excellent cosmetic outcome. An alternative is the use of 1% to 5% fluorouracil creams once a day for 2 to 3 weeks until the lesions become crusted over. As another alternative, 5% fluorouracil cream can be used once a day for 1 day to 2 consecutive days weekly for 7 to 10 weeks. This will yield a similar therapeutic outcome without crusting or discomfort. Treatment of skin cancers usually involves removal of the lesion. Further therapy is guided by the histologic diagnosis.

DISCUSSION SOURCES

Britton, I, and Hektor Dunphy, L. (2004). Skin disorders. In Hektor Dunphy: Management Guidelines for Nurse Practitioners Working with Adults. Philadelphia: F. A. Davis.

Schleve, M. (2001). Common cutaneous malignancies. In Fitzpatrick, J., and Aeling, J. (eds.). Dermatology Secrets (2nd ed., pp. 313–320) Philadelphia: Hanley & Belfus.

QUESTIONS

66. Which of the following is the most frequent cause of stasis ulcers?

    A. arterial insufficiency
    B. venous insufficiency
    C. diabetes mellitus
    D. fungal dermatitis

67. You examine the left lower extremity of a patient and find an ulcerated lesion with irregular borders and edema with brown discoloration of the surrounding tissue. The best treatment option at this time is:

    A. compression therapy.
    B. referral for surgical débridement.
    C. daily use of a topical antibiotic cream.
    D. application of a dry, sterile dressing.

68. A 70-year-old man presents with absent popliteal pulses and a cool, hairless foot with a 2-cm ulcer that has a "punched-out" appearance on the dorsum of the second toe. The appropriate next measure is to:

    A. arrange for evaluation by a vascular surgeon.
    B. apply wet to dry dressings.

C. start the patient on a peripheral vasodilator.

D. advise the patient to elevate his feet for 15 minutes three times a day.

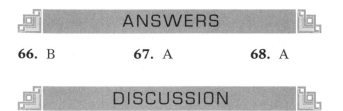

ANSWERS

66. B   **67.** A   **68.** A

DISCUSSION

Stasis ulcers are most commonly caused by venous insufficiency. They are also caused far less commonly by arterial insufficiency, diabetes mellitus, and fungal infections. Because poor venous return causes lower extremity edema, which leads to decreased tissue perfusion and the resulting risk of ulcer, compression therapy is key to successful therapy. Débridement is needed only when necrotic tissue is present, and antimicrobial therapy is needed when there are signs of infection. Venous stasis ulcers usually respond well to occlusive hydroactive dressings such as hydrocolloid gel (Duoderm). In addition, an Unna boot can help but it necessitates weekly changing. If the wound does not respond, treatment with becalermin (Regranex) or grafting may be necessary. Regardless of the treatment chosen, venous stasis ulcers necessitate long-term care, including good nutrition and expert wound management. Involving home help care and wound care management nursing experts greatly enhances success.

The description of the lesion in Question 68 is consistent not with peripheral venous disease but rather with peripheral arterial disease. The treatment of choice is revascularization of the limb to enhance circulation. This is the only treatment option that will result in resolution of the lesion (see Chapter 9 for additional information).

DISCUSSION SOURCES

Berger, A. (2003). Skin, hair, and nails. In Tierney, L., McPhee, S., and Papadakis, M. (eds.). Current Medical Diagnosis and Treatment (pp. 80–145). Philadelphia: Lange Medical Books/McGraw-Hill.

Britton, J. and Hektor Dunphy, L. (2004). Skin disorders. In Hektor Dunphy: Management Guidelines for Nurse Practitioners Working with Adults. Philadelphia: F. A. Davis.

QUESTIONS

69. Which of the following do you expect to find in the assessment of the person with urticaria?

A. eosinophilia
B. depressed sedimentation rate
C. elevated thyroid-stimulating hormone level
D. leukopenia

70. A 24-year-old woman presents with hive-form linear lesions that form over areas where she has scratched. These resolve within a few minutes. They most likely represent:

A. dermographism.
B. contact dermatitis.
C. angioedema.
D. allergic reaction.

71. An urticarial lesion is usually described as a:

A. wheal.
B. plaque.
C. patch.
D. papule.

ANSWERS

69. A   **70.** A   **71.** A

DISCUSSION

Urticaria is a condition in which eruptions of wheals or hives occur most often in response to allergen exposure. The most common cause is a type I hypersensitivity reaction. This type of reaction is caused when IgE antibodies occupy receptor sites on mast cells. This causes a degradation of the mast cell and subsequent release of histamine, vasodilatation, mucous gland stimulation, and tissue swelling. Treatment of type I hypersensitivity includes avoidance of the provoking agent, as well as antihistamines and steroids. Type I hypersensitivity reactions consist of two subgroups: atopy and anaphylaxis.

Urticarial lesions often develop as groups of intensely itchy wheals or hives. The lesions usually last less than 24 hours and often only 2 to 4 hours. However, new lesions may form, extending the outbreak to 1 to 2 weeks.

Within the atopy subgroup are a number of common clinical conditions such as allergic rhinitis, atopic dermatitis, allergic gastroenteropathy, and allergy-based asthma. Atopic diseases have a strong familial component and tend to cause localized rather than systemic reactions. The person with atopic disease is often able to identify allergy-inducing agents. In addition to avoidance of offending agents, treatment for systemic atopic disease includes antihistamines, corticosteroids, leukotriene modifiers (zafirlukast [Accolate], montelukast [Singulair]) and mast cell stabilizers such as cromolyn sodium (Intal, NasalCrom).

Anaphylaxis typically causes a systemic IgE-mediated reaction to exposure to an allergen, often a drug (e.g., penicillin) insect venom (e.g., bee sting), or food (e.g., peanuts). Anaphylaxis is characterized by widespread vasodilatation, urticaria, angioedema, and bronchospasm, creating a life-threatening condition of airway obstruction coupled with circulatory collapse. First-line treatment includes avoiding or discontinuing use of the offending agent. Simultaneously, maintaining airway patency as well as adequate circulation is critical. Angioedema and urticaria are subcutaneous anaphylactic reactions but are not life-threatening unless tissue swelling impinges on the airway (see Table 3–5).

DISCUSSION SOURCES

Berger, A. (2003). Skin, hair, and nails. In Tierney, L., McPhee, S., and Papadakis, M. (eds.). Current Medical Diagnosis and Treatment (pp. 80–145). Philadelphia: Lange Medical Books/McGraw-Hill.

Britton, I, and Hektor Dunphy, L. (2004). Skin disorders. In Hektor Dunphy: Management Guidelines for Nurse Practitioners Working with Adults. Philadelphia: F. A. Davis.

QUESTIONS

72. When counseling a person who has a 2-mm verruca on the hand, you advise that:

A. bacteria are the most common cause of these lesions.

B. most lesions will resolve without therapy in 12 to 24 months.

C. there is a significant risk for future dermatologic malignancy.

D. surgical excision is the treatment of choice.

73. Imiquimoid's mechanism of action is as:

A. immunomodulator.

B. antimitotic.

C. keratolytic.

D. irritant.

ANSWERS

72. B   **73.** A

DISCUSSION

Verruca vulgaris lesions are also known as warts. The majority of them are caused by human papillomavirus, which is passed through direct person-to-person contact. Over a 12- to 24-month period, nearly all of these lesions resolve without therapy. Surgical excision is rarely indicated. Intervention is warranted if warts interfere with function, such as with painful plantar warts on the soles of the feet, or if they are cosmetically problematic (Table 3–7).

DISCUSSION SOURCES

Berger, A. (2003). Skin, hair, and nails. In Tierney, L., McPhee, S., and Papadakis, M. (eds.). Current Medical Diagnosis and Treatment (pp. 80–145). Philadelphia: Lange Medical Books/McGraw-Hill.

Britton, I, and Hektor Dunphy, L. (2004). Skin disorders. In Hektor Dunphy: Management Guidelines for Nurse Practitioners Working with Adults. Philadelphia: F. A. Davis.

TABLE 3–7.
TREATMENT OPTIONS FOR WARTS

Treatment	Instructions for use	Comments
Liquid nitrogen	Apply to achieve a thaw time of 20–45 sec Two freeze-thaw cycles may be given every 2–4 weeks until lesion is gone	Usually good cosmetic results Can be painful, requires multiple treatments
Keratolytic agents (Occlusal, Duofilm, DuoPlant, others)	Apply as directed until lesions resolve	May need long-term therapy before resolution Well tolerated With plantar warts, pare down lesion; then apply 40% salicylic acid plaster, changing every 5 days
Podophyllum resin (podofilox)	Patient applies 3 times a week for 4–6 weeks	Multiple cycles may be needed Skin irritation common
Tretinoin	Apply BID to flat warts for 4–6 weeks	Needs consistent treatment for optimal results
Imiquimod (Aldara)	Frequency and duration of use are dependent on wart location	Immunomodulator Low rate of wart recurrence
Laser therapy	Used to dissect lesions	Needs 4–6 weeks to granulate tissue Best reserved for treatment-resistant warts

Britton, I, and Hektor Dunphy, L. (2004). Skin disorders. In Hektor Dunphy: Management Guidelines for Nurse Practitioners Working with Adults. Philadelphia: F. A. Davis.

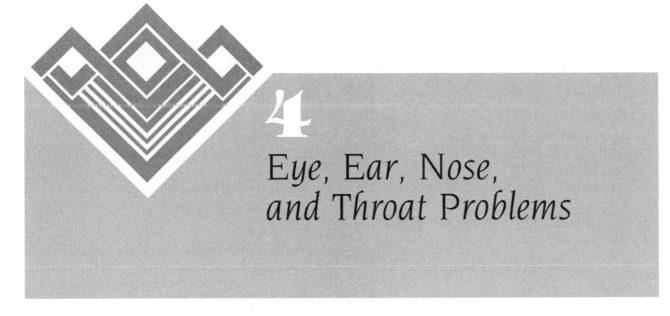

4

Eye, Ear, Nose, and Throat Problems

QUESTIONS

1. A 74-year-old woman has hypertension that is normally well controlled by hydrochlorothiazide. She presents with a 3-day history of unilateral throbbing headache with difficulty chewing because of pain. On physical examination, you find a tender, noncompressible temporal artery. Blood pressure (BP) is 160/88, apical pulse is 98, and respiratory rate is 22, and she is visibly uncomfortable. The most likely diagnosis is:

    A. giant cell arteritis.
    B. impending transient ischemic attack.
    C. migraine headache.
    D. temporal mandibular joint dysfunction.

2. Therapeutic interventions for the patient in Question 1 should include:

    A. corticosteroids for a number of months.
    B. addition of a dihydropyridine calcium channel blocker to her antihypertensive regimen.
    C. warfarin therapy.
    D. carbamazepine.

3. Concomitant disease seen with giant cell arteritis includes:

    A. polymyalgia rheumatica.
    B. pancreatitis.
    C. psoriatic arthritis.
    D. Reiter syndrome.

4. One of the most serious complications of giant cell arteritis is:

    A. hemiparesis.
    B. arthritis.
    C. blindness.
    D. uveitis.

ANSWERS

1. A   2. A
3. A   4. C

DISCUSSION

Giant cell or temporal arteritis is most common in patients who are 50 to 85 years old; average age at onset is 70 years. The headache is classically described as unilateral, surrounding the affected artery, and distressing.

Giant cell arteritis is a systemic disease affecting medium- and large-sized vessels. It also causes inflammation of the temporal artery because extracranial branches of the carotid artery are often involved; this is often a site of tenderness or a nodular, pulseless vessel. However, the temporal artery may be normal. Giant cell arteritis and polymyalgia rheumatica may represent two parts of a spectrum of disease and are often found together.

Apart from relieving pain, treatment of giant cell arteritis helps minimize the risk of blindness, which is the most serious complication of the disease. As soon as the diagnosis is made, corticosteroid therapy should be initiated; this therapy typically lasts 6 months to 2 years.

In the absence of symptoms of polymyalgia rheumatica, diagnosis of giant cell arteritis includes temporal artery biopsy and measurement of the erythrocyte sedimentation rate. At least 3 to 5 cm of artery is needed because the disease frequently skips portions of the vessel. Erythrocyte sedimentation rate, although it is a nonspecific test of inflammation, is usually markedly elevated.

The BP of the patient in Question 1 is probably elevated because of pain response. Analgesia should be given, and then BP response should be noted again. Adding a second antihypertensive agent to this patient's treatment ignores the most likely underlying cause of her BP elevation.

DISCUSSION SOURCES

Hellman, D., and Stone, J. (2003). Arthritis and musculoskeletal disorder. In Tierney, L., McPhee, S., and Papadakis, M. (eds.). Current Diagnosis and Treatment (42nd ed., pp. 783–836). New York: Lange Medical Books/McGraw-Hill.

Riordan-Eva, P. (2003). Eye. In Tierney, L., McPhee, S., and Papadakis, M. (eds.). Current Diagnosis and Treatment (42nd ed., pp. 147–177). New York: Lange Medical Books/McGraw-Hill.

Brinker Lester, P. (2004). Head and neck disorders. In Hektor Dunphy, L: Management Guidelines for Nurse Practitioners Working with Adults (2nd ed). Philadelphia: F.A. Davis, pp. 146–214.

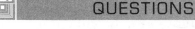

QUESTIONS

5. An 88-year-old community-dwelling man who lives alone has limited mobility because of osteoarthritis. Since his last office visit 2 months ago, he has lost 5% of his body weight and has developed angular cheilitis. You expect to find the following on examination:

   A. fissuring and cracking at the corners of the mouth
   B. marked erythema of the hard and soft palates
   C. white plaques on the lateral borders of the buccal mucosa
   D. raised, painless lesions on the gingiva

6. First-line therapy for angular cheilitis therapy includes the use of:

   A. metronidazole gel.
   B. hydrocortisone cream.
   C. topical nystatin.
   D. oral ketoconazole.

ANSWERS

5. A   **6.** C

DISCUSSION

A variety of oral infections are caused by *Candida* species, including angular cheilitis. The primary risk factor for oral candidiasis is immunocompromise, whether caused by advanced age and apparent malnutrition or as seen in human immunodeficiency virus infection.

Topical antifungals such as nystatin offer a reasonable first-line treatment for oral candidiasis. With particularly recalcitrant conditions and failure of topical therapy, systemic antifungals may be needed. Treatment of the underlying condition is critical.

DISCUSSION SOURCES

Jackler, R., and Kaplan, M. (2003). Ear, nose and throat. In Tierney, L., McPhee, S., and Papadakis, M. (eds.). Current Diagnosis and Treatment (42nd ed., pp. 179–215). New York: Lange Medical Books/McGraw-Hill.

Brinker Lester, P. (2004). Head and neck disorders. In Hektor Dunphy, L: Management Guidelines for Nurse Practitioners Working with Adults (2nd ed). Philadelphia: F.A. Davis, pp. 146–214.

QUESTIONS

7. A 19-year-old man presents with a chief complaint of a red, irritated right eye for the past 48 hours with eyelids that were "stuck together" this morning when he awoke. Examination reveals injected palpebral and bulbar conjunctiva; reactive pupils; vision screen with the Snellen chart of 20/30 in the right eye (OD), right eye (OS), and both eyes (OU); and purulent eye discharge on the right. This presentation is most consistent with:

  A. suppurative conjunctivitis.
  B. viral conjunctivitis.
  C. allergic conjunctivitis.
  D. mechanical injury.

8. A 19-year-old woman presents with conjunctivitis. She complains of bilaterally itchy, red eyes with tearing that occurs intermittently throughout the year and is often accompanied by a ropelike eye discharge and clear nasal discharge. This is most consistent with conjunctival inflammation caused by a(n):

  A. bacterium.
  B. virus.
  C. allergen.
  D. injury.

9. Common causative organisms of acute suppurative conjunctivitis include all of the following except:

  A. *Staphylococcus aureus.*
  B. *Haemophilus influenzae.*
  C. *Streptococcus pneumoniae.*
  D. *Pseudomonas aeruginosa.*

10. Treatment options in suppurative conjunctivitis include all of the following ophthalmic preparations except:

  A. bacitracin–polymyxin B.
  B. ciprofloxacin.
  C. erythromycin.
  D. penicillin.

11. Treatment options in acute and recurrent allergic conjunctivitis include all of the following except:

  A. cromolyn ophthalmic drops.
  B. oral antihistamines.
  C. ophthalmologic antihistamines.
  D. corticosteroid ophthalmic drops.

ANSWERS

7. A   **8.** C   **9.** D
10. D   **11.** D

DISCUSSION

Because therapy in conjunctivitis is in part aimed at eradicating or eliminating the underlying causes, accurate diagnosis is critical. The patient with a presumptive diagnosis of suppurative conjunctivitis requires antimicrobial therapy, whereas the person with allergic conjunctivitis benefits from therapy focused on identifying and limiting exposure to specific allergens, as well as the appropriate use of antiallergic agents (Table 4–1).

DISCUSSION SOURCES

Gilbert, D., Moellering, R., and Sande, M. (2004). The Sanford Guide to Antimicrobial Therapy (34th ed.). Hyde Park, VT: Antimicrobial Therapy.

Riordan-Eva, P. (2003). Eye. In Tierney, L., McPhee, S., and Papadakis, M. (eds.). Current Diagnosis and Treatment (42nd ed., pp. 147–177). New York: Lange Medical Books/McGraw-Hill.

QUESTIONS

12. Anterior epistaxis is usually caused by:

  A. hypertension.
  B. bleeding disorders.
  C. localized nasal mucosa trauma.
  D. a foreign body.

TABLE 4–1

TREATMENT OF COMMON BACTERIAL EENT INFECTION

Site of Infection	Common Pathogens	Recommended Antimicrobial	Comment
Suppurative conjunctivitis (non-gonococcal, non-chlamydial)	S. aureus, S. pneumoniae, H. influenzae	Primary: Ophthalmic treatment with bacitracin-polymixin B or trimethoprim or FQ (levofloxacin, ciprofloxacin, ofloxacin) or erythromycin Alternative: Ophthalmic gentamicin or tobramycin	Bacterial and viral conjunctivitis often self-limiting
Otitis externa (swimmer's ear)	Pseudomonas, Proteus, Enterobacteriaceae	Otitic drops with ofloxacin or ciprofloxacin with hydrocortisone or polymyxin B with neomycin and hydrocortisone	Ear canal cleansing important. Decrease risk of reinfection by use of eardrops of 1:2 mixture of white vinegar and rubbing alcohol after swimming. For acute disease, consider suprainfection w/ S. aureus; treat for dicloxacillin 500 mg QID.
Malignant otitis externa in person w/ DM	Pseudomonas	Oral ciprofloxacin for early disease suitable for outpatient therapy	Surgical débridement usually needed. MRI or CT imaging to evaluate for osteomyelitis may be indicated. Parenteral antimicrobial therapy may be warranted for severe disease.
Acute otitis media	S. pneumoniae, H. influenzae, M. catarrhalis, viral	If no antimicrobial therapy in the past month: Amoxicillin at high dose (HD) (3–4 g/d) in adults or usual doses (1.75–3 g/d) If antimicrobial therapy in past month: HD amoxicillin with or without clavulanate, cefdinir, cefpodoxime, cefprozil, cefuroxime If treatment failure >72 h of therapy and no antimicrobial therapy in past month: HD amoxicillin with clavulanate, cefdinir, cefpodoxime, cefprozil, cefuroxime, or IM ceftriaxone (ceftriaxone daily $\times$ 3 days) If treatment failure >72 h of therapy and antimicrobial therapy in past month: IM ceftriaxone qd $\times$ 3 d, clindamycin or tympanocentesis	Consider drug-resistant S. pneumoniae (DRSP) risk; Antimicrobial therapy in 3 months, age < 2 years, day care attendance. HD amoxicillin effective in DRSP. Length of therapy; < 2 y = 10 days, > 2 y 5–7 days If allergy to β-lactam drugs: TMP-SMX, clarithromycin, azithromycin; all less effective against DRSP when compared with other options If penicillin allergy history is unclear or rash (no hive-form lesions), cephalosporins likely OK. Clindamycin effective against DRSP, ineffective against H. influenzae, M. catarrhalis

Site of Infection	Common Pathogens	Recommended Antimicrobial	Comment
Exudative pharyngitis	Group A, C, G streptococcus, viral, HHV-6, *M. pneumoniae*	1st line: Penicillin V PO × 10 d or benzathine penicillin IM × 1 dose if adherence an issue Alternative: Erythromycin × 10 d, 2 d generation cephalosporin × 4–6 d, azithromycin × 5 d, clarithromycin × 10 d	Vesicular, ulcerative pharyngitis usually viral No treatment recommended for asymptomatic group A streptococcus carrier. For recurrent, culture-proven group A streptococcus, consider coinfection w/ beta-lactamase producing organism, treat w/ amoxicillin w/ clavulanate or clindamycin

Gilbert, D, Moellering, R, Sande, M. (2004). The Sanford Guide to Antimicrobial Therapy, 34th ed. Hyde Park, VT: Antimicrobial Therapy, Inc.

13. First-line intervention for anterior epistaxis includes:

   A. nasal packing.
   B. application of topical thrombin.
   C. firm pressure to the area superior to the nasal alar cartilage.
   D. chemical cauterization.

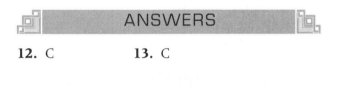

ANSWERS

12. C   **13.** C

DISCUSSION

Anterior epistaxis is usually the result of localized nasal mucosa dryness and trauma and is rarely a result of other causes. Most episodes can be easily managed with simple pressure. If this is ineffective, second-line therapies include nasal packing and cautery. If epistaxis is seen in the presence of a bleeding disorder, topical thrombin should be used.

DISCUSSION SOURCE

Jackler, R., and Kaplan, M. (2003). Ear, nose and throat. In Tierney, L., McPhee, S., and Papadakis, M. (eds.). Current Diagnosis and Treatment (42nd ed., pp. 179–215). New York: Lange Medical Books/McGraw-Hill.

QUESTIONS

14. A 58-year-old woman presents with a sudden left-sided headache that is worse in her left eye. Her vision is blurred, and the left pupil is slightly dilated and poorly reactive. The left conjunctiva is markedly injected, and the eyeball is firm. Vision screen with the Snelling chart is 20/30 OD and 20/90 OS. The most likely diagnosis is:

   A. unilateral herpetic conjunctivitis.
   B. open-angle glaucoma.
   C. angle-closure glaucoma.
   D. anterior uveitis.

15. In caring for this patient, the most appropriate next action is:

   A. prompt referral to an ophthalmologist.
   B. to provide analgesia and repeat the evaluation once the patient is more comfortable.
   C. to instill a corticosteroid ophthalmic solution.
   D. to patch the eye and arrange for follow-up in 24 hours.

16. A 48-year-old man presents with a new-onset vision change in the right eye. The right pupil is small, irregular, and poorly reactive. Vision screen with the Snelling chart is 20/30 OS and 20/80 OD. The most likely diagnosis is:

    A. unilateral herpetic conjunctivitis.
    B. open-angle glaucoma.
    C. angle-closure glaucoma.
    D. anterior uveitis.

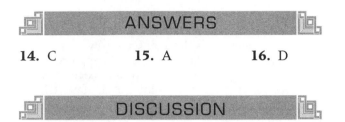

ANSWERS

14. C   **15.** A   **16.** D

DISCUSSION

The components of an ophthalmologic emergency are a painful, red eye with a visual disturbance. In the case of angle-closure glaucoma, the patient usually presents with all of these findings, and without intervention, blindness ensues in 3 to 5 days. Prompt referral to expert ophthalmologic care focused on relieving acute intraocular pressure is needed; laser peripheral iridectomy after reduction of intraocular pressure with appropriate medications is usually curative. In contrast, open-angle glaucoma is a slowly progressive disease that seldom produces symptoms. In anterior uveitis, another cause of an occasionally dully painful red eye with visual change, the pupil is usually constricted, nonreactive, and irregularly shaped. Treatment includes medications to assist in pupillary dilatation, as well as corticosteroids, administered topically, by periocular injection, and/or systemically.

DISCUSSION SOURCE

Riordan-Eva, P. (2003). Eye. In Tierney, L., McPhee, S., and Papadakis, M. (eds.). Current Diagnosis and Treatment (42nd ed., pp. 147–177). New York: Lange Medical Books/McGraw-Hill.

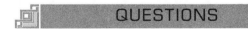

QUESTIONS

17. Which of the following is a common vision problem in the person with untreated open-angle glaucoma?

    A. peripheral vision loss
    B. blurring of near vision
    C. difficulty with distant vision
    D. need for increased illumination

18. Which of the following is most likely to be found on the funduscopic examination in a patient with untreated open-angle glaucoma?

    A. excessive cupping of the optic disk
    B. arteriovenous nicking
    C. papilledema
    D. flame-shaped hemorrhages

19. Risk factors for open-angle glaucoma include all of the following except:

    A. African ancestry.
    B. type 2 diabetes mellitus.
    C. advanced age.
    D. blue eye color.

20. Treatment options for open-angle glaucoma include all of the following topical agents except:

    A. beta-adrenergic antagonists.
    B. alpha$_2$-agonists.
    C. prostaglandin analogs.
    D. mast cell stabilizers.

ANSWERS

17. A   **18.** A
19. D   **20.** D

DISCUSSION

Although the etiology of open-angle glaucoma is not completely understood, the result is elevated intraocular pressure caused by abnormal drainage of aqueous humor through the trabecular meshwork. Risk factors for angle-closure glaucoma include African ancestry, diabetes mellitus, family history of glaucoma, history of certain eye trauma and uveitis, and advancing age. A gradual-onset peripheral vision loss is most specific for open-angle glaucoma. Although all of these changes may be seen in patients with advanced open-angle glaucoma, changes in near vision are common as part of the aging process because of hardening of the lens (i.e., presbyopia) and the need for increased illumination. New onset of difficulty with distance vision can be found in patients with cataracts.

Glaucoma, whether open-angle or angle-closure, is primarily a problem with excessive intraocular pressure. Tonometry reveals intraocular pressure greater than 25 mm Hg; in angle-closure glaucoma, the abnormal measurement is usually documented on more than one occasion. As a result, the optic disk and cup are "pushed in," creating the classic finding often called glaucomatous cupping. This creates a cup-disk ratio of greater than 0.3 or asymmetry of cup-disk ratio of 0.2 or more. Papilledema, in which the optic disk bulges and the margins are blurred, is seen when there is excessive pressure behind the eye, as in increased intracranial pressure (Fig. 4–1).

Medical treatment options for angle-closure glaucoma include topical beta-adrenergic agonists such as timolol, alpha$_2$ agonists such as brimonidine, carbonic anhydrase inhibitors such as dorzolamide, or prostaglandin analogs such as latanoprost. Pilocarpine is now seldom used because it causes pupillary constriction. Laser trabeculoplasty and surgical trabeculectomy are additional treatment options.

DISCUSSION SOURCES

Brinker Lester, P. (2004). Head and neck disorders. In Hektor Dunphy, L: Management Guidelines for Nurse Practitioners Working with Adults (2nd ed). Philadelphia: F.A. Davis, pp 146–214.

Riordan-Eva, P. (2003). Eye. In Tierney, L., McPhee, S., and Papadakis, M. (eds.). Current Diagnosis and Treatment (42nd ed., pp. 147–177). New York: Lange Medical Books/McGraw-Hill.

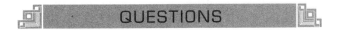

QUESTIONS

21. A 17-year-old woman presents with a "pimple" on her right eyelid. Examination

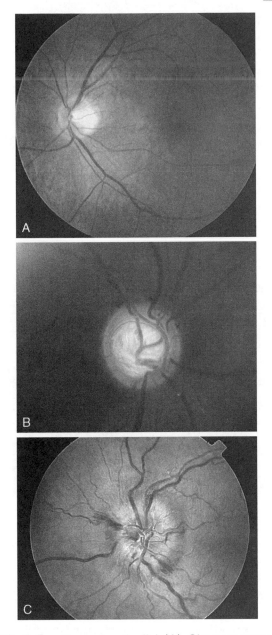

FIG. 4–1.   Normal optic disk (A). Glaucomatous cupping (B). Bulging optic disk in papilledema (C).

reveals a 2-mm pustule on the lateral border of the right eyelid margin. This is most consistent with:

A. a chalazion.
B. a hordeolum.
C. blepharitis.
D. cellulitis.

22. A 17-year-old woman presents with a "bump" on her right eyelid. Examination reveals a 2-mm hard, nontender swelling on the lateral border of the right eyelid margin. This is most consistent with:

   A. a chalazion.
   B. a hordeolum.
   C. blepharitis.
   D. cellulitis.

23. Treatment options for uncomplicated hordeolum include all of the following except:

   A. erythromycin ophthalmic ointment.
   B. warm compresses to the affected area.
   C. incision and drainage.
   D. oral antimicrobial therapy.

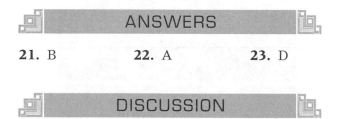

ANSWERS

21. B   **22.** A   **23.** D

DISCUSSION

A hordeolum is often called a stye and is usually caused by a staphylococcal infection of a hair follicle on the eyelid. An internal hordeolum points towards the conjunctival eye surface, whereas an external hordeolum is found on the lid margin. A chalazion is an inflammatory eyelid condition that may not involve infection but can follow hordeolum and is characterized by a hard, nontender swelling of the upper or lower lid. Because treatment regimens for each of these differ significantly, accurate diagnosis is critical. Cellulitis is a serious complication of a hordeolum and is evidenced by widespread redness and edema over the eyelid.

Treatment for a simple hordeolum, or stye, includes warm compresses to the affected eye for 10 minutes 3 to 4 times a day. Local antimicrobial therapy with erythromycin or bacitracin ophthalmic ointment along the lid margin may accelerate resolution. In rare instances, incision and drainage are needed. Oral antimicrobial therapy for an uncomplicated hordeolum is not warranted. However, an infrequently encountered complication of a hordeolum is cellulitis of the eyelid. If this occurs, ophthalmic consultation should be obtained and appropriate antimicrobial therapy promptly initiated, Because *S. aureus* is the most common pathogen, treatment options include the use of an antibiotic with gram-positive coverage and beta-lactamase stability, such as dicloxacillin, a cephalosporin, or selected fluoroquinolones. Antimicrobial therapy for chalazion is not warranted, because this is an inflammatory but not infectious disease. Treatment includes warm soaks of the area. If this is not helpful, referral to an ophthalmologist for intralesion corticosteroid injection or excision is recommended, particularly if the chalazion impairs lid closure or presses on the cornea.

DISCUSSION SOURCES

Gilbert, D., Moellering, R., and Sande, M. (2004). The Sanford Guide to Antimicrobial Therapy (34th ed.). Hyde Park, VT: Antimicrobial Therapy.

Riordan-Eva, P. (2003). Eye. In Tierney, L., McPhee, S., and Papadakis, M. (eds.). Current Diagnosis and Treatment (42nd ed., pp. 147–177). New York: Lange Medical Books/McGraw-Hill.

QUESTIONS

24. Which of the following is true concerning Menière disease?

   A. Neuroimaging helps locate the offending cochlear lesion.
   B. Associated high-frequency hearing loss is common.
   C. It is largely a diagnosis of exclusion.
   D. Tinnitus is rarely reported.

25. Prevention and prophylaxis in Menière disease include all of the following except:

   A. avoiding ototoxic drugs.
   B. protecting the ears from loud noise.
   C. limiting sodium intake.
   D. restricting fluid intake.

26 to 29. Match the following to the lettered descriptions:

26. dizziness

    A. perception that the person or the environment is moving

27. vertigo

    B. subjective perception of altered equilibrium

28. nystagmus

    C. rhythmic oscillations of the eyes

29. tinnitus

    D. perception of abnormal hearing or head noises

ANSWERS

24. C	**25.** D	**26.** B
27. A	**28.** C	**29.** D

DISCUSSION

Both Menière disease, an idiopathic condition, and Menière syndrome, with symptoms identical to those of Menière disease but whose cause is known, are believed to result from increased pressure within the endolymphatic system. In health, two fluids, one potassium rich and the other potassium poor, separated by a thin membrane, fill the chambers of the inner ear: endolymph and perilymph. Housed within the separating membrane is the nervous tissue of hearing and balance. Normally, the pressure exerted on these fluids is constant, allowing for normal balance and hearing. If the pressure of these fluids varies, the nerve-rich membranes are stressed, which causes disturbance in hearing, ringing in the ears, imbalance, and a pressure sensation in the ear as well as vertigo. The reason for the pressure changes varies, but most often they are caused by an increase in endolymphatic pressure that causes a break in the membrane separating the two fluids. When these fluids mix, the vestibular nerve receptors are bathed in the new, abnormal chemical mix, which leads to depolarization blockade and sudden change in the vestibular nerve firing rate. This creates an acute vestibular imbalance and the resulting sense of vertigo. Symptoms improve after the membrane is repaired and normal sodium and potassium concentrations are restored.

A distinction needs to be made between Menière disease, usually idiopathic in origin, and Menière syndrome, usually secondary to various processes that interfere with normal production or resorption of endolymph, such as endocrine abnormalities, trauma, electrolyte imbalance, autoimmune dysfunction, medications, parasitic infections, and hyperlipidemia. Menière disease is largely a diagnosis of exclusion: diagnosis is made after other possible causes for the recurrent and often debilitating symptoms of dizziness, tinnitus, and low-frequency hearing loss have been ruled out. A distinct causative lesion cannot be identified. It is more common with repeat attacks and more frequent in persons who use ototoxic drugs and have exposure to loud noise.

Clinical presentation of Menière disease and Menière syndrome usually involves a history of episodes of vertigo with a sensation that the room is whirling about, often preceded by decreased hearing, low-tone roaring tinnitus, and a feeling of increased ear pressure. Particularly severe episodes are accompanied by nausea and vomiting. Attacks can last minutes to hours, with exhaustion often reported once the most severe symptoms have passed. Duration and frequency of attacks can vary, although common triggers include certain foods and drinks, mental and physical stress, and variations in the menstrual cycle.

Examination of the person with Menière disease typically reveals significant nystagmus or rhythmic oscillations of the eyes and slow movement toward one side, usually the side of the affected ear, with a rapid correction to the midline. The Weber tuning test result usually lateralizes to the unaffected ear, whereas the Rinne test shows that air exceeds bone conduction, a normal finding. Pneumatic otoscopy in the affected ear may elicit symptoms or cause nystagmus, whereas the same maneuver to the unaffected ear yields little response. Objective measures of hearing often reveal diminished hearing. The Romberg test is positive, with the patient demonstrating increased swaying and difficulty staying balanced when standing with the eyes closed. Additional findings include a positive Fukuda marching step test, in which a directional drift, usually toward the affected ear, can be noted when the patient is asked to perform a march step with the eyes closed. This latter maneuver may not be possible for the patient with the most severe symptoms. The result of the Dix-Hallpike test (i.e., observation of nystagmus while moving a patient from sitting to supine with the head angled 45 degrees to one side and then to the other) may be positive, indicating coexisting benign positional vertigo. Neuroimaging is not warranted unless the examination reveals additional findings or the diagnosis is unclear.

Treatment of Menière disease is aimed largely at minimizing or preventing symptoms. Antihistamines such as meclizine or antiemetics such as chlorpromazine can minimize symptoms. Benzodiazepines can be used to help reinforce rest and minimize anxiety associated with severe symptoms; these options do not treat the underlying condition. Diuretics decrease fluid pressure load in the inner ear and can be used to prevent but not treat attacks, but they do not help once the attack has been triggered. Corticosteroids also have been shown to be helpful, likely because of their anti-inflammatory properties, causing a reduction in endolymph pressure and potentially ameliorating vertigo, tinnitus, and hearing loss. In Menière syndrome, symptomatic treatment is warranted, as well as intervention for the underlying cause.

DISCUSSION SOURCES

Devinsky, O., and Feldmann, E. (2000). Neurological Pearls. Philadelphia: F. A. Davis.

Jackler, R., and Kaplan, M. (2003). Ear, nose and throat. In Tierney, L., McPhee, S., and Papadakis, M. (eds.). Current Diagnosis and Treatment (42nd ed., pp. 179–215). New York: Lange Medical Books/McGraw-Hill.

Brinker Lester, P. (2004). Head and neck disorders. In Hektor Dunphy, L: Management Guidelines for Nurse Practitioners Working with Adults (2nd ed). Philadelphia: F.A. Davis, pp 146–214.

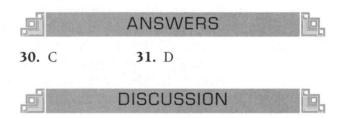

QUESTIONS

30. You inspect the oral cavity of a 69-year-old man who has a 100–pack-year cigarette smoking history. You find a lesion suspect for malignancy and describe it as:

A. raised, red, and painful.
B. a denuded patch with a removable white coating.
C. an ulcerated lesion with indurated margins.
D. a vesicular-form lesion with macerated margins.

31. A firm, painless, relatively fixed submandibular node will most likely be seen in the diagnosis of:

A. herpes simplex.
B. acute otitis media (AOM).
C. bacterial pharyngitis.
D. oral cancer.

ANSWERS

30. C   **31.** D

DISCUSSION

Oral cancer, most often squamous cell cancer, is usually characterized by a relatively painless, firm ulceration or raised lesion. Risk factors for oral cancer include tobacco and alcohol abuse. In addition, the lymphadenopathy associated with oral cancer consists of relatively immobile nodes that are not tender when palpated. Self-limiting oral lesions such as herpes simplex, oral candidiasis, and aphthous stomatitis usually cause discomfort. With infection, the associated lymphadenopathy that follows drainage tracts is characterized by tenderness and mobility.

DISCUSSION SOURCE

Jackler, R., and Kaplan, M. (2003). Ear, nose and throat. In Tierney, L., McPhee, S., and Papadakis, M. (eds.). Current Diagnosis and Treatment (42nd ed., pp. 179–215). New York: Lange Medical Books/McGraw-Hill.

QUESTIONS

32. A 45-year-old man has otitis externa. Likely causative pathogens include all of the following except:

   A. fungal agents.
   B. *P. aeruginosa*.
   C. *S. aureus*.
   D. *M. catarrhalis*.

33. Appropriate oral antimicrobial therapy for malignant otitis externa includes the:

   A. macrolides.
   B. cephalosporins.
   C. fluoroquinolones.
   D. penicillins.

34. Physical examination findings in otitis externa include:

   A. tympanic membrane immobility.
   B. increased ear pain with tragus pull.
   C. tympanic membrane erythema.
   D. tympanic membrane bullae.

35. A risk factor for malignant external otitis is:

   A. diabetes mellitus.
   B. age of younger than 15 years.
   C. recent upper respiratory tract infection (URI).
   D. serous otitis media.

ANSWERS

32. D   **33.** C
34. B   **35.** A

DISCUSSION

Risk factors for otitis externa include a history of recent ear canal trauma, usually with a cotton swab or other item used to clean the canal, and conditions in which moisture is frequently held in the ear canal, such as cerumen impaction and swimming. Otitis externa can be caused by a number of infectious agents, including a variety of gram-positive organisms and fungi. However, *P. aeruginosa* is the most common causative agent and the most likely organism in refractory otitis externa or auricular cellulitis. Effective topical therapies include otic suspension of an antimicrobial such as an aminoglycoside, fluoroquinolone, or neomycin, with or without hydrocortisone solution and the combination of 2% nonaqueous acetic acid and hydrocortisone (V̄oSol HC Otic 2%). The preferred oral antipseudomonal therapy is a fluoroquinolone such as ciprofloxacin or levofloxacin, usually reserved for severe cases (see Table 4–1).

DISCUSSION SOURCES

Gilbert, D., Moellering, R., and Sande, M. (2004). The Sanford Guide to Antimicrobial Therapy (34th ed.). Hyde Park, VT: Antimicrobial Therapy.
Jackler, R., and Kaplan, M. (2003). Ear, nose and throat. In Tierney, L., McPhee, S., and Papadakis, M. (eds.). Current Diagnosis and Treatment (42nd ed., pp. 179–215). New York: Lange Medical Books/McGraw-Hill.

QUESTIONS

36. Likely causative organisms in AOM include:

   A. select gram-positive and gram-negative bacteria.
   B. gram-negative bacteria and pathogenic viruses.
   C. rhinovirus and *S. aureus*.
   D. predominantly beta-lactamase–producing organisms.

37. Expected findings in AOM include:

   A. prominent bony landmarks.
   B. tympanic membrane immobility.
   C. itchiness and crackling in the affected ear.
   D. submental lymphadenopathy.

38. A 25-year-old woman has a 3-day history of left ear pain after a week of URI symptoms. On physical examination, you find that she has AOM. She is allergic to penicillin (it causes a hive-form reaction). The most appropriate antimicrobial option for this patient is:

A. ciprofloxacin.
B. clarithromycin.
C. amoxicillin.
D. cephalexin.

39. A reasonable treatment option for AOM that does not respond to amoxicillin therapy is:

A. cefuroxime.
B. erythromycin.
C. cephalexin.
D. sulfamethoxazole.

40. Characteristics of *M. catarrhalis* include:

A. high rate of beta-lactamase production.
B. antimicrobial resistance resulting from altered protein-binding sites.
C. often being found in middle ear exudate in recurrent otitis media.
D. gram-positive organisms.

41. Characteristics of *H. influenzae* include:

A. rare beta-lactamase production.
B. antimicrobial resistance resulting from altered protein-binding sites.
C. organisms that are most commonly isolated from mucoid middle ear effusion in recurrent otitis media.
D. gram-positive organisms.

42. Characteristics of *S. pneumoniae* include:

A. beta-lactamase production, commonly.
B. antimicrobial resistance as a result of altered protein-binding sites.
C. organisms most commonly isolated from mucoid middle ear effusion.
D. gram-negative organisms.

43. Clindamycin is most effective against:

A. *S. pneumoniae.*
B. *H. influenzae.*
C. *M. catarrhalis.*
D. Adenovirus.

44. Which of the following is absent in otitis media with effusion?

A. fluid in the middle ear
B. otalgia
C. fever
D. itch

45. Treatment of otitis media with effusion usually includes:

A. symptomatic treatment.
B. antimicrobial therapy.
C. an antihistamine.
D. a mucolytic.

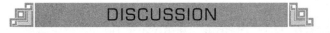

ANSWERS

36. A	37. B	38. B
39. A	40. A	41. C
42. B	43. A	
44. C	45. A	

DISCUSSION

Although often considered a disease limited to childhood, AOM still ranks among the most frequent diagnoses noted in office visits in adults. *S. pneumoniae, H. influenzae, M. catarrhalis*, and a variety of viruses contribute to the infectious and inflammatory process of the middle ear. Eustachian tube dysfunction usually precedes the development of AOM, allowing negative pressure to be generated in the middle ear and pharyngeal pathogens to be aspirated. As a result, avoiding conditions that can cause eustachian tube dysfunction, such as upper respiratory infection, untreated or undertreated allergic rhinitis, cigarette smoking, and exposure to air pollution, can lead to a reduction in the occurrence of AOM.

S. pneumoniae causes 40% to 50% of AOM; it is the least likely of the three major causative bacteria to resolve without antimicrobial intervention, and it causes the most significant symptoms. This organism has exhibited resistance to a number of antibiotic agents, including amoxicillin, cephalosporins, and macrolides. The mechanism of resistance is an alteration of intracellular protein-binding sites, which can typically be overcome by using higher doses of amoxicillin and selected cephalosporins. The major risk factor for infection with drug-resistant *S. pneumoniae* is recent antimicrobial use.

H. influenzae and *M. catarrhalis* are gram-negative organisms capable of producing beta-lactamase. These two organisms have relatively high rates of spontaneous resolution in AOM (50% and 90%, respectively); however, *H. influenzae* is the organism most commonly isolated from mucoid and serous middle ear effusion. Beta-lactamase production by organisms probably contributes less to AOM treatment failure than does prescribing inadequate dosages of amoxicillin needed to eradicate drug-resistant *S. pneumoniae*. Common viral agents that cause AOM include human rhinovirus, respiratory syncytial virus, and coronavirus. AOM caused by these viral agents usually resolves in 7 to 10 days with supportive care alone.

Appropriate assessment is critical for arriving at the diagnosis of AOM. The tympanic membrane may be retracted or bulging and is typically reddened with loss of translucency and mobility on insufflation. With recovery, tympanic membrane mobility returns in about 1 to 2 weeks, but middle ear effusion typically persists for 4 to 6 weeks. Itching and crackling in the ear is common in patients with AOM, as well as in those with serous otitis, also known as otitis media with effusion. The bony landmarks usually appear prominent when the tympanic membrane is retracted, a condition usually seen with eustachian tube dysfunction that may not be present in patients with AOM. The submental node is not in the drainage tract of the middle ear and therefore is not enlarged in patients with AOM. Rather, the nodes within the anterior cervical chain on the ipsilateral side of the infection are often enlarged and painful.

Otalgia, fever, and other symptoms that persist beyond 3 days of therapy may indicate treatment failure. Repeat evaluation is in order. The organisms that cause recurrent otitis media are the same ones that cause acute disease. If amoxicillin fails to eradicate the infection, a drug-resistant pathogen such as drug-resistant *S. pneumoniae* might be the cause. Also, the contribution of a beta-lactamase–producing organism such as *H. influenzae* or *M. catarrhalis* should be considered. If there is treatment failure, the choice of a new antimicrobial is dependent on the initial medication that failed to eradicate the infection and patterns of recent antimicrobial use.

DISCUSSION SOURCES

Gilbert, D., Moellering, R., and Sande, M. (2004). The Sanford Guide to Antimicrobial Therapy (34th ed.). Hyde Park, VT: Antimicrobial Therapy.

Jackler, R., and Kaplan, M. (2003). Ear, nose and throat. In Tierney, L., McPhee, S., and Papadakis, M. (eds.). Current Diagnosis and Treatment (42nd ed., pp. 179–215). New York: Lange Medical Books/McGraw-Hill.

QUESTIONS

46. An 18-year-old woman has a chief complaint of a "sore throat and swollen glands" for the past 3 days. Her physical examination includes a temperature of 101°F, exudative pharyngitis, and tender anterior cervical lymphadenopathy. Right and left upper quadrant abdominal tenderness is absent. The most likely diagnosis is:

    A. *Streptococcus pyogenes* pharyngitis.
    B. infectious mononucleosis.
    C. viral pharyngitis.
    D. Vincent angina.

47. Treatment options for streptococcal pharyngitis for a patient with penicillin allergy include all of the following except:

    A. azithromycin.
    B. trimethoprim-sulfamethoxazole.

C. clarithromycin.

D. erythromycin.

48. You are seeing a 25-year-old man with *S. pyogenes* pharyngitis. He asks if he can get a "shot of penicillin" for therapy. You consider the following when counseling about the use of intramuscular penicillin:

A. There is nearly a 100% cure rate in streptococcal pharyngitis when it is used.

B. Treatment failure rates approach 20%.

C. It is the preferred agent in treating group G streptococcal infection.

D. Injectable penicillin has a superior spectrum of antimicrobial coverage in comparison with the oral version of the drug.

49. With regard to pharyngitis caused by group C streptococci, the NP considers that:

A. potential complications include glomerulonephritis.

B. appropriate antimicrobial therapy helps minimize symptoms.

C. infection with these organisms carries a significant risk of subsequent rheumatic fever.

D. hepatitis can occur if not treated with an appropriate antimicrobial.

50. Clinical presentation of peritonsillar abscess includes:

A. occipital lymphadenopathy.

B. congested cough.

C. "hot potato" voice.

D. abdominal pain.

51. Patients with "strep throat" can be cleared to return to work or school after ___ hours of antimicrobial therapy.

A. 12

B. 24

C. 36

D. 48

52. When advising a patient with scarlet fever, the NP considers that:

A. there is increased risk for poststreptococcal glomerulonephritis.

B. the rash often peels during recovery.

C. an injectable cephalosporin is the preferred treatment option.

D. throat culture is usually negative for group A streptococci.

53. The incubation period for *S. pyogenes* is usually:

A. 1 to 3 days.

B. 3 to 5 days.

C. 6 to 9 days.

D. 10 to 13 days.

54. The incubation period for *M. pneumoniae* is usually:

A. less than 1 week.

B. 1 week.

C. 2 weeks.

D. 3 weeks.

55. All of the following are common causes of penicillin treatment failure in streptococcal pharyngitis except:

A. infection with a beta-lactamase–producing *Streptococcus* strain.

B. failure to initiate or complete the antimicrobial course.

C. concomitant infection with a beta-lactamase–producing organism.

D. inadequate penicillin dosage.

ANSWERS

46. A	47. B	48. B
49. B	50. C	51. B
52. B	53. B	
54. D	55. A	

DISCUSSION

S. pyogenes, also known as group A beta-hemolytic streptococcus, is the causative pathogen in 15% to 40% of presenting sore throats in school-aged children but is less common before age 3 years and in the teenaged and adult populations. The organism is transmitted primarily via saliva and droplet contact.

Its inoculation period lasts an average of 3 to 5 days but can be up to 3 months. Clinical presentation of exudative pharyngitis caused by *S. pyogenes* includes complaint of sore throat and fever, as well as evidence of large, beefy tonsils, usually covered with exudate; palatial petechiae; and anterior cervical lymphadenopathy. Communicability gradually decreases over a period of weeks in untreated patients. Patients are no longer contagious within 24 hours of initiation of appropriate antimicrobial therapy. Asymptomatic nasopharyngeal carriage is common.

S. pyogenes is not the sole reason for bacterial exudative pharyngitis. Another causative pathogen implicated is *Mycoplasma pneumoniae*. Infection with this organism is uncommon in children age 5 or younger and is most often seen in teenagers and younger adults. Clinical presentation includes inflammatory exudate, pharyngeal edema and erythema, cervical lymphadenopathy, and tonsillar enlargement. Because this organism is also a cause of acute bronchitis, the person with *M. pneumoniae* pharyngitis often has a bothersome dry cough; rapid streptococcal screen and standard throat culture fail to reveal the presence of this organism and yield negative results. The incubation period for *M. pneumoniae* is approximately 3 weeks and is usually transmitted by cough. Signs and symptoms that point to viral pharyngitis include rhinorrhea, cough, and a report of scratchy throat.

Groups C and G streptococci cause pharyngitis, but infection with these organisms carries minimal risk for rheumatic fever or glomerulonephritis. The infection clears without antimicrobial therapy, but taking an appropriate antimicrobial helps minimize symptoms.

Complications of bacterial pharyngitis include peritonsillar abscess, rheumatic fever, and acute glomerulonephritis. Clinical presentation of peritonsillar abscess includes progressively worsening sore throat, often worse on one side; trismus (inability or difficulty in opening the mouth); drooling; a muffled, "hot potato" voice with an erythematous, swollen tonsil with contralateral uvular deviation; and cervical lymphadenopathy. Because airway compromise is a potential life-threatening consequence of peritonsillar abscess, ultrasonography or computed tomographic scan should confirm the diagnosis. Treatment with appropriate antimicrobial therapy, needle aspiration, and airway maintenance must be initiated promptly. Antimicrobial therapy initiated early in the course of the illness minimizes peritonsillar abscess risk.

Rheumatic fever is usually caused by *S. pyogenes* serotypes 1, 3, 5, 6, 14, 18, 19, and 24; on average, onset of symptoms of carditis and arthritis begins about 19 days (range, 7 to 35 days) after the onset of sore throat symptoms. Antimicrobial treatment is helpful in minimizing rheumatic fever risk. Acute glomerulonephritis is also a complication of *S. pyogenes*, usually serotypes 1, 3, 4, 12, and 25 when associated with pharyngitis and serotypes 2, 4, 9, 55, 57, 59, and 60 when associated with skin infection. Onset of glomerulonephritis symptoms is usually seen 1 to 3 weeks after pharyngeal or skin infection. Although poststreptococcal glomerulonephritis is usually a self-limiting condition, patients can develop renal scarring with chronic proteinuria or hematuria. Antimicrobial therapy does not minimize glomerulonephritis risk. Infrequently seen but potential purulent complications of streptococcal pharyngitis include otitis media, sinusitis, peritonsillar and retropharyngeal abscess, and suppurative cervical adenitis. Scarlet fever is the clinical condition seen when a scarlatiniform rash with a fine sandpaper-like texture erupts during streptococcal pharyngitis, usually on the second day of illness. The rash starts on the trunk and spreads widely, usually sparing the palms and soles. Peeling is common during recovery. Scarlet fever treatment is identical to that of streptococcal pharyngitis and carries no increased risk of complications or sequelae.

A positive throat culture for streptococcus is considered the standard for diagnosing streptococcal pharyngitis. A potential drawback is that a positive result does not distinguish between acute viral pharyngitis with group A streptococcus carriage and acute streptococcal pharyngitis. In spite of this, all patients with a positive throat culture should be treated with an appropriate antimicrobial. Rapid antigen detection tests detect the presence of the group A streptococcus carbohydrate antigen and can be completed in minutes but with lower sensitivity and specificity than standard throat culture. As a result, many advocate treating in the presence of a positive rapid streptococcal screen and following up negative studies with a throat culture in the patient in whom there is a high index of suspicion. If a rapid streptococcal test result is positive, antimicrobial treatment should be initiated immediately. If a throat culture is performed, the question is raised as to whether treatment should be initiated while results are awaited or once a positive throat culture is noted. In the former, some patients need to be notified of the need to discontinue antimicrobial therapy if the culture results are negative; some unneeded antibiotic will have been consumed, potentially contributing to the development of resistant pathogens. In the later case, treatment for patients with positive cultures is delayed by 2 days. This delay poses little risk in the otherwise well person.

In the treatment of bacterial pharyngitis caused by *S. pyogenes*, penicillin remains highly effective. When the total daily dose is given in equally divided BID doses, treatment outcomes are equivalent to TID or QID therapy with significantly improved adherence. A single dose of injectable penicillin given intramuscularly offers a one-time treatment option. Limitations include increased risk of serious reaction with penicillin allergy and a treatment failure rate similar to that of a completed course of oral therapy. Erythromycin or other macrolides offer effective treatment choices for the person with penicillin allergy. Advice on the use of symptomatic treatment with saltwater gargles, throat lozenges, and analgesics should also be given.

When penicillin therapy fails, seldom is the issue a resistant *S. pyogenes* strain; rather, the pharynx is colonized with a beta-lactamase–producing organism such as *H. influenzae*. The presence of beta-lactamase renders the penicillin ineffective. Treatment with an antimicrobial stable in the presence of beta-lactamase such as amoxicillin with clavulanate, a cephalosporin, or macrolide is effective. If the streptococcal test result is negative and the patient continues to have symptoms, infection with *M. pneumoniae* or *C. pneumoniae* should be considered, particularly if cough if present. A macrolide or fluoroquinolone should be prescribed, inasmuch as the beta-lactams (penicillins, cephalosporins) are ineffective.

The treatment of *S. pyogenes* carriage, defined as a positive throat culture in a person who is without symptoms, bears some mention. Antimicrobial therapy for *S. pyogenes* carriage is indicated only when an outbreak of rheumatic fever and/or glomerulonephritis is in process or when there is an outbreak of streptococcal pharyngitis in a closed or semiclosed environment such as a correctional facility or college dormitory. First-line therapy includes treatment with clindamycin or amoxicillin with clavulanate; rifampin with penicillin can also be used.

DISCUSSION SOURCES

Brinker Lester, P. (2004). Head and neck disorders. In Hektor Dunphy, L: Management Guidelines for Nurse Practitioners Working with Adults (2nd ed). Philadelphia: F.A. Davis, pp. 146–214.

Gilbert, D., Moellering, R., and Sande, M. (2004). The Sanford Guide to Antimicrobial Therapy (34th ed.). Hyde Park, VT: Antimicrobial Therapy.

Jackler, R., and Kaplan, M. (2003). Ear, nose and throat. In Tierney, L., McPhee, S., and Papadakis, M. (eds.). Current Diagnosis and Treatment (42nd ed., pp. 179–215). New York: Lange Medical Books/McGraw-Hill.

QUESTIONS

56. A 25-year-old woman who has seasonal allergic rhinitis likes to spend time outdoors. She asks you when the pollen count is likely to be the lowest. You respond:

A. "Early in the morning."
B. "During breezy times of the day."
C. "After a rain shower."
D. "When the sky is overcast."

57. You prescribe nasal corticosteroid spray for a patient with allergic rhinitis. What is the anticipated onset of symptom relief with its use?

    A. immediately with the first spray
    B. 1 to 2 days
    C. 1 to 2 weeks
    D. about 1 month

58. Which of the following medications is most appropriate for allergic rhinitis therapy in an acutely symptomatic 24-year-old machine operator?

    A. nasal cromolyn
    B. diphenhydramine
    C. flunisolide nasal spray
    D. loratadine

59. Antihistamines work primarily through:

    A. vasoconstriction.
    B. action on the histamine 1 (H_1) receptor sites.
    C. inflammatory mediation.
    D. peripheral vasodilatation.

60. Decongestants work primarily through:

    A. vasoconstriction.
    B. action on the H_1 receptor sites.
    C. inflammatory mediation.
    D. peripheral vasodilatation.

61. Which of the following medications affords the best relief of acute nasal itch?

    A. anticholinergic nasal spray
    B. oral decongestant
    C. corticosteroid nasal spray
    D. oral antihistamine

62. According to the ARIA guidelines, which of the following medications affords the best relief of acute nasal congestion?

    A. anticholinergic nasal spray
    B. decongestant nasal spray
    C. corticosteroid nasal spray
    D. oral antihistamine

63. According to the ARIA guidelines, which of the following medications affords the least control of rhinorrhea associated with allergic rhinitis?

    A. anticholinergic nasal spray
    B. antihistamine nasal spray
    C. corticosteroid nasal spray
    D. cromolyn nasal spray

64. Ipratropium bromide (Atrovent) helps control nasal secretions through:

    A. antihistaminic action.
    B. anticholinergic effect.
    C. vasodilatation.
    D. vasoconstriction.

65. Oral decongestant use should be discouraged in patients with:

    A. allergic rhinitis.
    B. migraine headache.
    C. cardiovascular disease.
    D. chronic bronchitis.

66. Cromolyn's mechanism of action is as:

    A. an anti–immunoglobulin E antibody.
    B. a vasoconstrictor.
    C. a mast cell stabilizer.
    D. a leukotriene modifier.

67. In the treatment of allergic rhinitis, leukotriene modifiers should be used as:

    A. an agent to relieve nasal itch.
    B. an inflammatory inhibitor.
    C. a rescue drug.
    D. an intervention in acute inflammation.

68. According to the Global Resources in Allergy (GLORIA) guidelines, which of the following is recommended for intervention in persistent allergic conjunctivitis?

    A. topical mast cell stabilizer with a topical antihistamine
    B. ocular decongestant
    C. topical nonsteroidal anti-inflammatory drug
    D. topical corticosteroid

69. Allergy immunotherapy is most successful in controlling allergies caused by:

    A. dust mites.
    B. molds.
    C. animal dander.
    D. air pollution.

ANSWERS

56. C	57. C	58. D
59. B	60. A	61. D
62. B	63. D	64. B
65. C	66. C	67. B
68. A	69. A	

DISCUSSION

The most important component of allergic rhinitis and allergic conjunctivitis therapy is avoidance of the allergen. In seasonal allergic rhinitis, pollens are often triggers. Pollen counts are generally the highest early in the morning because these substances are released during the night. After a rain shower, the air is relatively cleansed of the offending agent.

Because the mechanism of action of corticosteroid nasal spray in allergic rhinitis therapy is prevention of production of inflammatory substances, corticosteroid and mast cell stabilizer nasal sprays are effective at preventing, but not acutely controlling, symptoms of allergic rhinitis. Therefore, at least 1 to 2 weeks of use is needed before symptom relief is achieved. However, antihistamines prevent action of formed histamine, a potent inflammatory mediator, and therefore can be used to control acute allergic symptoms. A nonsedating second-generation antihistamine such as loratadine (Claritin) is the best choice for active adults. Diphenhydramine (Benadryl) is an example of a rapidly acting, sedating, first-generation antihistamine. All antihistamines work by blocking H_1 receptor sites. Decongestants act as vasoconstrictors, thus opening edematous nasal passages (Table 4–2).

TABLE 4–2

MEDICATIONS USED IN THE TREATMENT OF ALLERGIC RHINITIS

Therapeutic Goal	Intervention	Comment
Controller therapy to prevent formation of inflammatory mediators	• Corticosteroids (nasal spray) • Leukotriene modifiers (montelukast, zafirlukast) • Mast cell stabilizer (intranasal and optic cromolyn)	• Controller therapy usually needs to be used for 1–4 weeks prior to maximum effect noted; little effect on acute symptoms
Rescue therapy by inactivating formed inflammatory mediators	• Oral antihistamines (1st generation [chlorpheniramine, diphenhydramine], 2nd generation [loratadine, cetirizine, fexofenadine]) • Antihistamine nasal spray • Antihistamine optic drops • Short-term oral corticosteroids if needed for severe allergic symptoms	• Using only antihistamine rescue therapy usually not as effective on overall disease control as consistent use of controller therapy with rescue therapy as an adjunct
Rescue therapy and symptom relief by minimizing nasal discharge	• Anticholinergic nasal spray (Ipratropium bromide [Atrovent]) • Antihistamine nasal spray	• Helpful adjuncts as part of rescue therapy for the patient with bothersome profuse nasal discharge
Rescue therapy and symptom relief by minimizing nasal congestion	• Oral and nasal decongestants (alpha-adrenergic agonists [pseudoephedrine])	• Potential for vasoconstriction, increased BP, and HR; avoid or use with caution in HTN, cardiovascular disease.

Adapted from Bousquet J, Van Cauwenberge P, and Khaltaev N: Allergic rhinitis and its impact on asthma. J Allergy Clin Immunol 2001;108: S147–S334.

TABLE 4–3
ALLERGIC CONJUNCTIVITIS DEFINING TERMS

Seasonal, intermittent, allergic conjunctivitis (SAC)	• IgE-mediated diseases related to seasonal allergens • Common triggers: Dependent on time of year and geographic location (examples: April/May—Tree pollens; June/July—Grass pollens; July/August—Mold spores and weed pollens, others dependent on local environmental factors)
Perennial, persistent, allergic conjunctivitis (PAC)	• IgE-mediated diseases are related to perennial allergens • Common trigger — house dust mites (present in all geographic areas)

GLORIA Guidelines for the treatment of allergic rhinitis and allergic conjunctivitis, available at http://www.worldallergy.org/educational_programs/gloria/guidelines.pdf

The person with allergic rhinitis should also be evaluated for allergic conjunctivitis (Table 4–3). Often, the nasal symptoms are more distressing and the patient simply fails to mention that the eyes often itch and tear. The inflammatory mediator–filled tears from allergic conjunctivitis drain into the nose, making allergic rhinitis symptoms significantly worse. Allergic conjunctivitis treatment includes allergen avoidance and use of products that help prevent the formation of inflammatory mediators, such as ophthalmic mast cell stabilizers and antihistamines. Oral antihistamines can help with symptom management (Table 4–4 and 4–5 and Figures 4–2 and 4–3).

DISCUSSION SOURCES

Bousquet J, Van Cauwenberge P, and Khaltaev N. (2001). Allergic rhinitis and its impact on asthma. Journal of Allergy and Clinical Immunology 108(Suppl):S147–S334.

Gilbert, D., Moellering, R., and Sande, M. (2004). The Sanford Guide to Antimicrobial Therapy (34th ed.). Hyde Park, VT: Antimicrobial Therapy.

TABLE 4–4
ALLERGIC RHINITIS AND CONJUNCTIVITIS TREATMENT

Non-drug therapies for all classifications	• Non-drug therapies
	  • Avoidance
	  • Cool compresses
	  • Preservative-free artificial tears

For intermittent, seasonal allergic conjunctivitis	• Controller therapy with:
	  • Topical antihistamine &/or topical cromones *or*
	  • Topical antihistamine w/mast cell stabilizer *or*
	  • Topical antihistamine w/vasoconstrictor *or*
	  • Topical NSAIDs
	• If inadequate control for intermittent, seasonal
	  • Oral antihistamine

Persistent (mainly perennial) allergic rhinitis	• Controller therapy
	  • Topical mast cell stabilizer w/wo topical/oral antihistamine
	• If inadequate control
	  • Allergy immunotherapy
	  • Topical corticosteroids (nasal only)

GLORIA Guidelines for the treatment of allergic rhinitis and allergic conjunctivitis, available at http://www.worldallergy.org/educational_programs/gloria/guidelines.pdf, accessed 9.10.04.

TABLE 4–5

MEDICATIONS FOR ALLERGIC RHINITIS PER ARIA

	Sneezing	*Rhinorrhea*	*Nasal obstruct*	*Nasal itch*	*Eye*
HI-Antihistamines					
Oral	+ + +	+ + +	0 to +	+ + +	+ +
Intranasal	+ +	+ + +	+	+ +	0
Intraocular	0	0	0	0	+ + +
Corticosteroids	+ + +	+ + +	+ +	+ +	+
Cromolyn					
Intranasal	+	+	+	+	0
Intraocular	0	0	0	0	+ +
Decongestants					
Intranasal	0	0	+ +	0	0
Oral	0	0	+	0	0
Anticholinergics	0	+ + +	0	0	0
Antileukotrienes	+	+ +	+ +	?	+ +

Bousquet J, Van Cauwenberge P, Khaltaev N: Allergic rhinitis and its impact on asthma. J Allergy Clin Immunol 2001;108(Suppl): S147–S334.

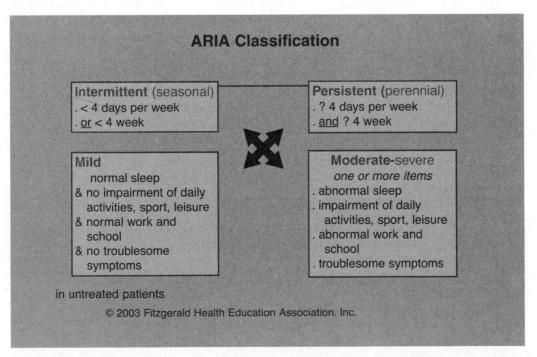

ARIA Classification

Intermittent (seasonal)
. < 4 days per week
. or < 4 week

Persistent (perennial)
. ? 4 days per week
. and ? 4 week

Mild
  normal sleep
& no impairment of daily
  activities, sport, leisure
& normal work and
  school
& no troublesome
  symptoms

Moderate-severe
one or more items
. abnormal sleep
. impairment of daily
  activities, sport, leisure
. abnormal work and
  school
. troublesome symptoms

in untreated patients

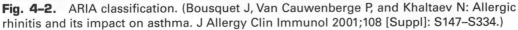
© 2003 Fitzgerald Health Education Association, Inc.

Fig. 4–2. ARIA classification. (Bousquet J, Van Cauwenberge P, and Khaltaev N: Allergic rhinitis and its impact on asthma. J Allergy Clin Immunol 2001;108 [Suppl]: S147–S334.)

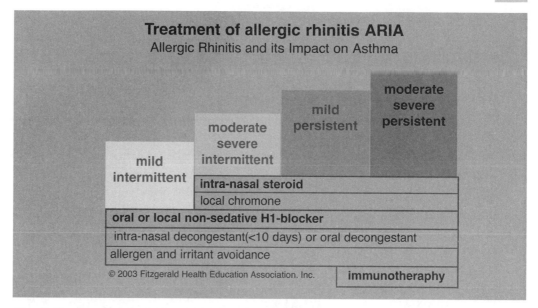

Fig. 4–3. Treatment of allergic rhinitis according to ARIA recommendations. (Bousquet J, Van Cauwenberge P, Khaltaev N: Allergic rhinitis and its impact on asthma. J Allergy Clin Immunol 2001;108 [Suppl]: S147–S334.)

GLORIA Guidelines for the treatment of allergic rhinitis and allergic conjunctivitis. Available at http://www.worldallergy.org/educational_programs/gloria/guidelines.pdf, accessed 10/26/03.

Jackler, R., and Kaplan, M. (2003). Ear, nose and throat. In Tierney, L., McPhee, S., and Papadakis, M. (eds.). Current Diagnosis and Treatment (42nd ed., pp. 179–215). New York: Lange Medical Books/McGraw-Hill.

QUESTIONS

70. The most specific finding for acute bacterial rhinosinusitis (ABRS) is:

    A. upper respiratory tract infections persisting beyond 7 to 10 days or worsening after 5 to 7 days.

    B. mild midfacial fullness and tenderness.

    C. preauricular lymphadenopathy.

    D. marked eyelid edema.

71. The most common causative pathogen in ABRS is:

    A. *M. pneumoniae.*

    B. *S. pneumoniae.*

    C. *M. catarrhalis.*

    D. *H. influenzae.*

72. Which of the following is not consistent with the diagnosis of ABRS?

    A. nasal congestion responsive to decongestant use

    B. maxillary toothache

    C. colored nasal discharge

73. Which of the following is a first-line therapy for the treatment of ABRS in an adult with no recent antimicrobial use?

    A. amoxicillin

    B. trimethoprim-sulfamethoxazole

    C. clarithromycin

    D. levofloxacin

74. Which of the following represents a therapeutic option for ABRS in a patient with no recent antimicrobial care with treatment failure after 72 hours of appropriate-dose amoxicillin therapy?

    A. clindamycin

    B. clarithromycin

    C. ofloxacin

    D. amoxicillin/clavulanate

75. A 34-year-old man with penicillin allergy presents with ABRS. Three weeks ago, he was treated with penicillin for "bronchitis." You now prescribe:

    A. clarithromycin.
    B. levofloxacin.
    C. cephalexin.
    D. amoxicillin.

76. The most appropriate pharmacologic intervention for treating ABRS in a 45-year-old with a 35–pack-year cigarette smoking history is:

    A. erythromycin.
    B. amoxicillin with clavulanate.
    C. cephalexin.
    D. ciprofloxacin.

ANSWERS

70. A	**71.** B	**72.** A
73. A	**74.** D	
75. B	**76.** B	

DISCUSSION

ABRS is a clinical condition caused by an inflammation of the lining of the membranes of the paranasal sinuses. Risk factors include any condition that alters the normal cleansing mechanism of the sinuses, including viral infection, allergies, tobacco use, and abnormalities in sinus structure. Cigarette smoking disturbs normal sinus mucociliary action and drainage, causing secretions to pool and increasing the risk of superimposed bacterial infection. In addition, viral URI causes similar dysfunction, thus increasing ABRS risk. The observation of purulent discharge from one of the nasal turbinates is a highly sensitive finding in ABRS. Midfacial fullness is common in patients with uncomplicated URI, and anterior cervical lymphadenopathy is often found in a number of infectious and inflammatory conditions involving the head and pharynx. Marked eyelid edema is found only when the infection has extended beyond the sinuses and an orbital cellulitis has formed, a potentially life-threatening complication of ABRS.

S. pneumoniae causes the majority of ABRS; it is the least likely of the three major causative bacteria to resolve without antimicrobial intervention, and it causes the most significant symptoms. This organism has exhibited resistance to a number of antibiotic agents, including lower dose amoxicillin, cephalosporins, and macrolides. The mechanism of resistance is alterations of intracellular protein-binding sites, which can typically be overcome by using higher doses of amoxicillin, selected cephalosporins, and respiratory fluoroquinolones (levofloxacin, gatifloxacin, moxifloxacin). Recent antimicrobial use is the major risk for infection with drug-resistant *S. pneumoniae*. *H. influenzae* and *M. catarrhalis* are gram-negative organisms capable of producing beta-lactamase. Although these two organisms have relatively high rates of spontaneous resolution without antimicrobial intervention in AOM, infections caused by these pathogens seldom resolve without antimicrobial therapy in ABRS. Antimicrobial therapy in ABRS should be aimed at choosing an agent with significant activity against gram-positive (*S. pneumoniae*) and gram-negative organisms (*H. influenzae, M. catarrhalis*), with consideration for drug-resistant *S. pneumoniae* risk and stability in the presence of beta-lactamase. If there is treatment failure, the choice of a new antimicrobial is dependent on the initial medication that failed to eradicate the infection and patterns of recent antimicrobial use (Table 4–6).

DISCUSSION SOURCES

Antimicrobial treatment guidelines for acute bacterial rhinosinusitis. Sinus and Allergy Health Partnership (2004). Otolaryngology—Head and Neck Surgery 123(1, Pt 2):1–31.

Jackler, R., and Kaplan, M. (2003). Ear, nose and throat. In Tierney, L., McPhee, S., and Papadakis, M. (eds.). Current Diagnosis and Treatment (42nd ed., pp. 179–215). New York: Lange Medical Books/McGraw-Hill.

TABLE 4–6

ACUTE BACTERIAL RHINOSINUSITIS: ADULT TREATMENT

Patient Characteristics	Initial Therapy	No Improvement or Worsening After 72 Hours
Adults with mild disease and no prior antimicrobial use in the past 4–6 weeks	• Amoxicillin (1.5–4 g/d) or • Amoxicillin/clavulanate (1.75–4 g/250 mg/d) or • Cefpodoxime proxetil or • Cefuroxime axetil or • Cefdinir	• Respiratory fluoroquinolone such as levofloxacin or moxifloxacin or • Amoxicillin/clavulanate (4g/250 mg/d) or • Ceftriaxone or • Rifampin plus clindamycin
Adults with mild disease *and* β-lactam allergy and *no* prior antimicrobial use in the past 4–6 weeks	• TMP/SMX or • Doxycycline or • A macrolide such as azithromycin, clarithromycin, erythromycin, or telithromycin	• Respiratory fluoroquinolone such as levofloxacin or or • Rifampin plus clindamycin
Adults with mild disease with a history of prior antimicrobial use in the past 4–6 weeks *or* adults with moderate disease with or without prior antimicrobial use	• Respiratory fluoroquinolone such as levofloxacin or moxifloxacin or • Amoxicillin/clavulanate (4g/250 mg/d) • Ceftriaxone or • Rifampin plus clindamycin	• Re-evaluate patient
Adults with mild disease *with* prior antimicrobial use in the past 4–6 weeks *and* β-lactam allergy *or* adults with moderate disease with or without prior antibiotic use *and* β-lactam allergy	• Respiratory fluoroquinolone such as gatifloxacin, levofloxacin, or moxifloxacin or • Rifampin plus clindamycin	• Re-evaluate patient

Sinus and Allergy Health Partnership Treatment Guidelines. Otolaryngol Head Neck Surg 2004:130, 1–45.

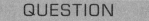

QUESTION

77. Which of the following best describes hearing loss associated with presbycusis?

   A. rapidly progressing and often asymmetric, and in all frequencies
   B. slowly progressive, usually symmetric, and predominantly high frequency
   C. variable in progress, usually unilateral, in the midrange frequencies
   D. primarily conductive and bilateral with slow progress

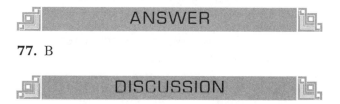

ANSWER

77. B

DISCUSSION

Presbycusis is a progressive, fairly symmetric, high-frequency, age-related sensory hearing loss likely caused by cochlear deterioration. Speech discrimination is usually the primary problem.

DISCUSSION SOURCES

Hektor Dunphy, L. (2004). Management Guidelines for Nurse Practitioners Working with Adults. Philadelphia: F.A. Davis.

Kennedy-Malone L, Fletcher K, and Plank, L. (2004). Management Guidelines for Nurse Practitioners Working with Older Adults (2nd ed). Philadelphia: F.A. Davis.

QUESTIONS

78. A 78-year-old woman has early bilateral senile cataracts. Which of the following situations would likely pose the greatest difficulty?

    A. reading the newspaper
    B. distinguishing between the primary colors
    C. following extraocular movements
    D. reading road signs while driving

79. Which of the following is consistent with the visual problems associated with presbyopia?

    A. bilateral peripheral vision loss
    B. blurring of near vision
    C. difficulty with distant vision
    D. loss of the central vision field

80. Which of the following is consistent with the visual problems associated with macular degeneration?

    A. peripheral vision loss
    B. blurring of near vision
    C. difficulty with distant vision
    D. loss of the central vision field

81. All of the following are consistent with normal age-related vision changes except:

    A. need for increased illumination.
    B. increasing sensitivity to glare.
    C. washing out of colors.
    D. gradual loss of peripheral vision.

ANSWERS

78. D   79. B
80. D   81. D

DISCUSSION

Distance vision poses the greatest problem for individuals with senile cataracts. As the lens becomes more opaque, near vision also deteriorates. Other visual changes of age-related cataracts include loss of ability to distinguish contrasts and progressive dimming of vision. Close vision is usually retained, and there are occasional improvements in reading ability.

Presbyopia is age-related vision changes caused by a progressive hardening of the lens. Patients most often complain of close vision problems, usually first manifested by difficulty with reading smaller print. Other normal age-related vision changes include a progressive yellowing of the lens and decreased flexibility of the sclera, in part leading to the perception of washing out of colors, difficulty seeing under low illumination, and increased sensitivity to glare.

Macular degeneration is the most common cause of blindness and vision loss in elderly persons. Vision changes seen in macular degeneration include loss of the central vision field. This disease is more often seen in women of European descent. A history of cigarette smoking and a family history of the disease are often found as well. A history of excessive sun exposure has been implicated as a risk factor for macular degeneration. The ophthalmologic examination reveals hard drusen or yellow deposits in the macular area. Soft drusen may also be seen. These appear larger, paler, and less distinct.

DISCUSSION SOURCES

Hektor Dunphy, L. (2004). Management Guidelines for Nurse Practitioners Working with Adults. Philadelphia: F.A. Davis.

Kennedy-Malone L, Fletcher K, and Plank, L. (2004). Management Guidelines for Nurse Practitioners Working with Older Adults (2nd ed). Philadelphia: F.A. Davis.

5

Chest Disorders

1. Which of the following best describes asthma?

   A. intermittent airway inflammation with occasional bronchospasm
   B. a disease of bronchospasm that leads to airway inflammation
   C. chronic airway inflammation with superimposed bronchospasm
   D. relatively fixed airway constriction

2. The patient you are evaluating is having an asthma flare. You have assessed that his condition is appropriate for office treatment. You expect to find the following on physical examination:

   A. tripod posture
   B. inspiratory crackles
   C. increased vocal fremitus
   D. hyperresonance on thoracic percussion

3. A 44-year-old man has a long-standing history of moderate persistent asthma that is normally well controlled by fluticasone with salmeterol (Advair) via metered-dose inhaler, 1 puff twice a day, and the use of albuterol 1 to 2 times a week as needed for wheezing. Three days ago, he developed a sore throat, clear nasal discharge, body aches, and a dry cough. In the past 24 hours, he has had intermittent wheezing, which necessitated the use of albuterol, 2 puffs every 3 hours, which produced partial relief. Your next most appropriate action is to obtain a:

   A. chest radiograph.
   B. measurement of oxygen saturation (SaO_2).
   C. peak expiratory flow (PEF) measurement.
   D. sputum smear for white blood cells (WBCs).

4. You examine a 24-year-old woman who has an acute asthma flare. She is using budesonide (Pulmicort) and albuterol as directed and continues to have difficulty with coughing and wheezing. Her PEF is 55% of predicted level. Her medication regimen should be adjusted to include:

   A. theophylline.
   B. salmeterol (Serevent).
   C. prednisone.
   D. montelukast (Singulair).

5. Which of the following is most likely to appear on a chest radiograph of a person during an acute asthma attack?

A. hyperinflation
B. atelectasis
C. consolidation
D. Kerley B signs

6. A 36-year-old man with asthma also needs antihypertensive therapy. Which product would you avoid prescribing?

    A. hydrochlorothiazide
    B. propranolol
    C. nicardipine
    D. enalapril

7. Which of the following is not consistent with the diagnosis of asthma?

    A. a troublesome nocturnal cough
    B. cough or wheeze after exercise
    C. morning sputum production
    D. colds that "go to the chest" or take more than 10 days to clear

8. The cornerstone of moderate persistent asthma drug therapy is the use of:

    A. oral theophylline.
    B. mast cell stabilizers.
    C. short-acting beta agonists.
    D. inhaled corticosteroids.

9. Sharon is a 29-year-old woman with moderate intermittent asthma. She is not using prescribed inhaled corticosteroids but is using albuterol PRN to relieve her cough and wheeze. Currently she uses about 2 albuterol metered-dose inhalers per month and is requesting a prescription refill. You respond that:

    A. albuterol use may continue.
    B. excessive albuterol use is a risk factor for asthma death.
    C. she should also use salmeterol (Serevent) to reduce her albuterol use.
    D. theophylline should be added to her treatment plan.

10. In the treatment of asthma, leukotriene inhibitors should be used as a/an:

    A. long-acting bronchodilators.
    B. inflammatory inhibitors.
    C. rescue drugs.
    D. intervention in acute inflammation.

11. According to the National Asthma Education and Prevention Program Expert Panel Report 2 (NAEPP EPR-2) guidelines, which of the following is not a risk for asthma death?

    A. hospitalization or an emergency department visit for asthma in the past month
    B. current use of systemic corticosteroids or recent withdrawal from systemic corticosteroids
    C. difficulty perceiving airflow obstruction or its severity
    D. rural residence

12. A 18-year-old high school senior presents, asking for a letter stating that he should not participate in gym class because he has asthma. The most appropriate response is to:

    A. write the note, because gym class participation may trigger an asthma flare.
    B. excuse him from outdoor activities only in order to avoid pollen exposure.
    C. remind him that with appropriate asthma care, he should be capable of participating in gym class.
    D. excuse him from indoor activities only in order to avoid dust mite exposure.

13. After inhaled corticosteroid or leukotriene modifier therapy is initiated, clinical effects will be seen:

    A. immediately.
    B. within the first week.
    C. in about 1 to 2 weeks.
    D. in about 1 to 2 months.

14. In comparison with albuterol, levalbuterol (Xopenex) has:

    A. a different mechanism of action.
    B. the ability to provide greater bronchodilation with a lower dose.
    C. an anti-inflammatory effect similar to that of an inhaled corticosteroid.
    D. a contraindication to use in elderly patients.

ANSWERS

1. C	**2.** D	**3.** C	**4.** C	**5.** A
6. B	**7.** C	**8.** D	**9.** B	**10.** B
11. D	**12.** C	**13.** C	**14.** B	

DISCUSSION

Asthma is a chronic inflammatory airway disease involving an increase in bronchial hyperresponsiveness with superimposed bronchospasm and a resulting decrease in the ratio of forced expiratory volume in 1 second (FEV_1) to forced vital capacity (FVC). Although the condition ranks second after allergic rhinitis as the most common chronic respiratory disease in North America, many persons with asthma continue to be undiagnosed and therefore untreated (see Table 5–1).

According to the NAEPP EPR-2, the goals of asthma care are as follows, with a brief explanation of the rationale for each objective:

- minimal or, ideally, no chronic symptoms such as cough and wheeze, including nocturnal symptoms

  Asthma symptoms typically following a circadian rhythm, in which bronchospasm is worse during the night sleep hours. Therefore, a marker of effective airway inflammation control is minimal nocturnal symptoms.

TABLE 5–1

MAKING THE DIAGNOSIS:
IS IT ASTHMA?

- Attack or recurrent attacks of wheezing?
- Troublesome cough at night?
- Cough or wheeze after exercise?
- Cough, wheeze, chest tightness after exposure to airborne allergens or pollutants?
- Do colds "go to the chest" or take more than 10 days to clear?
- Does the person use anti-asthma medication? How often?
- — If patient answers "yes" to any question, asthma diagnosis is likely.

National Asthma Education and Prevention Program. Expert Panel Report Guideline for the Diagnosis and Management of Asthma. Available at www.nhbli.nih.gov, accessed 9.10.04.

- no emergency room or emergency visits

  When airway inflammatory control is poor, patients with asthma typically use emergency services for treatment of frequent acute flares. With appropriate asthma instruction to help the patient with management of acute and chronic airway inflammation and its resulting symptoms, emergency visits can be minimized or eliminated.

- minimal (ideally, no) use of PRN short-acting $beta_2$ agonist (certainly two or fewer uses of $beta_2$ agonist/week)

  Asthma is a disease of airway inflammation with superimposed bronchospasm. The need for short-acting $beta_2$ agonist use as a rescue drug should be viewed as failure to provide adequate airway inflammatory control. Excessive $beta_2$ agonist use is a risk factor for asthma death (see Table 5–1).

- no limitations on activities, including exercise

  When airway inflammation control is inadequate, asthma symptoms such as cough or wheeze can accompany or immediately follow physical activity. The person with well-controlled asthma should be able and encouraged to participate in fitness and leisure activities.

- PEF circadian variation of less than 20%

  The body's normal circadian rhythm provides a variation from awakening PEF to late evening PEF of 10% to 15%. With asthma, this variation increases to more than 15%, reflecting the nocturnal bronchospasm that is a part of the disease.

- (near) normal PEF

  With asthma treatment that focuses on the prevention of airway inflammation and bronchospasm, the PEF can be normal or near normal.

- no or minimal side effects while receiving optimal medications

  Because of the wide range of asthma medications currently available, the nurse practitioner (NP), patient, and family can work together to find a lifestyle and treatment regimen that provide optimal care with minimal to few adverse medication effects.

The backbone of mild persistent, moderate persistent, or severe persistent asthma therapy is the use of an inflammatory controller drug such as inhaled corticosteroids, mast cell stabilizers such as nedocromil or cromolyn, and leukotriene modifiers such as montelukast or zafirlukast. Although all these products afford anti-inflammatory capability, the inhaled corticosteroids have proved to be the most effective in preventing airway inflammation and are recognized as the preferred asthma controller drug (Fig. 5–1). Rescue medications that relieve acute superimposed bronchospasm include short-acting $beta_2$ agonists such as albuterol, levalbuterol, and pirbuterol. In comparison with albuterol and pirbuterol, some of levalbuterol's therapeutic advantages include greater bronchodilation with fewer side effects and at a lower dose. Long-acting $beta_2$ agonists such as salmeterol and formoterol provide bronchospasm protection. In moderate or severe persistent asthma, adding a long-acting $beta_2$ agonist to the inhaled corticosteroid is more effective in achieving symptom control than is increasing the inhaled corticosteroid dose. Adding a leukotriene modifier to an inhaled corticosteroid or doubling the dosage of inhaled corticosteroids also improves asthma outcomes, but the evidence is not as substantial as that for adding a long-acting $beta_2$ agonist. It is important to remember that the clinical effects of the inhaled corticosteroid and leukotriene modifier take at least 1 to 2 weeks to be seen. Theophylline remains helpful in preventing bronchospasm; as a narrow therapeutic index medication, the theophylline dose must be closely titrated and monitored with serial measurements of serum drug levels, which significantly limits the drug's usefulness.

When acute asthma flare-up is present and the PEF is less than 50% to 80% of predicted, rapidly acting, higher potency anti-inflammatory therapy with an oral corticosteroid is needed. Adding more bronchodilators, such as theophylline and salmeterol, does not reverse the cause of the bronchospasm: significant airway inflammation. The leukotriene modifiers are helpful in preventing, but not acutely treating, inflammation (Table 5–2).

Here are memory aids that may be useful for developing a plan of care for patients with asthma:

- Antagonists are drugs that block activity of a receptor site; agonists stimulate activity of a receptor site.
- $Beta_1$ receptors predominate in the heart; the $beta_2$ receptors predominate in the lungs. (One easy way to remember: You have $beta_1$ receptors in your one heart and $beta_2$ receptors in your two lungs.)
- Names of $beta_2$ agonists have a "-terol" suffix. Medications such as albuterol stimulate $beta_2$ receptor sites and cause bronchodilation. These medications are available in quick-onset, shorter acting forms (albuterol, levalbuterol, pirbuterol) and in longer acting forms (salmeterol, formoterol).
- Beta-adrenergic antagonists (beta blockers) block adrenergic (adrenaline-like) activity. Examples include medications whose names have the "-lol" suffix, such as atenolol and propranolol. Whereas cardioselective beta blockers such as metoprolol focus activity in the heart, mixed or noncardioselective $beta_1$ and $beta_2$ blockers such as propranolol antagonize activity at receptors in the heart and lungs. Using beta blockers, particularly a nonselective agent such as propranolol, in the presence of asthma can precipitate bronchospasm. If a beta blocker is needed, using a low dosage of a cardioselective agent is likely the best choice.
- Names of corticosteroids have an "-one" or "-ide" suffix. Fluticasone (Flovent), prednisone, and budesonide (Pulmicort) are examples of corticosteroids used in the treatment of asthma.
- Leukotriene receptor antagonists, also known as leukotriene modifiers, include medications whose names have the "-lukast" suffix. These products attenuate the effects of a group of inflammatory mediators known as the leukotrienes, thus helping to

Stepwise Approach for Adults and Children (>5 years)

Severity Class	Symptoms/Day Symptoms/Night	PEF or FEV$_1$ PEF Variability	Daily Medications

Step 4
Severe
Persistent
	Continual
	Frequent
		≤60%
		>30%
			• Preferred treatment:
			   High-dose ICS + LABA AND, if needed,
			   corticosteroid tablets or syrup long term

Step 3
Moderate Persistent
	Daily
	>1 night/week
		>60% – <80%
		>30%
			• Preferred treatment:
			   Low-to-medium dose ICS + LABA
			
			• Alternative treatment: increase ICS dose
			   within med-dose range OR low-to-med dose
			   ICS + LTM OR theophylline
			
			If needed:
			• Preferred treatment: increased medium-dose
			   ICS + LABA
			• Alternative treatment: increased medium-
			   dose ICS + LTM OR theophylline

Step 2
Mild Persistent
	>2/week but <1x/day
	>2 nights/month
		≥80%
		20%–30%
			• Preferred treatment:
			   Low-dose inhaled corticosteroid
			
			• Alternative treatment: cromolyn, LTM,
			   nedocromil OR theophylline SR (serum
			   concentration of 5–15 mcg/mL)

Step 1 Mild Intermittent	≤2 days/week ≤2 nights/month	≥80% <20%	• No daily medication needed

Guidelines for the Diagnosis and Management of Asthma—Update on Selected Topics 2002. NIH, NHLBI. June 2002.
NIH publication no. 02–5075

Stepwise Approach for Managing Infants and Young Children (≤5 Years)

Severity Class	Symptoms/Day Symptoms/Night	Daily Medications

Step 4
Severe Persistent
	Continual
	Frequent
		• Preferred treatment:
		   High-dose ICS + LABA AND, if needed, corticosteroid
		   tablets or syrup long term

Step 3 Moderate Persistent	Daily >1 night/week	• Preferred treatment: Low-dose ICS + LABA OR medium-dose ICS
		• Alternative treatment: Low-dose ICS + LTRA OR theophylline If needed: • Preferred treatment: Medium-dose ICS + LABA • Alternative treatment: Medium-dose ICS + LTRA OR theophyllin
Step 2 Mild Persistent	>2/week but <1x/day >2 nights/month	• Preferred treatment: Low-dose inhaled corticosteroid • Alternative treatment: Cromolyn OR LTRA
Step 1 Mild Intermittent	≤2 days/week ≤2 nights/month	• No daily medication needed

Guidelines for the Diagnosis and Management of Asthma—Update on Selected Topics 2002. NIH, NHLBI June 2002,
NIH publication no 02–5075.

FIG. 5–1. Stepwise approach for adults and children. FEV$_1$, forced expiratory volume in 1 second; ICS, intercostal space; LABA, long-acting beta$_2$ agonist; LTM, leukotriene modifier; LTRA, leukotriene receptor antagonist; PEF, peak expiratory flow (Source: National Asthma Education and Prevention Program, Expert Panel Report 2. Guidelines for the Diagnosis and Management of Asthma. Available at http://www.nhlbi.nih.gov/guidelines/asthma/asthgdln.htm, accessed 9.10.04.)

TABLE 5–2

MEDICATIONS USED FOR TREATING PATIENTS WITH ASTHMA
AND CHRONIC OBSTRUCTIVE PULMONARY DISEASE

Medication	Mechanism of Action	Indication	Comment
Inhaled corticosteroids	Inhibit eosinophilic action and other inflammatory mediators, potentate effects of beta$_2$ agonists	Controller drug, prevention of inflammation	Need consistent use to be helpful
Cromolyn sodium (Intal), nedocromil (Tilade)	Halts degradation of mast cells and release of histamine and other inflammatory mediators (mast cell stabilizer)	Controller drug, prevention of inflammation	Need consistent use to be helpful Less clinical effect in comparison with inhaled corticosteroids
Leukotriene modifier (montelukast [Singulair], zafirlukast [Accolate])	Inhibit action of inflammatory mediator (leukotriene) by blocking select receptor sites	Controller drug, prevention of inflammation	Likely less effective than inhaled corticosteroids Particularly effective add-on medication when disease control is inadequate with inhaled corticosteroid, when asthma is complicated by allergic rhinitis
Oral corticosteroids	Inhibit eosinophilic action and other inflammatory mediators	Treatment of acute inflammation such as in asthma flare or COPD exacerbation	Indicated in treatment of acute asthma flare to reduce inflammation In higher dose and with longer therapy (>2 weeks), adrenal suppression may occur No taper needed if use is short term (<10 days) and at lower dose (prednisone, 40–60 mg/day or less) Potential for causing gastropathy, particularly gastric ulcer and gastritis
Albuterol (Ventolin, Proventil), pirbuterol (Maxair) Levalbuterol (Xopenex)	Beta$_2$ agonists; bronchodilation via stimulation of beta$_2$ receptor site	Rescue drugs for treatment of acute bronchospasm	Albuterol and pirbuterol • Onset of action, 15 min • Duration of action, 4–6 hr
Long-acting beta$_2$ agonists (salmeterol [Serevent], formoterol [Foradil])	Beta$_2$ agonists; bronchodilation through stimulation of receptor site beta$_2$	Prevention of bronchospasm	Salmeterol • Onset of action, 1 hr • Duration of action, 12 hr • Indicated for prevention rather than treatment of bronchospasm • Patient should also have short-acting beta$_2$ agonist as rescue drug Formoterol • Onset of action, 15–30 hr • Duration of action, 12 hr • Indicated for prevention rather than treatment of bronchospasm • Patient should also have short-acting beta$_2$ agonist as rescue drug

Medication	Mechanism of Action	Indication	Comment
Ipratropium bromide (Atrovent) Tiotropium bromide (Spiriva)	Anticholinergic and muscarinic antagonist, yielding bronchodilatation	Treatment and prevention of bronchospasm	Onset of action $\Rightarrow$ 30 minutes Best used to avoid rather than treat the bronchospasm associated with COPD and asthma Well tolerated
Theophylline	Mild bronchodilator, helps with diaphragmatic contraction	Prevention of bronchospasm, mild anti-inflammatory	Narrow therapeutic index drug with numerous drug interactions Monitor carefully for toxicity by checking drug levels and clinical presentation

COPD, chronic obstructive pulmonary disease.

prevent airway inflammation. Examples include montelukast (Singulair) and zafirlukast (Accolate).

Because this is a lower airway disease, the person with asthma has more of a problem with expiration, or getting air out, than with inspiration, or getting air in. This leads to findings characteristic of air trapping, such as decreased PEF rate, prolonged expiratory phase, thoracic hyperresonance on percussion, and hyperinflation as seen on chest radiographs. Oxygen desaturation is a late finding in an acute asthma flare.

DISCUSSION SOURCES

Muzik, J. (2004). Chest disorders. In Hektor Dunphy, L. (2004). Management Guidelines for Nurse Practitioners Working with Adults (2nd ed). Philadelphia: F.A. Davis, pp 215–276.
National Asthma Education and Prevention Program, Expert Panel Report 2 (2002). Guidelines for the Diagnosis and Management of Asthma. Available at http://www.nhlbi.nih.gov/guidelines/asthma/asthgdln.htm, accessed 9.10.04.

QUESTIONS

15. Ipratropium bromide (Atrovent), when used in treating chronic obstructive pulmonary disease (COPD), is prescribed to achieve which of the following therapeutic effects?
    A. increase mucociliary clearance
    B. reduce alveolar volume
    C. bronchodilation
    D. mucolytic action

16. What is the desired therapeutic action of inhaled corticosteroids when used in treating COPD?
    A. reversal of fixed airway obstruction
    B. improvement of central respiratory drive
    C. reduction of airway inflammation
    D. mucolytic activity

17. Which is most consistent with the diagnosis of COPD?
    A. FEV$_1$/FVC ratio of less than 0.70
    B. dyspnea on exhalation
    C. elevated diaphragms noted on x-ray
    D. polycythemia noted on complete blood cell count

18. Which of the following characteristics is found in the early stages of chronic bronchitis?
    A. enlargement of air spaces distal to the terminal bronchiole
    B. excessive mucus production
    C. alveolar fibrosis
    D. dyspnea at rest

19. Which of the following characteristics is typically found in patients with emphysema?

    A. alpha₁ antiprotease deficiency
    B. enlargement of air spaces distal to the terminal bronchiole
    C. alveolar fibrosis
    D. hypertrophy of the larger airways

20. According to the Global Initiative for Chronic Obstructive Lung Disease (GOLD) COPD guidelines, the following medications are indicated for all patients with stages II to IV COPD:

    A. short-acting inhaled bronchodilators
    B. inhaled corticosteroid
    C. mucolytic agent
    D. theophylline

21. According to the GOLD COPD guidelines, the goal of inhaled corticosteroid use in stage III COPD is to:

    A. minimize the risk of repeated exacerbations.
    B. improve cough function.
    C. reverse alveolar hypertrophy.
    D. help mobilize secretions.

22. Which of the following corticosteroid doses is most potent?

    A. methylprednisolone, 8 mg
    B. triamcinolone, 10 mg
    C. prednisone, 15 mg
    D. hydrocortisone, 18 mg

23. Which of the following pathogens is often found in the sputum during an acute exacerbation of chronic bronchitis?

    A. *Klebsiella pneumoniae*
    B. *Streptococcus pyogenes*
    C. *Haemophilus influenzae*
    D. *Staphylococcus aureus*

24. Which is the most appropriate choice of antimicrobial therapy in acute bacterial COPD for a 72-year-old man with heart failure who has failed amoxicillin therapy?

    A. azithromycin
    B. cefprozil
    C. doxycycline
    D. levofloxacin

25. Which is the most appropriate choice of antimicrobial therapy in acute bacterial COPD exacerbation for a 52-year-old man with stage II COPD?

    A. azithromycin
    B. amoxicillin
    C. trimethoprim-sulfamethoxazole
    D. levofloxacin

26. The most likely causative organism in acute bronchial suppuration association with acute bacteria COPD exacerbation is:

    A. *Pseudomonas aeruginosa.*
    B. *Chlamydia pneumoniae.*
    C. *Streptococcus pneumoniae.*
    D. *Haemophilus influenzae.*

ANSWERS

15. C	**16.** C	**17.** A	**18.** B
19. B	**20.** A	**21.** A	**22.** C
23. C	**24.** D	**25.** A	**26.** A

DISCUSSION

COPD is a disease state characterized by airflow limitation that is not fully reversible. The airflow limitation is usually both progressive and associated with an abnormal inflammatory response of the lungs to noxious particles or gases. This results in a decrease in FEV_1/FVC ratio. Chronic bronchitis and emphysema are two conditions that are part of COPD. The diagnosis of chronic bronchitis is made clinically, with the patient reporting the presence of excessive mucus production for 3 or more months per year for at least 2 consecutive years in the absence of other causes. Emphysema is characterized by permanent enlargement of the air spaces distal to the terminal bronchiole without fibrosis.

Patients with COPD typically present for care in the fifth and sixth decades of life after having some symptoms, particularly excessive sputum production and dyspnea on exertion, for more than a decade. Late in the disease, dyspnea at rest may be reported.

Because 80% of all cases of COPD can be attributed directly to tobacco use, smoking cessation is the goal. In spite of symptoms, many patients continue to smoke. Raising the issue of smoking cessation with every visit and offering assistance with this is an important part of the ongoing care of the person with COPD. Counseling about general respiratory hygiene should also be supplied, including information on minimizing exposure to passive smoking, allergens, and air pollution, as well as advice on hydration and nutrition. Annual influenza and appropriate antipneumococcal vaccination should be encouraged.

Tiotropium bromide (Spiriva) and ipratropium bromide (Atrovent) are anticholinergic agents considered backbone drugs in treatment of patients with stages II to IV COPD (Table 5–3). An atropine analog with these medications act as a muscarinic antagonist. Muscarinic receptor sites are located in organs innervated by the parasympathetic nervous system. When these sites are stimulated, bronchoconstriction occurs. Ipratropium and tiotropium act as a bronchodilator but have no sympathomimetic effects or action at beta$_2$ receptors sites, such as with albuterol. In contrast to albuterol, the muscarinic antagonists have a long onset of action (>1/2 hour) and are best used to avoid rather than treat the bronchospasm associated with COPD. In addition, the use of these medications may help reduce the volume of secretions produced in COPD. If a patient with COPD continues to have symptoms despite consistent use of a full therapeutic dose of ipratropium or tiotropium, a beta$_2$ agonist should be added to provide additional bronchodilation through another mechanism of action.

Theophylline, which has mild bronchodilation and anti-inflammatory action, is used as a

---

TABLE 5–3
MANAGEMENT OF COPD

For all states of COPD, the following should be advised:
- Avoidance of noxious agents
- Smoking cessation
- Reduction of indoor pollution
- Reduction of occupational irritant exposure
- Annual influenza vaccination, antipneumococcal vaccine as appropriate

Stage	Characteristics	Treatment
Stage 0	• Cough • Sputum production • No spirometric abnormalities	• COPD risk reduction
Stage I Mild	• FEV$_1$:FVC ratio <0.70 • FEV$_1$ >80% of predicted • With/without symptoms	• Short-acting bronchodilator PRN • Albuterol, pirbuterol, levalbuterol
Stage II Moderate	• FEV$_1$:FVC ratio <0.70 • 50%> FEV$_1$ <80% of predicted • With/without symptoms	• Regular use of => 1 long-acting bronchodilator • Tiotropium bromide • Salmeterol or formoterol • Short-acting bronchodilator PRN • Albuterol, pirbuterol, levalbuterol • Inhaled corticosteroid if repeated exacerbations • Pulmonary rehabilitation

(continued)

TABLE 5–3

MANAGEMENT OF COPD *(continued)*

Stage	Characteristics	Treatment

Stage III Severe	• FEV_1:FVC ratio <0.70
	• 30%> FEV_1 <50% of predicted
	• With/without symptoms
		• Regular use of => 1 long-acting bronchodilator
		  • Tiotropium bromide
		  • Salmeterol or formoterol
		• Short-acting bronchodilator PRN
		  • Albuterol, pirbuterol, levalbuterol
		• Inhaled corticosteroid if repeated exacerbations
		• Pulmonary rehabilitation

Stage IV Very severe	• FEV_1:FVC ratio <0.70
	• FEV_1 <30% of predicted or presence of respiratory failure or heart failure
		• Regular use of => 1 long-acting bronchodilator
		  • Tiotropium bromide
		  • Salmeterol or formoterol
		• Short-acting bronchodilator PRN
		  • Albuterol, pirbuterol, levalbuterol
		• Inhaled corticosteroid if repeated exacerbations
		• Pulmonary rehabilitation
		• Treatment of complications
		• Long-term oxygen therapy if respiratory failure
		• Consider surgical options

NHLBI/WHO Global Initiative for Chronic Obstructive Lung Disease. Global Strategy for the Diagnosis, Management, and Prevention of Chronic Obstructive Pulmonary Disease. Bethesda, MD: National Institutes of Health; available at www.goldcopd.org, accessed 9.27.04.

third-line agent in treating COPD. Corticosteroids are also used to minimize airway inflammation and possibly limit the frequency and severity of acute exacerbations of chronic bronchitis (see Tables 5–2 and 5–3).

Exacerbations of respiratory symptoms that necessitate treatment are important clinical events in COPD. The most common causes of an exacerbation are infection of the tracheobronchial tree and air pollution, but the cause of about one third of severe exacerbations cannot be identified. Inhaled bronchodilators (beta$_2$ agonists and/or anticholinergics), theophylline, and systemic, preferably oral corticosteroids are effective for the treatment of COPD exacerbations. In COPD exacerbations with clinical signs of airway infection (e.g., increased volume and change of color of sputum, and/or fever), patients may benefit from antimicrobial treatment, with antibiotic chosen according to patient characteristics and likely causative organisms (Tables 5–4 and 5–5). Noninvasive intermittent positive pressure ventilation in acute exacerbations improves blood gases and pH, reduces in-hospital mortality, decreases the need for invasive mechanical ventilation and intubation, and decreases the length of hospital stay.

DISCUSSION SOURCES

Emerman, C. (2002). Acute Exacerbations of Chronic Obstructive Pulmonary Disease (AE-COPD): Outcome-Effective Antimicrobial Selection and Recent Advances in Outpatient Management. Available at http://www.ahcpub.com/ahc_root_html/hot/sponsored/emr101199.htm, accessed 7/29/03.

Global Initiative for Chronic Obstructive Lung Disease (2003): Workshop Report. Available at www.goldcopd.org, accessed 5/04/04.

TABLE 5–4

CORTICOSTEROIDS: RELATIVE POTENCY

Higher potency corticosteroids (equipotent doses)	Betamethasone, 0.6–0.75 mg Dexamethasone, 0.75 mg	$T^1/_2 = 36–54$ hr
Medium potency corticosteroids (equipotent doses)	Methylprednisolone, 4 mg Triamcinolone, 4 mg Prednisolone, 5 mg Prednisone, 5 mg	$T^1/_2 = 18–36$ hr
Lower potency (equipotent doses)	Hydrocortisone, 20 mg Cortisone, 25 mg	$T^1/_2 = 8–12$ hr

Drug Facts and Comparisons (2002). St. Louis: Facts and Comparisons.
$T^1/_2$, half-life.

TABLE 5–5

GUIDELINES FOR ACUTE BACTERIAL EXACERBATION OF COPD AND CHRONIC BRONCHITIS

	Infectious Etiology	*Treatment Options*
COPD exacerbation with evidence of bacterial infection (fever, increased sputum volume/purulence)	Gram-positive and gram-negative respiratory pathogens, atypical pathogens	Amoxicillin *or* Doxycycline *or* Newer macrolide (azithromycin, clarithromycin, telithromycin) *or* Cephalosporin (cefuroxime, cefpodoxime, cefprozil) *If antimicrobial treatment failure:* respiratory fluoroquinolone (levofloxacin, moxifloxacin, gatifloxacin) *or* HD amoxicillin/clavulanate
Chronic bronchial suppuration risk, severely impaired lung function, chronic corticosteroid use	*P. aeruginosa*, other less common pathogens possible in addition to above organisms	Ciprofloxacin, levofloxacin, other antimicrobials as indicated by causative pathogen

American Thoracic Society, Standards for the Diagnosis and Management of Patients with COPD, 2004 Update, available at www.thoracic.org/COPD, accessed 9.27.04.

Hektor Dunphy, L. (2004). Management Guidelines for Nurse Practitioners Working with Adults (2nd ed). Philadelphia: F.A. Davis.

QUESTIONS

27. You examine a 28-year-old woman who has emigrated from a South American country. She has documentation of receiving bacille Calmette-Guérin vaccine as a child. With this information, you consider that:

   A. she will always have a positive tuberculin skin test (TST) result.
   B. biannual chest radiographs are needed to accurately assess her health status.
   C. a TST finding of 10 mm or more induration should be considered a positive result.
   D. isoniazid therapy should be given for 6 months before TST is undertaken.

28. A 33-year-old woman works in a small office with a man recently diagnosed with active pulmonary tuberculosis (TB). Which of the following best represents plan of care for this woman?

   A. She should receive TB chemoprophylaxis if her TST result is 5 mm or more in induration.
   B. Because of her age, TB chemoprophylaxis is contraindicated even in the presence of a positive TST result.
   C. If the TST result is positive but the chest radiograph is normal, no further evaluation or treatment is needed.
   D. Further evaluation is needed only if the TST result is 15 mm or more in induration.

29 to 32. For these questions, answer "yes" or "no" in response to the question "Does this patient have a reactive TST?"

29. a 45-year-old woman with type 2 diabetes mellitus and chest radiograph finding consistent with previous TB and a 7-mm induration (Yes/No)

30. a 21-year-old man with no identifiable TB risk factors and a 10-mm induration (Yes/No)

31. a 31-year-old man with human immunodeficiency virus (HIV) and a 6-mm induration (Yes/No)

32. a 45-year-old woman from a country where TB is endemic who has an 11-mm induration (Yes/No)

33. Risk factors for active TB in patients with latent TB infection include all of the following except:

   A. diabetes mellitus.
   B. immunocompromise.
   C. chronic oral corticosteroid therapy.
   D. male gender.

34. Clinical presentation of progressive primary TB includes all of the following except:

   A. malaise.
   B. fever.
   C. dry cough.
   D. frank hemoptysis.

ANSWERS

27. C	**28.** A	**29.** Yes
30. No	**31.** Yes	**32.** Yes
33. D	**34.** D	

DISCUSSION

Pulmonary TB is a chronic bacterial infection, caused by *Mycobacterium tuberculosis* and transmitted through droplets. With an estimated 20% to 43% of the world's population infected, the disease occurs disproportionately in disadvantaged populations such as homeless persons, malnourished persons, and those living in overcrowded and substandard housing. In the immunocompetent host, once the organism is acquired, an immune reaction ensues to help contain the infection within granulomas. This stage, known as primary TB, is usually without symptoms. However, viable organisms can lie dormant within the granulomas for years; this stage is known as latent TB infection. The person with latent TB infection does not have active disease and is not contagious. Without treatment, 10% of patients with latent TB infection go on to develop active disease; this number skyrockets in the presence of HIV infection, other immunocompromise (corticosteroid or other immunosuppressive drug use, many chronic illnesses), or diabetes mellitus. After primary infection, about 5% do not mount a containing immune response and develop progressive primary TB.

Public health measures to ensure adequate shelter, hygiene, and nutrition for the vulnerable public is an important primary prevention measure against the spread of TB infection. TST with purified protein derivative containing 5 tuberculin units is an effective method of identifying those infected with *M. tuberculosis*.

This test, when performed on an asymptomatic patient, is an example of secondary prevention or health screening. Any patient with a positive TST result needs to be carefully evaluated for evidence of active disease, including malaise, weight loss, fever, night sweats, and chronic cough. Although blood-tinged sputum is occasionally reported, the cough associated with TB is often dry; frank hemoptysis is rarely reported. The chest examination is usually within normal limits, with dyspnea seldom reported unless disease is extensive.

A positive TST result is usually noted within 2 to 10 weeks of acquiring the organism. The test is performed by injecting 0.1 mL of purified protein derivative transdermally. The results should be checked within 48 to 72 hours, with the transverse measurement of any change in the test site measured in millimeters of induration, not simply redness. The interpretation of the test is the same in the presence or absence of bacille Calmette-Guérin vaccination history. Thresholds for a positive TST result are as follows:

- 5-mm or larger induration in those with suspected or known HIV infection or other immunosuppression, including organ transplant; those receiving the equivalent of prednisone, 15 mg or more daily; close contact with a person with active pulmonary TB; and those with radiographic changes consistent with old disease
- 10-mm or larger induration in those with high risk, such as immigrants from countries where TB is endemic; injection drug users; health care providers; residents of group housing, including long-term care facilities, correctional facilities, and homeless shelters; and persons with select health conditions that increase TB risk (diabetes mellitus, chronic renal failure, select hematologic conditions, and malignancies; children younger than 4 years)
- 15-mm or larger induration in all others, including those who appear to have no TB risk

In select circumstances, two-step testing and anergy testing should be considered. The

TABLE 5–6
GLOSSARY OF TERMS: TUBERCULOSIS (TB)

Term	Definition
Anergy testing	Giving skin tests of substances other than TB to determine whether person does not react to PPD because of weakened immune system
Bacille Calmette-Guerin	Vaccine against TB infection given in many countries; low risk of causing false-positive TST result
Booster phenomenon	Often seen in elderly patients, who, even if infected long ago, have an initial negative TST result but a positive test result when retested up to 1 year later; this occurs as the first test "boosts" the immune response
Two-step testing	Strategy used to distinguish a booster reaction (caused by TB infection that occurred many years ago) from a reaction caused by recent infection; a person with a negative TST result is retested in 1–3 weeks; a positive reaction with test 2 likely represents a boosted reaction, not recent infection

www.cdc.gov/hchstp/tb/htm, accessed 9.27.04.
PPD, purified protein derivative; TST, tuberculin skin test.
TB Guidelines, available www.cdc.gov/nchstp/tb/pubs/ mmwr html/mai_guide/ list_categories.htm, accessed 9.28.04.

booster phenomenon can be seen with repeated testing (Table 5–6).

Chemoprophylaxis therapy with isoniazid and other agents to prevent the development of active pulmonary TB should be considered for asymptomatic patients with positive TST results but negative chest radiograph results. Although the risk of liver toxicity with anti-TB drug use rises with age, age alone is not a contraindication to its use, particularly in the higher risk individual. In the presence of active pulmonary TB, multiple antimicrobial therapies are given that are aimed not only at eradicating the infection but also at minimizing the risk of developing a resistant pathogen. In this era of multidrug-resistant TB, it is prudent to consult with local TB experts to ascertain the local patterns of susceptibility.

DISCUSSION SOURCES

Chesnutt, M., and Prendergast, T. (2003). Lung. In Tierney, L., McPhee, S., and Papadakis, M. (eds.). Current Medical Diagnosis and Treatment (42nd ed., pp. 216–311). New York: Lange Medical Books/McGraw-Hill.

TB Guidelines, available www.cdc.gov/nchstp/tb/pubs/mmwr html/mai_guide/list_categories.htm, accessed 9.28.04.

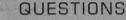

QUESTIONS

35 to 39. Which of the following is the most appropriate antimicrobial for treatment of community-acquired pneumonia (CAP) in:

35. a 42-year-old man with no comorbidity and no recent antimicrobial use?

    A. azithromycin
    B. cefpodoxime
    C. trimethoprim-sulfamethoxazole
    D. ciprofloxacin

36. a 46-year-old well woman who cannot take a macrolide?

    A. clarithromycin
    B. amoxicillin
    C. doxycycline
    D. fosfomycin

37. a 78-year-old woman with COPD?

    A. clindamycin
    B. amoxicillin with a macrolide
    C. nitrofurantoin
    D. ceftriaxone

38. a 69-year-old man with heart failure and type 2 diabetes?

    A. respiratory fluoroquinolone
    B. amoxicillin with beta-lactamase inhibitor
    C. cephalosporin
    D. a macrolide

39. a 58-year-old woman who has a dry cough, headache, malaise, no recent antimicrobial use, and no comorbidity?

    A. clarithromycin
    B. amoxicillin
    C. levofloxacin
    D. trimethoprim-sulfamethoxazole

40. Which of the following is a quality of the respiratory fluoroquinolones?

    A. activity against drug-resistant *S. pneumoniae* (DRSP)
    B. inferior efficacy against atypical pathogens
    C. predominantly renal metabolism
    D. absence of photosensitizing action

41. DRSP's mechanism of resistance is through:

    A. beta-lactamase production.
    B. hypertrophy of cell membrane.
    C. alteration in protein-binding sites.
    D. failure of DNA gyrase reversal.

42. *H. influenzae's* primary mechanism of antimicrobial resistance is through:

    A. beta-lactamase production.
    B. hypertrophy of cell membrane.
    C. alteration in protein binding sites.
    D. failure of DNA gyrase reversal.

43. Which of the following characteristics apply to the macrolides?

    A. consistent activity against DRSP
    B. contraindicated in pregnancy
    C. effective against atypical pathogens
    D. unstable in the presence of beta-lactamase

44. The American Thoracic Society guidelines recommend considering which of the following as length of antimicrobial therapy for the treatment of CAP for outpatients?

A. less than 5 days
B. 5 to 7 days
C. 7 to 10 days
D. 10 to 14 days

45. Modifying factors for *P. aeruginosa* include all of the following except:

A. corticosteroid use.
B. structural lung disease.
C. malnutrition.
D. day care attendance.

46. Which of the following best describes the mechanism of transmission in an atypical pneumonia?

A. microaspiration
B. cough
C. surface contamination
D. aerosolized contaminated water

47. Risk factors for pneumonia death include:

A. viral origin.
B. history of allergy.
C. renal insufficiency.
D. polycythemia.

48. All of the following antimicrobial strategies help facilitate the development of resistant pathogens except:

A. longer course of therapy.
B. lower antimicrobial dosage.
C. higher antimicrobial dosage.
D. prescribing a broader spectrum product.

49. Findings of increased tactile fremitus and dullness to percussion at the right base lung in the person with CAP likely indicate an area of:

A. atelectasis.
B. pneumothorax.
C. consolidation.
D. cavitation.

50. Which of the following represents findings in an acceptable sputum specimen for Gram staining?

A. many squamous epithelial cells and few WBCs
B. three or more stained organisms
C. few squamous epithelial cells and many WBCs
D. motile bacteria with monocytes

51. You are caring for a 52-year-old smoker with CAP. It is the third day of his therapy, and he is without fever, is well hydrated, and is feeling somewhat better. Which of the following represents the best schedule for ordering a chest radiograph for this patient?

A. No chest radiograph is needed, because he is recovering.
B. A chest radiograph should be taken today to confirm resolution of pneumonia.
C. He should have a chest radiograph taken in 7 to 12 weeks.
D. A computed tomography scan of the thorax is needed now.

52. While seeing a 62-year-old who is hospitalized with CAP, the NP considers that:

A. antipneumococcal vaccine should be given once antimicrobial therapy has been completed.
B. antipneumococcal vaccine can be given today and influenza vaccine in 2 weeks.
C. influenza vaccine can be given today and antipneumococcal vaccine in 2 weeks.
D. influenza and antipneumococcal vaccines should be given today.

ANSWERS

35. A	36. C	37. B
38. A	39. A	40. A
41. C	42. A	43. C
44. B	45. D	46. B
47. C	48. C	49. C
50. C	51. C	52. D

DISCUSSION

Pneumonia remains the most common cause of infectious disease death and is the sixth leading cause of overall mortality in the United States. Although pneumonia is often considered a disease primarily of older adults and chronically ill persons, the majority of episodes occur in immunocompetent community-dwelling individuals; about 20% of children develop pneumonia by age 5 years. Most often caused by bacteria or virus, pneumonia is an acute lower respiratory tract infection involving lung parenchyma, interstitial tissues, and alveolar spaces. The term community-acquired pneumonia is used to describe the onset of disease in a person who resides within the community, not in a nursing home or other care facility, with no recent (<2 weeks') hospitalization.

Patients with pneumonia usually present with cough (more than 90%), dyspnea (66%), sputum production (66%), and pleuritic chest pain (50%), although nonrespiratory symptoms may also be noted. Elderly patients may report fewer symptoms. Chest x-ray is helpful in the assessment of the person with CAP. Characteristic infiltrate patterns are typically seen with certain pathogens, such as interstitial infiltrates with atypical pathogens and areas of consolidation with *S. pneumoniae* (Table 5–7). However, therapy should be based on patient characteristics and risk factors rather than the pattern of the infiltrate. In cigarette smokers, a chest radiograph should be taken 7 to 12 weeks after initiation of pneumonia therapy to check for the presence of lung cancer.

Although a number of organisms are capable of causing pneumonia, relatively few are seen with frequency. *S. pneumoniae*, the pneumococcal organism, is a gram-positive diplococcus, is the most common CAP pathogen in adults, and is found in the majority of CAP deaths. Pneumonia caused by *H. influenzae* is predominantly a disease of tobacco users. After many years of smoking, the tracheobronchial tree becomes colonized with this gram-negative coccobacillus. *Mycoplasma pneumoniae* and *C. pneumoniae* are among the most common pathogens causing CAP. These organisms are cough-transmitted and are often found among people living in closed communities, such as households, college dormitories, military barracks, and residential centers, including long-term care facilities. Risk factors for *Legionella* species, a group of atypical pathogens, include tobacco use, airway disease, and diabetes. With airway impairment, pneumonia is often caused

---

TABLE 5–7

AMERICAN THORACIC SOCIETY GUIDELINES FOR THE TREATMENT OF COMMUNITY-ACQUIRED PNEUMONIA

Patient Category	Empirical Therapy
No comorbidity	**Macrolide:** Azithromycin, clarithromycin • Activity against *Streptococcus pneumoniae, Haemophilus influenzae, atypical pathogens* **Alternative:** Doxycycline • If macrolide intolerant
Comorbidity: congestive heart failure, chronic obstructive lung disease	**Beta-lactam:** Cefpodoxime, cefuroxime, high-dose amoxicillin, amoicillin with clavulanate, or ceftriaxone + cefpodoxime *Plus* **macrolide or doxycycline** *Or* **respiratory fluoroquinolone:** Gatifloxacin, levofloxacin, moxifloxacin

Adapted from www.thoracic. org/statements, accessed 9.10.04.
DRSP, drug-resistant *Streptococcus pneumoniae.*

by anaerobic gram-negative bacilli or mixed gram-negative organisms.

Successful community-based care of the person with pneumonia requires a number of factors. The patient must have intact gastrointestinal function and be able to take and tolerate oral medications as well as adequate amounts of fluids. A competent caregiver must be available. Also, the patient should be able to return for follow-up examination and evaluation.

Certain patient characteristics increase the likelihood of death from pneumonia and should alert the NP to consider hospitalization and aggressive therapy. These include age of more than 65 years and severe electrolyte and/or hematologic disorder, such as serum sodium concentration of less than 130 mEq/L, hematocrit below 30%, or absolute neutrophil count of less than 1000/mm³. The presence of a comorbid disease such as impaired renal function, diabetes mellitus, congestive heart failure, immunosuppression, and airway dysfunction poses increased risk, as do abnormalities in vital signs, such as fever, tachycardia, tachypnea, and hypotension. The pathogen responsible for the pneumonia needs to also be considered, because pneumonia death risk is increased when *S. aureus,* often seen in post-influenza pneumonia, or gram-negative rods such as *K. pneumoniae,* found frequently in pneumonia in alcohol abusers, cause infection. Risks for CAP by *P. aeruginosa* include structural lung disease, corticosteroid therapy (prednisone, ≥10 mg/day, or its equivalent) and broad-spectrum antibiotic therapy in the previous month, and malnutrition.

Sputum gram staining and culture are helpful in ascertaining the pathogen in fewer than 50% of persons with CAP. Most often, the sputum specimen is inadequate, coming from the oropharynx rather than the chest. Clues to an inadequate specimen are the presence of a large number of epithelial cells with few WBCs. Conversely, if a large number of WBCs and few epithelial cells are found, the specimen is from the chest.

Because definitive identification of the organism is unlikely, the choice of antimicrobial agent for the treatment of pneumonia is largely empirical, directed at the most likely causative organism in view of patient characteristics, such as age and comorbidity. Because pneumococcal pneumonia carries a significant risk for mortality, the chosen antimicrobial should always be effective against this pathogen, regardless of patient presentation. Choosing an antimicrobial with activity against both atypical organisms (*M. pneumoniae, C. pneumoniae, Legionella* species) and gram-positive and negative organisms (*S. pneumoniae, H. influenzae*) helps ensure optimal outcome. An additional consideration is antimicrobial resistance. Factors that facilitate the development of resistant microbes include repeated exposure to a given agent, underdosing (eradicating more sensitive organisms, leaving more resistant pathogens untouched), and an unnecessarily prolonged period of treatment. Shorter course high-dose therapy maximizes and exploits concentration-dependent killing by achieving higher maximum concentration and area under the curve/minimal inhibitory concentration values; allowing treatment of difficult pathogens, increased tissue penetration, and improved patient adherence to the regimen; and minimizing the development of resistance.

S. pneumoniae has demonstrated increasing resistance to beta-lactams (penicillins, cephalosporins) and macrolides (erythromycin, clarithromycin, azithromycin) or multidrug resistant (known as DRSP). DRSP's mechanism resistance is caused by alteration of intracellular protein-binding sites. Risk factors for DRSP include antimicrobial therapy in the previous 3 months, exposure to children in day care, age older than 65, alcohol abuse, multiple comorbidity (e.g., COPD, coronary heart disease, diabetes mellitus) and immunosuppressive state, including use of corticosteroids and chronic illness. Respiratory fluoroquinolones provide enhanced activity against DRSP, as well as atypical organism coverage and beta-lactamase stability. High-dose amoxicillin (⇒3g/d) and select cephalosporins are

al treatment options, whereas the
les and tetracyclines do not consis-
xhibit activity against DRSP and may
lead atment failure.

H. influenzae has the capacity to produce beta-lactamase, rendering the penicillins ineffective; this varies regionally but averages approximately 40% nationwide. Antimicrobials stable in the presence of beta-lactamase include the macrolides, respiratory fluoroquinolones, and cephalosporins; adding clavulanate to amoxicillin (Augmentin) inactivates beta-lactamase and also provides effective activity against *H. influenzae.*

Because the atypical pathogens do not have a true cell wall, beta-lactams are ineffective. The macrolides, tetracyclines, and respiratory fluoroquinolones provide activity against these pathogens.

The American Thoracic Society and the Infectious Disease Society of America offer guidelines for the assessment and treatment of CAP. Factors influencing the choice of antimicrobial agent include patient comorbidity and risk if treatment fails. All treatment options offer activity against *S. pneumoniae, H. influenzae,* and the atypical pathogens, the most common organisms implicated in CAP.

NPs are ideally positioned to help minimize risk for pneumonia through immunization and hygienic measures. Nearly two thirds of all fatal cases of pneumonia are caused by *S. pneumoniae,* the pneumococcal organism. Although available for more than 20 years, pneumococcal vaccine continues to be underutilized. The use of influenza vaccine can help minimize the risk of post-influenza pneumonia, an often debilitating and potentially fatal condition. Both vaccines can be given together and in the presence of moderately severe illness. Ensuring adequate ventilation, reinforcing cough hygiene, and proper hand washing can help minimize pneumonia risk.

DISCUSSION SOURCES

American Thoracic Society (2001). Guidelines for the Management of Adults with Community-Acquired Pneumonia. Available at http://www.thoracic.org/statements/default.asp, accessed 9.10.04.

Baer, R. W. (2002). Community-Acquired Pneumonia (CAP) Prognostic Calculator. Available at http://ursa.kcom.edu/CAPcalc/default.htm, accessed 7/27/03.

Chesnutt, M., and Prendergast, T. (2003). Lung. In Tierney, L., McPhee, S., and Papadakis, M. (eds.). Current Medical Diagnosis and Treatment (42nd ed., pp. 216–311). New York: Lange Medical Books/McGraw-Hill.

Hektor Dunphy, L. (2004). Management Guidelines for Nurse Practitioners Working with Adults (2nd ed). Philadelphia: F.A. Davis.

Infectious Disease Society of American (2003). Initial Empiric Therapy for Suspected Bacterial Community-Acquired Pneumonia (CAP) in Immunocompetent Adults. Available at http://www.journals.uchicago.edu/IDSA/guidelines, accessed 5/4/04.

QUESTIONS

53. You examine a 38-year-old obese woman who has presented for an initial examination and Papanicolaou test. She has no complaint. Her blood pressure (BP) is 144/98 mm Hg bilaterally. The rest of her physical examination is unremarkable. Your next best action is to:

    A. initiate antihypertensive therapy.
    B. arrange for at least two additional BP measurements during the next 2 weeks.
    C. order blood urea nitrogen, creatinine, and potassium ion measurements and urinalysis.
    D. advise her to reduce her sodium intake.

54. You see a 68-year-old woman who has systolic hypertension that is currently treated with hydrochlorothiazide. Her BP is usually within a satisfactory range. Today she presents with a 8-lb weight gain and BP of 152/82 mm Hg. The rest of her history and examination is unremarkable. Your next best action is to:

A. prescribe low-dose captopril.

B. have her return for a BP check in 1 week.

C. obtain blood urea nitrogen, creatinine, and potassium ion measurements and urinalysis.

D. review dietary sodium, fat, and caloric reduction.

55. You examine an elderly woman with long-standing, poorly controlled hypertension. When evaluating her for hypertensive target organ damage, you look for evidence of:

   A. lipid abnormalities.

   B. hyperinsulinemia and insulin resistance.

   C. left ventricular (LV) hypertrophy.

   D. clotting disorders.

56. Diagnostic testing for a patient with newly detected hypertension should include all of the following except:

   A. hematocrit.

   B. uric acid.

   C. creatinine.

   D. potassium.

57. In the person with hypertension, which of the following yields the greatest potential reduction in BP in a patient with BMI = 30?

   A. 10-kg weight loss

   B. dietary sodium restriction to 2.4 g (6 g NaCl) per day

   C. regular aerobic physical activity such as 30 minutes of brisk walking most days of the week

   D. moderate alcohol consumption

58. Which of the following medications is a dihydropyridine calcium channel blocker?

   A. lisinopril

   B. verapamil

   C. amlodipine

   D. prazosin

59. Which of the following medications is a nondihydropyridine calcium channel blocker?

   A. lisinopril

   B. diltiazem

   C. amlodipine

   D. prazosin

60. Which of the following medications is an alpha-adrenergic antagonist?

   A. enalapril

   B. diltiazem

   C. felodipine

   D. doxazosin

61. Which of the following medications is an angiotensin-converting enzyme inhibitor (ACEI)?

   A. trandolapril

   B. clonidine

   C. felodipine

   D. doxazosin

62. Which of the following medications is an angiotensin receptor antagonist?

   A. trandolapril

   B. methyldopa

   C. telmisartan

   D. atenolol

63. Which of the following medications is a beta-adrenergic receptor antagonist?

   A. clonipine

   B. spironolactone

   C. hydrochlorothiazide

   D. pindolol

64 to 69. According to information found in the Seventh Report of the Joint National Committee on the Prevention, Detection, Evaluation, and Treatment of Hypertension (JNC-7), which of the following medications has a compelling indication for use in the following patient conditions? (The medications listed can be used more than once. A given condition may have more than one medication indicated.)

—**64.** heart failure

—**65.** diabetes mellitus

—**66.** chronic renal disease

—**67.** high risk for coronary artery disease

—**68.** after myocardial infarction (MI)

—**69.** recurrent stroke

    A. thiazide diuretic

    B. beta blocker

    C. ACEI

    D. angiotensin receptor blocker (ARB)

    E. aldosterone antagonist

    F. calcium channel blocker

ANSWERS

53. B	**54.** D	**55.** C
56. B	**57.** A	**58.** C
59. B	**60.** D	**61.** A
62. C	**63.** D	
64. A, B, C, D, E	**65.** A, B, C, D, F	
66. C, D	**67.** A, B, C, F	
68. B, C, E	**69.** A, C	

DISCUSSION

The JNC-7 report provides evidence-based guidance for the diagnosis, prevention, and treatment of hypertension. Here are some highlights from the JNC-7:

- When a BP reading of 115/75 is used as a starting point, cardiovascular disease risk doubles with each increment of 20/10 mm Hg. Hypertension control leads to a reduction of stroke incidence by 35% to 40%, MI by 20% to 25%, and heart failure by 50%.
- People with systolic BP of 120 to 139 mm Hg and/or diastolic BP of 80 to 89 mm Hg should be considered prehypertensive. Lifestyle modification to prevent cardiovascular disease is indicated. In adults older than 50, systolic BP higher than 140 mm Hg is a more important risk for cardiovascular disease than diastolic BP.
- Proper measurement of BP is emphasized. The patient should be seated in a chair, not on an examination table with feet dangling, with arm supported at heart level, for at least 5 minutes. The BP cuff should cover more than 80% of the upper arm.
- BP goals are less than 140/90, with less than 130/80 for those with diabetes mellitus and/or chronic renal disease.
- In stage 1 hypertension (140 to 159/90 to 99 mm Hg), a thiazide diuretic is indicated for most, alone or in combination with an ACEI, an ARB, a beta-blocker, or a calcium channel blocker. In stage 2 hypertension ($\geq 160/\geq 100$ mm Hg), a combination of two or more drugs, one usually a thiazide diuretic, is needed by most patients. Most patients need multidrug therapy to meet these goals. Lifestyle modification yields significant improvement in BP reading (see table).
- Many conditions provide compelling indications to use certain drugs. See Tables 5–8 and 5–9 for details.
- Along with the traditional risks, microalbuminuria (MA), or glomerular filtration rate of less than 60 mL/minute is identified in the JNC-7 as a cardiovascular risk factor. In one study, when adjusted for other risk factors, the relative risk of ischemic heart disease associated with MA was 2.3 (95% confidence interval, 1.3 to 3.9; $p = 0.002$), and the 10-year disease-free survival rate decreased from 97% to 91% ($p < 0.0001$) when MA was present. An interaction between MA and smoking was observed, and the presence of MA more than doubled the predictive effect of the conventional atherosclerotic risk factors for development of ischemic heart disease. MA not only is an independent predictor of ischemic heart disease but also substantially increases the risk associated with other established risk factors. Because the person with MA has significant cardiovascular disease risk, JNC-7 recommendations for hypertension treatment include the thiazide diuretics, beta blockers, ACEIs, and calcium channel blockers; in the presence of chronic renal disease, as manifested by MA, recommendations also include the use of an ACEI and an ARB.
- People of African ancestry demonstrate somewhat reduced BP responses to monotherapy with ACEIs, ARBs, and beta

TABLE 5–8

JNC-7 COMPELLING INDICATIONS FOR INDIVIDUAL DRUG CLASSES

	Diuretic	β-blocker	ACE inhibitor	AEB	Calcium antagonist	Aldosterone antagonist
Heart failure	√	√	√	√		√
Post MI		√	√			√
High coronary disease risk	√	√	√		√	
Diabetes	√	√	√	√	√	
Chronic renal disease			√	√		
Recurrent stroke prevention	√		√			

blockers in comparison with diuretics or calcium channel blockers. Although the complete explanations for these racial differences are not known, what is known is that hypertension is the most common cause of renal failure in African Americans. As a result, an ACEI or an ARB should be prescribed to minimize renal disease risk. Using an ACEI or an ARB as part of a multidrug therapy, including a CCB and thiazide diuretic, will likely be needed. The nondihydropyridine calcium channel blockers (vera-pamil, diltiazem) are particularly helpful for BP control and renal protection.

TABLE 5–9

LIFESTYLE MODIFICATION

Modification	Approximate SBP reduction (range)
Weight reduction	5–20 mm Hg/10 kg weight loss
Adopt DASH eating plan	8–14 mm Hg
Dietary sodium reduction	2–8 mm Hg
Physical activity	4–9 mm Hg
Moderation of alcohol	2–4 mm Hg

DISCUSSION SOURCES

Hektor Dunphy, L. (2004). Management Guidelines for Nurse Practitioners Working with Adults (2nd ed). Philadelphia: F.A. Davis.

Massie, B. (2003). Hypertension, In Tierney, L., McPhee, S., and Papadakis, M. (eds.). Current Medical Diagnosis and Treatment (42nd ed., pp. 409–435). New York: Lange Medical Books/ McGraw-Hill.

National Institutes of Health (2003). The Seventh Report of the Joint National Committee on Prevention, Detection, Evaluation, and Treatment of High Blood Pressure (JNC 7). Available at http://www.nhlbi.nih.gov/guidelines/hypertension/index.htm, accessed 9.10.04.

United States Renal Data System (USRDS) (2000). Annual Data Report. National Institutes of Health, National Institute of Diabetes and Digestive and Kidney Diseases—Division of Kidney, Urologic and Hematologic Diseases. USRDS Coordinating Center operated by the Minneapolis Medical Research Foundation. Available at www.usrds.org, accessed 9.10.04.

70. You examine a 24-year-old woman with mitral valve prolapse (MVP). Her physical examination findings may also include:

    A. pectus excavatum.
    B. obesity.
    C. petite stature.
    D. hyperextendible joints.

71. In performing a cardiac examination in the person with MVP, you expect to find:

    A. an early to midsystolic, crescendo-decrescendo murmur.
    B. a pansystolic murmur.
    C. a low-pitched, diastolic rumble.
    D. a middle to late systolic murmur.

72. Additional findings in MVP include:

    A. an opening snap.
    B. a midsystolic click.
    C. a paradoxical splitting of the second heart sound (S_2).
    D. a fourth heart sound (S_4).

73. Intervention for patients with MVP may include:

    A. restricted activity because of low cardiac output.
    B. control of fluid intake to minimize risk of volume overload.
    C. routine use of beta-adrenergic antagonists to control palpitations.
    D. encouragement of a regular program of aerobic activity.

74. When a heart valve fails to open to its normal orifice size, it is:

    A. stenotic.
    B. incompetent.
    C. sclerotic.
    D. regurgitant.

75. When a heart valve fails to close properly, it is:

    A. stenotic.
    B. incompetent.
    C. sclerotic.
    D. regurgitant.

76. You are evaluating a patient who has rheumatic heart disease. When assessing her for mitral stenosis, you look for the following murmur.

    A. systolic with wide radiation over the precordium
    B. localized diastolic with little radiation
    C. diastolic with radiation to the neck
    D. systolic with radiation to the axilla

77. In evaluating mitral valve incompetency, you expect to find the following murmur:

    A. systolic with radiation to the axilla
    B. diastolic with little radiation
    C. diastolic with radiation to the axilla
    D. localized systolic

78. In evaluating the person with aortic stenosis (AS), the NP anticipates finding 12-lead electrocardiogram (ECG) changes consistent with:

    A. right bundle branch block.
    B. extreme axis deviation.
    C. right atrial enlargement.
    D. LV hypertrophy.

79. Of the following patients, who is in greatest need of endocarditis prophylaxis with dental work?

    A. a 22-year-old woman with MVP with trace mitral regurgitation (MR) noted on echocardiogram
    B. a 54-year-old woman with a prosthetic aortic valve
    C. a 66-year-old man with cardiomyopathy
    D. a 58-year-old woman who had a three-vessel coronary artery bypass graft 1 year ago

80. Of the following, who has no significant risk for developing bacterial endocarditis?

    A. a 43-year-old woman with a bicuspid aortic valve
    B. a 55-year-old man who has undergone three-vessel coronary artery bypass grafting

C. a 45-year-old woman with a history of endocarditis

D. a 75-year-old man with dilated cardiomyopathy

81. You are examining an elderly woman and find a grade 3/6 crescendo-decrescendo systolic murmur with radiation to the neck. This is most likely caused by:

A. aortic stenosis

B. aortic regurgitation.

C. anemia.

D. mitral stenosis.

82. Aortic stenosis in a 15-year-old is most likely:

A. a sequela of rheumatic fever.

B. a result of a congenital defect.

C. calcific in nature.

D. found with atrial septal defect.

83. A physiologic murmur has which of the following characteristics?

A. occurs late in systole

B. is noted in a localized area of auscultation

C. becomes softer when the patient moves from supine to standing

D. frequently obliterates S_2

84. You are examining an 18-year-old man who is seeking a sports clearance physical examination. You note a midsystolic murmur that gets louder when he stands. This may represent:

A. aortic stenosis.

B. hypertrophic cardiomyopathy.

C. a physiologic murmur.

D. a Still murmur.

85. Which of the following is the American Heart Association's (AHA's) recommended agent for endocarditis prophylaxis in patients who are allergic to penicillin?

A. erythromycin

B. dicloxacillin

C. azithromycin

D. ofloxacin

70. A	**71.** D	**72.** B	**73.** D
74. A	**75.** B	**76.** B	**77.** A
78. D	**79.** B	**80.** B	**81.** A
82. B	**83.** C	**84.** B	**85.** C

DISCUSSION

Heart murmurs are the sounds of turbulent blood flow. Blood traveling through the chambers and great vessels is usually a silent event. When the flow is sufficient to generate turbulence in the wall of the heart or great vessel, a murmur occurs.

Murmurs may be benign, in that the examiner simply hears the blood flowing through the heart but no cardiac structural abnormality exists. However, certain cardiac structural problems, such as valvular and myocardial disorders, can contribute to the development of a murmur (Table 5–10).

Normal heart valves allow one-way, unimpeded, forward blood flow through the heart. The entire stroke output is able to pass freely during one phase of the cardiac cycle (diastole with the atrioventricular [AV] valves, systole with the others), and there is no backflow of blood. When a heart valve fails to open to its normal orifice, it is stenotic. When it fails to close appropriately, the valve is incompetent, causing regurgitation of blood to the previous chamber or vessel. Both of these events place a patient at significant risk for embolic disease.

Physiologic murmurs are found in the absence of cardiac pathology. The term physiologic implies that the reason for murmur is something other than obstruction to flow and that the murmur is present with a normal gradient across the valve. This murmur may be heard in up to 80% of thin adults or children if the cardiac examination is performed in a soundproof booth, and it is best heard at the left sternal border. It occurs in early to middle systole, leaving the two heart sounds intact. In addition, the person with a benign systolic ejection murmur denies having cardiac symptoms and has an otherwise normal cardiac

TABLE 5–10

ASSESSMENT OF COMMON CARDIAC MURMURS IN ADULTS

When evaluating the adult with cardiac murmur:

- Ask about major symptoms of heart disease: chest pain, CHF symptoms, palpitations, syncope, activity intolerance.
- The bell of the stethoscope is most helpful for auscultating lower-pitched sounds and the diaphragm for higher pitch.
- Systolic murmurs are graded on a 1–6 scale, from barely audible to audible with stethoscope off the chest. Diastolic murmurs are usually graded on the same scale but abbreviated to grades 1–4, as these murmurs are not loud enough to reach grades 5 and 6.
- A critical part of the evaluation of a person with a heart murmur is a decision to offer antimicrobial prophylaxis. No prophylaxis is needed with benign murmurs. Please refer to the American Heart Association's Guideline for the latest advice (www.americanheart.org)

Murmur	Important Cardiac Exam Findings	Additional Findings	Comments
Physiologic (AKA innocent, functional)	Gr 1–3/6 early to midsystolic murmur; heard best at LSB but usually audible over precordium	No radiation beyond precordium; softens or disappears with standing, increases in intensity with activity, fever, anemia; S1, S2 intact, normal PMI	Etiology probably flows over aortic valve; may be heard in +/– 80% of thin adults if examined in soundproof room; asymptomatic with no report of chest pain, CHF symptoms, palpitations, syncope, activity intolerance
Aortic stenosis	Gr 1–4/6 harsh systolic murmur, usually crescendo-decrescendo pattern, heard best at 2nd RICS, apex, softens with standing	Radiates to carotids, may have diminished S2, slow filling carotid pulse, narrow pulse pressure, loud S4, heaving PMI; greater the degree of stenosis, later the peak of murmur	In younger adults, usually congenital bicuspid valve; in older, usually calcific, rheumatic in nature; dizziness, syncope ominous signs, pointing to severely decreased cardiac output
Aortic sclerosis	Gr 2–3/6 systolic ejection murmur heard best at 2nd RICS	Carotid upstroke full, not delayed, no S4, absence of symptoms	Benign thickening and/or calcification of aortic valve leaflets; no change in valve pressure gradient; AKA "50 over 50" murmur as found in >50% those over 50 years
Aortic regurgitation	Gr 1–3/4 high-pitched blowing diastolic murmur heard best at 3rd LICS	May be enhanced by forced expiration, leaning forward; usually with S3, wide pulse pressure, sustained thrusting apical impulse	More common in men, usually from rheumatic heart disease but occasionally due to 3rd-degree syphilis
Mitral stenosis	Gr 1–3/4 low-pitched late diastolic murmur heard best at the apex, localized; short crescendo-decrescendo rumble, like a bowling ball rolling down an alley or distant thunder	Often with opening snap, accentuated S1 in the mitral area; enhanced by left lateral decubitus position, squat, cough, immediately post-Valsalva	Nearly all rheumatic in origin. Protracted latency period, then gradual decrease in exercise tolerance leading to rapid downhill course due to low cardiac output; AF common

Murmur	Important Cardiac Exam Findings	Additional Findings	Comments
Atrial septal defect (uncorrected)	Gr 1–3/6 systolic ejection murmur at the pulmonic area	Widely split S2, right ventricular heave	Typically without symptoms until middle age, then present with CHF; persistent ostium secundum in mid septum
Pulmonary hypertension	Narrow splitting S2, murmur of tricuspid regurgitation	Report of shortness of breath nearly universal	Seen with RVH, RAH as identified by ECG, echo. Secondary PH may be a consequence of Redux, "phen/fen" use
Mitral regurgitation	Gr 1–4/6 high-pitched blowing systolic murmur, often extending beyond S2. Sounds like long "haaa," "hooo"; heard best at RLSB	Radiates to axilla, often with laterally displaced PMI; decreased with standing, Valsalva maneuver; increased by squat, hand grip	Found in ischemic heart disease, endocarditis, RHD; with RHD, often with other valve abnormalities (AS, MS, AR)
Mitral valve prolapse	Gr 1–3/6 late systolic crescendo murmur with honking quality heard best at apex; murmur follows midsystolic click	With Valsalva or standing, click moves forward into earlier systole, resulting in a longer-sounding murmur; with hand grasp, squat, click moves back further into systole, resulting in a shorter murmur	Often seen with minor thoracic deformities such as pectus excavatum, strait back, and shallow AP diameter; chest pain is sometimes present, but there is quest on whether MVP itself is cause

© 2005 Fitzgerald Health Education Associates, Inc.

examination, including an appropriately located point of maximum impulse and full pulses. Because no cardiac pathology is present with a physiologic murmur, no endocarditis prophylaxis is needed.

AS is the inability of the aortic valves to open to optimum orifice. The aortic valve normally opens to 3 cm²; AS usually does not cause significant symptoms until the valvular orifice is limited to 0.8 cm². The disease is characterized by a long symptom-free period with rapid clinical deterioration at the onset of symptoms, including dyspnea, syncope, chest pain, and congestive heart failure (CHF). Low pulse pressure is a characteristic of severe AS.

When AS is present in adults who are middle-aged and older, it is most often the acquired form. In the older adult, the problem is usually calcification, leading to the inability of the valve to open to its normal orifice. Valvular changes in middle-aged adults without congenital AS are usually the sequelae of rheumatic fever and represent about 30% of valvular dysfunction seen in rheumatic heart disease.

AS may be present in children and younger adults and is usually caused by a congenital bicuspid (rather than tricuspid) valve or by a three-cusp valve with leaflet fusion. This defect is most often found in boys and young men and is commonly accompanied by a long-standing history of becoming excessively short of breath with increased activity such as running. The physical examination is usually normal except for the associated cardiac findings.

The heart murmur of MR arises from mitral valve incompetency or the inability of the mitral valve to close properly. This allows a retrograde flow from a high-pressure area (left ventricle) to an area of lower pressure (left atrium). MR is most often caused by the degeneration of the mitral valve, most commonly by rheumatic fever, endocarditis, calcific annulus, rheumatic heart disease, ruptured chordae, or papillary muscle dysfunction. In MR from rheumatic heart disease, there is usually some degree of mitral stenosis. After the person is symptomatic, the disease progresses

in a downhill course of CHF over the next 10 years.

MVP is likely the most common valvular heart problem, present in perhaps 10% of the population. The degree of distress (chest pain, dyspnea) may depend in part on the degree of MR, although some studies have failed to reveal any difference in the rates of chest pain in patients with or without MVP. Potentially the greatest threat is the rupture of chordae, usually seen only in those with connective tissue disease, especially Marfan syndrome.

The majority of patients with MVP have a benign condition in which one of the valve leaflets is unusually long and buckles or prolapses into the left atrium, usually in midsystole. At that time, a click occurs that is followed by a short murmur caused by regurgitation of blood into the atrium. Cardiac output is usually uncompromised, and the event goes unnoticed by the patient. However, the clinician may detect this on examination. Echocardiography fails to reveal any abnormality, simply noting the valve buckling followed by a small-volume MR. If there are no cardiac complaints and the rest of the cardiac examination, including the ECG, is within normal limits, no further evaluation is needed.

One way of describing this variation from the norm is to inform the patient that one leaflet of the mitral valve is a bit longer than usual. However, the "holder" (valve orifice) is of average size. This causes the valve to buckle a bit, just as a person's foot would if forced into a shoe that is one or two sizes too small. As a result, the heart makes an extra set of sounds (click and murmur) but is not diseased or damaged. MVP is often found in patients with minor thoracic deformities such as pectus excavatum, a dish-shaped concave area at T1, and scoliosis. The exact nature of this correlation of findings is not understood.

The second and much smaller group of patients with MVP has systolic displacement of one or both of the mitral leaflets into the left atrium alone with valve thickening and redundancy, usually accompanied by mild to moderate MR. This group typically has additional health problems such as Marfan syndrome or other connective tissue disease. There is a risk of bacterial endocarditis in this group because structural cardiac abnormality is present.

Barring other health problems, patients with MVP usually have normal cardiac output and tolerate a program of aerobic activity. This activity should be encouraged to promote health and well-being. The degree of valve prolapse is increased, thus increasing intensity of the murmur, when circulating volume is low. Maintaining a high level of fluid intake should be encouraged for patients with MVP. Treatment with a beta-adrenergic antagonist (beta blocker) is indicated only when symptomatic recurrent tachycardia or palpitations is an issue.

Hypertrophic cardiomyopathy is a disease of the cardiac muscle. The ventricular septum is thick and asymmetric, leading to potential outflow track block. Patients often exhibit symptoms of cardiac outflow tract blockage with activity because the hypertrophic ventricular walls better approximate with the increased force of myocardial contraction associated with exercise. Unfortunately, the presentation of hypertrophic cardiomyopathy may be sudden cardiac death. Idiopathic hypertrophic subaortic stenosis is a type of cardiomyopathy. Because it is an autosomal dominant disorder, a strong family history is often present. Patients with this disorder are usually young adults with a history of dyspnea with activity, but they may also be asymptomatic.

According to the AHA guidelines for Prevention of Bacterial Endocarditis, patients with prosthetic heart valves have the highest risk for endocarditis. Thus, these patients are at greatest need for endocarditis prophylaxis. Whereas the presence of cardiomyopathy places the person at moderate risk, coronary bypass grafting for these patients has no greater endocarditis risk than for the general public. MVP without significant regurgitation carries no endocarditis risk. Trace MR may be found in patients without valvular heart problems (see Table 5–11 for more information).

TABLE 5–11

AMERICAN HEART ASSOCIATION GUIDELINES FOR BACTERIAL ENDOCARDITIS PROPHYLAXIS

Dental, oral, respiratory tract, or esophageal procedures One hour before procedure • Adults: Amoxicillin 2 g 1 h before procedure • Children: Amoxicillin 50 mg/kg 1h before procedure *If Amoxicillin-allergic* 1 h before procedure • Adult: Clindamycin 600 mg; children: 20 mg/kg OR • Adult: Cephalexin or cefadroxil 2 g; Children: 50 mg/kg OR • Adult: Azithromycin or clarithromycin 500 mg; Children: 50 mg/kg *Endocarditis recommended prophylaxis high-risk category* • Prosthetic heart valves • Previous bacterial endocarditis • Complex cyanotic congenital heart disease • Surgically constructed systemic pulmonary shunts or conduits	*Moderate risk category* • Most other congenital cardiac deformities • RHD and other acquired cardiac defects, even after repair • Hypertrophic cardiomyopathy • MVP with valvular regurgitation and/or thickened valves *Who does not need prophylaxis?* • Isolated secundum atrial septal defect • Surgical repair of ASD, VSD, PDA without residual problems • MVP without regurgitation • Physiologic, function, or innocent heart murmurs • Previous Kawasaki's disease without valvular dysfunction • Previous rheumatic fever without valvular dysfunction • Cardiac pacemakers (intravascular and epicardial)

Source: Dajani, AS, et al. Prevention of Bacterial Endocarditis, Recommendations of the American Heart Association. JAMA 277 (22) pp. 1794–1801.

DISCUSSION SOURCES

Dajani, A. S., Taubert, K. A., Wilson, W., et al. (1997). Prevention of bacterial endocarditis. Recommendations by the American Heart Association. JAMA 277(22):1734–1801.

Jarvis, C. (2000). Physical Examination and Health Assessment (3rd ed.). Philadelphia: W. B. Saunders.

Massie, B., and Amidon, T. (2003). Heart, In Tierney, L., McPhee, S., and Papadakis, M. Current Medical Diagnosis and Treatment (42nd ed., pp. 312–408). New York: Lange Medical Books/McGraw-Hill.

QUESTIONS

86. Causes of unstable angina include all of the following except:

    A. ventricular hypertrophy.
    B. vasoconstriction.
    C. nonocclusive thrombus.
    D. inflammation or infection.

87. Which of the following is most consistent with a person presenting with unstable angina?

    A. a 5-minute episode of chest tightness brought on by stair climbing and relieved by rest
    B. a severe, searing pain that penetrates the chest and lasts about 30 seconds
    C. chest pressure lasting 20 minutes that occurs at rest
    D. "heartburn" relieved by position change

88. In assessing a woman with or at risk for acute coronary syndrome (ACS), the NP considers that the patient will likely present:

    A. in a manner similar to that of a man with equivalent disease.
    B. at the same age as a man with similar health problems.
    C. more commonly with angina and less commonly with acute MI.
    D. less commonly with CHF.

89. The cardiac finding most commonly associated with unstable angina is:

    A. physiologic split S_2.
    B. S_4.
    C. opening snap.
    D. summation gallop.

90. Which of the following changes on the 12-lead ECG do you expect to find in a patient with ACS?

    A. flattened T wave
    B. R wave larger than 25 mm
    C. ST segment deviation ($\geq$0.05 mV)
    D. fixed Q wave

91. Beta-adrenergic antagonists are used in ACS therapy because of their ability to:

    A. reverse obstruction-fixed vessel lesions.
    B. reduce myocardial oxygen demand.
    C. enhance myocardial vessel tone.
    D. stabilize cardiac rhythm.

92. Nitrates are used in ACS therapy because of their ability to:

    A. reverse fixed vessel obstruction.
    B. reduce myocardial oxygen demand.
    C. cause vasodilatation.
    D. stabilize cardiac rhythm.

93. Which of the following is most consistent with a patient presenting with acute MI?

    A. a 5-minute episode of chest tightness brought on by stair climbing
    B. a severe, localized pain that penetrates the chest and lasts about 3 hours
    C. chest pressure lasting 20 minutes that occurs at rest
    D. retrosternal diffuse pain for 30 minutes accompanied by diaphoresis

94. Which of the following changes on the 12-lead ECG would you expect to find in a patient with history of acute transmural MI 6 months ago?

    A. 2-mm ST segment elevation
    B. R wave larger than 25 mm
    C. T wave inversion
    D. deep Q waves

95. Which of the following changes on the 12-lead ECG would you expect to find in a patient with myocardial ischemia?

    A. 2-mm ST segment elevation
    B. S wave larger than 10 mm
    C. T wave inversion
    D. deep Q waves

96. Thrombolytic therapy is indicated in patients with chest pain and ECG changes such as:

    A. 1-mm ST segment depression in leads V1 and V3.
    B. physiologic Q waves in leads aVF, V5, and V6.
    C. 3-mm ST segment elevation in leads V1 to V4.
    D. T wave inversion in leads aVL and aVR.

97. Which of the following is the most sensitive marker for myocardial damage?

    A. aspartate aminotransferase
    B. creatine phosphokinase (CPK)
    C. troponin I (cTnI)
    D. lactate dehydrogenase

98. All of the following should be prescribed during therapy for ACS except:

    A. aspirin.
    B. atenolol.
    C. lisinopril.
    D. nisoldipine.

99. Which of the following is an absolute contraindication to the use of thrombolytic therapy?

    A. history of hemorrhagic stroke
    B. BP of 160/100 or more at presentation
    C. current use of warfarin
    D. active peptic ulcer disease

100. According to the Adult Treatment Panel III guidelines, the low-density lipoprotein goal for a 64-year-old man who had an MI 2 years ago should be less than:

    A. 100 mg/dL.
    B. 110 mg/dL.
    C. 130 mg/dL.
    D. 160 mg/dL.

101. Which of the following is least likely to be reported in ACS?

    A. new rales
    B. transient MR murmur
    C. hypotension
    D. pain reproduced with palpation

ANSWERS

86. A	**87.** C	**88.** C	**89.** B
90. C	**91.** B	**92.** C	**93.** D
94. D	**95.** C	**96.** C	**97.** C
98. D	**99.** A	**100.** A	**101.** D

DISCUSSION

ACS (acute MI, unstable angina) and angina pectoris, most often caused by atherosclerosis, result from an imbalance in the ability to supply the myocardium with sufficient oxygen to meet its metabolic demands. Patterns of symptom provocation are usually predictable (stable angina), with exertion often causing discomfort that is promptly relieved with rest, use of sublingual nitroglycerin, or both. Unstable angina is defined as a new onset of symptoms at rest or worsening symptoms with previously provoking activities. Certain characteristics increase or decrease the ACS likelihood (Tables 5–12 to 5–15).

Treatment of stable angina pectoris includes reduction of cardiovascular disease risk factors. In addition, beta-adrenergic blockers are among first-line therapy because these agents reduce myocardial workload through lowering heart rate and stroke volume. Nitrates are used to enhance myocardial perfusion through peripheral and central vasodilatation. The clinical presentation of unstable angina (ACS) represents an emergency and should be handled accordingly.

The S_4 is often heard with myocardial ischemia and poorly controlled angina pectoris. This sound of poor myocardial relaxation

TABLE 5–12

Chest Pain, Typical of Myocardial Ischemia or Myocardial Infarction

- Substernal compression or crush
- Pressure, tightness, heaviness, cramping, aching sensation
- Unexplained indigestion, belching, epigastric pain
- Radiating pain to neck, jaw, shoulders, back, or one or both arms
- Dyspnea, nausea and/or vomiting, diaphoresis

ACC/AHA Guidelines for the Management of Patients with Unstable Angina and Non-ST-Segment Elevation Myocardial Infarction. Available at www.american-heart.org, accessed 9.10.04.

(compliance) and diastolic dysfunction may potentially cause decreased cardiac output. The third heart sound (S_3) is the sound of poor myocardial contractility and systolic dysfunction and usually leads to decreased cardiac output.

Women usually have onset of coronary heart disease at significantly older ages and are likely to present differently than men. For example, dyspnea may be an anginal equivalent in older women. Women usually present first with angina pectoris that may lead to MI. Men often have their first manifestation of coronary heart disease in the form of MI. However, women younger than 60 years often have a presentation similar to that of men, and atypi-

TABLE 5–13

LIKELIHOOD THAT SIGNS AND SYMPTOMS REPRESENT ACUTE CORONARY SYNDROME SECONDARY TO CORONARY ARTERY DISEASE

Feature	High Likelihood: Any of the Following Present	Intermediate Likelihood. Absence of High-likelihood Features and Presence of any of the Following	Low Likelihood: Absence of High- or Intermediate-likelihood Features but Many Have the Following
History	Chest or left arm pain or discomfort as chief symptom producing documented angina	Chest or left arm pain or discomfort as chief symptom Age > 70 yr Male sex Diabetes mellitus	Probable ischemic symptoms in absence of any of the intermediate-likelihood characteristics Recent cocaine use
Examination	Pulmonary edema New rales Transient mitral regurgitation murmur Hypotension	Extracardiac vascular disease	Chest discomfort reproduced by palpation
ECG findings	New or presumable new transient ST segment deviation (≥0.05 mV) or T wave inversion (≥0.2 mV) with symptoms	Fixed Q waves Abnormal ST segments or E waves not documented as new	T wave flattening or inversion in leads with dominant R waves Normal ECG
Cardiac markers	Elevated cTnT, cTnI, or CPK-MB	Normal	Normal

ACC/AHA Guidelines for the Management of Patients with Unstable Angina and Non-ST-Segment Elevation Myocardial Infarction. Available at www.americanheart.org, accessed 9.10.04.
CPK-MB, creatine phosphokinase isoenzyme MB; ECG, electrocardiogram; cTnI, troponin I; cTnT, troponin T.

TABLE 5–14

PRINCIPAL PRESENTATIONS OF UNSTABLE ANGINA

Rest angina	Angina occurring at rest, prolonged, usually >20 min
New-onset angina	New-onset angina that occurs walking ≤ 1–2 blocks on the level and climbing 1 flight of stairs under normal conditions and at a normal pace (CCS classification III)
Increasing angina	Previously diagnosed angina that has become distinctly more frequent, longer in duration, or lower in threshold (i.e., increased by greater than or equal to CCS class to a less CCS Class III severity)

CCS, Canadian Cardiovascular Society.

TABLE 5–15

GRADING OF ANGINA PECTORIS ACCORDING TO
CANADIAN CARDIOVASCULAR SOCIETY CLASSIFICATION

Class	Description of Stage
I	Ordinary physical activity such as walking or climbing stairs does not cause angina. Symptoms occur with strenuous, rapid, or prolonged exertion at work or recreation.
II	Slight limitations in ordinary activity. Angina occurs on walking or climbing stairs rapidly, walking uphill, walking or stair climbing after meals, in cold, in wind, or in emotional distress. Symptoms occurs on walking >2 blocks on the level and climbing >1 flight of ordinary stairs at a normal pace and under normal conditions.
III	Marked limitation of ordinary physical activity. Angina occurs on walking 1–2 blocks on the level and climbing 1 flight of stairs under normal conditions and at a normal pace.
IV	Inability to carry out any physical activity without discomfort. Symptoms may be present at rest.

ACC/AHA Guidelines for the Management of Patients with Unstable Angina and Non-ST-Segment Elevation Myocardial Infarction. Available at www.americanheart.org, accessed 9.10.04.

cal MI presentation is often noted in both sexes when patients are more than 80 years old.

MI/ACS most commonly occurs when an atherosclerotic plaque ruptures, leading to the formation of an occlusive thrombus. Coronary artery spasm may also occur, adding to the vessel obstruction. The patient with a suspected ACS needs to be assessed promptly and accurately because therapy to reinstitute vessel patency (thrombolysis, percutaneous angio-plasty, coronary artery bypass grafting, and the like) should be initiated early in the process to limit myocardial damage. The 12-lead ECG should be assessed for changes consistent with myocardial ischemia, injury, and infarction.

In 75% of patients admitted for MI, this condition is ruled out. At the same time, 25% of all MIs are clinically silent. In order to reduce unneeded hospitalization and detect asymptomatic MI/ACS, diagnostic tests that are highly sensitive and specific for myocardial damage are needed.

Creatine phosphokinase (CK) isoenzyme MB (CK-MB) has long been used as a serum marker of myocardial damage. Its level increases within 6 to 12 hours of MI, begins to decrease within 24 to 48 hours and usually returns to normal in about 60 hours. Because CK-MB clears quickly, its use in late detection of MI is limited. In addition, false-positive and false-negative results are noted.

Troponin is a regulatory protein of the myofibril with three major subtypes: C, I, and T. Subtypes I (cTnI) and T (cTnT) are released in presence of myocardial damage. Both increase rapidly within the first 12 hours after MI, with cTnT typically remaining elevated for about 168 hours, whereas cTnI remains elevated for about 192 hours. cTnI is the more cardiac-specific measure and is sensitive for small-volume myocardial damage. cTnT levels can be elevated in chronic renal failure, muscle trauma, and rhabdomyolysis. cTnI is more sensitive and specific than ECG and CK-MB in diagnosing unstable angina and non–Q wave MI. In addition, cTnI results are available quickly through a rapid assay.

Protracted elevation of cTnI after MI or unstable angina may be a predictor of increased mortality. Angina patients without documented MI have a significantly higher risk of death within 42 days if cTnI is persistently elevated.

The AHA has published Guidelines for the Management of Patients with ST—Elevation Myocardial Infarction, Unstable Angina, and Non-ST-Segment-Elevation Myocardial Infarction Developed from consensus of nursing and medical experts as well as evidence-based health care, the AHA recommends the following ventral therapy:

- Nitroglycerin via spray or sublingual tablet, followed by parenteral nitroglycerin.
- Supplemental oxygen for patients with cyanosis, respiratory distress, pulse oximetry, or arterial blood gas determination to confirm adequate arterial SaO_2 (>90%).

- Adequate analgesia with morphine sulfate intravenously when symptoms are not immediately relieved by nitroglycerin or when pulmonary congestion and/or severe agitation is present.
- A beta blocker if there are no contraindications. The first dose should be administered intravenously. An ACEI should be given if no contraindications exist.
- Aspirin, 160 to 325 mg orally in a chewable nonenteric form. Other antiplatelet agents such as clopidogrel may be used if aspirin allergy or intolerance is present.
- A history, physical examination, 12-lead ECG, and cardiac marker tests should be performed promptly.

With a diagnosis of ACS and ST-segment elevation, the patient should be evaluated for reperfusion; the examiner should look for greater than 1-mm ST-segment elevation in contiguous leads. The presence of these changes usually indicates acute coronary artery occlusion, usually from thrombosis. In addition, clinically significant ST-segment elevation largely dictates reperfusion therapy with the use of thrombolytic therapy, primary percutaneous transluminal coronary angioplasty, or other revascularization options. These therapies have the best effect on clinical outcomes if used within 6 hours after onset of chest pain but may be helpful as much as 7 to 12 hours or more after MI symptoms begin. When thrombolysis is used, heparin is usually given for at least 48 hours to ensure continued vessel patency.

Before giving a product such as tissue plasminogen activator or streptokinase, the prescriber must be aware of absolute and relative contraindications to thrombolytic therapy. See Table 5–16a.

If left bundle branch block is evident on ECG and the clinical scenario is consistent with acute MI, standard acute MI care should be offered. Patients with a presentation suggestive of MI but without ST segment changes should not receive thrombolysis. These patients should be hospitalized and placed on continuous ECG monitoring for rhythm disturbances;

TABLE 5–16a

CONTRAINDICATIONS AND CAUTIONS FOR FIBRINOLYSIS IN STEMI*

Absolute Contraindications	Any prior intracranial hemorrhage
	Known structural cerebral vascular lesion (e.g., arteriovenous malformation)
	Known malignant intracranial neoplasm (primary or metastatic)
	Ischemic stroke within 3 months EXCEPT acute ischemic stroke within 3 hours
	Suspected aortic dissection
	Active bleeding or bleeding diathesis (excluding menses)
	Significant closed-head or facial trauma within 3 months
Relative Contraindications	History of chronic, severe, poorly controlled hypertension
	Severe uncontrolled hypertension on presentation (SBP greater than 180 mm Hg or DBP greater than 110 mm Hg)†
	History of prior ischemic stroke greater than 3 months, dementia, or known intracranial pathology not covered in contraindications
	Traumatic or prolonged (greater than 10 minutes) CPR or major surgery (within less than 3 weeks)
	Recent (within 2 to 4 weeks) internal bleeding
	Noncompressible vascular punctures
	For streptokinase/anistreplase: prior exposure (more than 5 days ago) or prior allergic reaction to these agents
	Pregnancy
	Active peptic ulcer
	Current use of anticoagulants: the higher the INR, the higher the risk of bleeding

STEMI =S T-elevation myocardial infarction; SBP = systolic blood pressure; DBP = diastolic blood pressure; INR = International normalized ratio.
*Viewed as advisory for clinical decision making and may not be all-inclusive or definitive.
†Could be an absolute contraindication in low-risk patients with STEMI (see Section 6.3.1.6.3.2 in the full-text guidelines).

disturbances that are noted should be appropriately treated. Serial 12-lead ECGs should be obtained and results correlated with clinical measures of myocardial necrosis such as CPK or CK isoenzymes and troponin. Aspirin therapy should be continued, and consideration should be given to heparin use, particularly in the presence of a large anterior MI or LV mural thrombus because of increased risk of embolic stroke.

If no contraindications are present, beta blocker therapy and ACEI therapy should be initiated promptly because the use of these products is associated with reduced mortality and morbidity after MI. Beta blocker therapy and ACEI should be continued indefinitely.

Before hospital discharge, patients should undergo standard exercise testing to assess functional capacity, efficacy of current medical regimen, and risk stratification for subsequent cardiac events.

Ongoing care includes a goal of reducing low-density lipoprotein cholesterol to less than 100 mg/dL, and in some very high-risk patients to less than 70 mg/dL, and using diet, exercise, and, as is typically needed, drug therapy. This is in keeping with an overall plan to reduce or eliminate all cardiac risk factors, including inactivity, smoking, and obesity (Table 5–17 and Fig. 5–2).

DISCUSSION SOURCES

Abrams, J., et. al. (2002) ACC/AHA 2002 Guideline update for the management of patients with chronic stable angina: A Report of the American College of Cardiology/American Heart Associa-

TABLE 5–17
ADULT TREATMENT PANEL III
LIPID AND LIPOPROTEIN
CLASSIFICATION

Total Cholesterol (TC) (mg/dL)	<200: Desirable 200–239: Borderline high ≥240: High
LDL-C (mg/dL)	<100: Optimal 100–129: Near optimal 130–159: Borderline high 160–189: High ≥190: Very high
HDL-C (mg/dL)	<40: Low ≥60: High
Triglycerides (TG)	Normal: <150 mg/dL Borderline high: 150–199 mg/dL High: 200–499 mg/dL Very high: ≥500 mg/dL

Adult Treatment Panel III (ATP III). Guidelines National Cholesterol Education Program Adult Treatment Panel III Guidelines for Lipid Goals. Available at www.nhlbi.nih.gov/guidelines/cholesterol/index.htm, accessed 8/15/03.
HDL-C, high-density lipoprotein cholesterol; LDL-C, low-density lipoprotein cholesterol.

Risk Categories that Modify LDL-Cholesterol Goals

Risk Category	LDL Goal
CHD, at very high risk	<70 mg/dL
CHD and CHD risk equivalents	<100 mg/dL
Multiple (2+) risk factors	<130 mg/dL
Zero to one risk factor	<160 mg/dL

FIG. 5–2. Risk categories that modify low-density lipoprotein (LDL) cholesterol goals. CHD, coronary heart disease. (Source: National Cholesterol Education Program Adult Treatment Panel III [ATP III] Guidelines. Available at www.nhlbi.nih.gov/ncep, accessed 8.12.04.

tion Task Force on Practice Guidelines, available at http://www.americanheart.org/downloadable/heart/1044991838085StableAnginaNew Figs.pdf. Accessed 8/12/04.
Antman, E. M., et al. (2004). ACC/AHA guidelines for the management of patients with ST-elevation myocardial infarction: A report of the American College of Cardiology/American Heart Association Task Force on Practice Guidelines, available at http://www.americanheart.org/downloadable/heart/1090338315100STEMIFinalFinalforposting.pdf. Accessed 8/12/04.
Braunwald, E., et al, (2002)ACC/AHA Guideline update for the management of patients with unstable angina and non–ST-segment elevation myocardial infarction: A report of the American College of Cardiology/American Heart Association Task Force on Practice Guidelines. Available at http://circ.ahajournals.org/cgi/content/full/106/14/1893. Accessed 8/12/04.
Expert Panel on Detection, Evaluation, and Treatment of High Blood Cholesterol in Adults. (2001). Executive summary of the third report of the National Cholesterol Education Program (NCEP) Expert Panel on Detection, Evaluation, and Treatment of High Blood Cholesterol in Adults (Adult Treatment Panel III). Journal of the American Medical Association 285:2486–2497.
Grundy, S. (2004) NCEP Report: Implications of recent clinical trials for the National Cholesterol Education Program Adult Treatment Panel III Guidelines, available at http://circ.ahajournals.org/cgi/content/full/110/2/227. Accessed 8/12/04.
Hektor Dunphy, L. (2004). Management Guidelines for Nurse Practitioners Working with Adults (2nd ed). Philadelphia: F.A. Davis.

QUESTIONS

102. You examine an 82-year-old woman who has a history of CHF. She is in the office because of increasing shortness of breath. When auscultating her heart, you note a tachycardia with a rate of 104 beats per minute and an extra heart sound early in diastole. This sound most likely represents:

A. summation gallop.
B. S_3.
C. opening snap.
D. S_4.

103. You examine a 65-year-old man with dilated cardiomyopathy and CHF. On examination, you expect to find all of the following except:

A. jugular venous distention.
B. tenderness on right upper abdominal quadrant palpation.
C. point of maximum impulse at the fifth intercostal space, midclavicular line.
D. peripheral edema.

104. One of the most underutilized classes of drugs for the treatment of heart failure is:

A. beta blockers.
B. ACEIs.
C. calcium channel blockers.
D. loop diuretics.

105. The rationale for using beta blocker therapy in treating a patient with CHF is to:

A. increase myocardial contractility.
B. reduce the effects of circulating catecholamines.
C. relieve concomitant angina.
D. stabilize cardiac rhythm.

106. ECG findings in a patient who is taking digoxin in a therapeutic dose typically includes:

A. shortened PR interval.
B. slightly depressed, cupped ST segments.
C. widened QRS complex.
D. tall T waves.

107. A potential adverse effect of ACEIs when used with spironolactone therapy is:

A. hypotension.
B. hyperkalemia.
C. renal insufficiency.
D. proteinuria.

108. ECG findings in a patient with digoxin toxicity will most likely include:

A. AV heart block.
B. T wave inversion.
C. sinus tachycardia.
D. pointed P waves.

109. Patients reporting digoxin toxicity are most likely to include:

A. anorexia.
B. disturbance in color perception.
C. blurred vision.
D. diarrhea.

110. Which of the following is among the most common causes of CHF?

A. dietary indiscretion
B. COPD
C. hypertensive heart disease
D. anemia

111. Which of the following medications is an aldosterone antagonist?

A. clonipine
B. spironolactone
C. hydrochlorothiazide
D. furosemide

112. Which of the following best describes orthopnea?

A. shortness of breath with exercise
B. dyspnea that develops when the person is recumbent and is relieved with elevation of the head
C. shortness of breath that occurs at night, characterized by a sudden awakening after a couple of hours of sleep, with a feeling of severe anxiety, breathlessness, and suffocation
D. dyspnea at rest

113. Which of the following is unlikely to be noted in the person in heart failure?

A. elevated serum B-type natriuretic peptide (BNP)
B. Kerley B lines on chest x-ray
C. LV hypertrophy on ECG
D. evidence of hemoconcentration on hemogram

ANSWERS			
102. B	103. C	104. A	105. B
106. B	107. B	108. A	109. A
110. C	111. B	112. B	113. D

DISCUSSION

CHF occurs as a result of altered cardiac function that leads to inadequate cardiac output and a resulting inability to meet the oxygen and metabolic demands of the body. Hypertensive heart disease and atherosclerosis are the leading causes of CHF. Less common causes include pneumonia (as a result of increased right-sided heart workload), anemia (because of the resulting decreased oxygen-carrying capability of the blood), and increased sodium intake (because of the resultant increase in circulating volume).

Clinical presentation of an acute exacerbation of CHF includes dyspnea, or shortness of breath, (SOB) that increases in severity, seen in a spectrum from exertional dyspnea (SOB with exercise), orthopnea (SOB that develops when the person is recumbent and is relieved with elevation of the head), paroxysmal nocturnal dyspnea (SOB that occurs at night, characterized by a sudden awakening after a couple hours of sleep, with a feeling of severe anxiety, breathlessness, and suffocation), and dyspnea at rest to acute pulmonary edema. Additional reported history often includes nocturia, fatigue, and weakness. Except for the mildest cases, crackles heard over the lung bases are characteristic; in severe cases, there is wheezing and expectoration of frothy, blood-tinged sputum. An S_3 is usually noted, typically disappearing upon resolution of the acute event. Additional findings usually include tachycardia, diaphoresis, pallor, and peripheral cyanosis with pallor. Although edema is considered a classic finding in CHF, a substantial gain of extracellular fluid volume (i.e., a minimum of 5 L in adults) must occur before peripheral edema is manifested. As a result of liver engorgement from elevated right-sided heart pressures, hepatojugular reflux, hepatic engorgement, and tenderness are typically noted. The point of maximum impulse is normally at the fifth intercostal space, midclavicular line. It is shifted laterally and perhaps over more than one intercostal space in the presence of dilated cardiomyopathy and its resultant increase in cardiac size.

Radiographic findings demonstrate cardiomegaly (in patients with underlying CHF) and alveolar edema with pleural effusions and bilateral infiltrates in a butterfly pattern and Kerley B lines; the chest x-ray may appear normal for up to 12 hours after onset of symptoms.

The ECG helps to identify the presence of left atrial enlargement, LV hypertrophy, and dysrhythmias often noted in CHF but not specific to the diagnosis. ECG changes consistent with acute myocardial ischemia or MI as the cause of heart failure may also be revealed.

Laboratory testing in CHF usually includes evaluation to rule in or rule out potential underlying causes (e.g., anemia, infection, renal insufficiency). BNP is an amino acid structure common to all natriuretic peptides. The major source of plasma BNP is the cardiac ventricles; the amount in circulation is in proportion to ventricular volume expansion and pressure overload. As part of the evaluation of a patient with dyspnea and suspected CHF, an elevated BNP level helps to support the diagnosis. The increased circulating volume found in heart failure can occasionally lead to evidence of hemodilution on hemogram; this corrects as circulating volume is normalized.

The goal of CHF therapy is threefold: reduction of preload, reduction of systemic vascular resistance (afterload reduction), and inhibition of the renin and sympathetic nervous system. Because ACEIs and ARBs cause central and peripheral vasodilatation, they result in a reduction in cardiac workload and improvement in cardiac output. Although ACEIs and ARBs are the cornerstone of CHF therapy, their use can be associated with adverse effects. Most common is hypotension, particularly when one of these agents is prescribed for a person who is currently taking a diuretic or vasodilator. In order to avoid this, ACEI or ARB therapy should be started at low dosages and increased slowly to achieve a therapeutic response. Renal insufficiency can be precipitated by ACEI or

ARB therapy; this usually occurs only in the presence of renal artery stenosis or underlying renal disease. Hyperkalemia with ACEI or ARB use is usually seen only with concurrent use of a potassium-sparing diuretic such as spironolactone or in advancing renal disease.

Diuretics assist with circulating volume and preload reduction. Unless contraindicated, a potassium-sparing diuretic such as spironolactone should be used because of its neurohumoral effects, allowing sodium excretion and enhanced vasodilatation. These effects are achieved by the drug's ability to competitively bind at receptors found in aldosterone-dependent sodium-potassium exchange sites in the renal tubule. Beta-adrenergic blockers are used to inhibit chronotropic, inotropic, and vasodilatory responses to beta-adrenergic stimulation. Digoxin has a positive inotropic effect and slows conduction through the AV node. A prolongation of the PR interval and cupping of the ST segment are typically seen in ECGs of patients taking a therapeutic dose of digoxin. With digoxin toxicity, a number of cardiac effects can be seen; AV block is the most common. Anorexia is the most common patient report during digoxin toxicity. Visual changes are rarely reported.

DISCUSSION SOURCES

Antman E. M., et al (2004) ACC/AHA guidelines for the management of patients with ST-elevation myocardial infarction: A report of the American College of Cardiology/American Heart Association Task Force on Practice Guidelines, available at http://www.americanheart.org/downloadable/heart/1090338315100STEMIFinalFinalforposting.pdf. Accessed 8/12/04.

Barker, D., et al. (2001) ACC/AHA guidelines for the evaluation and management of chronic heart failure in the adult: A report of the American College of Cardiology/American Heart Association Task Force on Practice Guidelines, available at http://www.americanheart.org/downloadable/heart/1013201138293HFGuidelineFinal.pdf. Accessed 8/12/04.

Hektor Dunphy, L. (2004). Management Guidelines for Nurse Practitioners Working with Adults (2nd ed). Philadelphia: F. A. Davis.

Massie, B., and Amidon, T. (2003). Heart. In Tierney, L., McPhee, S., and Papadakis, M. (eds.). Current Medical Diagnosis and Treatment (42nd ed., pp. 312–408). New York: Lange Medical Books/McGraw-Hill.

6

Abdominal Disorders

1. You examine a 59-year-old man with a chief complaint of new onset of rectal pain after a bout of constipation. On examination, you note an ulcerated lesion on the posterior midline of the anus. The most likely diagnosis is:

   A. perianal fistula.
   B. anal fissure.
   C. external hemorrhoid.
   D. Crohn proctitis.

2. Rectal bleeding associated with hemorrhoids is usually described as:

   A. streaks of bright red blood on the stool.
   B. dark brown to black in color and mixed in with normal appearing stool.
   C. a large amount of brisk red bleeding.
   D. significant blood clots and mucus mixed with stool.

3. Therapy for hemorrhoids includes all of the following except:

   A. weight control.
   B. low-fiber diet.
   C. topical corticosteroids.
   D. stool softener.

1. B   **2.** A   **3.** B

In anal fissure, there is an ulcer or tear of the margin of the anus. Most fissures occur posteriorly. Risk factors include constipation, diarrhea, recent childbirth, and anal intercourse or other anal insertion practices. The best treatment for anal fissure is avoidance of the condition through adequate fiber and fluid intake, avoiding constipation, and minimizing or eliminating activity that triggers the condition.

Whereas the superior hemorrhoidal veins form internal hemorrhoids, the inferior hemorrhoidal veins form external hemorrhoids. Both forms are actually normal anatomic findings but cause discomfort when there is an increase in the venous pressure and resulting dilatation and inflammation, such as in childbirth, obesity, constipation, and prolonged sitting. Over time, tissue and vessel redundancy develop, resulting in rectal protrusion and increased risk for bleeding. With chronically protruding or prolapsing hemorrhoids, the patient often reports itch, mucous leaking, and staining of undergarments with streaks of stool.

125

Manual reduction of the protruding hemorrhoid after evacuation can be helpful.

As with anal fissure, prevention of hemorrhoidal engorgement and inflammation is the best treatment. Strategies include weight control, high-fiber diet, regular exercise, and increased fluid intake. Treatment for acute hemorrhoid flare-ups includes the use of astringents and topical corticosteroids, as well as sitz baths and analgesics. Surgical intervention is warranted when more conservative therapy fails to yield clinical improvement. These therapies are also used in treating patients with anal fissure.

DISCUSSION SOURCES

McQuaid, K. R. (2003). Alimentary tract. In Tierney, L., McPhee, S., and Papadakis, M. (eds.). Current Diagnosis and Treatment (42nd ed., pp. 522–627). New York: Lange Medical Books/McGraw-Hill.

Thompson, M, and Hektor Dunphy, L: Abdominal disorders. In Hektor Dunphy, L. (2004). Management Guidelines for Nurse Practitioners Working with Adults. Philadelphia: F.A. Davis, pp 215–276.

QUESTIONS

4. All of the following are often found in patients with the diagnosis of acute appendicitis except:

   A. epigastric pain.
   B. obturator sign.
   C. rebound tenderness.
   D. marked febrile response.

5. A 26-year-old man presents with acute abdominal pain. As part of the evaluation for appendicitis, you order a white blood cell (WBC) count with differential and anticipate the following results:

   A. total WBCs, 4500; neutrophils, 35%; bands, 2%; lymphocytes, 45%
   B. total WBCs, 14,000; neutrophils, 55%; bands, 3%; lymphocytes, 38%
   C. total WBCs, 16,500; neutrophils, 66%, bands; 8%, lymphocytes; 22%
   D. total WBCs, 18,100; neutrophils, 55%, bands, 3%; lymphocytes, 28%

6. In evaluating a patient with suspected appendicitis, the nurse practitioner (NP) considers that:

   A. the presentation may differ according to the anatomic location of the appendix.
   B. this is a common reason for acute abdominal pain in the elderly.
   C. vomiting before onset of abdominal pain is often seen.
   D. the presentation is markedly different from that of pelvic inflammatory disease.

7. The psoas sign can be best described as abdominal pain elicited by:

   A. passive extension of the hip.
   B. passive flexion and internal rotation of the hip.
   C. deep palpation.
   D. asking the patient to cough.

8. The obturator sign can be best described as abdominal pain elicited by:

   A. passive extension of the hip.
   B. passive flexion and internal rotation of the hip.
   C. deep palpation.
   D. asking the patient to cough.

9. To support the diagnosis of acute appendicitis with suspected appendiceal rupture, you consider obtaining the following abdominal imaging study:

   A. magnetic resonance image
   B. computed tomography (CT) scan
   C. ultrasound
   D. flat plate

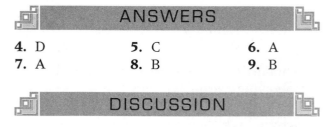

ANSWERS

4. D	**5.** C	**6.** A
7. A	**8.** B	**9.** B

DISCUSSION

Appendicitis is an inflammatory disease of the vermiform appendix caused by infection or obstruction. The peak age of patients with appendicitis is between 10 and 30 years; it is rather uncommon in infants and elderly persons. However, at either end of the lifespan, there is often a delay in diagnosis of appendicitis because providers may not consider appendicitis a possibility.

There is no true classic presentation of appendicitis. However, vague epigastric or periumbilical pain often heralds its beginning, with the discomfort shifting to the right lower quadrant over the next 12 hours. Pain may be aggravated by walking or coughing. Nausea and vomiting are late symptoms that invariably occur a number of hours after the onset of pain; this late onset helps to differentiate appendicitis from gastroenteritis, in which vomiting usually precedes abdominal cramping. The presentation of appendicitis also differs significantly according to the anatomic position of the appendix, with pain being reported in the epigastrium, flank, or groin. The obturator and psoas signs indicate inflammation of the respective muscles and strongly suggest peritoneal irritation and the diagnosis of appendicitis. Rebound tenderness indicates the likelihood of peritoneal irritation and helps with the diagnosis of acute appendicitis.

A total WBC count and differential are obtained as part of the evaluation of patients with suspected appendicitis. The most typical WBC count pattern found in this situation is the "left shift." A "left shift" is usually seen in the presence of severe bacterial infection, such as appendicitis and pneumonia. The following are typically noted:

- Leukocytosis: an elevation in the total WBC.
- Neutrophilia: an elevation in the number of neutrophils in circulation. Neutrophilia is defined as more than 7000 neutrophils/mm³. Neutrophils are also known as "polys" or "segs," both referring to the polymorph shape of the segment nucleus of this WBC.
- "Bandemia": an elevation in the number of bands or young neutrophils in circulation. Usually fewer than 4% of the total WBCs in circulation are bands. When this percentage is exceeded and the absolute band count is greater than 500/mm³, bandemia is present. This indicates that the body has called up as many mature neutrophils as were available

in the storage pool and is now accessing less mature forms. This further reinforces the seriousness of the infection. Other reasons for an increase in circulating bands include pneumonia, meningitis, septicemia, and tonsillitis when caused by bacterial infection.

There are other neutrophil forms that do not belong in circulation even with severe infection. These include myelocytes and metamyelocytes, immature neutrophil forms that are typically found in the granulopoiesis pool. The presence of these cells is an ominous marker of life-threatening infection and may be found in appendiceal rupture.

In addition to the WBC differential, an abdominal or transvaginal ultrasound reveals the inflamed appendix with a diagnostic accuracy of greater than 85%. CT of the abdomen is usually indicated when there is a suspicion of appendiceal perforation because this study reveals periappendiceal abscess formation or when an atypical presentation raises the issue of another possible diagnosis.

Surgical removal of the inflamed appendix via laparoscopy or laparotomy is indicated. If there is evidence of rupture with localized abscess and peritonitis, CT-directed abscess aspiration may be indicated first, with an appendectomy after appropriate antimicrobial therapy.

DISCUSSION SOURCES

McQuaid, K. R. (2003). Alimentary tract. In Tierney, L., McPhee, S., and Papadakis, M. (eds.). Current Diagnosis and Treatment (42nd ed., pp. 522–627). New York: Lange Medical Books/McGraw-Hill. New York: Lange Medical Books/Mcgraw-Hill

Thompson, M, and Hektor Dunphy, L: Abdominal disorders. In Hektor Dunphy, L. (2004). Management Guidelines for Nurse Practitioners Working with Adults. Philadelphia: F.A. Davis, pp 215–276.

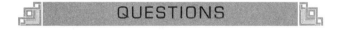

QUESTIONS

10. Which of the following is not a risk factor for bladder cancer?

A. occupational exposure to textile dyes
B. cigarette smoking
C. occupational exposure to heavy metals
D. chronic aspirin use

11. A 68-year-old man presents with suspected bladder cancer. You consider that its most common presenting sign or symptom is:

   A. painful urination.
   B. fever and flank pain.
   C. hematuria.
   D. palpable abdominal mass.

12. In a person diagnosed with superficial bladder cancer without evidence of metastases, you realize that:

   A. the prognosis for 2-year survival is poor.
   B. a cystectomy is indicated.
   C. despite successful initial therapy, local recurrence is common.
   D. systemic chemotherapy is the treatment of choice.

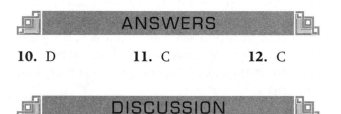

ANSWERS

10. D   **11.** C   **12.** C

DISCUSSION

Bladder cancer is the second most common urologic malignancy after prostate cancer. It is usually a disease of later in life; the mean age at diagnosis is 65 years, and it is more common in men. Risk factors include cigarette smoking, accountable for the majority of cases, and exposure to industrial chemicals, including paints, dyes, and solvents. Primary prevention of bladder cancer through risk reduction is critically important.

Gross or microscopic hematuria is the most common presenting sign of bladder cancer. Irritative voiding symptoms and frequency without fever are reported occasionally. Abdominal mass is palpable only with advanced disease.

The majority of patients with newly diagnosed bladder cancer have superficial disease, which allows for effective treatment through bladder-sparing surgery and intravesical chemotherapy. Meticulous follow-up is critical because recurrence is often seen, necessitating repeat chemotherapy and other therapies. Long-term survival is the norm with this noninvasive form of the disease. With invasive disease, treatment is dictated by type of tumor, degree of invasion, and presence of metastatic disease; long-term survival is based on numerous factors.

DISCUSSION SOURCES

Stoller, M., and Carrol, P. (2003). Urology. In Tierney, L., McPhee, S., and Papadakis, M. (eds.). Current Medical Diagnosis and Treatment (42nd ed., pp. 903–945). New York: Lange Medical Books/McGraw-Hill.

Thompson, M, and Hektor Dunphy, L: Abdominal disorders. In Hektor Dunphy, L. (2004). Management Guidelines for Nurse Practitioners Working with Adults. Philadelphia: F.A. Davis, pp 215–276.

QUESTIONS

13. A 43-year-old woman has a 12-hour history of sudden onset of right upper quadrant abdominal pain with radiation to the shoulder, fever, and chills. She has had similar, milder episodes in the past. Examination reveals marked tenderness to right upper quadrant abdominal palpation. Her most likely diagnosis is:

   A. hepatoma.
   B. acute cholecystitis.
   C. acute hepatitis.
   D. cholelithiasis.

14. Which of the following is not seen in the diagnosis of acute cholecystitis?

   A. elevated lactic dehydrogenase level
   B. increased alkaline phosphatase level
   C. leukocytosis
   D. elevated aspartate aminotransferase (AST) level

15. Murphy's sign can be best described as abdominal pain elicited by:

    A. right upper quadrant abdominal palpation.
    B. asking the patient to stand on tiptoes and then letting body weight fall quickly onto the heels.
    C. asking the patient to cough.
    D. percussion.

16. Risk factors for cholelithiasis include all of the following except:

    A. genetics.
    B. rapid weight loss.
    C. obesity.
    D. high-fiber diet.

17. Imaging in a patient with suspected symptomatic cholelithiasis usually includes obtaining an abdominal:

    A. magnetic resonance image.
    B. CT scan.
    C. ultrasound (right upper quadrant).
    D. flat plate.

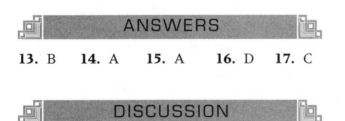

ANSWERS

13. B **14.** A **15.** A **16.** D **17.** C

DISCUSSION

Cholelithiasis is the formation of calculi or gallstones. The most common form of stones is cholesterol; major risk factors include obesity, rapid weight loss, pregnancy, and genetics. About 75% of all patients with cholelithiasis have no symptoms and become aware of the condition only when it is found during evaluation for another health problem. About 10% to 25% of those initially without symptoms become symptomatic over the next decade. Prophylactic cholecystectomy is not indicated. However, the remainder of patients with cholelithiasis have intermittent right upper quadrant abdominal pain. Ultrasound usually reveals the problem. Cholecystectomy is then

indicated. Stone-dissolving medications such as ursodeoxycholic acid are available but take up to 2 years to dissolve stones, and 50% of patients have a return of stones within 5 years. As a result, the use of this therapy has largely fallen out of favor.

Acute cholecystitis is an acute inflammation of the gallbladder, nearly always caused by gallstones. Right upper quadrant or epigastric pain and tenderness are present along with fever and vomiting; vomiting often affords temporary symptom relief. Tenderness on palpating right upper quadrant of the abdomen significant enough to cause inspiratory arrest (Murphy's sign) is nearly always present. Leukocytosis is usually present with typical total WBC count of 12,000 to 15,000, and levels of the hepatic enzymes, including gamma glutamyl transferase (GGT) and alkaline phosphatase (ALP), often rise (Table 6–1). ALP is an enzyme found in rapidly dividing or metabolically active tissue such as the liver, bone, intestine, and placenta. Elevated levels can reflect damage or accelerated cellular division in any of these areas, but the majority of circulating ALP is of hepatic origin. ALP level increases in response to any obstruction in the biliary systems; it is a sensitive indicator of intrahepatic or extrahepatic cholestasis. GGT, an enzyme involved in the transfer of amino acids across cell membranes, is found primarily in the liver and kidneys. In liver disease, its increased level usually parallels changes in ALP, which makes it a useful marker of hepatic disease in obstructive jaundice, hepatic metastasis to the liver, and intrahepatic cholestasis. In addition, GGT can serve as a backup marker with elevated ALP. For example, if the ALP level is elevated and the GGT level is normal, ALP elevation is likely caused by its bone, not hepatic, fraction. Other laboratory abnormalities include mildly elevated total serum bilirubin and amylase levels. Right upper quadrant abdominal ultrasound usually reveals stones; a hepato-iminodiacetic acid (HIDA) scan is more sensitive and specific at revealing an obstructed cystic duct.

Acute cholecystis symptoms usually subside

TABLE 6–1

HEPATIC ENZYME ELEVATIONS AND THEIR SIGNIFICANCE

Enzyme Elevation	Associated Condition	Comment
ALT rises higher than AST	Hepatitis A, B, C, D, E, etc.; drug or industrial chemical–associated hepatitis	A memory jog for recalling reasons for rise is that **ALT** symbolizes **A**vandia (rosiglitazone) and **A**ctos (pioglitazone), **L**iver infection, **T**herapeutic agents and select toxins
AST rises higher than ALT	Alcohol-related hepatic injury (2× norm), with HMG-CoA reductase inhibitor (-statin) use (rare finding in < 1% statin users), acetaminophen overdose or excessive use	A memory jog for recalling reasons for rise is that **AST** symbolizes **A**lcohol, **S**tatin, **T**ylenol
AST/ALT elevation 1–5 times norm	Alcohol use; skeletal muscle injury secondary to seizure, protracted immobilization	Example: 38-year-old man with a 10-year history of increasingly heavy alcohol use: AST = 83 U/L (NL = 0–31 U/L) ALT = 50 U/L (NL = 0–31 U/L) AST:ALT ratio >1
AST/ALT elevation >5 times norm	Infectious hepatitis	Example: 22-year-old woman with acute hepatitis A: AST = 678 U/L (NL = 0–31 U/L) ALT = 828 U/L (NL = 0–31 U/L) AST:ALT ratio <1
Gamma glutamyl transferase (GGT)	Enzyme involved in the transfer of amino acids across cell membranes; found primarily in the liver and kidney; in liver disease, usually parallels changes in alk phos Useful marker of hepatic disease in the following conditions, with marked elevation often noted in obstructive jaundice, hepatic metastasis, intrahepatic cholestasis. In response to binge drinking, GGT leaks out of cells in greater amounts than other hepatic enzymes; GGT elevation marked, sustained in high alcohol intake; will elevate modestly with lower alcohol consumption	Example: 40-year-old woman with cholecystitis: AST = 45 U/L (0–31) ALT = 55 U/L (0–31) U/L = 175 (0–125) GGT = 245 U/L (0–45) In alcohol abuse Example: 38-year-old man with a 10-year history of heavy alcohol use with recent binge AST = 83 U/L (0–31) ALT = 50 U/L (0–31) GGT = 150 U/L (0–45)

with conservative therapy such as a low-fat, clear-liquids diet and analgesics. Antimicrobial therapy may be indicated with evidence of infection. Cholecystectomy, usually performed via laparoscope, should be considered because of the likelihood of recurrence. In the person who is seriously ill with other health problems and considered too fragile to undergo cholecystectomy, ultrasound-guided gallbladder aspiration or percutaneous cholecystostomy can delay or occasionally eliminate the need for further surgical intervention.

DISCUSSION SOURCES

Friedman, L. (2003). Liver, biliary tract and pancreas. In Tierney, L., McPhee, S., and Papadakis, M. (eds.). Current Diagnosis and Treatment (42nd ed., pp. 628–673). New York: Lange Medical Books/McGraw-Hill.

Thompson, M, and Hektor Dunphy, L: Abdominal disorders. In Hektor Dunphy, L. (2004). Management Guidelines for Nurse Practitioners Working with Adults. Philadelphia: F.A. Davis, pp 215–276.

QUESTIONS

18. Which of the following is true concerning colorectal cancer?

    A. The majority are found during rectal examination.
    B. Rectal carcinoma is more common than cancers involving the colon.
    C. Early manifestations include abdominal pain and cramping.
    D. Later disease presentation often includes iron deficiency anemia.

19. According to the American Cancer Society recommendations, which of the following is the preferred method for annual colorectal cancer screening in a 51-year-old man?

    A. digital rectal examination
    B. fecal occult blood test
    C. colonoscopy
    D. barium enema study

20. A patient with colorectal cancer typically presents with:

    A. gross rectal bleeding.
    B. weight loss.
    C. few symptoms.
    D. nausea and vomiting.

21. Which of the following does not increase a patient's risk of developing colorectal cancer?

    A. family history of colorectal cancer
    B. familial polyposis
    C. personal history of neoplasm
    D. chronic aspirin therapy

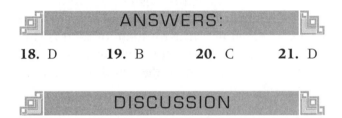

ANSWERS:

18. D   **19.** B   **20.** C   **21.** D

DISCUSSION

Colorectal cancer is second leading cause of cancer death in the United States, with 5% of the population developing the disease. Most such cancers are adenocarcinomas, with about 70% found in the colon and 30% in the rectum. Risk factors include a history of inflammatory bowel disease, personal history of neoplasia, age older than 50 years, a family history of colorectal cancer, and familial polyposis syndrome. In addition, an autosomal dominant condition known as hereditary nonpolyposis colorectal cancer has been identified. Although this accounts for about 3% of all colorectal cancers, persons with this risk factor tend to develop disease earlier and have as much as a 70% likelihood of colon cancer by age 65 years. A thorough family history is important in assessing an individual's risk of colorectal cancer. In addition, a high-fat, high-meat, low-calcium diet has also been implicated as a contributing factor. The use of antioxidants, calcium supplements, and low-dose aspirin may reduce colorectal cancer rates.

A patient with colorectal cancer is usually asymptomatic until disease is advanced. At that time, vague abdominal complaints coupled with iron deficiency anemia (as a result of chronic low-volume blood loss) may be found. The offending mass is most often beyond the examining digit. As a result, digital rectal examination is an ineffective method of colorectal cancer screening. In an effort to detect colorectal cancer, the American Cancer Society recommends an annual fecal occult blood test for all adults age 50 years and older. However, this has a high rate of both false-positive and false-negative results. Periodic additional tests such as colonoscopy are recommended. Individuals with increased risk for colorectal cancer have special screening needs. Treatment of colorectal cancer usually includes surgery and adjunctive chemotherapy. Long-term survival depends on a number of factors, including the size and depth of the tumor, the presence of positive nodes, and the overall health of a patient.

DISCUSSION SOURCES

American Cancer Society (2004). Colorectal Cancer Detection Guidelines. Available at www.cancer. org, accessed 11/26/04.

McQuaid, K. R. (2003). Alimentary tract. In Tierney, L., McPhee, S., and Papadakis, M. (eds.). Current Diagnosis and Treatment (42nd ed., pp. 522–627). New York: Lange Medical Books/ McGraw-Hill.

QUESTIONS

22. Which of the following is most consistent with the presentation of a patient with diverticulosis?

   A. diarrhea and leukocytosis
   B. constipation and fever
   C. few symptoms
   D. frank blood in the stool with reduced stool caliber

23. Which of the following is most consistent with the presentation of a patient with diverticulitis?

   A. cramping, diarrhea, and leukocytosis
   B. constipation and fever

   C. left-sided abdominal pain
   D. frank blood in the stool with reduced stool caliber

24. One of the preferred antibiotics in the treatment of diverticulitis is:

   A. metronidazole.
   B. azithromycin.
   C. clarithromycin.
   D. cefprozil.

25. Prevention of diverticulitis includes:

   A. use of antidiarrheal agents.
   B. avoiding gas-producing foods.
   C. high-fiber diet.
   D. low-dose antibiotic therapy.

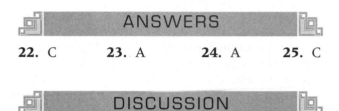

ANSWERS

22. C   **23.** A   **24.** A   **25.** C

DISCUSSION

Diverticulosis is a condition in which bulging pockets are present in the intestinal wall. However, inflammation is not present, and the patient is usually asymptomatic; the finding of diverticulosis is often made during studies done for other reasons, such as colorectal cancer screening. The major risk factor for the condition is long-term low-fiber diet. When symptoms are present, left-sided abdominal cramping, increased flatus, and a pattern of constipation alternating with diarrhea are often reported. Intervention includes a high-fiber diet and/or use of fiber supplements such as bran, psyllium, or methylcellulose. The treatment goal is to minimize the risk of complications such as diverticulitis.

In diverticulitis, the diverticula are inflamed, which causes fever, leukocytosis, diarrhea, and abdominal pain. Intestinal perforation can occur, from pinpoint lesions that cause local infection and respond to conservative management to major tears that necessitate surgical repair and are often complicated by intra-abdominal abscess or peritonitis. Imaging is important to assess disease severity. A plain abdominal film for free air, indicated diverticular perforation, or bowel obstruction should be obtained; if either of these findings is in evidence, particularly if coupled with peritoneal signs on physical examination, prompt surgical consultation is indicated. In the absence of these findings, conservative management, including increased fluid intake, rest, a low-residue diet for the duration of the illness, and antimicrobial therapy, should be initiated. If the patient fails to respond within 2 to 3 days or becomes significantly worse during that time, particularly if peritoneal signs develop, an abdominal CT should be obtained and specialty consultation should be considered during the course of illness.

The organisms most often implicated in diverticulitis are *Bacteroides* species and enterococci. Metronidazole is one of the antibiotics of choice because it has excellent activity against anaerobic organisms such as *Bacteroides* species. A second agent with strong gram-negative activity such as ciprofloxacin, ofloxacin, or trimethoprim-sulfamethoxazole (TMP-SMX) should be added because the infection is often polymicrobial.

Prevention of diverticulosis and diverticulitis includes actions, such as regular aerobic exercise, adequate hydration, and a high-fiber diet, that increase bowel motility.

DISCUSSION SOURCES

Gilbert, D., Moellering, R., and Sande, M. (2004). The Sanford Guide to Antimicrobial Therapy (34th ed.). Hyde Park, VT: Antimicrobial Therapy.
McQuaid, K. R. (2003). Alimentary tract. In Tierney, L., McPhee, S., and Papadakis, M. (eds.). Current Diagnosis and Treatment (42nd ed., pp. 522–627). New York: Lange Medical Books/ McGraw-Hill.

QUESTIONS

26. The gastric parietal cells produce:

   A. hydrochloric acid.
   B. a protective mucosal layer.
   C. prostaglandins.
   D. prokinetic hormones.

27. Antiprostaglandin drugs cause stomach mucosal injury primarily by:

   A. direct irritative effect.
   B. altering the thickness of the protective mucosal layer.
   C. decreasing peristalsis.
   D. modifying stomach pH level.

28. A 24-year-old man presents with a 3-month history of upper abdominal pain. He describes it as an intermittent, centrally located "burning" feeling in his upper abdomen, most often occurring 2 to 3 hours after meals. His presentation is most consistent with the diagnosis of:

   A. acute gastritis.
   B. gastric ulcer.
   C. duodenal ulcer.
   D. cholecystitis.

29. When choosing pharmacologic intervention to prevent recurrence of duodenal ulcer in a middle-aged man, you prescribe:

   A. a proton pump inhibitor (PPI).
   B. timed antacid use.
   C. antimicrobial therapy.
   D. a histamine 2 receptor antagonist (H_2RA).

30. The H_2RA most likely to cause drug interactions with phenytoin and theophylline is:

   A. cimetidine.
   B. famotidine.
   C. nizatidine.
   D. ranitidine.

31. Which of the following is least likely to be found in a patient with gastric ulcer?

   A. history of long-term naproxen use
   B. age younger than 50 years
   C. previous use of H_2RA or antacids
   D. cigarette smoking

32. Nonsteroidal anti-inflammatory (NSAID)–induced peptic ulcer can be best limited by the use of:

   A. antacids.
   B. HR_2As.

C. taking the medication with food.

D. misoprostol.

33. Cyclooxygenase-1 (COX-1) contributes to:

A. inflammatory response.

B. pain transmission.

C. maintenance of gastric protective mucosal layer.

D. renal arteriole constriction.

ANSWERS

26. A	**27.** B	**28.** C	**29.** C
30. A	**31.** B	**32.** D	**33.** C

DISCUSSION

Gastrointestinal (GI) irritation and ulcer occur when there is an imbalance between gastric protective mechanisms and irritating factors such as hydrochloric acid and other digestive juices. Gastric parietal cells secrete hydrochloric acid, mediated by histamine 2 receptor sites.

The normal stomach pH is about 2, which kills many swallowed bacteria and viruses. Gastric acid production is about 1 to 2 mEq/hour in the resting, empty stomach and increases to 30 to 50 mEq/hour after a meal. The stomach is protected by a number of mechanisms, including a mucus coat with a gel layer. This layer provides mechanical protection from shearing as a result of ingestion of rough substances. In addition, bicarbonate is held within the protective layer and helps maintain pH to protect the mucosa from stomach acidity. Endogenous prostaglandins stimulate and thicken the mucus layer as well as enhance bicarbonate secretion and promote cell renewal and blood flow. Endogenous prostaglandin levels normally decrease with age, which places older adults at increased risk for gastric damage. As part of the stress response, there is an increase in endogenous gastric acid and pepsin production and the potential for gastric mucosa injury and gastritis. Exogenous reasons for damage to the stomach's protective mechanism include the use of standard (non–COX-1-sparing) NSAIDs, corticosteroid use, tobacco use, and infection with *Helicobacter pylori*.

Peptic ulcer disease is located in areas, such as the duodenum, stomach, esophagus, and small intestine, that are exposed to peptic juices such as acid and pepsin. Peptic ulcer disease usually includes loss of mucosal surface, extending to muscularis mucosae, that is at least 5 mm in diameter, with most being two to five times this size. Whereas an upper GI series identifies more than 80% of all ulcers larger than 0.5 cm, upper GI endoscopy identifies nearly all of them. Ulcers are capable of brisk bleeding, scarring, and perforation. GI erosion is usually seen in patients with gastritis. These are superficial mucosal lesions, usually less than 5 mm in diameter, that ooze rather than bleed. With healing, there is no scarring (Table 6–2).

The clinical presentation of peptic ulcer disease differs according to the location of the lesion. Symptoms associated with acute gastritis and gastric ulcer often become worse with eating because of the increase in irritating stomach acid on top of the lesion. The symptoms may become somewhat lessened within an hour because food buffers the acid. In contrast, duodenal ulcer symptoms often become worse as the stomach pH decreases when emptying after a meal, resulting in a sensation of stomach burning around 2 hours after a meal.

Duodenal ulcer is more common than gastric ulcer. The most potent risk factor for this condition is most likely infection with *H. pylori*, a gram-negative, spiral-shaped organism with sheathed flagella found in at least 90% of patients with duodenal ulcer. The pathogen is also found in about 40% to 70% of those with gastric ulcer. *H. pylori* has an oral-fecal and oral-oral route of transmission, and rates of infection approach 100% in developing nations with impure water supplies. In developed nations with pure water supplies, at least 75% of the population older than 50 years has been infected at some time. Eradication of the or-

TABLE 6-2

ASSESSING A PATIENT WITH PEPTIC ULCER DISEASE

Location and Type of Peptic Ulcer Disease	Risk and Contributing Factors	Presenting Signs and Symptoms	Diagnostic Testing
Duodenal ulcer	*Helicobacter pylori* infection (most common), NSAID use, corticosteroid use (much less common)	Epigastric burning, gnawing pain about 2–3 hr PC; relief with foods, antacids Clusters of symptoms with periods of feeling well; awakening at 1 to 2 AM with symptoms common, morning waking pain rare Tender at the epigastrium, left upper quadrant abdomen; slightly hyperactive bowel sounds	*H. pylori* testing: anti–*H. pylori* antibodies present in the serum with acute infection and take up to decades to decline. Stool antigen testing is also available. If *H. pylori* test is positive and PUD history, assume active infection and treat Cost of treatment less than endoscopy Urea breath test establishes presence of acute infection Endoscopy with biopsy and urease testing of biopsy or staining, looking for *H. pylori* organisms, is diagnostic gold standard
Gastric ulcer	NSAID and corticosteroid use (potent risk factor) Cigarette smoking Male:female ratio equal Peak incidence in fifth and sixth decades of life; nearly all found in those without *H. pylori* infection are caused by NSAID use	Pain often reported with or immediately after meals Nausea, vomiting, weight loss common	Difficulty distinguishing gastric ulcer from stomach cancer through UGI Upper GI endoscopy with biopsy vital Need confirmation of presence of *H. pylori* before treatment, as is present in some of cases
Nonerosive gastritis, chronic type B (antral) gastritis	Most likely caused by *H. pylori* infection	Nausea Burning and pain limited to upper abdomen without reflux symptoms	Upper endoscopy is helpful diagnostic test
Erosive gastritis	Usually secondary to alcohol and NSAID use, ASA use, stress *H. pylori* infection usually not a factor	Nausea Burning and pain limited to upper abdomen without reflux symptoms; bleeding common	Upper endoscopy is helpful diagnostic test

ASA, acetylsalicylic acid; NSAID, nonsteroidal anti-inflammatory drug; PC, after meals; PUD, peptic ulcer disease; UGI, upper gastrointestinal.

TABLE 6–3

TREATMENT OPTIONS IN *HELICOBACTER PYLORI*-INFECTION ASSOCIATED WITH PEPTIC ULCER DISEASE

Antimicrobials and Acid-Suppressing Medication	*Duration of Therapy*	*Comments*
Bismuth, 2 tabs QID; metronidazole, 250 mg TID; tetracycline, 500 mg QID; omeprazole, 20 mg BID	14 days	Less effective if doxycycline is substituted for tetracycline; about 95% effective
Amoxicillin, 1 g BID; clarithromycin, 500 mg BID; omeprazole, 20 mg BID	14 days	Well tolerated 85%–95% effective if taken as directed

Gilbert, D., Moellering, R., and Sande, M. (2004). The Sanford Guide to Antimicrobial Therapy (34th ed.). Hyde Park, VT: Antimicrobial Therapy, FDA, Food and Drug Administration.

ganism dramatically alters the risk of relapse. A number of antimicrobial combinations are effective (Table 6–3).

Serologic titers and stool antigen testing are the most cost-effective methods of diagnosing *H. pylori* infection, particularly when coupled with a clinical presentation consistent with peptic ulcer disease. One limitation is that titers may take years to decline after effective treatment, although 50% of patients have undetectable titers 12 to 18 months after therapy. Correlating elevated titers with acute symptoms is helpful and ensures the most accurate diagnosis. The organism produces urease, which then breaks down urea into ammonia and CO_2. This allows the organism to control pH in its local environment in the stomach by neutralizing H^+ ions in gastric acid. Therefore, urea breath testing is a helpful diagnostic procedure when attempting to establish the presence of *H. pylori* infection but significantly less convenient and more expensive than the serologic tests. The use of a PPI can limit the sensitivity and specificity of stool and urea breath testing but not serologic testing.

In the past, the adage "no stress, no extra acid, no ulcer" was often quoted. Treatment for peptic ulcer disease often included the use of psychotropic medications for relief of stress, according to the hypothesis that this would reduce the acid production. In reality, only 30%

to 40% of those with duodenal ulcer have higher–than average acid secretion rates. In addition, coffee drinking and occasional alcohol use are not ulcer risk factors. However, alcohol abuse with cirrhosis remains a risk factor. *H. pylori* is also found in those with asymptomatic gastritis and dyspepsia without ulceration; eradication of the organism does not appear to make a difference in symptoms in patients with these conditions.

Suppression or neutralization of gastric acid is a critical part of peptic ulcer disease therapy. The H_2RAs (whose names have the "-tidine" suffix) competitively block the binding of histamine to the H_2 receptor site, thus reducing the secretion of gastric acid. Whereas in prescription dosages these products suppress approximately 90% of hydrochloric acid production, the over-the-counter dosages suppress about 80%. These products are generally well tolerated. Cimetidine is the only H_2RA that significantly inhibits cytochrome P-450, thus slowing metabolism of certain drugs. As a result, drug interactions between cimetidine and warfarin, diazepam, phenytoin, quinidine, carbamazepine, theophylline, imipramine, and other medications may occur.

Omeprazole (Prilosec) and lansoprazole (Prevacid) are examples of PPIs. These drugs inhibit gastric acid secretion by inhibiting the final step in acid secretion by altering the activity of the "proton pump" (H = K + -ATPase). As a result, there is a virtual cessation of stomach hydrochloric acid production. PPI use is indicated in the treatment of peptic ulcer disease and gastroesophageal reflux disease (GERD) when an H$_2$RA is ineffective, as well as in refractory erosive esophagitis and Zollinger-Ellison syndrome.

A significant amount of peptic ulcer disease, particularly gastric ulcer, acute gastritis, and NSAID-induced gastropathy, is caused by use of NSAIDs. This is partly because of the action of these products against cyclooxygenase. Cyclooxygenase-1 (COX-1) is an enzyme found in gastric mucosa, small and large intestine mucosa, kidneys, platelets, and vascular epithelium. It contributes to the health of these organs through a number of mechanisms, including the maintenance of the protective gastric mucosal layer and proper perfusion of the kidneys. Cyclooxygenase-2 (COX-2) is an enzyme that produces prostaglandins important in inflammatory cascade and pain transmission. The standard NSAIDs and steroids inhibit the synthesis of COX-1 and COX-2, thus controlling pain and inflammation but producing gastric and renal complications. NSAIDs such as celecoxib (Celebrex) that spare COX-1 and are more COX-2-selective afford control of the potential for arthritis symptoms but carry potentially less risk of gastric and renal problems.

Besides the use of a non–COX-1-sparing NSAID, major risk factors for gastric ulcer include age older than 60 years, history of peptic ulcer disease (especially gastric ulcer), and previous use of H$_2$RA or antacids for GI symptoms. Additional, less potent risk factors include cigarette smoking, cardiac disease, and alcohol use; taking more than one NSAID; and the concurrent use of NSAIDs and anticoagulants.

H$_2$RAs likely offer protection against NSAID-induced duodenal ulcer and perhaps gastritis, but not against gastric ulcer. PPIs afford better protection against peptic ulcer disease. A prostaglandin analog, misoprostol, is a drug specifically designed for gastric protection with NSAIDs. It may be helpful in preventing renal injury secondary to NSAID use.

DISCUSSION SOURCES

Gilbert, D., Moellering, R., and Sande, M. (2004). The Sanford Guide to Antimicrobial Therapy (34th ed.). Hyde Park, VT: Antimicrobial Therapy.

McQuaid, K. R. (2003). Alimentary tract. In Tierney, L., McPhee, S., and Papadakis, M. (eds.). Current Diagnosis and Treatment (42nd ed., pp. 522–627). New York: Lange Medical Books/ McGraw-Hill.

Thompson, M, and Hektor Dunphy, L: Abdominal disorders. In Hektor Dunphy, L. (2004). Management Guidelines for Nurse Practitioners Working with Adults. Philadelphia: F.A. Davis, pp 215–276.

QUESTIONS

34. An obese 45-year-old man presents, complaining of periodic "heartburn." Examination reveals epigastric tenderness without rebound. As first-line therapy, you advise:

    A. avoiding high-fat foods.
    B. the use of a prokinetic agent.
    C. a daily dose of a PPI.
    D. increased fluid intake with meals.

35. You see a 62-year-old man diagnosed with esophageal columnar epithelial metaplasia. You realize he is at increased risk for:

    A. esophageal stricture.
    B. adenocarcinoma.
    C. gastroesophageal reflux.
    D. *H. pylori* colonization.

36. In caring for a patient with symptomatic gastroesophageal reflux, you prescribe a PPI in order to:

    A. enhance motility.
    B. raise the stomach's pH level.
    C. reduce lower esophageal pressure.
    D. help limit *H. pylori* growth.

37. Which of the following represents the optimal dosing schedule for sucralfate (Carafate)?

    A. Each tablet should be taken with a snack.
    B. The medication should be taken with a full meal for buffering effect.
    C. The drug must be taken on an empty stomach.
    D. Sucralfate should be taken with other prescribed medications to enhance compliance.

38. Which of the following is most likely to be found in a patient with erosive gastritis?

    A. NSAID use
    B. weight gain
    C. melena
    D. *H. pylori* infection

39. Which of the following is likely to be reported in a patient with severe GERD?

    A. hematemesis
    B. chronic sore throat
    C. diarrhea
    D. melena

40. A 58-year-old man recently began taking an antihypertensive medication and reports that his "heartburn" has become much worse. He is most likely taking:

    A. atenolol.
    B. trandolapril.
    C. amlodipine.
    D. losartan.

ANSWERS

34. A	**35.** B	**36.** B
37. C	**38.** A	
39. B	**40.** C	

DISCUSSION

GERD is a common but troublesome condition. Reflux of stomach contents occurs regularly. Most is asymptomatic with no resulting esophageal injury. GERD is present when there are symptoms or evidence of tissue damage. Presentation of GERD includes dyspepsia, chest pain at rest, and postprandial fullness. In addition, chronic hoarseness, sore throat, nocturnal cough, and wheezing are often reported, occasionally in the absence of more classic GERD symptoms.

Reflux-induced esophageal injury, also known as reflux esophagitis, is present in 40% of patients with GERD. Erosions and ulcerations in squamous epithelium of esophagus are present and are most common in elderly patients. Complications of reflux esophagitis include esophageal stricture and columnar epithelial metaplasia, also known as Barrett esophagus. This is a risk factor for adenocarcinoma of the esophagus. Decreased lower esophageal sphincter tone and the resulting reflux of gastric contents cause GERD. Esophageal mucosal irritation results from exposure to hydrochloric acid and pepsin.

In GERD, there is often delayed esophageal peristalsis and gastric emptying. Certain medications can cause a decrease in lower esophageal sphincter pressure and worsen GERD; these include estrogen, progesterone, theophylline, calcium channel blockers, and nicotine. The use of an antacid can enhance lower esophageal sphincter pressure and help ameliorate GERD.

Initial therapy for patients with GERD includes reducing intake of offending medications and of GERD-enhancing foods such alcohol, tomato-based products, chocolate, peppermint, colas, and citrus juices. Behavioral intervention includes avoiding assuming the supine position within 3 hours of a meal, not overeating, and abstaining from high-fat meals. Because abdominal obesity contributes to GERD, weight loss can be helpful. Elevation of the head of the bed on 4-inch blocks may also offer some relief.

The use of antacids after meals and at bedtime is often sufficient to control milder, particularly intermittent, GERD symptoms. Antacids neutralize secreted acids and inactivate pepsin and bile salts. They are most effective when used 1 and 3 hours after meals and at bedtime. Antacids interact with many other medications and should therefore be used at least 2 hours apart.

If the use of antacids and lifestyle modification are inadequate to control symptoms of GERD, a H$_2$RA at full prescription strength BID should be added. If there is no improvement in 4 weeks, the patient should be referred for upper GI endoscopy, if possible, and the diagnosis of esophagitis should be entertained. With moderate to severe esophagitis symptoms that do not respond to a prescription dosage of H$_2$RA, a PPI such as omeprazole (Prilosec) or lansoprazole (Prevacid) should be prescribed. Adding sucralfate, 1 g QID, on an empty stomach should be considered in the presence of esophagitis. Sucralfate's mechanism of action is as a mucosal protective agent that acts by forming an adhesive gel that binds to the site of an ulcer. A small amount adheres to normal mucosa. It has no effect on acid formation but does inactivate pepsin while stimulating the formation of prostaglandins. Because it can inactivate many other drugs, sucralfate should be taken at least 2 hours before or after any other medication. In addition, it should be taken on an empty stomach. Prokinetic agents are emerging that should offer additional treatment options.

If this treatment regimen is unsuccessful, expert consultation with a gastroenterology specialist should be sought. GI referral should also be considered if there is concurrent anemia or weight loss. Patients with GERD symptoms for more than 5 years should be referred for upper GI endoscopy to rule out Barrett esophagus.

DISCUSSION SOURCES

McQuaid, K. R. (2003). Alimentary tract. In Tierney, L., McPhee, S., and Papadakis, M. (eds.). Current Diagnosis and Treatment (42nd ed., pp. 522–627). New York: Lange Medical Books/ McGraw-Hill.

Thompson, M, and Hektor Dunphy, L: Abdominal disorder. In Hektor Dunphy, L. (2004). Management Guidelines for Nurse Practitioners Working with Adults. Philadelphia: F.A. Davis, pp 215–276.

QUESTIONS

41. You are caring for a woman from a developing country. She reports that she had "yellow jaundice" as a young child. Her physical examination is unremarkable. Her laboratory studies are as follows: AST, 22 U/L (norm, 0 to 31); alanine aminotransferase (ALT), 25 U/L (norm, 0 to 50); hepatitis A virus (HAV) immunoglobulin G, positive. Laboratory testing reveals:

A. chronic hepatitis A.
B. no evidence of prior or current hepatitis A infection.
C. resolved hepatitis A infection.
D. prodromal hepatitis A.

42. The most common source of hepatitis A infection is:

A. sharing intravenous drug equipment.
B. cooked seafood.
C. contaminated water supplies.
D. sexual contact.

43. In addition to the laboratory work described, results reveal the following for the above-mentioned patient: hepatitis B surface antigen (HBsAg), positive. These findings are most consistent with:

A. no evidence of hepatitis B infection.
B. resolved hepatitis B infection.
C. chronic hepatitis B.
D. evidence of effective hepatitis B immunization.

44. A 28-year-old man with a long-standing history of injection drug use presents with malaise, nausea, fatigue, and "yellow eyes" for the past week. After ordering diagnostic tests, you confirm the diagnosis of acute hepatitis B. Anticipated laboratory results include:

A. hepatitis B surface antibody (HBsAb).
B. neutrophilia.

C. lymphopenia.

D. HBsAg.

45. Clinical findings in patients with acute hepatitis B likely include all of the following except:

    A. rebound tenderness.
    B. scleral icterus.
    C. a smooth, tender, palpable hepatic border.
    D. report of myalgia.

46. You see a woman who has been sexually involved with a man newly diagnosed with acute hepatitis B. You advise her to:

    A. start hepatitis B immunization series.
    B. limit the number of sexual partners.
    C. be tested for HBsAb.
    D. receive hepatitis B immune globulin and hepatitis B immunization series.

47. Which of the following is true concerning hepatitis C infection?

    A. It usually presents with jaundice, fever, and significant hepatomegaly.
    B. Among health care workers, it is most commonly found in nurses.
    C. More than 50% of those with hepatitis C infection go on to develop chronic infection.
    D. Interferon therapy is consistently curative.

48. Which of the following is predictive of severity of chronic liver disease in a patient with chronic hepatitis C?

    A. female gender, age younger than 30
    B. coinfection with hepatitis B, daily alcohol use
    C. acquisition of virus through intravenous drug use, history of hepatitis A infection
    D. frequent use of aspirin, nutritional status

49. When answering questions about hepatitis A vaccine, you consider that it:

    A. contains live virus.
    B. should be offered to those who frequently travel to developing countries.

C. usually is a required immunization for health care workers.

D. is given as a single dose.

50. In order to prevent an outbreak of hepatitis D infection, a NP plans to:

    A. promote a campaign for clean food supplies.
    B. immunize the population against hepatitis B.
    C. offer antiviral prophylaxis against the agent.
    D. encourage frequent hand washing.

51. Which of the following is true concerning hepatitis B vaccine?

    A. The vaccine contains live hepatitis B virus.
    B. The NP should consider checking postvaccination HBsAb titers for those at highest risk for infection.
    C. The vaccine is contraindicated in the presence of human immunodeficiency virus infection.
    D. Postvaccination arthralgias are often reported.

52. Hyperbilirubinemia can cause all of the following except:

    A. displacement of highly protein-bound drugs.
    B. scleral icterus.
    C. cola-colored urine.
    D. reduction in urobilinogen.

53. Monitoring for hepatoma in a patient with chronic hepatitis B or C often includes periodic evaluation of:

    A. erythrocyte sedimentation rate.
    B. HBsAb.
    C. alpha-fetoprotein.
    D. urobilinogen.

54. Which of the following is an expected laboratory result in a patient with acute hepatitis A infection (Norms: AST, 0 to 31 U/L; ALT, 0 to 31 U/L)

    A. AST, 55 U/L; ALT, 50 U/L
    B. AST, 320 U/L; ALT, 190 U/L

C. AST, 320 U/L; ALT, 300 U/L
D. AST, 440 U/L; ALT, 670 U/L

55. Which of the following is most likely to be reported in a patient taking a 3-hydroxy-3-methylglutaryl–coenzyme A (HMG-CoA) reductase inhibitor?

  A. AST, 55 U/L; ALT, 28 U/L
  B. AST, 320 U/L; ALT, 190 U/L
  C. AST, 32 U/L; ALT, 120 U/L
  D. AST, 440 U/L; ALT, 670 U/L

ANSWERS

41. C	**42.** C	**43.** C
44. D	**45.** A	**46.** D
47. C	**48.** B	**49.** B
50. B	**51.** B	**52.** D
53. C	**54.** D	**55.** A

DISCUSSION

A number of infective agents cause viral hepatitis (Table 6–4). Hepatitis A infection is caused by HAV, a small RNA virus. Transmitted primarily by fecally contaminated drinking water and food supplies, hepatitis A is typically a self-limiting infection with a very low mortality rate. In developing countries with limited pure water, the majority of the children contract this disease by age 5 years. In North America, adults ages 20 to 39 account for nearly 50% the reported cases.

The hepatitis A vaccine, which contains inactivated virus, consists of two injections 6 months apart. Candidates include those who reside or travel to areas where disease is endemic, such as developing nations with impure water supplies. Consideration should be given to offering this vaccine to food handlers, day care and long-term care workers, and military and laboratory personnel. Injection drug users may also benefit from the vaccine. However, hepatitis A is rarely transmitted sexually or from needle sharing; rather, intravenous drug users often live in conditions that facilitate the oral-fecal transmission of the hepatitis A virus. All patients with chronic hepatitis B and/or C should be immunized against hepatitis A, because the addition of yet another hepatic insult can result in hepatic failure.

TABLE 6–4
VIRAL HEPATITIS: KEY POINTS

Type	Route of Transmission	IZ Available? Postexposure prophylaxis?	Sequelae	Disease Marker
Hepatitis A	Fecal-oral	IZ: yes Postexposure prophylaxis with IG for close contacts	None; Complete recovery or death	Acute disease marker: • HAV IgM Disease in the past, Hx IZ: • Total anti-HAV (HAV IgG)
Hepatitis B	Blood, body fluids	IZ: yes Postexposure prophylaxis with HBIG for intimate contacts	Chronic hepatitis B, hepatocellular carcinoma, hepatic failure	Acute disease markers: • HBsAg with elevated hepatic enzymes ≥10 ULN • HBeAg: intensely contagious Chronic disease marker: • HBsAg with NL or slight elevated hepatic enzymes Hepatitis B in the past; history of IZ: • HBsAb with normal hepatic enzymes

(continued)

TABLE 6–4

VIRAL HEPATITIS: KEY POINTS *(Continued)*

Type	*Route of Transmission*	*IZ Available? Postexposure prophylaxis?*	*Sequelae*	*Disease Marker*
Hepatitis C	Blood, body fluids	IZ: no Postexposure prophylaxis: no	Chronic hepatitis C, hepatocellular carcinoma, hepatic failure	Acute disease marker: • Anti-HCV with HCV viral RNA, elevated hepatic enzymes Chronic disease marker: • Anti-HCV with HCV viral RNA, normal to slightly elevated hepatic enzymes Disease in the past: • Anti-HCV, HCV RNA absent, and normalized hepatic enzymes
Hepatitis D	Blood, body fluids	No, but prevent B and you can prevent D	Hepatic failure	Acute or chronic hepatitis B markers plus hepatitis D IgM

www.cdc.gov/ncidod/diseases/hepatitis accessed 12/1/03.
HAV, hepatitis A virus; HBeAg, hepatitis B early antigen; HBIG, hepatitis B immune globulin; HBsAb, hepatitis B surface antibody; HBsAg, hepatitis B surface antigen; HCV, hepatitis C virus; IG, immune globulin; IgG, immunoglobulin G; IgM, immunoglobulin M; IZ, immunization; NL, normal; ULN, upper limit of normal.

A small, double-stranded DNA virus that contains the inner core protein of hepatitis B core antigen and an outer surface of HBsAg causes hepatitis B. The virus is transmitted through exchange of body fluids such as blood and sexual fluids. Hepatitis B infection can be prevented by limiting exposure to blood and body fluids, as well as through immunization. Recombinant hepatitis B vaccine, which does not contain live virus, is well tolerated. About 90% to 95% of persons who receive the vaccine develop HBsAb after three doses, which implies protection from the virus. The NP should consider HBsAb testing to confirm the development of hepatitis B virus protection in those with high risk for infection (e.g., health care workers with extensive blood and body fluid exposure, such as emergency workers, operating room personnel, injection drug users, sex workers), as well as those at risk for poor immune response (e.g., dialysis recipients, immunosuppressed patients).

The presentation of viral hepatitis, regardless of the agent, usually includes malaise, myalgia, fatigue, nausea, and anorexia. Aversion to cigarette smoking is often reported. Occasionally, arthritis-like symptoms and skin rash are also noted. Mild fever is occasionally found. Hepatomegaly with usually mild right upper quadrant abdominal tenderness without rebound is found in about 50% of patients, with splenomegaly in about 15%. Jaundice typically occurs about 1 week after the onset of symptoms. However, jaundice is not found in most cases. The course of the illness is typically 2 to 3 weeks. During this period, a gradual increase in energy, appetite, and well-being is reported.

Laboratory findings common to all forms of viral hepatitis include leukopenia with lymphocytosis. Atypical lymphocytes are often found. Bilirubin in the urine is usually found in the absence of icterus. Hepatic enzyme elevation is universal.

The test of liver enzymes is an evaluation of the degree of hepatic inflammation. General rules on the cause of the hepatic inflammation are as follows.

AST/ALT rise in viral hepatitis (A, B, C, D, E)
- AST > 100 U/L
- ALT > 300 U/L
- ALT/AST ratio > 1

AST/ALT rise in selected prescription drugs and alcohol abuse
- AST < 300 U/L (typically <150 U/L)
- ALT < 100 U/L
- AST/ALT ratio >1

Hepatitis C infection is transmitted through the exchange of blood and body fluids. A single-strain RNA virus causes the infection. Although it is the most frequent cause of blood transfusion–associated hepatitis, only 4% of all cases of hepatitis C can be attributed to this cause. Since the advent of screening of the blood supply for hepatitis C virus (HCV), the risk of transfusion-associated hepatitis C has decreased from 10% in the early 1980s to 0.1% today. More than 50% of cases of HCV infection are caused by intravenous drug use with needle sharing. Transmission through sexual contact is possible, but this risk appears relatively low. Maternal-fetal transmission is also uncommon and is usually limited to women with high circulating HCV levels. Transmission through breast-feeding has not been reported.

The HCV incubation period is about 6 to 7 weeks, and the infection rarely causes a serious acute illness. Diagnosis is made by the presence of anti-HCV, an antibody that persists in the presence of the virus and is not protective. At least 50% to 80% of those with hepatitis C go on to develop chronic infection and exhibit anti-HCV along with a positive hepatitis C viral load. Progression to cirrhosis occurs in about 20% of people infected with chronic hepatitis C after 20 years of disease. HCV-related cirrhosis risk is increased in men, with disease acquisition after age 40 years, and in those who drink the equivalent of 50 g or more of alcohol per day. If anti-HCV persists in the absence of a positive hepatitis C viral load, this suggests that active infection is not present.

Because the hepatitis D virus is an RNA virus that can occur only concurrently in the presence of hepatitis B virus, it is found only in persons with acute or chronic hepatitis B. A patient with hepatitis B and D acute coinfection has a course of illness similar to that in a patient with only hepatitis B infection. If a patient with chronic hepatitis B becomes superinfected with hepatitis D virus, a fulminant or severe acute hepatitis often results. Prevention of hepatitis B through immunization also prevents hepatitis D.

Hepatic enzymes are found in circulation because of hepatic growth and repair. The AST level increases in response to hepatocyte injury, as may occur in alcohol abuse, the therapeutic use of HMG-CoA reductase inhibitors (lipid-lowering drugs whose names have the "-statin" suffix, such as lovastatin), and acetaminophen overdose. This enzyme is also found in skeletal muscle, myocardium, brain, and kidneys in smaller amounts, and so damage to these areas may also cause an AST rise.

AST has a circulatory half-life of approximately 12 to 24 hours; therefore, levels rise in response to hepatic damage and clear quickly after damage ceases. AST elevation is generally found in only about 10% of problem drinkers. However, if the AST level is elevated with normal ALT level and mild macrocytosis (mean corpuscular volume > 100 fL, seen in about 30% to 60% of men who drink five or more drinks per day and in women at a threshold of three or more drinks per day), long-standing alcohol abuse is the likely cause.

ALT (formerly known as serum glutamate pyruvate transaminase [SGPT]) is more specific to the liver, having limited concentration in other organs. This enzyme has a longer half-life than AST, at 37 to 57 hours. Therefore, elevation of ALT levels persists longer after hepatic damage has ceased. This enzyme's greatest elevation is likely seen in hepatitis caused by infection or inflammation. This enzyme is unlikely to increase in the presence of alcohol abuse. When evaluating a patient with suspected substance abuse causing hepatic dysfunction, the NP must note both the degree of AST or ALT elevation and the AST/ALT ratio.

An increase in bilirubin level is typically found in patients with viral hepatitis. Clinical jaundice is found when the total bilirubin level exceeds 2.5 mg. Bilirubin is the degradation product of heme, with 85% to 90% arising from hemoglobin and a smaller percentage from myoglobin. About 4 mg/kg/day of bilirubin is produced in healthy individuals, and because the rate of excretion usually matches rate of production, the levels stay low and stable. Reticuloendothelial cells take in haptoglobin, a protein that binds with hemoglobin from aged red blood cells (RBCs). The reticuloendothelial cells remove the iron from hemoglobin for recycling. The remaining substances are then degraded to bilirubin in its unconjugated, or indirect, form. This form is not water soluble.

When unconjugated bilirubin is released into circulation, it binds to albumin and is transported to the liver. When unconjugated bilirubin arrives at the liver, hepatocytes detach bilirubin from the albumin. It is then in a water-soluble form, also known as conjugated, or direct, bilirubin. Conjugated bilirubin loosely attaches to albumin and is easily detached in the kidney. The passing of small amounts of conjugated bilirubin through the kidney gives urine its characteristic yellow color.

Conjugated bilirubin not excreted by the kidney is reabsorbed by the small intestine and converted to urobilinogen by bacterial action in the gut. This can be reabsorbed into circulation, and excess amounts can appear in the urine. Small amounts of urobilinogen may also be found in fecally contaminated urine because urobilinogen is normally found in the large intestine.

When there is an excess of urinary excretion of bilirubin, as found in patients with viral hepatitis, urine develops a characteristic brown color, often described by a patient as looking like "cola." Also, bilirubin in excess may displace drugs with high propensity for protein (albumin) binding, thus increasing free drug and possibly causing drug toxicity.

Treatment of acute viral hepatitis is largely supportive. Corticosteroids, antiviral agents, and interferon are used on occasion, often with equivocal outcomes. Because of the seriousness of hepatitis B and C sequelae, considerable research is under way to develop effective, well-tolerated therapies. Currently, ribavirin and recombinant human interferon have shown clinical utility in inducing remission in some patients with chronic hepatitis B and C. Because of the rapid advances being made in this area, the NP must be aware of the most up-to-date treatment options.

Chronic hepatitis B and C are potent risk factors for hematoma or primary hepatocellular carcinoma. Consultation with a hepatitis specialist and awareness of the latest recommendation for ongoing monitoring is critical. Periodic monitoring for alpha-fetoprotein is often used, to look for an increase in the level that indicates hepatic tumor growth.

DISCUSSION SOURCES

Desai, S. (2004). Clinician's Guide to Laboratory Medicine (3rd ed.). Hudson, OH: Lexi-comp.

The National Center for Infectious Disease. Viral Hepatitis. Available at www.cdc.ogv/ncidod/diseases/hepatitis/, accessed 12/8/03.

Friedman, L. (2003). Liver, biliary tract and pancreas. In Tierney, L., McPhee, S., and Papadakis, M. (eds.). Current Diagnosis and Treatment (42nd ed., pp. 628–673). New York: Lange Medical Books/McGraw-Hill.

QUESTIONS

56. Which of the following is an expected finding in a patient with chronic renal failure?

    A. hypokalemia
    B. hypotension
    C. constipation
    D. anemia

57. The use of which of the following medications can precipitate acute renal failure in a patient with renal artery stenosis?

    A. corticosteroids
    B. angiotensin II receptor antagonists

C. beta-adrenergic antagonists

D. cephalosporins

58. A 78-year-old man presents with fatigue and difficulty with bladder emptying. Examination reveals a distended bladder but is otherwise unremarkable. The blood urea nitrogen (BUN) level is 88 mg/dL; the creatinine level is 2.8 mg/dL. The most likely diagnosis is:

A. prerenal azotemia.

B. acute glomerulonephritis.

C. tubular necrosis.

D. postrenal azotemia.

59. A 68-year-old woman with congestive heart failure presents with tachycardia, S₃ heart sounds, and basilar crackles bilaterally. Blood pressure is 90/68 mm Hg; BUN level is 58 mg/dL; creatinine level is 2.4 mg/dL. The most likely diagnosis is:

A. prerenal azotemia.

B. acute glomerulonephritis.

C. tubular necrosis.

D. postrenal azotemia.

60. Which of the following is found early in the development of chronic renal failure?

A. proteinuria

B. elevated creatinine level

C. uremia

D. hyperkalemia

61. Angiotensin-converting enzyme inhibitors can limit the progress of some forms of renal disease by:

A. increasing intraglomerular pressure.

B. lowering efferent arteriolar resistance.

C. enhancing afferent arteriolar tone.

D. increasing urinary protein excretion.

62. Objective findings in patients with glomerulonephritis include all of the following except:

A. edema.

B. urinary RBC casts.

C. proteinuria.

D. hypotension.

ANSWERS

56. D	57. B	58. D
59. A	60. A	
61. B	62. D	

DISCUSSION

Renal failure can occur either acutely or chronically. In acute renal failure, a precipitating event or cause is often easily identifiable. With prerenal azotemia, the most common cause of acute renal failure, the kidneys are hypoperfused, which often leads to acute tubular necrosis, the cause of 85% of all cases of acute renal failure. Reasons for this include decreased circulating volume, as seen in patients with dehydration and acute blood loss; decreased cardiac output, as seen in patients with congestive heart failure; or excessive sequestering of fluid, as seen in patients with burns. Postrenal azotemia, caused by obstruction to urine flow, accounts for about 5% of all cases of renal failure. Intrinsic renal failure is found when there is disease within the kidney at the levels of the renal tubules, glomerularis, interstitium, or vessels. Etiologies include glomerulonephritis and acute interstitial nephritis. Laboratory findings in these more common forms of acute renal failure vary (Table 6–5).

Typical findings in renal failure include increased serum creatinine and BUN levels. Creatinine is the end product of creatine metabolism, which arises from skeletal muscle. Its measurement is a surrogate marker of kidney function because creatinine excretion by the healthy kidney is very efficient, so that production equals excretion. As the kidney fails, the creatinine level increases. BUN is derived from the breakdown of protein from dietary or other sources. The BUN level typically increases (uremia) more rapidly than the creatinine level in response to decreased renal perfusion and can increase from the prerenal, renal, and postrenal causes of kidney failure. In particular, elevated BUN level with a nor-

TABLE 6–5

ETIOLOGY OF AND FINDINGS IN ACUTE RENAL FAILURE

Disease Causing Acute Renal Failure	Typical Etiology	Laboratory Findings
Acute glomerulonephritis	Post-streptococcal infection, autoimmune diseases	BUN:Cr ratio: >20:1 Urinalysis: renal casts, RBCs
Acute interstitial nephritis	Allergic reaction, drug reaction	BUN:Cr ratio: <20:1 Urinalysis: WBC casts, eosinophils
Acute tubular necrosis	Hypotension, nephrotoxins	BUN:Cr ratio: <20:1 Urinalysis: granular casts, renal tubular cells

BUN, blood urea nitrogen; Cr, creatinine; RBC, red blood cell; WBC, white blood cell.

mal creatinine level may be found in patients with healthy kidneys but with severe dehydration. In addition, GI bleeding usually causes a marked increase in BUN level as the gut digests and absorbs proteins found in the blood.

Anemia is typically seen in patients with chronic renal failure. Erythropoietin, a glycoprotein growth factor produced primarily by the kidneys, influences the undifferentiated stem cell to form the RBC precursor. With end-stage renal disease, there is reduced erythropoietin response because of limited supply; that is, as the kidney fails, erythropoietin production declines. In addition, as is common in chronic illness, RBC lifespan is shortened. These factors result in a normocytic, normochromic anemia in the presence of a low reticulocyte count. This can be treated by the use of recombinant erythropoietin and transfusion.

DISCUSSION SOURCES

Fitzgerald, M. (1999). Hematologic disorders. In Youngkin E., Sawin, K., Kissinger, J., and Israel, D. (eds.). Pharmacotherapeutics: A Primary Care Clinical Guide (pp. 605–620). Stamford, CT: Appleton & Lange.

National Kidney Foundation (2003). Kidney Disease Outcomes Quality Initiative. Available at www.kidney.org/professionals/kdoqi/index.cfm, accessed 12/8/03.

Thompson, M, and Hektor Dunphy, L: Abdominal disorders. In Hektor Dunphy, L. (2004). Management Guidelines for Nurse Practitioners Working with Adults. Philadelphia: F.A. Davis, pp 215–276.

Watnick, S., and Morrison, G. (2003). Kidney. In Tierney, L., McPhee, S., and Papadakis, M. (eds.). Current Diagnosis and Treatment (42nd ed., pp. 867–903). New York: Lange Medical Books/ McGraw-Hill.

QUESTIONS

63. Which of the following is most likely to be part of the clinical presentation of an otherwise healthy woman with uncomplicated lower urinary tract infection (UTI)?

  A. urinary frequency and urgency
  B. fever
  C. suprapubic tenderness
  D. nausea and vomiting

64. A 36-year-old afebrile woman without health problems presents with dysuria and frequency of urination. Her urinalysis findings include results positive for nitrites and leukocyte esterase. You evaluate these results and consider that she likely has:

  A. purulent vulvovaginitis.
  B. a gram-negative UTI.

C. cystitis caused by *Staphylococcus saprophyticus.*

D. urethral syndrome.

65. The most likely causative organism in community-acquired UTI is:

   A. *Klebsiella* species.
   B. *Proteus mirabilis.*
   C. *Escherichia coli.*
   D. *S. saprophyticus.*

66. Preferred therapy for an uncomplicated UTI in an otherwise healthy woman includes:

   A. TMP-SMX.
   B. amoxicillin.
   C. azithromycin.
   D. cephalexin.

67. The notation of alkaline urine in a patient with a UTI may point to infection caused by:

   A. *Klebsiella* species.
   B. *P. mirabilis.*
   C. *E. coli.*
   D. *S. saprophyticus.*

68. Which of the following is most accurate information in caring for a 40-year-old man with cystitis?

   A. This is a common condition in men of this age.
   B. A gram-positive organism is the likely causative pathogen.
   C. A urologic evaluation should be considered.
   D. Pyuria is rarely found.

69. A 44-year-old woman presents with pyelonephritis. The report of her urinalysis is least likely to include:

   A. WBC casts.
   B. positive nitrites.
   C. 3+ protein.
   D. rare RBCs.

70. An example of a first-line therapeutic agent for the treatment of pyelonephritis is:

   A. ampicillin.
   B. sulfamethoxazole.
   C. levofloxacin.
   D. nitrofurantoin.

71. Length of antimicrobial therapy for uncomplicated pyelonephritis is typically:

   A. 5 to 7 days.
   B. 1 to 2 weeks.
   C. 2 to 3 weeks.
   D. 3 to 4 weeks.

ANSWERS

63. A	**64.** B	**65.** C	**66.** A
67. B	**68.** C	**69.** C	**70.** C
71. B			

DISCUSSION

The urinary tract, adjacent to the bacteria-rich lower GI tract, produces and stores urine. The periurethral area is typically colonized with gut and other flora, some capable of causing UTI. Although the process of urination flushes bacteria from the urethral orifice, periurethral pathogens on occasion enter the urethra and ascend, reaching the bladder and resulting in UTI; this is the most common route for UTI acquisition. On rare occasion, hematogenous UTI occurs when a pathogen is delivered to the urinary tract via the bloodstream from a distant source of infection, such as the lungs in a patient with pneumonia.

UTIs can involve mucosal tissue (cystitis) or soft tissue (pyelonephritis, prostatitis). Anatomically, the infection can be limited to the lower urinary tract (cystitis involving the bladder and urethra) or the upper tract (pyelonephritis). Complicated UTI can occur in either the upper or lower urinary tract but is accompanied by an underlying condition that increases the risk for failing therapy, such as obstruction, urologic dysfunction, or resistant pathogens. Most UTIs occur via an ascending route.

UTI is typically diagnosed by clinical presentation and a limited number of physical examination findings. In the otherwise healthy woman, history of the present illness usually reveals a complaint of dysuria, often reported as an internal discomfort, with urinary frequency and urgency but without fever or constitutional symptoms. Although suprapubic tenderness and pain are often considered part of the clinical presentation, they are found in only about 20% of women with an uncomplicated UTI. Back pain, fever, nausea, and vomiting are more often associated with pyelonephritis and, in rare cases, with cystitis; many patients with pyelonephritis also report lower UTI symptoms. Although vaginal infection and irritation can cause dysuria, most women who have dysuria without vaginal discharge have a UTI, not vaginitis·

Hemorrhagic cystitis is characterized by large quantities of visible blood in the urine. Its etiology can be bacterial or adenovirus types 1 to 47 infection, or it can be a result of radiation, cancer chemotherapy, or select immunosuppressive medication. Clinical presentation usually depends on its origin; with all causes, irritative voiding symptoms are typically reported. When the disease is infectious in origin, signs and symptoms of infection may also be encountered. Adenovirus is a common cause and is self-limiting in nature. Hemorrhagic cystitis is often confused with glomerulonephritis, but hypertension and abnormal renal function are absent in the former.

Acute pyelonephritis is an infection of the renal parenchyma and renal pelvis, caused by an ascending cystitis; most episodes are uncomplicated and not accompanied by risk of treatment failure such as obstruction, urologic dysfunction, or a multidrug-resistant uropathogen. Irritative voiding symptoms similar to those of cystitis are usually reported, along with fever and flank pain and often with vomiting. Clinical findings usually include an acutely ill appearance, costovertebral tenderness, and pyuria.

Urine dipstick testing is commonly done in the office setting when UTI is suspected, because it is simple and convenient and yields immediate results. Leukocyte esterase, nitrites, protein, and blood are the important features in evaluating for UTI. The presence of leukocyte esterase on a urine dipstick is equivalent to 4 WBCs or more per high-power field. Nearly all (≥96%) patients with UTI have pyuria equivalent to more than 10 WBCs per high-power field. Some uropathogens are capable of reducing dietary nitrates in the urine to nitrite; this is an indirect test for bacteriuria. When this finding is coupled with a leukocyte esterase response, the likely offending organism is a gram-negative pathogen (*E. coli*, *Proteus* species, *Klebsiella pneumoniae*). The nitrite test result may be falsely negative in UTI with a low colony count or in recently voided or dilute urine. In addition, this test does not detect organisms unable to reduce nitrate to nitrite, such as enterococci, staphylococci, or adenovirus. Small amounts of protein and RBCs may also be positive on dipstick testing in cases of UTI (Table 6–6).

Urine culture is important when diagnosis is not clear or UTI is recurrent. The presence of more than one organism may indicate a contaminated urine specimen, and collection and testing should be repeated. The presence of 10^5 or more colony-forming units (CFU) per milliliter of bacteria is the traditional diagnostic indicator for UTI. However, in the presence of dysuria and other symptoms for UTI, 10^2 CFU/mL confirms diagnosis.

Certain factors protect against or increase the risk for UTI. Male sex is recognized as a potent protective factor, in part because of the longer urethral length than in women; women with a shorter urethra-to-anus length appear to be at increased UTI risk. Unlike the periurethral area in women, the male periurethral area does not support bacterial growth. Zinc-rich prostatic secretions are antibacterial, further discouraging pathogen growth.

In either sex, efficient emptying helps prevent urine stagnation and minimizes UTI risk. Factors that can alter efficient bladder emptying, such as cystocele, rectocele, and benign prostatic hyperplasia, increase UTI risk. In ad-

TABLE 6–6

COMMON URINALYSIS DIPSTICK FINDINGS IN URINARY TRACT INFECTION

Finding	Significance	Comment
COLOR	Typically pale yellow to colorless	Change in urine color is not synonymous with urinary tract infection or disease
CLARITY	Typically clear	Pyuria causes urinary turbidity
ODOR	Mild characteristic odor	Rancid or ammonia odor in urea-splitting organism
SPECIFIC GRAVITY (SG)	Dilute urine = SG = <=1.008 Concentrated urine = SG >1.020	Dilute or concentrated urine may influence the results of urine chemstrip testing
LEUKOCYTE ESTERASE	Test for enzyme present in white blood cells (WBCs)	Positive results indicate presence of neutrophils >5 WBCs/HPF, an indicator of urinary tract infection, reported sensitivity of 75% to 90%; results not valid in neutropenic patient; decreased sensitivity with increased urinary glucose concentration, high urinary SG, and presence of antimicrobial in urine
NITRITES	Surrogate marker for bacteriuria; presence indicates bacterial reduction of dietary nitrates to nitrites by select gram-negative uropathogens including *E. coli, Proteus* spp. Normally absent in sterile urine and infection caused by enterococci, staphylococci	Best done on well-concentrated urine such as first AM void; for nitrites to be present, urine should be held in bladder for at =>1 h for nitrate-to-nitrite conversion to take place; dietary nitrate intake must be adequate; false-negative result possible with low colony–count infections
PROTEIN	Dipstick testing most sensitive for albumin	Common in febrile response or represents presence of protein-containing substance such as WBCs, bacteria, mucus; in UTI, usually trace to 30 mg/dL (1+), seldom => 100 mg/dL
pH	Average pH = 5–6 Acid pH = 4.5–5.5 Alkaline pH = 6.5–8	If alkaline urine is found in presence of UTI symptoms and positive leukocyte esterase, likely that a urea splitting such as *Proteus*, allowing urea to be split into CO^2 and ammonia, causing a rise in the urine's normally acid pH.
RED BLOOD CELLS (RBCs)	Low number of RBCs noted Gross hematuria rare in uncomplicated UTI but may be present in infection complicated by nephrolithiasis	Microscopic hematuria common with urinary tract infection but not in urethritis or vaginitis

dition, robust fucosyltransferase activity discourages bacterial adherence; the presence of relatively few bacterial adhesion receptor sites in the bladder and urethra has a similar effect. Women with these receptors who do not have mucosal secretion of the fucosyltransferase enzyme to help block bacterial adherence are more likely to have colonization with *E. coli* and other coliforms from the rectum and less likely to have lactobacilli in the periurethral area; this situation results in frequent episodes of cystitis. The uroepithelial receptors can also be found in the upper urinary tract, increasing the risk of pyelonephritis. Women who are nonsecretors of ABH blood group antigens show enhanced adherence of pathogenic *E. coli* to uroepithelial cells in comparison with women who are secretors; this becomes a major UTI risk factor when coupled with spermicide use or frequent vaginal sexual intercourse.

The woman who is exposed to the spermicide nonoxynol-9, either through vaginal use or with a male partner who uses condoms with this spermicide, is at increased risk of UTI. The proposed mechanism of this risk is the spermicide's antibacterial effect: reducing lactobacilli, a normal component of the periurethral flora. Lactobacilli produce hydrogen peroxide and lactic acid, providing the periurethral area and vagina with a pH that inhibits bacterial growth and blocks potential sites of attachment, as well as being toxic to uropathogens. Voiding at regular intervals with efficient bladder emptying, wiping patterns, and postcoital voiding have not been shown to provide UTI protection; hot tubs, pantyhose, douching, and obesity have not been demonstrated to increase UTI risk.

In postmenopausal women, estrogen deficiency leads to a marked reduction in lactobacilli colonization in the vaginal-perineal areas; topical estrogen use results in reestablishment of the normal protective flora and a reduction of UTI risk. Recent antimicrobial use potentially increases UTI risk by the same mechanism. In children and elderly persons, constipation has been noted to contribute to bladder instability and may encourage UTI.

Most episodes of community-acquired cystitis in women, the most commonly encountered UTI, are caused by enteric gram-negative rods from the Enterobacteriaceae group, such as *E. coli* and *P. mirabilis*, as well as the less commonly encountered *K. pneumoniae*. *S. saprophyticus*, a gram-positive organism, and *E. coli* accounted for more than 90% of the uropathogens in one study of 4324 urine isolates obtained from women with cystitis during a 5-year period; nearly all of these isolates were sensitive to ciprofloxacin and nitrofurantoin, whereas up to 18% were resistant to TMP-SMX and at least 28% were resistant to beta-lactams (cephalothin and ampicillin).

Because *E. coli* is by far the most common uropathogen, developments in TMP-SMX–resistant strains bear mention. Factors influencing the development of multidrug-resistant *E. coli* strains include liberal use of TMP-SMX to treat UTI in adults and to provide prophylaxis against *Pneumocystis carinii* pneumonia in patients with human immunodeficiency virus. In children, attendance at day care, age younger than 3 years, and repeated TMP-SMX use for respiratory infections are risk factors for infection with a resistant uropathogen; child-to-child and child-to-parent transmission of this organism may then take place.

The Sanford Guide advises a 3-day course of TMP-SMX for acute cystitis treatment in the well woman in regions where *E. coli* TMP-SMX resistance is less than 20%. Alternative therapies in the presence of sulfa allergy or when *E. coli* TMP-SMX resistance rates exceed 20% include a fluoroquinolone. Other alternative therapies include an oral cephalosporin, amoxicillin with clavulanate, doxycycline, or nitrofurantoin, all for 3 days (Table 6–7).

Although *E. coli* remains the most common uropathogen in the community and in long-term care–dwelling elderly persons, *P. mirabilis* and *K. pneumoniae* account for approximately one third of all infections in this age group.

TABLE 6–7

URINARY TRACT INFECTION (UTI) TREATMENT

Type of Infection	Usual Pathogens	Regimens
Acute, uncomplicated urinary tract infection (cystitis, ureteritis) in nonpregnant women	E. coli, S. saprophyticus, enterococci	**Primary** • If local E. coli resistance to TMP-SMX <20%, then use TMP-SMX DS, BID × 3 days • If local E. coli resistance to TMP-SMX ≥20%, then use ciprofloxacin, 250 mg BID; levofloxacin, 250 mg QD; gatifloxacin, 200–400 mg QD; and ofloxacin, 200 mg BID, all for 3 days **Alternative** • TMP-SMX DS, BID × 3 days • Other options: nitrofurantoin, oral cephalosporin, amoxicillin with clavulanate, doxycycline, usually for 3 days
Recurrent UTI (3 or more/year)	E. coli, S. saprophyticus, enterococci, other pathogens possible	Eradicate organisms; then TMP-SMX DS, QD long term For recurrent UTI in postmenopausal women, consider use of estrogen cream
Acute uncomplicated pyelonephritis suitable for outpatient therapy	E. coli, Enterococci	**Primary** • Ciprofloxacin, 500 mg BID; levofloxacin, 250 mg QD; gatifloxacin, 400 mg QD; and ofloxacin, 400 mg BID, all for 7 days **Alternative** • Amoxicillin with clavulanate, cephalosporin, TMP-SMX DS, all for 14 days

Gilbert, D., Moellering, R., and Sande, M. (2004). The Sanford Guide to Antimicrobial Therapy (34th ed.). Hyde Park, VT: Antimicrobial Therapy. TMP-SMX DS, trimethoprim-sulfamethoxazole double-strength.

Length of antimicrobial treatment in elderly persons with uncomplicated UTI should be 7 to 10 days for women and 10 to 14 days for men; short-course therapy is not recommended. First-line therapy includes TMP-SMX or fluoroquinolones; nitrofurantoin should not be used in elderly patients, because its safe use requires a minimum creatinine clearance of 40 mL/minute. In the elderly patient with impaired renal function, TMP-SMX and fluoroquinolone dosages need adjustment as well.

UTI prophylaxis may be indicated for women who experience two or more symptomatic UTIs within 6 months or three or more UTIs over 12 months and for those with fewer infections but with severe discomfort. Both continuous prophylaxis, in which an antimicrobial is taken daily for 6 months or more, and postcoital prophylaxis, in which an antimicrobial is taken with each act of coitus, have been demonstrated to be effective in the management of recurrent uncomplicated cystitis. Before UTI prophylaxis is initiated, resolution of the previous UTI should be confirmed by a negative urine culture 1 to 2 weeks after treatment. The method prescribed is dependent upon the frequency and pattern of recurrences and on patient preference.

Choice of an antimicrobial agent for recurrent UTI should be based on susceptibility patterns of the strains causing the patient's previous UTIs and on patient history of drug allergies or intolerance. Long-term TMP-SMX or nitrofurantoin therapy has been used successfully for many years. In comparison with TMP-SMX, nitrofurantoin has the advantage of lower rates of resistance by the more common UTI pathogens. The use of a fluoroquinolone for UTI prophylaxis has gained some popularity; concern about emerging resistance is an issue. UTI prophylaxis in the postmenopausal woman should also include the use of a topical estrogen to encourage lactobacilli recolonization.

Cranberry and blueberry juice intake has been touted as a helpful measure to reduce the rate of recurrent infections. These juices were initially believed to cause high levels of benzoic acid that resulted in urinary acidification and bacteriostatic action; however, further study failed to support this hypothesis, with mixed results on efficacy in UTI prevention.

DISCUSSION SOURCES

Gilbert, D., Moellering, R., and Sande, M. (2004). The Sanford Guide to Antimicrobial Therapy (34th ed.). Hyde Park, VT: Antimicrobial Therapy.

O'Donnell, J., Gelone, S., and Abrutyne, E. (2002). Selecting drug regimens for urinary tract infection: Current recommendations. Infections in Medications 19:14–22. Available at http://www.medscape.com/viewarticle/423482, accessed 9/29/03.

Stoller, M., and Carrol, P. (2003). Urology. In Tierney, L., McPhee, S., and Papadakis, M. (eds.). Current Medical Diagnosis and Treatment (42nd ed., pp. 903–945). New York: Lange Medical Books/McGraw-Hill.

Thompson, M, and Hektor Dunphy, L: Abdominal disorders. In Hektor Dunphy, L. (2004). Management Guidelines for Nurse Practitioners Working with Adults. Philadelphia: F.A. Davis, pp 215–276.

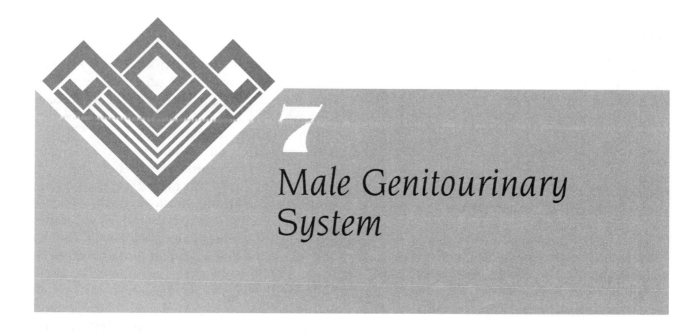

7
Male Genitourinary System

1. Which of the following is not consistent with the description of benign prostatic hyperplasia (BPH)?

   A. obliterated median sulcus
   B. size larger than 2.5 cm × 3 cm
   C. sensation of incomplete emptying
   D. boggy gland

2. When prescribing antihypertensive therapy for the man with BPH and hypertension, the nurse practitioner (NP) considers that:

   A. loop diuretics are the treatment of choice.
   B. an alpha$_1$ antagonist should not be used as a solo or first-line therapeutic agent.
   C. angiotension receptor antagonist use is contraindicated.
   D. beta-adrenergic antagonist use may enhance urinary flow.

3. When assessing a 78-year-old man with suspected BPH, the NP considers that:

   A. prostate size does not correlate well with severity of symptoms.
   B. BPH affects about 50% of men of this age.
   C. he is at increased risk for prostate cancer.
   D. limiting fluids is a helpful method of relieving severe symptoms.

4. Which of the following medications can cause acute urinary retention in a man with BPH?

   A. amitriptyline
   B. trimethoprim-sulfamethoxazole
   C. enalapril
   D. lorazepam

5. A 78-year-old man presents with fatigue and difficulty with bladder emptying. Examination reveals a distended bladder but is otherwise unremarkable. Blood urea nitrogen level is 88 mg/dL; creatinine = 2.8 mg/dL. The most likely diagnosis is:

   A. prerenal azotemia.
   B. acute glomerulonephritis.
   C. tubular necrosis.
   D. postrenal azotemia.

6. Surgical intervention in BPH should be considered with all of the following except:

   A. recurrent urinary tract infection.
   B. bladder stones.

C. persistent obstruction in spite of medical therapy.

D. acute tubular necrosis.

7. Finasteride is helpful in the treatment of BPH because of its effect on:

A. bladder contractility.

B. prostate size.

C. activity at bladder receptor sites.

D. bladder pressure.

ANSWERS

1. D	2. B	3. A	4. A
5. D	6. D	7. B	

DISCUSSION

BPH is a common disorder in older men, with a prevalence of approximately 50% by age 60 years and 90% by age 85 years. This benign enlargement of the prostate can lead to bladder outlet obstruction. There are both an enlargement in prostatic connective tissue and an increase in the number of epithelial and smooth muscle cells. The cause of BPH is not fully understood but may be in response to androgenic hormones.

BPH can lead to bladder outlet obstruction from urethral narrowing. As a result, men with BPH develop symptoms of increased frequency of urination, decreased force of urinary stream, nocturia, and the sensation of incomplete emptying. Postrenal azotemia accounts for about 5% of all renal failure and is characterized by urea nitrogen and creatinine elevation coupled with evidence of urinary outflow tract obstruction; other reasons for renal failure have been ruled out.

Patient education about BPH should include information on measures to avoid making symptoms worse. Drugs with anticholinergic effect, such as tricyclic antidepressants and first-generation antihistamines, can cause acute urinary retention in men with BPH. In addition, urinary frequency may become worse with ingestion of certain bladder irri-tants such as caffeine and artificial sweeteners. Although men with BPH may be tempted to limit fluid intake, this may yield a more concentrated and perhaps irritating urine, possibly leading to increased symptoms.

The prostate and bladder base contain numerous alpha$_1$ receptor sites. When these receptor sites are stimulated, the prostate contracts, increasing outflow track obstruction. As a result, medical therapy with alpha$_1$ receptor antagonists (alpha blockers) can be helpful in improving the symptoms of BPH. The use of alpha blockers as a solo or first-line antihypertensive agent has been associated with higher than expected rates of stroke and heart failure. Thus, alpha blockers should be considered as a desirable agent in treating the man with hypertension and BPH, but as medication added on to existing therapy. Finasteride, a 5α-reductase inhibitor that blocks the conversion of testosterone to dihydrotestosterone, helps to reduce the size of the prostate and ameliorate symptoms. Surgical intervention in BPH should be considered when any of the following are present and clearly secondary to the condition: recurrent urinary tract infection, recurrent or persistent gross hematuria, bladder stones, and/or renal insufficiency.

DISCUSSION SOURCES

Jen, K. (2004). Male genitalia disorders. In Hektor Dunphy, L. Management Guidelines for Nurse Practitioners Working with Adults (2nd ed., pp 350–378). Philadelphia: F.A. Davis.

Stoller, M., and Carrol, P. (2003). Urology. In Tierney, L., McPhee, S., and Papadakis, M. (eds.). Current Medical Diagnosis and Treatment (42nd ed., pp. 903–945). New York: Lange Medical Books/ McGraw-Hill.

QUESTIONS

8. You examine a 32-year-old man with chancroid and anticipate finding the following:

A. a verruciform lesion

B. a painful ulcer

C. a painless craterlike lesion

D. plaquelike lesion

9. The causative organism of chancroid is:

A. *Ureaplasma* spp.

B. *Chlamydia trachomatis.*

C. Mycoplasma *hominis.*

D. *Haemophilus ducreyi.*

10. Treatment options for chancroid include all of the following except:

A. azithromycin.

B. ciprofloxacin.

C. ceftriaxone.

D. amoxicillin.

11. When ordering laboratory tests to confirm chancroid, the NP considers that:

A. concomitant infection with herpes simplex is often found.

B. a disease-specific serum test is available.

C. a white blood cell count with differential is indicated.

D. dark-field examination is needed.

ANSWERS

8.	B	**9.**	D
10.	D	**11.**	A

DISCUSSION

The gram-negative bacillus *H. ducreyi* causes chancroid. The organism is most often contracted sexually. However, transmission to health care providers through direct contact with chancroid lesions has been documented. The chancroid lesion is typically found at the site of inoculation with a vesicular- to pustular-form lesion that forms a painful, soft ulcer with a necrotic base. Multiple lesions, acquired through autoinoculation, are usually found. A dense, matted lymphadenopathy can be found on the ipsilateral side of the lesion. The affected nodes may spontaneously rupture. Treatment options include azithromycin, ciprofloxacin, and ceftriaxone (Table 7–1).

As with all sexually transmitted infections (STIs), a critical part of care is discussion of prevention strategies, including condom use and limiting the number of sexual partners. The NP should offer and encourage testing for other STIs, including human immunodeficiency virus (HIV). Concomitant infection with syphilis, herpes simplex, and HIV is often found.

DISCUSSION SOURCES

Centers for Disease Control and Prevention (2002). 2002 guidelines for treatment of sexually transmitted diseases. Available at http://www.cdc.gov/STD/treatment/, accessed 9/10/04.

Chambers, H. (2003). Infectious disease: Bacterial and chlamydia. In Tierney, L., McPhee, S., and Papadakis, M. (eds.). Current Medical Diagnosis and Treatment (42nd ed., pp. 1346–1389). New York: Lange Medical Books/McGraw-Hill.

Jen, K. (2004). Male genitalia disorders. In Hektor Dunphy, L. Management Guidelines for Nurse Practitioners Working with Adults (2nd ed., pp 350–378). Philadelphia: F.A. Davis.

QUESTIONS

12. The most common causative organism of lymphogranuloma venereum is

A. *Ureaplasma.*

B. *C. trachomatis* types 1 to 3.

C. *Neisseria gonorrhoeae.*

D. *H. ducreyi.*

13. Physical examination findings in lymphogranuloma venereum include:

A. verruciform lesions.

B. lesions that fuse and create multiple draining sinuses.

C. a painless crater.

D. plaquelike lesions.

14. Treatment options for lymphogranuloma venereum include:

A. tetracycline.

B. penicillin.

C. ceftriaxone.

D. dapsone.

TABLE 7–1

GUIDELINES FOR ASSESSMENT AND TREATMENT OF MALE
GENITOURINARY INFECTION

Conditions	Causative Organism	Clinical Presentation	Treatment Options
Chancroid	*H. ducreyi*	Painful genital ulcer, multiple lesions common, inguinal lymphadenitis	Azithromycin 1 g orally in a single dose OR ceftriaxone 250 mg intramuscularly (IM) in a single dose, OR ciprofloxacin 500 mg orally twice a day for 3 days, OR erythromycin base 500 mg orally three times a day for 7 days.
Genital herpes	Human herpesvirus 2 (rarely human herpesvirus 1)	Painful ulcerated lesions, lymphadenopathy (particularly with primary outbreak)	For initial infection: Acyclovir 400 mg PO TID × 7–10 days or acyclovir 200 mg 5ID × 7–10 days or famciclovir 250 mg PO TID × 7–10 days or valacyclovir 1 g PO BID × 7–10 days; for episodic recurrent infection: Acyclovir 400 mg PO TID × 5 days or famciclovir 125 mg PO BID × 5 days or valacyclovir 1 g PO QD × 5 days or valacyclovir 500 mg PO BID × 5 days. For suppression of recurrent infection: Acyclovir 400 mg PO BID or famciclovir 250 mg PO BID or valacyclovir 1 g PO QD or valacyclovir 500 mg; 1 g PO for extended period of time
Lymphogranuloma venereum	Invasive serovar L1, L2, L3 of *C. trachomatis*	Vesicular or ulcerative lesion on the external genitalia with inguinal lymphadenitis or buboes.	Doxycycline 100 mg PO BID × 21 days or erythromycin 500 mg QID × 21 days
Nongonococcal urethritis and cervicitis	*C. trachomatis*	Cervicitis, irritative voiding symptoms, occasional mucopurulent discharge	Recommended therapy: Azithromycin 1 g PO as a single dose or doxycycline 100 mg PO BID × 7 days. Alternative therapy: Erythromycin 500 mg PO QID × 7 days or ofloxacin 300 mg BID × 7 days or levofloxacin 500 mg qd × 7 d
Gonococcal urethritis	*N. gonorrhoeae*	Irritative voiding symptoms, occasional purulent discharge	Recommended therapy: Single-dose therapy for uncomplicated infection. Cefixime 400 mg PO, ceftriaxone 125 mg IM or ciprofloxacin 500 mg or ofloxacin 400 mg or levofloxacin 250 mg. Concurrently treat with azithromycin 1 g as a single dose or doxycycline 100 mg BID × 7 days if chlamydial infection has not been ruled out. Alternative therapy: Spectinomycin 2 g IM as a single dose

Conditions	Causative Organism	Clinical Presentation	Treatment Options
Epididymitis Epididymoorchitis	N. gonorrhoeae, C. trachomatis, Gram-negative rods, others	Irritative voiding symptoms, fever and painful swelling of epididymis and scrotum	Recommended therapy: Ceftriaxone 250 mg IM as a single dose plus doxycycline 100 mg BID × 10 days. Alternative therapy: ofloxacin 300 mg PO bid or levofloxacin 500 mg PO qd mg × 10 days
Trichomoniasis	T. vaginalis	Dysuria (rare)	Recommended therapy: Metronidazole 2 g as a one-time dose. Alternative therapy: Metronidazole 500 mg PO BID × 7 days
Genital warts (Condyloma acuminata)	Human papilloma virus	Verruca-form lesions or may be subclinical or unrecognized	Recommended therapy: Patient-applied therapy: Podofilox 0.5% solution or imiquimod 5% cream. Provider-applied therapy: Liquid nitrogen or cryoprobe, trichloroacetic acid, podophyllin resin, or surgical removal
Acute bacterial prostatitis (men <35 y)	N. gonorrhoeae, C. trachomatis	Irritative voiding symptoms; suprapubic, perineal pain; fever; a tender, boggy prostate; leukocytosis	Ofloxacin 400 mg as one-time dose, then 300 mg BID × 10 d OR Ceftriaxone 250 mg IM as one-time dose, then doxycycline 100 mg PO BID × 10 d
Acute bacterial prostatitis (men >age 35 y)	Enterobacteriaceae (coliforms)	Irritative voiding symptoms; suprapubic, perineal pain; fever; a tender, boggy prostate; leukocytosis	Ciprofloxacin 500 mg PO bid or ofloxacin 200 mg PO qd mg × 10–14 days
Chronic bacterial prostatitis	Enterobacteriaceae (coliforms), P. aeruginosa	Irritative voiding symptoms; dull, poorly localized, suprapubic, perineal pain	Ciprofloxacin 500 mg PO bid × 4 weeks OR ofloxacin 300 mg PO qd mg × 6 weeks; Alternative: TMP-SMX DS 1 tab BID × 3 months

Center for Disease Control and Prevention (2002) Guidelines for Treatment of Sexually Transmitted Disease. Available at http://www.cdc.gov/STD/treatment/, accessed 12.19.04.

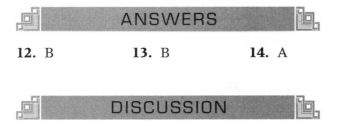

ANSWERS

12. B   **13.** B   **14.** A

DISCUSSION

Lymphogranuloma venereum is an STI caused by *C. trachomatis* types L1 to L3. The clinical presentation, usually occurring approximately 1 to 4 weeks after contact with an infected host, consists of a vesicular or ulcerative lesion on the external genitalia, often not noted by the patient, that then progresses to cause inguinal lymphadenitis or buboes. These may fuse and then drain, forming multiple sinus tracts with resultant scarring. Treatment options include tetracycline, doxycycline, and erythromycin (see Table 7–1).

As with all STIs, a critical part of care is discussion of prevention strategies, including condom use and limiting the number of sexual partners. Offer and encourage testing for other STIs, including HIV.

DISCUSSION SOURCES

Centers for Disease Control and Prevention (2002). 2002 Guidelines for Treatment of Sexually Transmitted Disease. Available at http://www.cdc.gov/STD/treatment/, accessed 4/3/03.

Chambers, H. (2003). Infectious disease: Bacterial and chlamydia. In Tierney, L., McPhee, S., and Papadakis, M. (eds.). Current Medical Diagnosis and Treatment (42nd ed., pp. 1346–1389). New York: Lange Medical Books/McGraw-Hill.

Jen, K. (2004). Male genitalia disorders. In Hektor Dunphy, L. Management Guidelines for Nurse Practitioners Working with Adults (2nd ed., pp 350–378). Philadelphia: F.A. Davis.

QUESTIONS

15. The presentation of acute epididymitis includes:

    A. the presence of a positive Prehn sign.
    B. low back pain.
    C. absent cremasteric reflex.
    D. diffuse abdominal pain.

16. The most likely causative pathogens in a 26-year-old man with acute epididymitis include:

    A. *Escherichia coli.*
    B. Enterobacteriaceae.
    C. *C. trachomatis.*
    D. *Pseudomonas* species.

17. Which of the following is a reasonable treatment option for a 30-year-old man with acute epididymitis?

    A. ofloxacin
    B. amoxicillin
    C. metronidazole
    D. clindamycin

ANSWERS

15. A   16. C   17. A

DISCUSSION

Acute epididymitis is an infectious disease caused by a variety of pathogens. In men younger than 40 years, it is usually caused by *C. trachomatis* or *N. gonorrhoeae;* the organism is acquired through sexual contact. In older men, acute epididymitis is often seen secondary to prostatitis and is typically caused by a gram-negative organism. This condition presents with irritative voiding symptoms; fever; and an acutely painful, enlarged epididymis. Pain may radiate up the spermatic cord to the ipsilateral lower abdomen. The Prehn sign, a reduction in pain when the scrotum is elevated above the symphysis pubis, is usually noted. Urethritis, scrotal swelling, and penile discharge are often found. As the disease progresses, the ipsilateral testis may become involved, swelling so that the two cannot be distinguished; this is known as epididymoorchitis.

Treatment options differ according to age and risk factors. In younger men with low risk for epididymoorchitis as a complication of urinary tract infection, particularly with risk for STI, antimicrobials effective against gonorrhea and chlamydia such as ceftriaxone followed by doxycycline or ofloxacin should be used (see Table 7–1). In men at risk for epididymoorchitis as a complication of urinary tract infection, the choice of an antimicrobial agent should be directed by urine culture. A fluoroquinolone such as ciprofloxacin will likely be effective.

As with all STIs, a critical part of care is discussion of prevention strategies, including condom use and limiting the number of sexual partners. Offer and encourage testing for other STIs, including HIV.

DISCUSSION SOURCES

Centers for Disease Control and Prevention (2002). 2002 Guidelines for Treatment of Sexually Transmitted Disease. Available at http://www.cdc.gov/STD/treatment/, accessed 4/3/03.

Jen, K. (2004). Male genitalia disorders. In Hektor Dunphy, L. Management Guidelines for Nurse

Practitioners Working with Adults (2nd ed., pp 350–378). Philadelphia: F.A. Davis.

Stoller, M., and Carrol, P. (2003). Urology. In Tierney, L., McPhee, S., and Papadakis, M. (eds.). Current Medical Diagnosis and Treatment (42nd ed., pp. 903–945). New York: Lange Medical Books/McGraw-Hill.

QUESTIONS

18. Gram stain of the urethral discharge of a 37-year-old man with dysuria reveals gram-negative cocci. This most likely represents:

    A. *C. trachomatis.*
    B. *Ureaplasma.*
    C. *N. gonorrhoeae.*
    D. *E. coli.*

19. Treatment options for uncomplicated gonococcal proctitis include:

    A. ceftriaxone, 125 mg intramuscularly as a single dose.
    B. erythromycin, 500 mg BID for 7 days.
    C. norfloxacin, 400 mg BID for 3 days.
    D. azithromycin, 1 g as a single dose.

20. Which of the following is recommended by the Centers for Disease Control and Prevention as single-dose therapy for uncomplicated urethritis caused by *N. gonorrhoeae?*

    A. cefixime
    B. metronidazole
    C. azithromycin
    D. amoxicillin

21. In gonococcal infection, which of the following is true?

    A. Risk of transmission from an infected woman to a male sexual partner is about 20% to 30% with a single coital act.
    B. Most men have symptomatic infection.
    C. The incubation period is about 2 to 3 weeks.
    D. The organism rarely produces beta-lactamase.

ANSWERS

18. C   19. A
20. A   21. A

DISCUSSION

Gonorrhea, caused by the gram-negative diplococcus *N. gonorrhoeae,* is one of the most common STIs. It has a short incubation period, 1 to 5 days, and is likely to cause infection in approximately 20% to 30% of men who have sexual contact with an infected woman and approximately 60% to 80% of women who have sexual contact with an infected man. Male-to-male and female-to-female rates of transmission are not well documented.

In men, presentation typically includes dysuria with a milky, occasionally blood-tinged penile discharge. However, the majority of men are asymptomatic. With anal-insertive sex, rectal infection leading to proctitis is often seen. Because the organism frequently produces beta-lactamase, the choice of a therapeutic agent should include agents with beta-lactamase stability and include a cephalosporin such as ceftriaxone and cefixime (see Table 7–1). Increasing prevalence of fluoroquinolone-resistant GC limits the usefulness of these medications.

As with all STIs, a critical part of care is discussion of prevention strategies, including condom use and limiting the number of sexual partners. Offer and encourage testing for other STIs, including HIV.

DISCUSSION SOURCES

Centers for Disease Control and Prevention (2002). 2002 Guidelines for Treatment of Sexually Transmitted Disease. Available at http://www.cdc.gov/STD/treatment/, accessed 4/3/03.

Chambers, H. (2003). Infectious disease: Bacterial and chlamydia. In Tierney, L., McPhee, S., and Papadakis, M. (eds.). Current Medical Diagnosis and Treatment (42nd ed., pp. 1346–1389). New York: Lange Medical Books/McGraw-Hill.

Jen, K. (2004). Male genitalia disorders. In Hektor Dunphy, L. Management Guidelines for Nurse Practitioners Working with Adults (2nd ed., pp 350–378). Philadelphia: F.A. Davis.

QUESTIONS

22. When choosing an antimicrobial agent for the treatment of chronic bacterial prostatitis, the NP considers that:

    A. gram-positive organisms are the most likely cause of infection.
    B. cephalosporins are the first-line choice of therapy.
    C. choosing an antibiotic with gram-negative coverage is critical.
    D. length of antimicrobial therapy is typically 10 days.

23. All of the following are likely to be reported by patients with acute bacterial prostatitis except:

    A. perineal pain.
    B. irritative voiding symptoms.
    C. penile discharge.
    D. fever.

24. During acute bacterial prostatitis, the digital rectal examination usually reveals a gland described as:

    A. boggy.
    B. smooth.
    C. irregular.
    D. cystic.

25. Symptoms in chronic bacterial prostatitis often include:

    A. fever.
    B. gastrointestinal upset.
    C. low back pain.
    D. penile discharge.

26. The most common causative organisms in chronic bacterial prostatitis include:

    A. gram-negative rods.
    B. gram-positive cocci.
    C. gram-negative cocci.
    D. gram-positive coccobacilli.

27. Which of the following is the best choice of therapy in chronic bacterial prostatitis?

    A. trimethoprim-sulfamethoxazole for 2 weeks
    B. amoxicillin for 4 weeks
    C. ciprofloxacin for 4 weeks
    D. gentamicin for 8 weeks

28. Diagnostic testing to identify the offending organism in acute bacterial prostatitis is best accomplished by obtaining:

    A. a urine culture.
    B. a urethral culture.
    C. antibody testing.
    D. a urine Gram stain.

ANSWERS

22. C	23. C	24. A
25. C	26. A	
27. C	28. A	

DISCUSSION

Gram-negative rods such as *E. coli* and *Pseudomonas* species usually cause acute bacterial prostatitis in older men. In younger men or men at risk for STIs, gonorrhea or chlamydia are most often implicated. Less often, gram-positive organisms such as enterococci are implicated. Irritative voiding symptoms are typically reported, as well as suprapubic and perineal pain. Objective findings include fever; a tender, boggy prostate; leukocytosis; and a urine culture positive for the causative organism. Urine Gram stain usually fails to identify the offending organism. Treatment options for acute bacterial prostatitis are similar to those of acute pyelonephritis: that is, an antimicrobial agent with activity against gram-negative organisms and excellent tissue penetration. In men younger than 35, ofloxacin or ceftriaxone followed by doxycycline is recommended. Length of therapy is usually 10 to 14 days.

In patients with chronic bacterial prostatitis, irritative voiding symptoms, low back and perineal pain, and a history of urinary tract infection are typically reported. Objective findings include a tender, boggy prostate. Urinalysis results are usually normal. Urinalysis and culture after prostatic massage typically yield leukocytes and the causative organism. Four to 12 weeks of antimicrobial therapy are usually required (see Table 7–1).

DISCUSSION SOURCES

Centers for Disease Control and Prevention (2002). 2002 Guidelines for Treatment of Sexually Transmitted Disease. Available at http://www.cdc.gov/STD/treatment/, accessed 4/3/03.

Gilbert, D., Moellering, R., and Sande, M. (2004). The Sanford Guide to Antimicrobial Therapy (34th ed.). Hyde Park, VT: Antimicrobial Therapy.

Stoller, M., and Carrol, P. (2003). Urology. In Tierney, L., McPhee, S., and Papadakis, M. (eds.). Current Medical Diagnosis and Treatment (42nd ed., pp. 903–945). New York: Lange Medical Books/McGraw-Hill.

QUESTIONS

29. You perform a rectal examination on a 72-year-old man and find a lesion suspicious for prostate cancer. The findings are described as:

    A. a rubbery, enlarged prostatic lobe.
    B. a prostatic induration.
    C. a tender, boggy gland.
    D. an asymmetric gland.

30. Which of the following prostate-specific antigen (PSA) results is most consistent with prostate cancer?

    A. a single elevated PSA result in a man recovering from prostatitis
    B. a doubling of PSA value in serial annual tests in the presence of a normal prostatic digital rectal examination
    C. an elevated, unchanged serial PSA level in a man with BPH
    D. a markedly abnormal PSA result immediately after cystoscopy

31. Risk factors for prostate cancer include all of the following except:

    A. African ancestry.
    B. history of genital trauma.
    C. family history of prostate cancer.
    D. high-fat diet.

32. The average American man has an approximately ____% lifetime risk of prostate cancer and an approximately ____% likelihood of clinical disease.

    A. 15, 5
    B. 25, 8
    C. 40, 10
    D. 60, 15

ANSWERS

29. B   30. B
31. B   32. C

DISCUSSION

Prostate cancer is the most common cancer in men in the United States. Although clinically detectable prostate cancer is a cause of considerable mortality and morbidity, the majority is likely occult and limited to the prostate with little risk of metastasis. Prostate cancer has been found on autopsy in two thirds of men age 80 to 89 years. The average American man has a 40% lifetime risk of latent prostate cancer, an approximate 10% risk of clinically significant disease, and an approximate 3% risk of dying of prostate cancer. Risk factors include advancing age, high-fat diet, family history of prostate cancer, and African ancestry. Vasectomy has been suggested as a prostate cancer risk factor.

Most men with prostate cancer are asymptomatic unless the disease is advanced. The prostate digital rectal examination can reveal a discrete lesion or induration but is often normal until disease is advanced. Measurement of PSA, a glycoprotein produced in benign and malignant prostate cells, is used to screen for prostate cancer. Whereas nearly two thirds of men with PSA levels of more than 10 ng/mL (normal PSA, <4 ng/mL) will have prostate cancer, about 25% of those with values between 4 and 10 ng/mL will have disease. Correlating an abnormal prostate examination finding with an abnormal PSA level increases the likelihood of a diagnosis of prostate cancer. PSA level is typically elevated during prostatitis or prostatic instrumentation such as cystoscopy. Levels may remain chronically elevated in patients with BPH. Serial increases even in the presence of a normal prostate examination should be further evaluated. Transrectal ultrasound should not be used as a first-line screening test for prostate cancer, because of its low sensitivity and specificity, but it can be helpful when coupled with PSA and digital rectal examination findings. Prostate cancer screening should begin at age 50 years in men with no risk factors and at age 40 years in those with one or more risk factors.

Pathology and disease staging guide prostate cancer treatment options. Watchful waiting is often a reasonable option for older men with local disease.

DISCUSSION SOURCES

Jen, K. (2004). Male genitalia disorders. In Hektor Dunphy, L. Management Guidelines for Nurse Practitioners Working with Adults (2nd ed., pp 350–378). Philadelphia: F.A. Davis.

Stoller, M., and Carrol, P. (2003). Urology. In Tierney, L., McPhee, S., and Papadakis, M. (eds.). Current Medical Diagnosis and Treatment (42nd ed., pp. 903–945). New York: Lange Medical Books/McGraw-Hill.

QUESTIONS

33. A 19-year-old man presents with sudden onset of left-sided scrotal pain and unilateral loss of the cremasteric reflex. This most likely represents:

    A. acute epididymitis.
    B. testicular torsion.
    C. testicular neoplasia.
    D. incarcerated hernia.

34. In assessing men with testicular torsion, the NP is most likely to note:

    A. relief of pain with scrotal elevation.
    B. white blood cells reported in urinalysis.
    C. a swollen, tender testicle.
    D. increased testicular blood flow by color-flow Doppler ultrasound.

35. Anticipated organ survival exceeds 85% with testicular decompression within how many hours of torsion?

    A. 1
    B. 6
    C. 16
    D. 24

36. In order to prevent a recurrence of testicular torsion, which of the following is recommended?

    A. use of a scrotal support
    B. avoidance of testicular trauma
    C. orchiopexy
    D. limiting the number of sexual partners

ANSWERS

33. B	**34.** C
35. B	**36.** C

DISCUSSION

Testicular torsion is a urologic emergency caused by a twisting of the testis and spermatic cord around a vertical axis. This results in arterial and venous compression, testicular swelling, and testicular death. Findings include severe unilateral scrotal pain and swelling, the affected testicle held high in the scrotum, absent cremasteric reflex, and lack of relief of pain with scrotal elevation. Radionuclide testicular scan and color-flow Doppler ultrasound may demonstrate reduction of blood flow.

Prompt referral to a urologic surgeon to detort the organ and restore testicular blood flow is indicated. If this is accomplished within 6 hours, testicular survival surpasses 85%. A bilateral orchiopexy, a procedure in which both testes are brought down and tacked lower in the scrotum, is usually performed in order to avoid subsequent torsion.

DISCUSSION SOURCE

Stoller, M., and Carrol, P. (2003). Urology. In Tierney, L., McPhee, S., and Papadakis, M. (eds.). Current Medical Diagnosis and Treatment (42nd ed., pp. 903–945). New York: Lange Medical Books/McGraw-Hill.

QUESTIONS

37. A 42-year-old man has a nontender "bag of worms" mass within the left scrotum that disappears when he is in the supine position. This is most consistent with:

    A. testicular neoplasm.
    B. varicocele.
    C. inguinal hernia.
    D. epididymitis.

38. Which of the following is a common finding in a man with varicocele?

    A. low sperm count with increased number of abnormal forms
    B. increased rate of testicular cancer
    C. recurrent scrotal pain
    D. BPH

ANSWERS

37. B   38. A

DISCUSSION

A varicocele is an abnormally dilated spermatic vein within the scrotum. Typically described as a "bag of worms" lesion and most often found in the left scrotum, the varicocele is present while the man is standing and disappears in the supine position. A decreased sperm count with an increase in abnormal forms is noted in

about two thirds of men with varicocele. Surgery is curative. A scrotal support may be helpful for relief of discomfort associated with varicocele.

DISCUSSION SOURCE

Stoller, M., and Carrol, P. (2003). Urology. In Tierney, L., McPhee, S., and Papadakis, M. (eds.). Current Medical Diagnosis and Treatment (42nd ed., pp. 903–945). New York: Lange Medical Books/McGraw-Hill.

QUESTIONS

39. How long after contact does the onset of clinical manifestations of syphilis typically occur?

    A. less than 1 week
    B. 1 to 3 weeks
    C. 2 to 4 weeks
    D. 4 to 6 weeks

40. Which of the following is not representative of the presentation of primary syphilis?

    A. a painless ulcer
    B. palpable inguinal nodes
    C. flulike symptoms
    D. a spontaneously healing lesion

41. Which of the following is not representative of the presentation of secondary syphilis?

    A. generalized rash
    B. chancre
    C. arthralgia
    D. aortic regurgitation

42. Which of the following is found in tertiary syphilis?

    A. arthralgia
    B. lymphadenopathy
    C. macropapular lesions involving the palms and soles
    D. gumma

43. Syphilis is most contagious at which of the following times?

A. before onset of signs and symptoms
B. during the primary stage
C. during the secondary stage
D. during the tertiary stage

44. First-line treatment options for syphilis include:

A. penicillin.
B. ciprofloxacin.
C. erythromycin.
D. ceftriaxone.

ANSWERS

39. C	**40.** C	**41.** B
42. D	**43.** C	**44.** A

DISCUSSION

Caused by the spirochete *Treponema pallidum*, syphilis is a complex, multiorgan disease. Sexual contact is the usual route of transmission. The initial lesion forms about 2 to 4 weeks after contact; contagion is greatest during the secondary stage. Treatment is guided by the stage of disease and clinical manifestation (Table 7–2).

As with all STIs, a critical part of care is discussion of prevention strategies, including condom use and limiting the number of sexual partners. Offer and encourage testing for other STIs, including HIV.

DISCUSSION SOURCES

Centers for Disease Control and Prevention (2002). 2002 Guidelines for Treatment of Sexually Transmitted Disease. Available at http://www.cdc.gov/STD/treatment/, accessed 4/3/03.

Jacobs, R. (2003). Infectious diseases: Spirochetal. In Tierney, L., McPhee, S., and Papadakis, M. (eds.). Current Medical Diagnosis and Treatment (42nd ed., pp. 1390–1410). New York: Lange Medical Books/McGraw-Hill.

QUESTIONS

45. Sequelae of genital human papillomavirus (HPV) infection in a man may include:

A. anorectal carcinoma.
B. low sperm count.
C. paraphimosis.
D. Reiter syndrome.

46. Which of the following best describes the lesions associated with condyloma acuminatum?

A. verruciform
B. plaquelike
C. vesicular
D. bullous

47. Treatment options for patients with condyloma acuminatum include:

A. imiquimod.
B. penicillin.
C. acyclovir.
D. metronidazole.

48. Which HPV types are most likely to cause colorectal carcinoma?

A. 1 and 3
B. 6 and 11
C. 16 and 18
D. 72 and 81

49. Which HPV types are most likely to cause condyloma acuminatum?

A. 1, 2, and 3
B. 6 and 11
C. 16 and 19
D. 22 and 24

ANSWERS

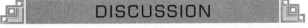

45. A	**46.** A	**47.** A
48. C	**49.** B	

DISCUSSION

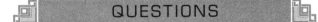

Condyloma acuminatum is a verruciform lesion seen in genital warts and is an STI. The causative agent is HPV, with multiple HPV types usually seen with genital infection. Anal, penile, and cervical carcinoma can be consequences of HPV infection. However, not all HPV types are correlated with malignancy.

━━━ **TABLE 7–2** ━━━

STAGES OF SYPHILIS, CLINICAL MANIFESTATIONS AND RECOMMENDED
TREATMENT

Stage of Syphilis	Clinical Manifestations	Treatment Options	Comment
Primary syphilis	Painless genital ulcer with a clean base and indurated margins, localized lymphadenopathy	Recommended therapy: • Benzathine penicillin G 2.4 million units IM Alternative therapy in penicillin allergy: • Doxycycline, 100 mg PO BID × 2 wk Or • Tetracycline, 500 mg PO QID × 2 wk	Also treatment for secondary syphilis or latent syphilis of <1 year's duration
Secondary syphilis	Diffuse maculopapular rash involving palms and soles, generalized lymphadenopathy, low-grade fever, malaise, arthralgias and myalgia, headache	Recommended therapy: • Benzathine penicillin G 2.4 million units IM as single dose Alternative therapy in penicillin allergy: • Doxycycline, 100 mg PO BID × 2 wk Or • Tetracycline, 500 mg PO QID × 2 wk	Also treatment for secondary syphilis or latent syphilis of <1 year's duration
Late or tertiary syphilis	Gumma (granulomatous lesions involving skin, mucous membranes, bone), aortic insufficiency, aortic aneurysm, Argyle Robertson pupil, seizures)	Recommended therapy: • Benzathine penicillin G, 2.4 million UIM weekly × 3 wk Alternative therapy: • Doxycycline, 100 mg PO BID × 4 wk or • Tetracycline, 500 mg PO QID × 4 wk	Also treatment for latent syphilis of >1 year's or unknown duration

From Centers for Disease Control and Prevention (2002). Guidelines for Treatment of Sexually Transmitted Disease. Available at http://www.cdc.gov/STD/treatment/, accessed 4/3/03. IM, intramuscularly; PO, orally.

HPV types with a high malignancy risk include types 16, 18, 31, 33, 35, 39, and 45, whereas low malignancy risk is seen with infection from types 6, 11, 40, 42, 43, 44, 54, 61, 70, 72, and 81. HPV types 6 and 11 most often cause genital warts. About 50% of patients have a spontaneous regression of warts without intervention. Treatment options include podofilox, imiquimod, trichloroacetic acid, and cryotherapy. Patient-administered therapies such as imiquimod (Aldara) or podofilox save on the cost and inconvenience of office visits. Surgical intervention is typically reserved for complicated, recalcitrant lesions (see Table 7–1).

As with all STIs, a critical part of care is discussion of prevention strategies, including condom use and limiting the number of sexual partners. The NP should offer and encourage testing for other STIs, including HIV.

DISCUSSION SOURCES

Centers for Disease Control and Prevention (2002). 2002 Guidelines for Treatment of Sexually

Transmitted Disease. Available at http://www.cdc.gov/STD/treatment/, accessed 4/3/03.

Jen, K. (2004). Male genitalia disorders. In Hektor Dunphy, L. Management Guidelines for Nurse Practitioners Working with Adults (2nd ed., pp 350–378). Philadelphia: F.A. Davis.

QUESTIONS

50. Which of the following is not a common risk factor for erectile dysfunction (ED)?

    A. diabetes mellitus
    B. hypertension
    C. cigarette smoking
    D. testosterone deficiency

51. Patient education about the use of sildenafil includes the following:

    A. A spontaneous erection occurs about 1 hour after taking the medication.
    B. This medication helps nearly all men who use it regain erectile function.
    C. With the use of the medication, sexual stimulation will also be needed to achieve an erection.
    D. Nitrates can be safely used concurrently.

52. When discussing ED with a 70 year-old man, the NP considers that:

    A. it is a consequence of aging.
    B. most cases have an underlying cause.
    C. although depression is common in older men, it is usually not correlated with increased rates of ED.
    D. treatment options for younger men are seldom effective in older men.

ANSWERS

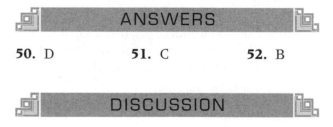

50. D   **51.** C   **52.** B

DISCUSSION

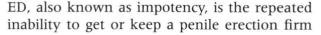

ED, also known as impotency, is the repeated inability to get or keep a penile erection firm enough for sexual intercourse. The spectrum of ED includes the total inability to achieve erection, an inconsistent ability to do so, and a tendency to sustain only brief erections. Achieving and sustaining a penile erection requires a precise sequence of events that depend on healthy nervous system function (brain, spinal column, penile innervation), appropriate muscle response, and intact blood flow via patent veins and arteries in and near the corpora cavernosa; therefore, any disorder that causes injury to the nerves or impairs blood flow in the penis has the potential to cause ED. Diabetes mellitus, kidney disease, chronic alcoholism, vascular disease, tobacco use, neuropathy, and urologic surgery such as radical prostatectomy are implicated in at least 70% of men with ED. Certain medications such as antihypertensives, antidepressants, and cimetidine can produce ED as a side effect. The presence of a mood disorder significantly contributes to the risk of ED. Hormonal disorders, particularly testosterone deficiency, pose a significant but uncommon ED risk. The incidence of ED increases with age, found in about 5% of 40-year-old men and 15% to 25% of 65-year-old men. However, this condition should not be thought to be an inevitable consequence of aging. Although most ED in older men has a physical cause, such as disease, injury, or side effects of drugs, treatment can often help the patient regain satisfactory sexual function.

Intervention in ED starts with treating or minimizing the underlying cause. With currently available therapies, effective ED treatment can be provided for the majority of affected men. Medications such as sildenafil and vardenafil work by enhancing the effects of nitric oxide, a chemical that relaxes smooth muscles in the penis during sexual stimulation and allows increased blood flow; its use does not trigger an automatic erection and should be taken about 1 hour before the anticipated onset of sexual activity. The concomitant use of a drug such as sildenafil with a nitrate is contraindicated because of the risk of profound hypotension. Drugs injected directly into the penis, such as alprostadil (Caverject), cause vasodilatation and are highly effective. An alprostadil pellet inserted into the urethra (Muse) can achieve the same effect.

Mechanical vacuum devices cause erection by creating a partial vacuum, which draws blood into the penis, engorging and expanding it. An elastic band is then placed around the base of the penis to maintain the erection after the cylinder is removed and during intercourse by preventing blood from flowing back into the body. This affords a mechanical method of ED treatment, particularly helpful when other methods fail to achieve desired results. Surgical options include vessel repair to treat the underlying ED; it should be borne in mind that atherosclerosis is a widespread disease and outcomes are unpredictable. Implantation of devices such as prostheses or pumps is another option, albeit with the associated risks and costs of any surgical procedure.

DISCUSSION SOURCES

Jen, K. (2004). Male genitalia disorders. In Hektor Dunphy, L. Management Guidelines for Nurse Practitioners Working with Adults (2nd ed., pp 350–378). Philadelphia: F.A. Davis.

Stoller, M., and Carrol, P. (2003). Urology. In Tierney, L., McPhee, S., and Papadakis, M. (eds.). Current Medical Diagnosis and Treatment (42nd ed., pp. 903–945). New York: Lange Medical Books/McGraw-Hill.

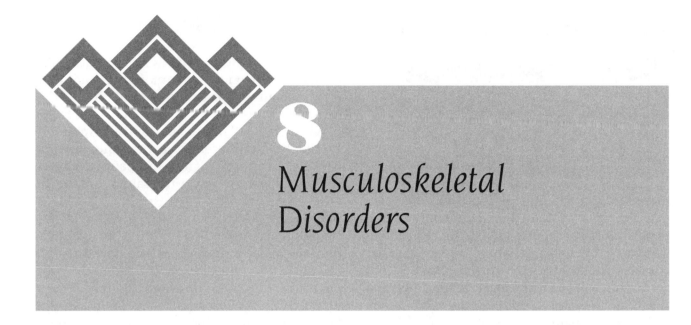

8

Musculoskeletal Disorders

1. The most common cause of bursitis is:

   A. inactivity.
   B. joint overuse.
   C. fibromyalgia.
   D. gonococcal infection.

2. First-line bursitis treatment options likely include:

   A. corticosteroid bursal injection.
   B. heat to area.
   C. weight-bearing exercises.
   D. nonsteroidal anti-inflammatory drugs (NSAIDs).

3. Patients with olecranon bursitis typically present with:

   A. swelling and redness over the affected area.
   B. limited elbow range of motion (ROM).
   C. nerve impingement.
   D. destruction of the joint space.

4. Patients with subscapular bursitis typically present with:

   A. limited shoulder ROM.
   B. heat over the affected area.
   C. localized tenderness under the supero-medial angle of the scapula.
   D. cervical nerve root irritation.

5. Patients with gluteus medius or deep trochanteric bursitis typically present with:

   A. increased pain from resisted hip abduction.
   B. limited hip ROM.
   C. sciatic nerve pain.
   D. heat over the affected area.

6. Likely sequelae of intrabursal corticosteroid injection include:

   A. irreversible skin atrophy.
   B. infection.
   C. inflammatory reaction.
   D. soreness at the site of injection.

7. First-line prepatellar bursitis therapy should include:

   A. bursal aspiration.
   B. intrabursal steroid injection.
   C. acetaminophen.
   D. knee splinting.

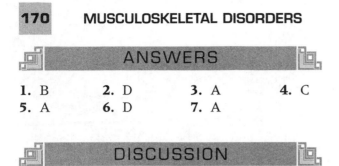

ANSWERS

1. B	**2.** D	**3.** A	**4.** C
5. A	**6.** D	**7.** A	

DISCUSSION

Bursitis, inflammation of the fluid-filled sacs that act as a cushion between tendons and bones, most commonly affects the subdeltoid, olecranon, ischial, trochanter, and prepatellar bursae. Unlike arthritis, bursitis typically has an abrupt onset with focal tenderness and swelling. The joint ROM is usually full but may be limited by pain (Table 8–1).

Risk factors for bursitis include joint overuse, trauma, infection, or arthritis conditions such as rheumatoid arthritis or osteoarthritis. Because recurrence is common, prevention of further joint overuse and trauma should be emphasized.

With prepatellar bursitis, bursal aspiration should be considered as a first-line therapy because it affords significant pain relief, as well as allows the bursa to reapproximate. In other sites, first-line bursitis therapy includes minimizing or eliminating the offending activity, applying ice to the affected area for 15 minutes at least four times per day, and the use of NSAIDs. If these conservative measures have not worked after approximately 4 to 8 weeks, intrabursal steroid injection should be given. Before injection, patients should be informed of the risks of this procedure, especially the most common problem: soreness

---

TABLE 8–1
CLINICAL PRESENTATION OF BURSITIS

Location of Bursitis	Clinical Presentation	Comments
Prepatellar (knee)	Knee swelling and pain in the front of the knee, normal ROM	Risk factors include frequent kneeling (housemaid's knee)
Olecranon (elbow)	Pain, swelling behind the elbow, swelling in same area, often described as ball or sac hanging from the elbow	Risk factors include prolonged pressure or trauma to the elbow (draftsman's elbow)
Trochanter (hip)	Gait disturbance, local trochanter tenderness, pain on hip rotation and resisted hip abduction with normal hip ROM	Risk factors include back disease, leg length discrepancy, and leg problems that lead to altered gait OA is seldom implicated
Subscapular (shoulder)	Local tenderness under the superomedial angle of the scapula over the adjacent rib, normal shoulder ROM, no nerve root impingement	Risk factors include repeated back-and-forth motion Common in assembly-line workers
Pre-Achilles (heel)	Pain and localized swelling behind the heel, minimal pain with dorsiflexion, normal ankle ROM	Usually not disabling and does not contribute to tendon rupture Often confused with Achilles tendonitis
Retrocalcaneal (heel)	Pain behind ankle made worse by walking Patient often runs fingers along both sides of Achilles tendon	Risk factors include wearing high-heeled shoes and repetitive ankle motion such as stair-climbing, running, jogging, and walking

OA, osteoarthritis; ROM, range of motion.

at the injection site. Infection, tissue atrophy, and inflammatory reaction are rarely encountered.

DISCUSSION SOURCES

Anderson, B. (1999). Office Orthopedics for Primary Care: Diagnosis and Treatment (2nd ed.). Philadelphia: W. B. Saunders.

Szoke-Halal, A.M. (2004). Musculoskeletal disorders. In Hektor Dunphy, L. Management Guidelines for Nurse Practitioners Working with Adults, pp 379–410. Philadelphia, F.A. Davis.

QUESTIONS

8. Patients with lateral epicondylitis typically present with:

    A. electric-like pain elicited by tapping over the median nerve.
    B. reduced joint range of motion.
    C. pain that is at its worst with elbow flexion.
    D. decreased hand grip strength.

9. Risk factors for lateral epicondylitis include all of the following except:

    A. repetitive lifting.
    B. playing tennis.
    C. hammering.
    D. gout.

10. Initial therapy for treatment of lateral epicondylitis includes:

    A. a long arm cast.
    B. a short arm cast with a thumb spica.
    C. a wrist splint with metal stays.
    D. a shoulder sling.

11. Patients with medial epicondylitis typically present with:

    A. forearm numbness.
    B. reduction in ROM.
    C. pain on elbow flexion.
    D. decreased grip strength.

12. Risk factors for medial epicondylitis include playing:

    A. tennis.
    B. golf.
    C. baseball.
    D. volleyball.

ANSWERS

8. D   **9.** D   **10.** C
11. D   **12.** B

DISCUSSION

The painful condition that arises as a result of injury to the extensor tendon at the lateral epicondyle is often called tennis elbow or lateral epicondylitis. Patients usually give a history of an aggravating activity followed by forearm weakness and point to tenderness over the inner aspect of the humerus (Table 8–2). Medial epicondylitis is often called golfer's elbow.

Conservative therapy in the first 3 to 4 weeks should include avoidance of the precipitating activity, application of appropriate splints, and use of NSAIDs. If symptoms persist, a short arm cast may be used to further limit arm movement. Local corticosteroid injection may be helpful if symptoms persist beyond 6 to 8 weeks or are particularly severe. The use of a tennis elbow band may help prevent recurrence.

DISCUSSION SOURCES

Anderson, B. (1999). Office Orthopedics for Primary Care: Diagnosis and Treatment (2nd ed.). Philadelphia: W. B. Saunders.

Szoke-Halal, A.M. (2004). Musculoskeletal disorders. In Hektor Dunphy, L. Management Guidelines for Nurse Practitioners Working with Adults, pp 379–410. Philadelphia, F.A. Davis.

QUESTIONS

13. Risk factors for gouty arthritis include:

    A. thiazide diuretic use.
    B. female gender.
    C. rheumatoid arthritis.
    D. joint trauma.

■■■■ **TABLE 8–2** ■■■■
CLINICAL PRESENTATION OF EPICONDYLITIS

Condition	Presentation	Comments
Medial epicondylitis	Patient complains of pain over medial epicondyle or inner aspect of lower humerus. Pain worsens with wrist flexion and pronation activities. Local epicondylar tenderness, elbow pain, forearm weakness, pain aggravated by wrist flexion, and pronation activities with decreased grip strength and full range of motion	Often called golfers' elbow; results from repetitive activity such as lifting, tooling, sports involving a tight grip. Prevent recurrence by using palm-up lifting, use of a tennis elbow band as well as avoiding precipitating causes, proper use of tools, proper body mechanics, flexibility and strength of the involved musculature.
Lateral epicondylitis	Patient complains of pain over the lateral epicondyle or outer aspect of the lower humerus, increases with resisted wrist extension, especially with elbow. Hand grip often weak on affected side. Elbow range of motion usually within normal limits.	Often called tennis elbow; results from repetitive activity such as lifting, tooling, sports involving a tight grip. Prevent recurrence by avoiding precipitating causes, proper use of tools, proper body mechanics, flexibility and strength of the involved musculature.

Gibbs, S. (2004). Medial epicondylitis, available at *http://www.emedicine.com/pmr/topic74.htm.* accessed 10/10/04.
Lorenzo, C. (2004). Lateral epicondylitis, available at *http://www.emedicine, com/PMR/topic64.htm,* accessed 10/10/04.

14. The clinical presentation of gouty arthritis affecting the great toe includes:

    A. slow onset of discomfort over a number of days.
    B. greatest swelling and pain along the median border of the joint.
    C. improvement of symptoms with joint rest.
    D. fever.

15. The most helpful diagnostic test to perform during acute gouty arthritis is:

    A. measurement of erythrocyte sedimentation rate (ESR).
    B. measurement of serum uric acid.
    C. analysis of joint aspirate.
    D. joint radiography.

16. First-line therapy for the treating patients with acute gouty arthritis includes:

    A. aspirin.
    B. naproxen sodium.
    C. allopurinol.
    D. probenecid.

17. Which of the following patients with acute gouty arthritis is the best candidate for local corticosteroid injection?

    A. a 66-year-old patient with a gastric ulcer
    B. a 44-year-old patient taking a thiazide diuretic
    C. a 68-year-old patient with type 2 diabetes mellitus
    D. a 32-year-old patient who is a binge drinker

18. The most common locations for tophi include all of the following except:

    A. the auricles.
    B. the elbows.
    C. the extensor surfaces of the hands.
    D. the shoulders

19. Dietary recommendations for the person with gouty arthritis include avoiding foods high in:

    A. artificial flavors and colors.
    B. purine.

C. vitamin C.

D. protein.

ANSWERS

13. A	**14.** B	**15.** C
16. B	**17.** A	
18. D	**19.** B	

DISCUSSION

Gout is an acute monoarticular arthritis usually caused by a disorder in uric acid excretion that allows an accumulation of urates in joints, bones, and subcutaneous tissues. About 90% of patients with primary gout are men; the condition is rarely seen in women before menopause. Risk factors include obesity and diabetes mellitus. Less often, gout is caused by excessive uric acid production, sometimes coupled with decreased urate excretion. The use of certain medications can precipitate a gouty episode (secondary gout) by this mechanism; alcohol use also precipitates gout by this mechanism. The use of other medications presents gout risk by causing hyperuricemia; these medications include thiazide diuretics, niacin, aspirin, and cyclosporine. Other causes of secondary gout include conditions characterized by increased catabolism and purine turnover, such as psoriasis, myeloproliferative and lymphoproliferative diseases, and chronic hemolytic anemia, as well as conditions with decreased renal uric acid clearance, such as intrinsic kidney disease.

This acutely painful condition typically affects the metacarpophalangeal joint of the great toe. The onset is sudden and is accompanied by significant distress. Patients report the inability to move the joint, walk, or even tolerate the weight of a bed sheet on the affected joint because of pain. The entire great toe is usually reddened and enlarged, and the greatest amount of swelling is noted along the median border of the joint; this usually is also the point of greatest discomfort. Although the presentation of gout can mimic that of an acutely infected joint, it is important to remember that gout is 100 times more common than monoarticular septic arthritis. With repeated episodes, tophic, nontender firm nodules can develop in soft tissue. Because the gouty crystals that fill tophi precipitate more easily in cooler areas of the body, these lesions often develop in the external ear; less common locations include nasal cartilage, extensor surfaces of the hands and feet, and over the elbows.

The diagnosis of acute gouty arthritis is usually straightforward, particularly in repeated episodes. With the first episode, uric acid levels may be obtained. However, uric levels may be reduced during the acute phase, or the etiology is largely one of poor urate excretion. Analysis of joint aspirate for urate crystals is diagnostic; the ESR is usually high, but this is neither sensitive nor specific for gout. Radiographs are not needed unless there are both a concurrent history of trauma and risk of fracture.

The treatment of acute gouty arthritis should include minimizing or removing contributing factors such as alcohol or thiazide diuretic use. Treatment should be aimed at reducing inflammation first and then treating hyperuricemia, trying to avoid a rapid reduction in serum uric acid, which may make the episode worse. A loading dose of an NSAID, such as naproxen, 750 mg, or indomethacin, 50 mg, followed by lower doses, can be helpful. Colchicine, 0.6 mg every hour up to 7.2 mg or when gastrointestinal symptoms occur, can be used. Because the use of aspirin can precipitate gout, it is contraindicated. Local injection with corticosteroids can provide significant relief and offers a treatment alternative to NSAIDs, particularly in the presence of warfarin use, renal failure, or peptic ulcer disease. Dietary modification to avoid foods with high purine content is an important and often overlooked intervention to minimize the risk of future gout episodes. Examples of high-purine foods include meats, seafood, beans, spinach, asparagus, and items containing yeast and yeast extracts.

After the acute flare has subsided, a 24-hour

urine collection for uric acid helps assess whether the patient overproduces or undersecretes uric acid. Long-term care to avoid future attacks is directed by the result: Undersecretors benefit from probenecid and overproducers from allopurinol.

DISCUSSION SOURCES

Anderson, B. (1999). Office Orthopedics for Primary Care: Diagnosis and Treatment (2nd ed.). Philadelphia: W. B. Saunders.

Hellman, D., and Stone, J. (2003). Arthritis and musculoskeletal disorders. In Tierney, L., McPhee, S., and Papadakis, M. (cds.). Current Diagnosis and Treatment (42nd ed., pp. 783–836). New York: Lange Medical Books/McGraw-Hill.

Szoke-Halal, A.M. (2004). Musculoskeletal disorders. In Hektor Dunphy, L. Management Guidelines for Nurse Practitioners Working with Adults, pp 379–410. Philadelphia, F.A. Davis.

QUESTIONS

20. Which of the following joints is most likely to be affected by osteoarthritis?

    A. the wrists
    B. the elbows
    C. the metacarpophalangeal joint
    D. the distal interphalangeal joint

21. Deformity of the proximal interphalangeal joints found in an elderly patient with osteoarthritis is known as:

    A. Heberden nodes.
    B. Bouchard nodes.
    C. Hallus valgus
    D. Dupuytren contracture

22. Which of the following best describes the presentation of a patient with osteoarthritis?

    A. worst symptoms in weight-bearing joints later in the day
    B. symmetric early morning stiffness
    C. sausage-shaped digits with associated skin lesions
    D. back pain with rest and anterior uveitis

23. As part of the evaluation of patients with osteoarthritis, the nurse practitioner (NP) anticipates finding:

    A. anemia of chronic disease
    B. elevated C-reactive protein level
    C. narrowing of the joint space on radiograph
    D. elevated antinuclear antibody (ANA) titer

24. First-line pharmacologic intervention for milder osteoarthritis should be a trial of:

    A. acetaminophen.
    B. naproxen.
    C. celecoxib.
    D. intra-articular corticosteroid injection.

25. In caring for a patient with osteoarthritis of the knee, you advise that:

    A. straight-leg raising should be avoided.
    B. heat should be applied to painful joints after exercise.
    C. quadriceps-strengthening exercises should be performed.
    D. exercise should be avoided.

26. Glucosamine and chondroitin are nutritional supplements that may help in the treatment of:

    A. rheumatoid arthritis.
    B. osteoarthritis.
    C. prevention of upper respiratory infections.
    D. insomnia.

ANSWERS

20. D	21. B	22. A
23. C	24. A	
25. C	26. B	

DISCUSSION

Osteoarthritis is the most common joint disease in the United States, affecting more than 20 million people. It is a degenerative disease without systemic manifestations or inflammation. The most problematic joint involvement is the hip and knee. Worst symptoms are reported with use of the joints, and there is minimum morning stiffness (in contrast to rheumatoid arthritis). Risk factors for osteoarthritis include a positive family history of osteoarthritis and contact sport participation. Obesity is also a risk factor, especially with hip and knee involvement.

In osteoarthritis, the articular cartilage becomes rough and wears away. Bone spurs may form, and the synovial membrane thickens. Consequently, the joint space narrows.

The clinical presentation in patients with osteoarthritis includes an insidious onset of symptoms, including use-related joint pain that is relieved by rest and joint stiffness that occurs with rest but resolves with less than 15 minutes of activity. Physical examination reveals smooth, cool joints and coarse crepitus. Particularly when the knee is affected, joint effusion is common and may be minimal to severe with up to 20 mL of fluid. Patients cannot achieve full knee flexion in the effused joint. The knee often locks or pops, which suggests a degenerative meniscal tear.

Radiologic findings in patients with osteoarthritis include narrowing of the joint space and increased density of subchondral bone. Bone cysts and osteophytes are often present. However, only about 50% of patients with radiologic findings have symptoms. Because osteoarthritis is typically a noninflammatory disease, ESR and C-reactive protein level, both markers of inflammation, are typically normal. In contrast to rheumatoid arthritis and systemic lupus erythematosus (SLE), ANAs are absent from the serum.

Therapeutic goals for those with osteoarthritis include preventing further articular cartilage destruction, minimizing pain, and enhancing mobility. Therapies for symptom control include lifestyle modification such as weight loss and minimum weight-bearing exercise such as swimming or water-based activities, as well as exercise to maintain joint flexibility and enhance strength in the surrounding muscles (Table 8–3). Application of heat to minimize pain and stiffness in the morning before activity can be helpful, but applying ice to the joint after activity can minimize discomfort. Acetaminophen and NSAIDs have long been used as arthritis drug treatments. These medications are helpful in controlling pain. Although NSAIDs also have potential anti-inflammatory activity, this is seldom needed in osteoarthritis therapy. Because of the gastropathy potential associated with long-term NSAID use, a trial of acetaminophen is warranted for symptom control in less severe cases of osteoarthritis; NSAIDs have superior analgesic effect. Long-acting opioids may be required if symptom control cannot be achieved.

Glucosamine, an amino acid, is usually used as first-line treatment for osteoarthritis in

TABLE 8–3

TREATMENT OF RHEUMATOID ARTHRITIS

Medication	Examples
Anti-inflammatory agents	NSAIDs, COX-2 inhibitors, corticosteroids.
Analgesics	NSAIDs, COX-2 inhibitors, acetaminophen, opioids, topical agents.
DMARDs (Disease-modifying anti-rheumatic drugs)	Anti-metabolites: methotrexate, leflunomide, azathioprine. Cytokine inhibitors: Cyclosporine, infliximab, etanercept, others. IL-1 receptor antagonist: anakinra. Miscellaneous DMARDs: Ridaura, injectable gold, hydroxychloroquine, penicillamine, sulfasalazine, minocycline, cyclophosphamide.

Hellman, D., and Stone, J. (2003). Arthritis and musculoskeletal disorder. In Tierney, L., McPhee, S., and Papadakis, M. Current Diagnosis and Treatment (42nd ed, p 783). New York: Lange Medical Books/McGraw-Hill, and American College of Rheumatology Guidelines for the management of rheumatoid arthritis, available at http://www.rheumatology.org/research/guidelines/raguidelines02.pdf, accessed 5/3/03.

many European nations and is available as an over-the-counter nutritional supplement in the United States. It appears to help rebuild damaged joint cartilage and results in reduction in pain, increased joint flexion, and articular function. Glucosamine must be used consistently for a minimum of 2 weeks and likely as long as 3 months before therapeutic effect is seen. Although no drug interactions or hepatotoxicity have been noted with its use, glucosamine should be used with caution because there is a risk of bronchospasm. Chondroitin is often used in conjunction with glucosamine because the two appear to have synergistic activity, although this has been disputed in limited study. Chondroitin's mechanism of action is not well understood. It is derived from bovine tracheal cartilage. Although chondroitin is generally well tolerated, it should be used with caution because of a potential anticoagulant effect.

Intra-articular corticosteroid joint injection may help when more conservative therapy has failed. In particular with osteoarthritis in the knee, corticosteroid injection can help when joint effusion is present. Hip injection is a technically challenging procedure that can be done with fluoroscopic guidance.

Joint replacement should be considered when pain is intractable, when function is severely compromised, or when more than 80% of the articular cartilage is worn away. Duration of prosthetic joint function is typically 10 to 15 years. As a result, the ideal candidate for joint replacement is older than 60 years and is able to tolerate a surgical procedure that lasts for several hours, followed by an aggressive postoperative course of rehabilitation. A patellar restraining brace, walker, or wheelchair may be needed for patients with advanced osteoarthritis of the knee and hip that cannot be surgically repaired.

DISCUSSION SOURCES

American College of Rheumatology (2002). Recommendations for the Medical Management of Osteoarthritis of the Hip and Knee. Available at http://www.rheumatology.org/ publications/guidelines/oa-mgmt/oa-mgmt.asp, accessed 5/3/03.

Anderson, B. (1999). Office Orthopedics for Primary Care: Diagnosis and Treatment (2nd ed.). Philadelphia: W. B. Saunders.

Hellman, D., and Stone, J. (2003). Arthritis and musculoskeletal disorder. In Tierney, L., McPhee, S., and Papadakis, M. (eds.). Current Diagnosis and Treatment (42nd ed., pp. 783–836). New York: Lange Medical Books/McGraw-Hill.

Szoke-Halal, A.M. (2004). Musculoskeletal disorders. In Hektor Dunphy, L. Management Guidelines for Nurse Practitioners Working with Adults, pp 379–410. Philadelphia, F.A. Davis.

QUESTIONS

27. Which of the following is not characteristic of rheumatoid arthritis?

   A. More common in women at a 3:1 ratio
   B. Family history of rheumatoid disease often reported by patient
   C. Peak age for disease onset from 50 to 70 years of age
   D. Wrists, ankles, and toes are often involved

28. Which of the following best describes the presentation of a person with rheumatoid arthritis?

   A. worst symptoms in weight-bearing joints later in the day
   B. symmetric early-morning stiffness
   C. sausage-shaped digits with skin lesions
   D. back pain with rest and anterior uveitis

29. NSAIDs cause gastric injury primarily by:

   A. direct irritative effect.
   B. slowing gastrointestinal motility.
   C. thinning of the protective mucosa.
   D. enhancing prostaglandin synthesis.

30. Of the following, who is at highest risk for NSAID-induced gastropathy?

   A. a 28-year-old man with an ankle sprain who has taken ibuprofen for the past week and who drinks four to six beers every weekend

B. a 40-year-old woman who smokes and takes about six doses of naproxen sodium per month to control dysmenorrhea

C. a 43-year-old man with dilated cardiomyopathy who uses ketoprofen one to two times per week for low back pain

D. a 72-year-old man who takes aspirin four times a day for pain control of osteoarthritis

31. Which of the following is the preferred method of preventing NSAID-induced gastric ulcer?

    A. a high-dose histamine 2 receptor antagonist
    B. timed antacid use
    C. sucralfate (Carafate)
    D. misoprostol (Cytotec)

32. Taking a high dose of aspirin or ibuprofen causes:

    A. an increase in the drug's half-life.
    B. enhanced renal excretion of the drug.
    C. a change in the drug's mechanism of action.
    D. a lowering of antiprostaglandin effect.

33. Which of the following is most accurate concerning rheumatoid arthritis?

    A. Joint erosions may be evident on radiographs.
    B. Men are affected more frequently than women.
    C. A butterfly-shaped facial rash is common.
    D. Parvovirus B_{19} infection may contribute to its development.

34. Principles of treating patients with rheumatoid arthritis include:

    A. using a stepwise approach to care.
    B. early use of disease-modifying antirheumatic drugs (DMARDs) to slow or stop joint damage.
    C. pain relief as the chief therapeutic goal.
    D. recognizing that joint splinting is seldom advisable.

35. Which of the following tests is most specific to the diagnosis of rheumatoid arthritis?

    A. elevated levels of rheumatoid factor
    B. elevated ESR
    C. depressed total white blood cell count
    D. elevated levels of ANA

36. A 52-year-old woman has rheumatoid arthritis. She now presents with decreased tearing, "gritty"-feeling eyes, and a dry mouth. You consider a diagnosis of:

    A. systemic lupus erythematosus (SLE).
    B. vasculitis.
    C. Sjögren syndrome.
    D. scleroderma.

37. Cyclooxygenase-1 (COX-1) contributes to:

    A. inflammatory response.
    B. pain transmission.
    C. maintenance of gastric protective mucosal layer.
    D. renal arteriole constriction.

38. Cyclooxygenase-2 (COX-2) contributes to all of the following except:

    A. inflammatory response.
    B. pain transmission.
    C. maintenance of gastric protective mucosal layer.
    D. renal arteriole constriction.

39. Which of the following special examinations should be periodically obtained during hydroxychloroquine sulfate use?

    A. ophthalmoscopy
    B. bone marrow biopsy
    C. pulmonary function tests
    D. exercise tolerance test

ANSWERS

27. C	**28.** B	**29.** C
30. D	**31.** D	**32.** A
33. A	**34.** B	**35.** A
36. C	**37.** C	
38. C	**39.** A	

DISCUSSION

Rheumatoid arthritis is a disease causing chronic systemic inflammation, including the synovial membranes of multiple joints. As with most autoimmune diseases, rheumatoid arthritis is more common in women, at a 3:1 ratio. Although new-onset rheumatoid arthritis can occur at any age, peak age at onset is from 20 to 40 years. A family history of rheumatoid disease is often noted. Initial presentation may be with acute polyarticular inflammation. However, a clinical picture of slowly progressive malaise, weight loss, and stiffness is more common (Table 8–4). The stiffness is symmetric, is typically worst upon arising, lasts about 1 hour, involves at least three joint groups, and can recur after a period of inactivity or exercise. The hands (with sparing of the distal interphalangeal joints), wrists, ankles, and toes are most often involved. Soft tissue swelling or fluid is also present, as are subcutaneous nodules. There are often periods of exacerbation and remission. Whereas in the past rheumatoid arthritis was noted to be a debilitating condition with little impact on longevity, it is now known to potentially shorten the lifespan while producing considerable disability, particularly without optimal treatment.

Common diagnostic tests in rheumatoid arthritis include the ANA, ESR, and rheuma-

TABLE 8–4

AMERICAN COLLEGE OF RHEUMATOLOGY CRITERIA
FOR DIAGNOSIS OF RHEUMATOID ARTHRITIS*

Criterion	Comment
Morning stiffness	Lasting ≥1 hr in and around joint
Symmetric arthritis	Simultaneous involvement of joint areas on both sides
Hands involved	Wrist, PIP, and MCP involvement with evidence of fluid, joint swelling
Rheumatoid nodules	Subcutaneous nodules over bony prominences, extensor surfaces, and/or juxta-articular regions
Arthritis of three or more joints	Simultaneous soft tissue swelling or fluid in up to 14 possible areas (right or left PIP, MCP, wrist, elbow, knee, ankle, MTP)
Serum rheumatoid factor	Abnormal amounts present in serum Although noted in approximately 85% with RA, false-positive and false-negative test results are possible
Radiographic changes	Include juxta-articular osteopenia, joint erosions, narrowing of joint space, most marked in involved joints

Adapted from American College of Rheumatology (2002). Fact Sheet on Rheumatoid Arthritis. Available at www.rheumatology.org/factsheet/ra.html, accessed 10/10/04; and from American College of Rheumatology (2002). Guidelines for the Management of Rheumatoid Arthritis. Available at http://www.rheumatology.org/publications/guidelines/raguidelines02.asp, accessed 5/3/03.
*Four of the seven criteria must be present for ≥6 weeks.
MCP, metacarpophalangeal; MTP, metatarsophalangeal; PIP, proximal interphalangeal; RA, rheumatoid arthritis.

toid factor measurements and radiographs. When interpreting results, the NP should bear in mind the following:

- Radiographs typically reveal joint erosion and loss of normal joint space.
- ESR is a nonspecific test of inflammation. In general, the higher the ESR, the greater the degree and intensity of the inflammatory process. Although it is frequently elevated in patients with rheumatoid arthritis, its presence is not diagnostic of this or other conditions. In addition, a single elevated ESR is seldom helpful; however, following trends during flare and regression of disease often aids in charting the therapeutic course and response.
- C-reactive protein measurement is also a nonspecific test of inflammation. The level tends to increase more rapidly than ESR in patients with rheumatoid arthritis but decreases an equivalent amount. Its usefulness and limitations are similar to those of ESR.
- Rheumatoid factor, an immunoglobulin M antibody, is present in approximately 50% to 90% of patients with rheumatoid arthritis. The level of the titer may correspond to the severity of disease.
- Hemogram may reveal anemia of chronic disease.
- ANAs are antibodies against cellular nuclear components that act as antigens. ANA is occasionally present in healthy adults, but its presence is usually found in those with systemic rheumatic or collagen vascular disease. ANA is the most sensitive laboratory marker for SLE, detected in approximately 95% of patients, but it is found in only 30% to 50% of those with rheumatoid arthritis. Patterns of immunofluorescence vary but have been given misplaced credence as to type of disease. Here are some examples of ANA patterns:
- homogeneous, diffuse, or solid pattern to DNA: high titers strongly associated with SLE
- peripheral or rim pattern: associated with anti–double-stranded DNA and strongly correlated with SLE
- nucleolar pattern: associated with antiribonucleoprotein and strongly correlated with scleroderma
- speckled pattern: further antigen testing should be ordered with this result; this additional testing may be required in those with a variety of collagen-vascular or rheumatic diseases

The program of treatment of patients with rheumatoid arthritis is to reduce inflammation and pain while preserving function and preventing deformity. Behavioral management is key because stress may precipitate a flare of rheumatoid arthritis. Allowing for proper rest periods is critical. Physical therapists can assist in the development of a reasonable activity plan. Maintenance of physical activity through appropriate exercise is of greatest importance. Water exercise in particular is helpful because it includes mild resistance as well as buoyancy. Splints may provide joint rest while maintaining function and preventing contracture.

As helpful as NSAIDs are in symptom control, these products do not alter the underlying disease process; joint destruction continues despite control of symptoms and reduction in swelling. The use of DMARDs helps minimize the risk of joint damage and disease progression and should be started as soon as the diagnosis of rheumatoid arthritis is made (see Table 8–3). As the number and types of DMARDs available increase, knowledge of current rheumatoid arthritis therapy is critical for providing optimal patient care.

If a patient fails to achieve control of pain or symptoms with an adequate trial of a DMARD and an NSAID, additional therapy should be added. One option is intra-articular steroid injection. This can be quite helpful but should be limited to not more than two to three injections per joint per year, to minimize risk of joint deterioration. Systemic corticosteroids can be most helpful in relieving inflammation, but use should not exceed 2 to 8 weeks, if possible, because of their adverse reaction profile.

Aspirin and other NSAIDs have been the backbone of rheumatoid arthritis drug treatment for years. These medications are helpful in controlling inflammation and pain, both worthy therapeutic goals. Aspirin and ibuprofen are two of the more commonly used products. With many of the NSAIDs, the half-life of the drug is increased as the dose is raised.

A significant amount of peptic ulcer disease, particularly gastric ulcer and gastritis, is caused by NSAID use. NSAIDs inhibit synthesis of prostaglandins from arachidonic acid, yielding an anti-inflammatory effect. This is partly caused by the action of these products against cyclooxygenase (cox). COX-1 is an enzyme found in gastric mucosa, small and large intestine mucosa, kidneys, platelets, and vascular epithelium. It contributes to the health of these organs through a number of mechanisms, including the maintenance of the protective gastric mucosal layer and proper perfusion of the kidneys. COX-2 is an enzyme that produces prostaglandins important in inflammatory cascade and pain transmission. The standard NSAIDs and corticosteroids inhibit the synthesis of COX-1 and COX-2, thus controlling pain and inflammation but with gastric and renal complications. NSAIDs such as celecoxib (Celebrex) that spare COX-1 and are more COX-2-selective afford control of the potential for arthritis symptoms but have less risk of gastric problems and minimal impact on platelet activity.

Sjögren syndrome is an autoimmune disease that usually occurs in conjunction with another chronic inflammatory condition such as rheumatoid arthritis or SLE. Complaints usually concern problems related to decreased oral and ocular secretions. In addition, mouth ulcers and dental caries are common, and ESR is elevated in more than 90% of patients. A salivary gland biopsy for presence of mononuclear cells infiltration is useful. Intervention for patients with Sjögren syndrome includes management of presenting symptoms with appropriate lubricants. Treating the underlying disease is critical.

DISCUSSION SOURCES

American College of Rheumatology (2002). Guidelines for the Management of Rheumatoid Arthritis. Available at http://www.rheumatology. org/publications/guidelines/raguidelines02.asp, accessed 5/3/03.

Hellman, D., and Stone, J. (2003). Arthritis and musculoskeletal disorder. In Tierney, L., McPhee, S., and Papadakis, M. (eds.). Current Diagnosis and Treatment (42nd ed., pp. 783–836). New York: Lange Medical Books/McGraw-Hill.

Szoke-Halal, A.M. (2004). Musculoskeletal disorders. In Hektor Dunphy, L. Management Guidelines for Nurse Practitioners Working with Adults, pp 379–410. Philadelphia, F.A. Davis.

QUESTIONS

40. In order to confirm the results of a McMurray test, you ask the patient to:

   A. squat.
   B. walk.
   C. flex the knee.
   D. rotate the ankle.

41. Which of the following best describes the presentation of a patient with complete median meniscus tear?

   A. joint effusion
   B. heat over the knee
   C. inability to kneel
   D. loss of smooth joint movement

42. In order to help prevent meniscal tear, you advise:

   A. limiting participation in sports.
   B. quadriceps-strengthening exercises.
   C. using a knee brace.
   D. applying ice to the knee before exercise.

43. Initial treatment for meniscal tear includes all of the following except:

   A. NSAIDs.
   B. applying ice.
   C. elevation.
   D. joint aspiration.

ANSWERS

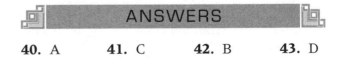

40. A   **41.** C   **42.** B   **43.** D

DISCUSSION

A meniscal tear is a disruption of the fibrocartilage pad located between the femoral condyles and the tibial plateaus. Because the purpose of the fibrocartilage pad is shock absorption and smooth joint mobility, patients with larger tears often report that the knee locks, pops, or gives out. Effusion is also common, with the patient reporting a sensation of knee tightness and stiffness. With certain positions, there is often sudden-onset, sharp, localized pain, usually on the median aspect of the knee. Over time, premature osteoarthritis is seen as the normal joint space is compromised.

Meniscal tears are often classified in a number of manners, including complex or partial; traumatic or degenerative; lateral, posterior, horizontal, or vertical; and radial, parrot-beak, or bucket-handle. Patients with partial, horizontal, and anterior tears may have relatively normal examination findings because the knee's mechanics are relatively unchanged even though these patients continue to have knee locking and pain with certain positions. The McMurray test, a palpable popping on the joint line, is highly specific but poorly sensitive for meniscal tear; the Apley grinding test gives similar results. Squatting or kneeling is nearly impossible for patients with a large, complete, or bucket-handle meniscal tear. Joint effusion is typical, with ROM being limited by discomfort.

Knee radiographs, which can reveal osteoarthritic changes and possible foreign bodies, are reasonable as initial diagnostic tests. Initial treatment includes rest, elevation, and ice application, as well as analgesia. Because joint effusion is nearly always present but is relatively mild, aspiration should be considered only if there is no improvement after 2 to 4 weeks of conservative therapy. Crutch walking should be encouraged, and a patellar stabilizer may be needed when significant knee instability is present. Straight-leg–raising exercises help strengthen the quadriceps and stabilize the joint.

Magnetic resonance imaging (MRI) can identify the type and extent of the tear and should be considered if milder symptoms do not resolve within 2 to 4 weeks or if severe symptoms do not resolve earlier. Arthroscopy, which provides the most accurate diagnosis with the possibility of concurrent treatment through débridement, should be considered at 4 to 6 weeks if there is no improvement and earlier if joint locking, giving out, and effusion are particularly problematic.

DISCUSSION SOURCES

Anderson, B. (1999). Office Orthopedics for Primary Care: Diagnosis and Treatment (2nd ed.). Philadelphia: W. B. Saunders.

Hellman, D., and Stone, J. (2003). Arthritis and musculoskeletal disorder. In Tierney, L., McPhee, S., and Papadakis, M. (eds.). Current Diagnosis and Treatment (42nd ed., pp. 783–836). New York: Lange Medical Books/McGraw-Hill.

Szoke-Halal, A.M. (2004). Musculoskeletal disorders. In Hektor Dunphy, L. Management Guidelines for Nurse Practitioners Working with Adults, pp 379–410. Philadelphia, F.A. Davis.

QUESTIONS

44. The Phalen sign is described as:

  A. reproduction of symptoms with forced flexion of the wrists.

  B. abnormal tingling when the median nerve is tapped.

  C. pain on internal rotation.

  D. palmar atrophy.

45. The Tinel sign is best described as:

  A. reproduction of symptoms with forced flexion of the wrists.

  B. abnormal tingling when the median nerve is tapped.

  C. pain on internal rotation.

  D. palmar atrophy.

46. Risk factors for carpal tunnel syndrome (CTS) include all of the following except:

  A. pregnancy.

  B. hypothyroidism.

C. repetitive motion.

D. multiple sclerosis.

47. Which of the following is least likely to be reported by patients with CTS?

A. worst symptoms during the day

B. burning sensation in the affected hand

C. tingling pain that radiates to the forearm

D. nocturnal numbness

48. Initial therapy for patients with CTS includes:

A. intra-articular injection.

B. joint splinting.

C. systemic corticosteroids.

D. referral for surgery.

49. Primary prevention of CTS includes:

A. screening for thyroid dysfunction.

B. treatment of osteoarthritis.

C. stretching and toning exercises.

D. wrist splinting.

ANSWERS

44. A	**45.** B	**46.** D
47. A	**48.** B	**49.** C

DISCUSSION

CTS is a painful syndrome caused by compression of the median nerve between the carpal ligament and other structures within the carpal tunnel. This leads to an entrapment neuropathy, causing symptoms in the distribution of the median nerve.

The most common risk factor is repetitive motion; the condition is common with protracted computer keyboard use, as well as in workers such as cake decorators and soldiers, who must continually grasp a small object. CTS may also be part of the manifestation of a systemic disease such as rheumatoid arthritis and sarcoidosis. Primary prevention of CTS includes limiting time spent in these activities, ensuring proper work breaks, and encouraging toning and stretching exercises.

Patients with CTS usually report a burning, aching, or tingling pain radiating to the forearm in the distribution of the median nerve, occasionally to the shoulder, neck, and chest. Symptoms are often worst at night. A classic finding is the report of acroparesthesia, awakening at night with numbness and burning pain in the fingers. Physical examination findings may include positive Tinel and Phalen signs, although the carpal compression test, in which symptoms are induced by direct application of pressure over the carpal tunnel, is likely a more sensitive and specific test. In later disease, muscle weakness and thenar atrophy are often noted. Diagnostic tests for patients suspected of having CTS include electromyography and nerve conduction studies that can confirm the median neuropathy.

Treatment of patients with CTS includes limiting the activity that caused the condition, elevating the affected extremity, and splinting the hand and forearm. Pain relief with NSAIDs or acetaminophen can be helpful. Corticosteroid injection into the carpal tunnel at 6-week intervals may reduce swelling and symptoms but should be attempted only by a skilled practitioner. Surgery to release the transverse carpal ligament provides symptom relief in the majority of patients who do not respond to conservative therapy. However, about 10% do not respond because of nerve damage or new pressure within the carpal tunnel that results from recurrent compression caused by scar formation. Vitamin B_6 and other nutraceutical therapy have been reported to be helpful in minimizing CTS symptoms, although some studies have not supported their use.

CTS is often noted transiently at the end of pregnancy and in patients with untreated hypothyroidism. Pregnancy-induced CTS usually resolves quickly after the woman gives birth, and thyroxine supplements quickly ameliorate CTS caused by hypothyroidism. In the interim, splinting and analgesia can be helpful.

DISCUSSION SOURCES

Anderson, B. (1999). Office Orthopedics for Primary Care: Diagnosis and Treatment (2nd ed.). Philadelphia: W. B. Saunders.

Hellman, D., and Stone, J. (2003). Arthritis and

musculoskeletal disorder. In Tierney, L., McPhee, S., and Papadakis, M. (eds.). Current Diagnosis and Treatment (42nd ed., pp. 783–836). New York: Lange Medical Books/McGraw-Hill.

Szoke-Halal, A.M. (2004). Musculoskeletal disorders. In Hektor Dunphy, L. Management Guidelines for Nurse Practitioners Working with Adults, pp 379–410. Philadelphia, F.A. Davis.

QUESTIONS

50. Most episodes of low back pain are caused by:

    A. an acute precipitating event.
    B. disk herniation.
    C. muscle or ligamentous strain.
    D. nerve impingement.

51. With the straight-leg–raising test, the NP is evaluating tension on which of the following nerve roots?

    A. L1 and L2
    B. L3 and L4
    C. L5 and S1
    D. S2 and S3

52. During acute lumbosacral strain, which of the following is the best advice to give about exercising?

    A. You should not exercise until you are free of pain.
    B. Back-strengthening exercises may cause mild muscle soreness.
    C. Electric-like pain is to be expected.
    D. Conditioning exercises should be started immediately.

53. Early neurologic changes in patients with lumbar radiculopathy include:

    A. loss of deep tendon reflexes.
    B. poor two-point discrimination.
    C. reduced muscle strength.
    D. foot drop.

54. In the evaluation of a patient with low back pain, the loss of bowel and bladder control most likely indicates:

    A. cauda equina syndrome.
    B. muscular spasm.
    C. vertebral fracture.
    D. sciatic nerve entrapment.

55. Loss of posterior tibial reflex may indicate a lesion at:

    A. L3.
    B. L4.
    C. L5.
    D. S1.

56. Loss of Achilles tendon reflex most likely indicates a lesion at:

    A. L1 to L2.
    B. L3 to L4.
    C. L5 to S1.
    D. S2 to S3.

57. Which test is demonstrated when the examiner applies pressure to the top of the head with the neck bending forward producing pain or numbness in the upper extremities?

    A. Spurling
    B. McMurray
    C. Lachman
    D. Newman

58. Which of the following tests will yield the greatest amount of information in a patient with acute lumbar radiculopathy?

    A. a lumbosacral radiograph series.
    B. ESR measurement.
    C. MRI.
    D. a bone scan.

59. The most common site for a cervical disk lesion is:

    A. C3 to C4.
    B. C4 to C5.
    C. C5 to C6.
    D. C6 to C7.

60. The most common sites for lumbar disk herniation are:

    A. L1 to L2 and L2 to L3
    B. L2 to L3 and L4 to L5
    C. L4 to L5 and L5 to S1
    D. L5 to S1 and S1 to S2

DISCUSSION

Low back pain is at least an occasional problem for nearly all adults, with a lifetime prevalence of 60% to 90%. In about 90% of patients with low back pain, symptoms are short-lived and resolve within 1 month without specific therapy. However, a small number have recurrent or chronic low back pain and significant disability.

Lumbosacral strain or disk herniation and its resulting lumbar radiculopathy and sciatica can cause musculoskeletal low back pain. Most often, contributing factors include muscle or ligamentous strain, degenerative joint disease, or a combination of these factors. Lumbosacral strain is the most common reason for a patient to present to primary care with acute low back pain. In the typical presentation, the patient complains of stiffness, spasm, and reduced ROM. The erector spinae muscle is most often implicated. Sitting usually aggravates the pain, but there may be some relief if the patient lies supine on a firm surface. A precipitating event is reported only by a small number of patients because lumbosacral strain is usually the culmination of a number of events, including repeated used of improperly stretched muscles in patients with overall poor conditioning. In addition, poor posture, scoliosis, and spinal stenosis can be predisposing factors. The physical examination usually reveals a straightening of the lumbosacral curve, paraspinal muscle tenderness, and spasm worst at the level of L3 to L4, as well as decreased lumbosacral flexion and lateral bending. The neurologic examination findings are typically within normal limits unless radiculopathy is present.

Diagnostic tests in lumbosacral strain vary according to the length and severity of symptoms. Radiographs can be of help if spondylolisthesis, scoliosis, or degenerative joint disease is suspected. However, in the absence of these, little will likely be revealed. Therefore, lumbosacral radiographs should not be routinely obtained. Computed tomographic scanning or MRI should be considered if radiculopathy is present, because these studies could reveal contributing factors such as spinal stenosis and disk herniation; MRI is a superior study for revealing soft tissue problems, whereas computed tomography provides superior information on bony structures.

Lumbosacral disk herniation usually occurs after years of episodes of back pain caused by repeated damage to the annular fibers of the disk and is less common than lumbosacral strain as a cause of low back pain. Lumbar disk herniation often leads to sciatica, neurologic changes, and significant distress. Because the intravertebral disks contain less water and are more fibrous, the risk of disk rupture decreases after age 50 years. The most common sites of lumbosacral disk herniation are L4 to L5 and L5 to S1, with the posterolateral aspect of the disk protruding.

Neuralgia along the course of the sciatic nerve is known as sciatica. The cause of sciatica is usually pressure on lumbosacral nerve roots from a herniated disk, spinal stenosis, or a compression fracture. On occasion, sciatica can be caused by external pressure on the sciatic nerve, such as that often found in people who carry a wallet in a rear pants pocket and develop symptoms after prolonged sitting. Patients with sciatica complain of shooting pain that starts over the hip and radiates to the foot, often accompanied by leg numbness and weakness. The degree of pain can vary according to the degree of nerve involvement; it ranges from mildly bothersome and occasionally reported to be more itchy than painful to incapacitating pain.

Neck pain, a common clinical complaint, can result from abnormalities in the soft tissues such as muscles, ligaments, and nerves, as well as in bones and joints of the spine. The most common causes of neck pain are soft tissue abnormalities caused by injury or prolonged wear and tear; rare causes of neck pain include infection and tumors. The most common site for a cervical disk lesion is C5 to C6.

In patients who have herniated disks, whether in the neck or back, the degree of neurologic involvement ranges from more minor symptoms of numbness to loss of extremity function. Deep tendon reflexes may be absent. With cauda equina involvement, there is compression of the lower portion of the nerve root inferior to the spinal cord, usually secondary to disk herniation. This leads to rectal or perineal pain and disturbance in bowel and bladder function. Signs of lumbosacral strain are present, and the straight-leg–raising maneuver yields reproduction of pain.

Management of patients with low back pain differs according to presentation. In the majority with acute low back pain and intact neurologic examination, a short course of 2 to 4 days of bed rest may be helpful; longer periods of immobilization may contribute to deconditioning and are potentially harmful. Intervention for acute neck pain is similar. Application of cold packs for 20 minutes three to four times a day can help with pain control, and heat applications may help before gentle stretching exercise. NSAIDs or acetaminophen should be prescribed for pain control. Muscle relaxers have been demonstrated to be of help in some patients. However, these medications are usually sedating and need to be used with caution. Treatment should also include initiation of aerobic and toning exercises and teaching the patient to minimize back stress through appropriate use of body mechanics.

Prompt referral to specialty care is needed when there is limb, bowel, or bladder dysfunction. Surgery is usually considered only if severe symptoms persist beyond 3 months. In addition, early referral is indicated in select conditions that are particularly worrisome (Table 8–5).

DISCUSSION SOURCES

Hellman, D., and Stone, J. (2003). Arthritis and musculoskeletal disorder. In Tierney, L., McPhee, S., and Papadakis, M. (eds.). Current Diagnosis and Treatment (42nd ed., pp. 783–836). New York: Lange Medical Books/McGraw-Hill.

Szoke-Halal, A.M. (2004). Musculoskeletal disorders. In Hektor Dunphy, L. Management Guidelines for Nurse Practitioners Working with Adults, pp 379–410. Philadelphia, F.A. Davis.

QUESTIONS

61. A 22-year-old man presents with new onset of pain and swelling in his feet and ankles, as well as conjunctivitis, oral lesions, and dysuria. The most important test to obtain is:

TABLE 8–5

LOW BACK PAIN: POTENTIALLY SERIOUS CONDITIONS

Possible Fracture	Possible Tumor or Infection	Cauda Equina Syndrome
History of recent trauma, particularly fall from significant height or motor vehicle accident In person with or at risk for osteoporosis, minor trauma or strenuous lifting	Age <20 years or >50 years Constitutional symptoms such as unexplained weight loss, fever Recent bacterial infection, injection drug use, immunosuppression Increased pain with rest History of cancer	Bladder dysfunction, perineal sensory loss, and/or anal laxity Neurologic deficit in lower extremities Lower extremity motor weakness

From the Agency for Health Care Policy and Research Guideline on Acute Low Back Problems in Adults/(2002). Available at http://text.nlm.nih.gov/ftrs/gateway, accessed 9/25/04.

A. ANA analysis.
B. ESR measurement.
C. rubella titer measurement.
D. urethral cultures.

62. Treatment for Reiter syndrome in a sexually active man usually includes:

A. antimicrobial therapy.
B. corticosteroid therapy.
C. antirheumatic medications.
D. immunosuppressive drugs.

63. In reference to Reiter syndrome, which of the following is false?

A. When the disease is associated with urethritis, the male:female ratio is about 9:1.
B. When the disease is associated with infectious diarrhea, the male and female incidences are approximately equal.
C. ANA analysis will reveal a speckled pattern.
D. Results of joint aspirate culture are usually unremarkable.

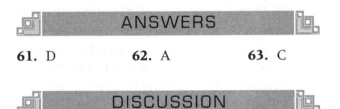

ANSWERS

61. D   62. A   63. C

DISCUSSION

Reiter syndrome, a reactive arthritis, is a generalized inflammatory condition. The classic tetrad of the disease consists of urethritis, conjunctivitis, mucocutaneous lesions, and arthritis. The knees and ankles are most often involved, and sacroiliitis is less common. Uveitis may also be seen. This condition is typically seen a number of days to weeks after an episode of acute bacterial diarrhea caused by *Shigella* species, *Salmonella* species, *Campylobacter* species, or a sexually transmitted infection such as *Chlamydia trachomatis* or *Ureaplasma urealyticum*. When seen with infectious diarrhea, the disease is found equally in both genders. When it is seen with urethritis, there is a male predominance of 9:1, the majority being

HLA-B27 positive. Cultures of joint aspirates in Reiter syndrome typically have negative results. Diagnostic testing is aimed at finding the underlying cause, such as urethral or stool cultures. Because this is an inflammatory condition, ESR is elevated, but this is not particularly sensitive or specific for the condition. Laboratory tests for rheumatic disease, such as ANA and rheumatoid factor analyses, are not affected by the disease.

Treatment includes the use of anti-inflammatory drugs such as NSAIDs. When Reiter syndrome occurs with urethritis, the use of a tetracycline shortens the duration of symptoms. Early antimicrobial treatment of infectious urethritis appears to limit a patient's risk of developing Reiter syndrome. No change in symptoms is usually seen with antibiotic use if infectious diarrhea was the precipitating event.

DISCUSSION SOURCE

Hellman, D., and Stone, J. (2003). Arthritis and musculoskeletal disorder. In Tierney, L., McPhee, S., and Papadakis, M. (eds.). Current Diagnosis and Treatment (42nd ed., pp. 783–836). New York: Lange Medical Books/McGraw-Hill.

QUESTIONS

64. During a preparticipation sports examination, you hear a grade 2/6 early to midsystolic ejection murmur, heard best at the second intercostal space of the left sternal border, in an asymptomatic young adult. This most likely represents:

A. an innocent flow murmur.
B. mitral valve incompetency.
C. aortic regurgitation.
D. mitral valve prolapse (MVP).

65. You are examining an 18-year-old man who is seeking a sports clearance physical examination. You note a midsystolic murmur that gets louder when he stands. This may represent:

A. aortic stenosis.
B. hypertrophic cardiomyopathy.

C. a physiologic murmur.

D. a Still murmur.

66. A Still murmur:

A. is an indication to selectively restrict sports participation.

B. has a buzzing quality.

C. is usually heard in patients who experience dizziness when exercising.

D. is a sign of cardiac structural abnormality.

67. A 22-year-old woman wants to know whether she can start a walking program. She has a diagnosis of MVP, with echocardiogram revealing trace mitral regurgitation. You respond that:

A. she should have an exercise tolerance test.

B. an electrocardiogram should be obtained.

C. she may proceed in the absence of activity intolerance symptoms.

D. running should be avoided.

68. You hear a fixed split second heart sound (S_2) in a 28-year-old man who wants to start an exercise program and consider that it is:

A. a normal finding in a younger adult.

B. occasionally found in uncorrected atrial septal defect.

C. the result of valvular sclerosis.

D. often found in patients with right bundle branch block.

69. A 19-year-old man presents with stage 1 hypertension. Which of the following is correct concerning sports participation?

A. Full activity should be encouraged.

B. Weight lifting is contraindicated.

C. An exercise tolerance test is advisable.

D. A beta-adrenergic antagonist should be prescribed.

70. A 25-year-old woman presents with sinus arrhythmia. Which of the following is correct concerning sports participation?

A. Full activity should be encouraged.

B. Weight lifting is contraindicated.

C. An exercise tolerance test is advisable.

D. A calcium channel antagonist should be prescribed.

ANSWERS

64. A	**65.** B	**66.** B
67. C	**68.** B	
69. A	**70.** A	

DISCUSSION

Cardiovascular evaluation is an important component of the sports participation evaluation. Reducing the risk of exercised-induced sudden cardiac death and the progression or deterioration of cardiovascular function caused by exercise are the primary goals of preparticipation evaluation. The precise lesions responsible for athletic field deaths differ considerably according to age. In victims younger than 35 years, the vast majority of sudden deaths are caused by several congenital cardiac malformations. Hypertrophic cardiomyopathy is the predominant abnormality in about one third of cases, and congenital coronary anomalies rank as the second most common etiology. Most of these deaths occur while the victims are playing team sports. In athletes aged 35 years or older, the majority of deaths are caused by atherosclerotic coronary artery disease, usually while the victims are participating in an individual endeavor such as long-distance running.

The preparticipation cardiovascular history should include questions about the following:

- prior occurrence of exertional chest pain/discomfort or syncope/near-syncope
- excessive, unexpected, and unexplained shortness of breath or fatigue associated with exercise
- past detection of a heart murmur or high blood pressure
- family history of the following: premature death (sudden or otherwise), significant dis-

ability from cardiovascular disease in one or more close relatives younger than 50 years, or specific knowledge of the occurrence of certain conditions (hypertrophic cardiomyopathy, dilated cardiomyopathy, long QT syndrome, Marfan syndrome, or clinically important arrhythmias)

The cardiovascular physical examination should include the following:

- precordial auscultation in both the supine and standing positions to identify heart murmurs consistent with dynamic left ventricular outflow obstruction
- assessment of the femoral artery pulses to exclude coarctation of the aorta
- recognition of the physical stigmata of Marfan syndrome
- blood pressure measurement in the sitting position

If any abnormalities in the history or physical examination are revealed, further evaluation and/or appropriate referral should follow. The ability to participate in athletic activities is determined by the results of these studies.

Hypertension is a common clinical problem. Because of the cardiovascular benefit of exercise, activity restriction is usually not advisable unless severely elevated hypertension or target organ damage is present. Certain antihypertensive agents may influence exercise tolerance. In general, the use of angiotensin-converting enzyme inhibitors, angiotensin receptor blockers, calcium channel antagonists, and alpha-adrenergic blockers has little to no impact on exercise tolerance. However, use of a beta-adrenergic antagonist may reduce the ability to exercise because of its ability to blunt the normal increase in heart rate in response to exercise. Diuretic use should be avoided if possible because of increased risk of dehydration and hypokalemia.

Cardiac rhythm disturbances are common and are usually benign. In particular, the presence of sinus arrhythmia in a younger adult is a normal finding and is not an indication for curtailing activity. Dysrhythmias associated with ischemic heart disease and certain supraventricular and ventricular rhythms may preclude sports participation.

A cardiac murmur may be benign, in that the examiner simply hears the blood flowing through the heart but no cardiac structural abnormality exists. However, certain cardiac structural problems, such as valvular and myocardial disorders, can contribute to the development of a murmur (Table 8–6).

Normal heart valves allow one-way, unimpeded forward blood flow through the heart. The entire stroke output is able to pass freely during one phase of the cardiac cycle (diastole with the atrioventricular valves, systole with the others), and there is no backward flow of blood. When a heart valve fails to open to its normal size, it is stenotic. When it fails to close appropriately, the valve is incompetent, causing regurgitation of blood to the previous chamber or vessel. Both of these events place patients at significant risk for embolic disease.

Physiologic murmurs, also known as functional or innocent flow murmurs, are present in the absence of cardiac pathology. There is no obstruction to flow, and there is a normal gradient across the valve. This type of murmur may be heard in up to 80% of thin adults or children if the cardiac examination is performed in a soundproof booth, and it is best heard at the left sternal border. It occurs in early to middle systole, leaving the two heart sounds intact. In addition, patients with a benign systolic ejection murmur deny having cardiac symptoms and have otherwise normal cardiac examination results, including an appropriately located point of maximum impulse and full pulses. Because no cardiac pathology is present in patients with a physiologic murmur, full activity should be encouraged.

Aortic stenosis is the inability of the aortic valves to open to optimum size. The aortic valve normally opens to 3 cm^2; aortic stenosis usually does not cause significant symptoms until the valvular orifice is limited to 0.8 cm^2. In children and younger adults, aortic stenosis is occasionally found, usually caused by a congenital bicuspid (rather than tricuspid) valve or by a three-cusp valve with leaflet

TABLE 8–6

CARDIAC CONDITIONS: FINDINGS AND IMPACT ON SPORTS PARTICIPATION

Cardiac Condition	Important Examination Findings	Additional Findings	Impact on Sports Participation
Hypertension	Elevated blood pressure	With target organ damage: S_3, S_4 heart sounds; PMI displacement; hypertensive retinopathy	With all but markedly elevated BP and/or evidence of target organ damage, full participation should be encouraged because of cardiovascular benefit of exercise
Physiologic murmur (also called innocent or functional murmur)	Grade 1–3/6 early to midsystolic murmur, heard best at LSB but usually audible over precordium	No radiation beyond precordium Softens or disappears with standing, increases in intensity with activity, fever, anemia S_1, S_2 intact, normal PMI	Full participation Patient should be asymptomatic, with no report of chest pain, CHF symptoms, palpitations, syncope, and activity intolerance
Aortic stenosis (AS)	Grade 1–4/6 harsh systolic murmur, usually crescendo-decrescendo pattern, heard best at 2nd RICS, apex	Radiates to carotids; may have diminished S_2, slow filling carotid pulse, narrow pulse pressure, loud S_4 Softens with standing The greater the degree of stenosis, later the peak of murmur	Impact in participation varies with degree of stenosis Mild: full participation Moderate: selected participation Severe: No participation In younger adults, usually congenital bicuspid valve In older adults, usually calcific, rheumatic in nature Dizziness, syncope are ominous signs, pointing to severely decreased cardiac output
Mitral stenosis (MS)	Grade 1–3/4 low-pitched late diastolic murmur heard best at the apex, localized Short crescendo-decrescendo rumble, like a bowling ball rolling down an alley or distant thunder	Often with opening snap, accentuated S_1 in the mitral area Enhanced by left lateral decubitus position, squat, cough, immediately after Valsalva maneuver	Impact in participation varies with degree of stenosis Mild: full participation Moderate: selected participation Mild with atrial fibrillation: selected participation Severe: no participation Nearly all cases rheumatic in origin Protracted latency period, then gradual decrease in exercise tolerance, leading to rapid downhill course as a result of low cardiac output Atrial fibrillation common

(continued)

TABLE 8–6

CARDIAC CONDITIONS: FINDINGS AND IMPACT ON SPORTS PARTICIPATION
(continued)

Cardiac Condition	Important Examination Findings	Additional Findings	Impact on Sports Participation
Mitral regurgitation (MR)	Grade 1–4/6 high-pitched blowing systolic murmur, often extending beyond S_2 Sounds like long "haaa," "hooo" Heard best at RLSB	Radiates to axilla, often with laterally displaced PMI Decreased with standing, Valsalva maneuver Increased by squat, hand grip	Impact in participation varies with ventricular size and function MR with normal LV size and function: full participation MR with mild LV enlargement but normal function at rest: selected participation MR with LV enlargement or any LV dysfunction at rest: no participation Origin: rheumatic, ischemic heart disease, endocarditis Often with other valve abnormalities (AS, MS, AR)
Aortic regurgitation (AR)	Grade 1–3/4 high-pitched blowing diastolic murmur heard best at third LICS	May be enhanced by forced expiration, leaning forward Usually with S_3, wide pulse pressure, sustained thrusting apical impulse	Impact in participation varies with ventricular size, function, and dysrhythmias AR with normal or mildly increased LV size and function: full participation AR with moderate LV enlargement, premature ventricular contractions at rest and with exercise: selected participation Mild to moderate AR with symptoms, severe AR, AR with progressive LVH: no participation More common in men, usually caused by rheumatic heart disease but occasionally by tertiary syphilis
Mitral valve prolapse (MVP)	Grade 1–3/6 late systolic crescendo murmur with honking quality, heard best at apex Murmur follows midsystolic click	With Valsalva maneuver or standing, click moves forward into earlier systole, resulting in a longer sounding murmur With hand grasp or squat, click moves back further into systole, resulting in a shorter murmur	Impact in participation varies with ventricular function and dysrhythmia MVP without: full participation MVP with mild to moderate regurgitation, dysrhythmias such as repetitive supraventricular tachycardia, complex ventricular dysrhythmias: selected participation Often seen with minor thoracic deformities such as pectus excavatum, straight back, and shallow AP diameter

Cardiac Condition	Important Examination Findings	Additional Findings	Impact on Sports Participation
Hypertrophic cardiomyopathy	Harsh midsystolic crescendo-de-crescendo murmur heard best at the lower left sternal border or at the apex	Murmur may increase with standing, squat, or Valsalva maneuver Triple apical impulse, loud S_4, bisferiens carotid pulse	Dyspnea, chest pain, postexertional syncope often reported Sports participation should be determined on an individual basis according to degree of ventricular function and symptoms
Still murmur (also called vibratory innocent murmur)	Grade 1–3/6 early systolic ejection, musical or vibratory, short, often buzzing, heard best midway between apex and LLSB	Softens or disappears when sitting or standing or with Valsalva maneuver Usual onset age, 2–6; may persist through adolescence Benign condition	Benign finding No limitation on sports participation
Atrial septal defect (without surgical intervention)	Grade 1–3/6 systolic ejection murmur heard best at the ULSB with widely split fixed S_2 May be accompanied by a mid-diastolic murmur heard at the 4th ICS LSB common, caused by increased flow across tricuspid valve	Twice as common in girls Child may be entirely well or present with CHF Often missed in the first few months of life or even entire childhood Watch for the child with easy fatigability	With correction, full sports participation is typical Without correction, sports participation should be determined on an individual basis according to degree of pulmonary hypertension, right-to-left shunt, and symptoms
Ventricular septal defect (without surgical intervention)	Grade 2–5/6 regurgitant systolic murmur heard best at LLSB Occasionally holosystolic, usually localized	Usually without cyanosis With small to moderate-sized left-to-right shunt and without pulmonary hypertension, likely to have minimal symptoms Larger shunts may result in CHF with onset in infancy	With correction, full sports participation is typical Without correction, sports participation should be determined on an individual basis according to degree of pulmonary hypertension, right-to-left shunt, and symptoms

Adapted from Constant, J. (1999). Essentials of Bedside Cardiology. Philadelphia: Lippincott Williams & Wilkins; and from Van Camp, S. (1999) Cardiology. In Sarafan, M., McKeag, D., and Van Camp, S. (eds.). Manual of Sports Medicine (pp 226–243). Philadelphia: Lippincott Williams & Wilkins.
BP, blood pressure; CHF, congestive heart failure; ICS, intercostal space; LICS, left intercostal space; LLSB, left sternal border; LSB, LV, left ventricular; LVH, left ventricular hypertrophy; PMI, point of maximum impulse; RICS, right intercostal space; RLSB, right lower sternal border; S_1, S_2, S_3, and S_4, first to fourth heart sounds; ULSB, upper left sternal border.

fusion. This defect is most often found in boys and men and is commonly accompanied by a long-standing history of becoming excessively short of breath with increased activity such as running. The physical examination results are usually normal except for the murmur. The ability to participate in sports or other vigorous activity is dictated by the degree of aortic stenosis and patient symptoms (see Table 8–6).

In older adults, calcification aortic stenosis leading to the inability of the valve to open to its normal size is usually the problem. In middle-aged adults without congenital aortic stenosis, the disease is usually a sequela of rheumatic fever, representing about 30% of cases of valvular dysfunction seen in patients with rheumatic heart disease. As with those who have congenital aortic stenosis, the ability to participate in sports or an exercise program is dictated by the degree of valvular dysfunction, ventricular enlargement, and patient symptoms.

The murmur of mitral regurgitation arises from mitral valve incompetency, or the inability of the mitral valve to close properly. This allows a retrograde flow from a high-pressure area (left ventricle) to an area of lower pressure (left atrium). Mitral regurgitation is most often caused by the degeneration of the mitral valve, most commonly by rheumatic fever, endocarditis, calcific annulus, rheumatic heart disease, ruptured chordae, or papillary muscle dysfunction. In mitral regurgitation from rheumatic heart disease, some mitral stenosis is usually present. After a patient becomes symptomatic, and without intervention, the disease progresses in a downhill course of chronic heart failure over the next 10 years. Sports or other vigorous activity participation is dictated by the degree of mitral regurgitation and ventricular chamber enlargement.

MVP is likely the most common valvular heart problem, present in perhaps 10% of the general population. The majority of patients with MVP have a benign condition in which one of the valve leaflets is unusually long and buckles or prolapses into the left atrium, usually in midsystole. At that time, a click occurs, followed by a short murmur caused by regurgitation of blood into the atrium. Cardiac output is usually not compromised, and the event goes unnoticed by patients. Echocardiography fails to reveal any abnormality, simply noting the valve buckling, followed by a small-volume or trace mitral regurgitation. If there are no cardiac complaints and the rest of the cardiac examination, including electrocardiogram, is within normal limits, no further evaluation is needed. One way of describing this variation from the norm is to inform patients that one leaflet of the mitral valve is a bit longer than usual. However, the "holder" (valve orifice) is of average size. This variation causes the valve to buckle a bit, just as a person's foot would if forced into a shoe that is one or two sizes too small. Therefore, the heart makes an extra set of sounds (click and murmur) but is not diseased or damaged. MVP is often found in people with minor thoracic deformities such as pectus excavatum, a dish-shaped concave area at T1, and scoliosis. The second and much smaller group with MVP has systolic displacement of one or more of the mitral leaflets into the left atrium along with valve thickening and redundancy, usually accompanied by mild to moderate mitral regurgitation. This group typically has additional health problems such as Marfan syndrome or other connective tissue disease. Because structural cardiac abnormality is present in this group, there is a risk of bacterial endocarditis.

Barring other health problems, patients with MVP usually have normal cardiac output and tolerate a program of aerobic exercise well. A program of regular aerobic activity should be encouraged in order to promote health and well-being. The mitral valve prolapses more, thus increasing the murmur, when circulating volume is low; thus, maintaining a high level of fluid intake should be encouraged in patients with MVP. Treatment with beta-adrenergic agonists (beta blockers) is indicated only when symptomatic recurrent tachycardia or palpitations are an issue. Although this degree of distress (i.e., chest pain, dyspnea) may depend in part on the degree of mitral regurgitation, some studies have failed to reveal any difference in the rates of chest pain in patients with or without MVP. The potentially biggest threat is the rupture of chordae, usually seen only in those with connective tissue diseases (especially Marfan syndrome).

Hypertrophic cardiomyopathy is a disease of the cardiac muscle. The ventricular septum is thick and asymmetric, leading to potential outflow tract block. Patients with hypertrophic cardiomyopathy often exhibit symptoms of cardiac outflow tract blockage with activity because the hypertrophic ventricular walls better approximate with the increased force of myocardial contraction associated with exercise. Unfortunately, the presentation of hypertrophic cardiomyopathy may be sudden cardiac death. Idiopathic hypertrophic subaortic stenosis is a type of cardiomyopathy. A strong family history is often present in those who have this autosomal dominant disorder. The typical patient is a young adult with a history of dyspnea with activity, but patients may also be asymptomatic.

In those with congenital heart disease such as atrial or ventricular septal defect, recommendations for sports participation vary according to patient presentation and surgical intervention. Most often, if the defect has been surgically repaired with little residual dysfunction, full sports participation is allowed. If the defect is uncorrected or if there is significant alteration in cardiac function despite repair, the degree of participation should be assessed on an individual basis.

DISCUSSION SOURCES

American Heart Association (1996). Cardiovascular Preparticipation Screening of Competitive Athletes: A Statement for Health Professionals From the Sudden Death Committee (Clinical Cardiology) and Congenital Cardiac Defects Committee (Cardiovascular Disease in the Young), American Heart Association. Available at www.americanheart.org, accessed 5/4/03.

Van Camp, S. (1999). Cardiology. In Sarafan, M., McKeag, D., and Van Camp, S. (eds.). Manual of Sports Medicine (pp. 226–243). Philadelphia: Lippincott-Raven.

71. All of the following are common sites of fracture in patients with osteoporosis except:

    A. the proximal femur.
    B. the distal forearm.
    C. the vertebrae.
    D. the clavicle.

72. Osteoporosis is more common in individuals:

    A. with type 2 diabetes mellitus.
    B. taking chronic corticosteroid therapy.
    C. who are obese.
    D. of African ancestry.

73. Osteoporosis screening tests include all of the following except:

    A. quantitative ultrasound measurement.
    B. dual-energy x-ray absorptiometry.
    C. qualitative computed tomography.
    D. wrist, spine, and hip radiographs.

74. Osteoporosis prevention measures include all of the following except:

    A. calcium supplementation.
    B. selective estrogen receptor modulator use.
    C. vitamin B_6 supplementation.
    D. weight-bearing exercise.

75. Early disease presentation in osteoporosis may include:

    A. greater than 1-inch loss in terminal adult height.
    B. hip fracture.
    C. kyphosis.
    D. back pain.

76. In counseling a postmenopausal woman, you advise her that hormone therapy users may experience:

    A. an increase in breast cancer rates with long-term use.
    B. reduction in high-density lipoprotein cholesterol.
    C. a 10% increase in bone mass.
    D. no change in the occurrence of osteoporosis.

77. When counseling a patient taking a bisphosphonate such as alendronate (Fosamax), you advise that the medication should be taken with:

   A. a bedtime snack.
   B. a meal.
   C. other medications.
   D. a large glass of water.

ANSWERS

71. D **72.** B **73.** D
74. C **75.** D
76. A **77.** D

DISCUSSION

Osteoporosis is a disorder of bone thinning in which bone absorption exceeds its formation to the degree that bone density is insufficient to meet skeletal needs. In addition, osteoporosis is defined as bone density more than 2.5 standard deviations below the average bone mass for women who are younger than 35 years. For every reduction of bone mass by 1 standard deviation, the relative risk of fracture rises by 1.5-fold to threefold.

Estrogen deficiency is a potent risk factor, and osteoporosis is most common in postmenopausal women; by age 80 years, the average woman has lost more than 30% of her premenopausal bone density. Men appear to be at significantly less risk; this is partly because of inherently greater bone density. Body habitus and ethnicity can influence the risk of osteoporosis; it is most common in petite women of Asian and European ancestry, who usually have lower bone density in adulthood. Obesity appears to minimize osteoporosis risk caused by highly endogenous estrogen production by fatty tissue. Additional risk factors for osteoporosis include disorders such as thyroid toxicosis, Cushing disease, and rheumatoid arthritis, as well as inactivity and prolonged therapy with select anticonvulsants, heparin, and corticosteroids.

In patients with osteoporosis, hip, wrist, and spinal fractures most commonly occur, but all bones are at risk. Early disease usually does not have symptoms, but backache may be reported. Although hip fracture is often the first clinical manifestation of osteoporosis, it usually indicates advanced disease, as does loss of terminal adult height.

In patients with osteoporosis, the bone lost is from the baseline bone density. A small amount of loss may be of great significance against poor bone density but of little consequence with greater density. Therefore, primary prevention of osteoporosis includes ensuring the development of maximum adult bone density. Because maximum bone density is achieved in the early adult years, encouraging adequate calcium intake and weight-bearing exercise throughout the teen and adult years is important. The calcium intake goal should be the equivalent of 1000 mg/day for men and premenopausal women, increased to 1200 to 1500 mg/day or more in postmenopausal women. Vitamin D, 600 to 900 IU daily, is also recommended. Foods should be the main source of nutrition; supplements may be used if dietary intake is inadequate.

A number of tests are available to evaluate osteoporosis risk or detect progress of the disease (Table 8–7). Dual-energy x-ray absorptiometry is considered one of the more reliable measures. Qualitative computed tomography is precise but uses more radiation than dual-energy x-ray absorptiometry. Quantitative ultrasound is relatively inexpensive and can be performed with portable equipment. Plain radiographic films should not be used for screening or evaluation of osteoporosis because disease detection is not possible until 40% to 50% of bone mass is lost.

When taken with calcium supplements, hormone therapy can help reduce the risk of postmenopausal fracture by as much as 50% by minimizing further bone loss; the benefit must be balanced against the noted increased risk of breast cancer and other problems with long-term use. A selective estrogen receptor modulator such as raloxifene (Evista) helps perserve bone density. Because it does not attach to es-

---
TABLE 8–7
OSTEOPOROSIS: RISKS, SCREENING GUIDELINES, AND TREATMENT

Risk Factors for Osteoporosis

- Gender: Women at greater risk due to less dense bones.
- Age: Increases steadily and substantially with age. Women => 65 years at greatest risk.
- Lower body weight is also consistently associated with osteoporosis, but to a lesser degree than age. Women weighing less than 132 pounds are at greatest risk; women 60 years and older who weigh less than 154 pounds are at increased risk.

Recommendations for Osteoporosis Screening

- All women =>65 years and older be screened routinely for osteoporosis:
  - For women at high risk for fractures, screening to begin at age 60 years.
  - No recommendation for or against screening women aged 60–64 years for osteoporosis if they are not at high risk for this condition.

Available Screening Tests for Osteoporosis

- Dual-energy x-ray absorptiometry (DXA) of the hip
  - Best predictor of hip fracture. Using DXA to measure bone density of the hand, wrist, forearm, and heel also appears to detect women who are at increased risk for fracture.
- Other tests to measure bone mineral density
  - Ultrasound, radiographic absorptiometry, single energy x-ray, absorptiometry, peripheral dual-energy x-ray absorptiometry, and peripheral quantitative computed tomography

Osteoporosis Treatment

- All to be used with appropriate calcium and vitamin D supplementation
  - Bisphosphonates, such as alendronate and risedronate
  - Selective estrogen-receptor modulators (SERMs), such as raloxifene
  - Calcitonin
  - Estrogen

Osteoporosis Risk Assessment Instrument (ORAI) to identify higher risk women <65 years who should be screened (2002), available at http://www.osteoed.org/faq/screening/orai/shtml, accessed 5/5/03. www.ahrq.gov/clinic/3rduspstf/osteoporosis/osteowh/htm, accessed 5/5/03.

trogen receptor sites in the breast or uterus, a selective estrogen receptor modulator may be an alternative to hormone therapy. The bisphosphonates such as alendronate (Fosamax) inhibit the resorptive activity of osteoclasts, can help modestly increase bone mass, and can significantly reduce fracture risk. In order to minimize the risk of drug-induced esophagitis, patients taking an oral bisphosphonate should be cautioned to take the medication in the morning with a full glass of water. At least 30 minutes must elapse before food, other liquids, or medications are ingested. In addition, patients should remain upright for at least 1 hour. Calcitonin is most helpful in building vertebral bone. Because it also has analgesic properties, calcitonin can help in the treatment of vertebral fracture pain and can help minimize the risk of future fracture. With all therapies, calcium supplements should be continued.

DISCUSSION SOURCES

Hellman, D., and Stone, J. (2003). Arthritis and musculoskeletal disorder. In Tierney, L., McPhee, S., and Papadakis, M. (eds.). Current Diagnosis and Treatment (42nd ed., pp. 783–836). New York: Lange Medical Books/McGraw-Hill.

Szoke-Halal, A.M. (2004). Musculoskeletal disorders. In Hektor Dunphy, L. Management Guidelines for Nurse Practitioners Working with Adults, pp 379–410. Philadelphia, F.A. Davis.

QUESTIONS

78. The most common site of sprain is the:

A. wrist.
B. shoulder.
C. ankle.
D. knee.

79. A grade II ankle sprain is best described as:

A. minor swelling and minimal joint instability.
B. moderate joint instability without swelling or ecchymosis.
C. moderate swelling, mild to moderate ecchymosis, and moderate joint instability.
D. complete ankle instability, significant swelling, and moderate to severe ecchymosis.

80. A person with a grade III ankle sprain will present with:

A. minor swelling and minimal joint instability.
B. moderate joint instability without swelling or ecchymosis.
C. moderate swelling, mild to moderate ecchymosis, and moderate joint instability.
D. complete ankle instability, significant swelling, and moderate to severe ecchymosis.

81. Patients with a grade III ankle sprain should be advised that full recovery will likely take:

A. a few days.
B. 2 to 3 weeks.
C. 4 to 6 weeks.
D. a number of months.

82. Which of the following is usually not part of treatment of a sprain?

A. immobilization
B. applying ice to the area
C. joint rest
D. local corticosteroid injection

ANSWERS

78. C   **79.** C   **80.** D
81. D   **82.** D

DISCUSSION

A sprain is a partial or complete injury of a ligament either within the ligament body or at its site of attachment to the bone. Inversion injuries of the ankle cause about 85% of all sprains. This is the most common injury that involves jumping or running. Sprains can also involve the wrist, elbow, and knee. Wearing appropriate footwear, improved conditioning, and preexercise warm-up exercises, as well as taping, can be helpful in avoiding sprains.

Sprains are often graded according to presentation and proposed underlying degree of ligamentous injury (Table 8–8). The ankle anterior draw test is used to assess for excessive laxity of the tibiotarsal joint. Excessive anterior motion is usually seen with a grade III sprain.

Immobilization is important in helping appropriate healing and minimizing sequelae. Grades II and III injuries are occasionally associated with joint laxity and a risk of future sprain.

DISCUSSION SOURCES

Hellman, D., and Stone, J. (2003). Arthritis and musculoskeletal disorder. In Tierney, L., McPhee, S., and Papadakis, M. (eds.). Current Diagnosis and Treatment (42nd ed., pp. 783–836). New York: Lange Medical Books/McGraw-Hill.

Szoke-Halal, A.M. (2004). Musculoskeletal disorders. In Hektor Dunphy, L. Management Guidelines for Nurse Practitioners Working with Adults, pp 379–410. Philadelphia, F.A. Davis.

Hektor Dunphy, L. (2004). Management Guidelines for Adult Nurse Practitioners (pp. 398–401). Philadelphia: F. A. Davis.

QUESTIONS

83. The diagnosis of tendonitis is usually made from:

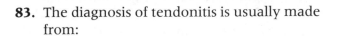

TABLE 8–8

LIGAMENTOUS SPRAINS: GRADING, PRESENTATION AND INTERVENTION

Grade of Injury	Pathology and Presentation	Intervention
Grade I	Partial tear No instability	RICE (rest, ice, compression, elevation) Immobilizer Limit weight bearing Analgesia Length of disability is usually limited to a few days
Grade II	Partial ligamentous tear Moderate joint instability Moderate swelling Mild to moderate ecchymosis	RICE Immobilizer Limit weight bearing Analgesia Length of disability is usually several weeks to a few months
Grade III	Complete ligamentous tear Complete ankle instability Significant swelling Moderate to severe ecchymosis	Orthopedic referral RICE Immobilizer Limit weight bearing Analgesia Length of disability may be many months

  A. clinical presentation.
  B. plain radiographic films.
  C. MRI.
  D. laboratory diagnosis.

84. Complications of Achilles tendonitis include:

  A. tendon rupture.
  B. neurologic sequelae.
  C. stress fracture.
  D. bursitis.

85. Which of the following is often found with rotator cuff tendonitis?

  A. osteoarthritis
  B. tendon rupture
  C. bursitis
  D. joint effusion

86. First-line therapy for biceps tendonitis usually includes:

  A. applying ice to the area.
  B. local steroid injection.
  C. orthopedic referral.
  D. nerve block.

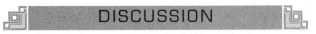

ANSWERS

83. A   **84.** A
85. C   **86.** A

DISCUSSION

The most common sites for tendonitis are the rotator cuff, elbow, biceps (shoulder), wrist, and heel. In the majority of cases, a microscopic tear causes tendon inflammation; the resulting swelling and inflammation in the tendon are a result of overuse. The clinical presentation usually includes report of reduced ROM caused by joint stiffness and discomfort, as well as a dull, aching pain over the affected tendon, especially with joint use. This pain can become sharp and acute when the tendon is squeezed. With rotator cuff involvement, abduction and elevation of the shoulder joint worsen symptoms.

The diagnosis of tendonitis is usually straightforward, with no special studies required. If it occurs with a history of recent trauma, plain radiographic films of the affected area may reveal calcium deposits on the tendon. Because bursitis and tendonitis often occur concurrently, assessment may reveal both conditions. If there is a question about accompanying soft tissue injury, MRI is the most helpful diagnostic test.

Treatment of tendonitis includes limiting or discontinuing the contributing activity. Applying ice to the region is helpful. When the hand or wrist is affected, splinting and NSAIDs are reasonable first-line therapies. Achilles tendonitis may necessitate treatment with a posterior splint to immobilize the heel, as well as heel cord stretching and orthotics after the acute phase to prevent recurrence. There is a 10% risk of tendon rupture with recurrent Achilles tendonitis; the risk can exceed 12% with biceps tendonitis. With rotator cuff involvement, the likelihood of concurrent bursitis is high; treatment includes limiting overhead movement as well as intrabursal corticosteroid injection.

DISCUSSION SOURCES

Anderson, B. (1999). Office Orthopedics for Primary Care: Diagnosis and Treatment (2nd ed.). Philadelphia: W. B. Saunders.

Szoke-Halal, A.M. (2004). Musculoskeletal disorders. In Hektor Dunphy, L. Management Guidelines for Nurse Practitioners Working with Adults, 2nd, pp 379–410. Philadelphia, F.A. Davis.

9
Peripheral Vascular Disease

1. Who is most likely to have new-onset primary Raynaud phenomenon?

   A. a 68-year-old man
   B. a 65-year-old woman
   C. a 25-year-old man
   D. an 18-year-old woman

2. All of the following are associated with secondary Raynaud phenomenon except:

   A. hypertension.
   B. scleroderma.
   C. repeated use of vibrating tools.
   D. use of beta-adrenergic antagonists.

3. Lifestyle modification for patients with Raynaud phenomenon includes:

   A. discontinuing cigarette smoking.
   B. increasing fluid intake.
   C. avoiding placing hands in warm water.
   D. discontinuing aspirin use.

4. Medications that may be helpful in treating patients with Raynaud phenomenon include:

   A. nonsteroidal anti-inflammatory drugs (NSAIDs).
   B. angiotensin-converting enzyme inhibitors.
   C. beta-adrenergic antagonists.
   D. diuretics.

5. Which of the following is the most common presentation in a patient with Raynaud phenomenon?

   A. digital ulceration
   B. gangrene of the tip of the second fingers bilaterally
   C. a period of intense itchiness after blanching
   D. unilateral symptoms

1. D   2. A   3. A   4. B   5. C

Raynaud phenomenon is characterized by paroxysmal digital vasoconstriction that results in bilateral symmetric pallor or cyanosis. The hands are nearly always involved; foot involvement is rare. A period of rubor follows this initial response. Primary Raynaud phenomenon, also known as Raynaud disease, is idiopathic in origin in most patients and is most often found in women. The condition usually appears between the ages of 15 and 45 years. Vasoconstriction triggers include exposure to cold relieved by warmth and, less commonly, emotional upset. Symptoms tend to be progressive, with vasospasm becoming more frequent and prolonged.

There are no specific studies to help diagnose primary Raynaud disease. The diagnosis is made if recurrent episodes occur for a period of more than 3 years without notation of associated disease or secondary cause.

Secondary Raynaud phenomenon is seen in the presence of an underlying condition such as atherosclerosis, collagen vascular disease, and select autoimmune disease such as scleroderma. In addition, the use of vibrating tools, repeated sharp digit movement such as piano playing or typing, frostbite, tobacco, ergotamine, and beta blocker use can be contributing factors. The presentation of secondary Raynaud phenomenon is the same as that of the idiopathic condition; the degree and length of vasospasm may be more severe. On rare occasions, distal digital ulceration may be seen.

Whatever the cause, Raynaud phenomenon intervention is aimed primarily at preventing vasospasm by avoiding cold and other known triggers. At the onset of an episode, submerging the hands in warm water may be helpful in limiting the length and severity of vasospasm; hot water should not be used, because of risk of burn. Because wound healing may be delayed and infection more common, the hands should be protected from even minor injury. Keeping the skin well lubricated can help avoid small fissures. Because tobacco use exacerbates vasospasm, it should be discontinued. Biofeedback can be helpful because the patient can be taught to envision warming the digits, thus reducing symptoms. Oral and topical nitrates, dihydropyridine calcium channel blockers ("-ipine" suffix), and angiotensin-converting enzyme inhibitors ("-pril" suffix) can be used for their vasodilator effect when lifestyle modification is inadequate. In patients with secondary Raynaud phenomenon, treatment of the associated condition is important and may help minimize episodes.

DISCUSSION SOURCES

Krupp, D., and Graber, M. (2004). Rheumatology: Raynaud's phenomenon. In Virtual Hospital: University of Iowa Family Practice Handbook. Available at *http://www.vh.org/Adult/Provider/familymedicine//FPHandbook/Chapter*07/11–7. html, accessed 8/8/04.

Scott, L. (2004). Peripheral vascular disorders. In Hektor Dunphy, L. Management Guidelines for Nurse Practitioners Working with Adults (2nd ed, pp 411–424). Philadelphia, F.A. Davis.

QUESTIONS

6. Which of the following does not directly contribute to the development of varicose veins?

   A. leg crossing
   B. pregnancy
   C. heredity
   D. Raynaud disease

7. When advising a woman with varicose veins about the use of support stockings, you consider that the preferred type:

   A. can be purchased in the hosiery section of a department store.
   B. is lightweight and available over the counter.
   C. is a medium- to heavy-weight prescription product.
   D. is used with a panty girdle.

8. In patients with varicose veins, which vessel is most often affected?

   A. femoral vein
   B. posterior tibial vein
   C. peroneal vein
   D. saphenous vein

9. Which of the following statements is most accurate in the assessment of a patient with varicose veins?

A. The degree of venous tortuosity is well correlated with the amount of leg pain reported.

B. As the number of affected veins increases, so does the degree of patient discomfort.

C. Symptoms are sometimes reported with minimally affected vessels.

D. Lower extremity edema is usually seen only with severe disease.

10. Spider varicosities are:

A. usually symptomatic.

B. a potential site for thrombophlebitis.

C. responsive to laser obliteration.

D. caused by sun exposure.

ANSWERS

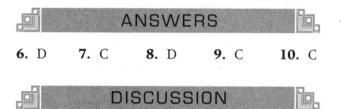

6. D   **7.** C   **8.** D   **9.** C   **10.** C

DISCUSSION

Seen in 15% of the adult population, varicose veins are most often found in the lower extremities. Tortuous, dilated, superficial veins are characteristic. An inherited venous defect of either a valvular incompetence or a weakness in the walls of the vessel likely plays a significant role. In addition, situations that cause high venous pressure, such as leg crossing, wearing of constricting garments, prolonged standing, heavy lifting, and pregnancy, contribute to their development. Women are affected twice as often as men.

The vessel most often affected is the great saphenous vein and its tributaries. Often asymptomatic, varicose veins may also be associated with leg aching but usually not severe pain. The degree of discomfort is poorly correlated with the number and appearance of the affected veins. Mild edema in the ankle area, particularly at the end of the day and in warm weather, is common. When palpated, the vein compresses easily and without pain. No specific diagnostic tests are needed with typical presentation.

With uncomplicated varicose veins, lifestyle modification usually helps minimize the symptoms and disease progress. Attaining and maintaining normal weight helps to reduce intravenous pressure and discourage the development and progress of varicose veins. Periodic leg elevation is helpful in minimizing edema and encouraging venous return. The use of medium- to heavy-weight elastic support hose such as Jobst stockings should be encouraged. Support hose purchased in a department or drug store do not supply enough compression. Wearing possibly constricting garments such as panty girdles and garters should be avoided. Surgery may be needed for symptomatic varicose veins that do not respond to conservative therapy. Sclerotherapy involves injecting a sclerosing agent into the affected vein, followed by a period of compression, which results in vessel obliteration.

Possible complications of varicose veins include superficial thrombophlebitis. Over time, varicose veins tend to dilate progressively. This can lead to secondary changes in the lower extremities, including chronic edema, skin hyperpigmentation, and the development of chronic venous insufficiency.

Spider varicosities are visible surface vessels usually seen with varicose veins. These vessels do not usually cause symptoms and pose no thromboembolic risk. Laser obliteration is helpful in reducing the appearance of spider varicosities and is considered a cosmetic procedure.

DISCUSSION SOURCE

Pak, L., Messina, L., and Tierney, L. (2003). Blood vessels and lymphatics. In Tierney, L., McPhee, S., and Papadakis, M. (eds.). Current Diagnosis and Treatment (42nd ed., pp. 435–468). New York: Lange Medical Books/ McGraw-Hill.

QUESTIONS

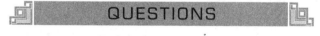

11. Which of the following is not a contributing factor to development of thrombophlebitis?

A. venous status
B. injury to vascular intima
C. malignancy-associated hypercoagulation states
D. isometric exercise

12. Presentation of superficial thrombophlebitis includes:

A. positive Homan sign.
B. diminished dorsalis pedis pulse.
C. a dilated vessel.
D. dependent pallor.

13. Treatment of superficial thrombophlebitis in a low-risk, stable patient includes use of:

A. compression stockings.
B. acetaminophen.
C. warfarin.
D. heparin.

14. In providing care for a patient with superficial thrombophlebitis, the nurse practitioner (NP) considers that:

A. it is a benign, self-limiting disease.
B. the linear pattern of induration can help differentiate the process from cellulitis or other inflammatory processes.
C. a chest radiograph should be obtained.
D. limited activity enhances recovery.

15. Which of the following is the most likely to be found in deep vein thrombophlebitis (DVT)?

A. unilateral leg edema
B. leg pain
C. warmth over the affected area
D. positive Homan sign

16. The NP considers that positive Homan sign is present in approximately what percentage of patients with DVT?

A. 25
B. 33
C. 50
D. 75

17. Diagnostic evaluation of a clinically stable patient with suspected DVT most often includes obtaining:

A. impedance plethysmography.
B. an iodine 125 fibrinogen scan.
C. contrast venography.
D. duplex ultrasonography.

18. Which of the following is the preferred medication used to reverse the anticoagulant effects of unfractionated heparin?

A. vitamin K
B. protamine sulfate
C. platelet transfusion
D. plasma components

19. Which of the following is the preferred medication used to reverse the anticoagulant effects of warfarin?

A. vitamin K
B. protamine sulfate
C. platelet transfusion
D. plasma components

20. Warfarin's onset of anticoagulation effect usually occurs how soon after the initiation of therapy?

A. immediately
B. 1 to 2 days
C. 3 to 5 days
D. 5 to 7 days

21. In comparison with unfractionated heparin, characteristics of low-molecular-weight heparin (LMWH) include all of the following except:

A. more antiplatelet effect.
B. decreased need for monitoring of anticoagulant effect.
C. longer half-life.
D. superior bioavailability.

22. Which of the following is least likely to be found in patients with pulmonary embolus (PE)?

A. pleuritic chest pain
B. tachypnea
C. DVT signs and symptoms
D. hemoptysis

23. The most commonly used method of preventing venous thromboembolism in higher risk surgical patients is:

A. antiplatelet therapy.
B. low-dose heparin.
C. vena cava filter.
D. warfarin.

24. When taken with warfarin, which of the following causes a possible increased anticoagulant effect?

    A. clarithromycin
    B. carbamazepine
    C. oral contraceptives
    D. sucralfate

25. When taken with warfarin, which of the following causes a possibly decreased anticoagulant effect?

    A. cholestyramine
    B. allopurinol
    C. cephalosporin
    D. chloral hydrate

26. What is the international normalized ratio (INR) range recommended for warfarin therapy during DVT treatment?

    A. 1.5 to 2.0
    B. 2.0 to 3.0
    C. 2.5 to 3.5
    D. 3.0 to 4.0

ANSWERS

11. D	**12.** C	**13.** A	**14.** B
15. A	**16.** B	**17.** D	**18.** B
19. A	**20.** C	**21.** A	**22.** D
23. B	**24.** A	**25.** A	**26.** B

DISCUSSION

Blood coagulation can be activated by a variety of pathways via the tissue factor (TF) pathway (formerly known as the extrinsic pathway) and the contact activation pathway (formerly known as the intrinsic pathway). Expressed by injured endothelial cells, TF is the clinically most significant initiator of coagulation. TF binds to and activates coagulation factor VII, and the TF/factor VIIa complex then activates factor X and factor IX to factors Xa and IXa, respectively. In the presence of factor XIIa, factor IXa can also convert factor X to factor Xa. The contact activation pathway is activated when factor XII comes in contact with a foreign surface. The resulting factor XIIa then activates factor XI, which in turn activates factor IX. Factor IXa then activates factor X. These pathways work together to provide maximum stimulation of factor X, which, in the presence of factor V, activates prothrombin to thrombin; this is also known as the common pathway.

Equally as important as blood coagulation is the blood's ability to avoid clot formation. In the larger arteries, clot risk is usually limited, because aggregating platelets are dislodged by high-velocity blood flow, and thrombus formation is avoided. In smaller arteries and veins, blood flow is slower, with platelet aggregation more likely to occur and clot risk higher. Working against thrombus formation, tissue factor pathway inhibitor binds to and inactivates the TF/factor VIIa/factor Xa complex. Antithrombin III inactivates circulating thrombin, whereas proteins C and S are contributors to a complex process that down-regulates thrombin activity by preventing the activation of factor V. If a clot does form, circulating plasminogen is incorporated into the thrombus; healthy endothelial cells adjacent to the vessel injury site release tissue plasminogen activator and activate plasminogen to plasmin, causing thrombolysis on the clot surface and minimizing thrombus size. At the same time, a number of factors, including plasminogen activator inhibitor, produced by the liver and endothelial cells, inhibit fibrin degradation by plasmin to limit thrombolysis.

The Virchow triad of stasis, injury to the vascular intima, and abnormal coagulation leading to clot usually contributes to the development of vessel inflammation and the resulting thrombophlebitis. The lower extremities are most often affected.

Thrombophlebitis can occur in superficial or deep veins. Risk factors for superficial thrombophlebitis include local trauma, prolonged travel or rest, presence of varicose veins, and history of prior episodes, as well as pregnancy and use of estrogen-containing hormonal contraceptives. Characteristics of superficial thrombophlebitis include a localized, tender, dilated, thrombosed vessel, usually causing a linear area of redness, often in the popliteal fossa. Homan sign is absent. Having the patient stand for 2 minutes before examination enhances the findings, because less severe cases may be missed on supine examination.

Superficial thrombophlebitis is often considered a benign condition. However, extension into a deep vein is typically present in 45% of patients with the condition. In particular, superficial thrombophlebitis in hospitalized patients is more likely to be associated with DVT and PE. Duplex ultrasound should be performed to help rule out concurrent DVT. Because superficial thrombophlebitis is often accompanied by DVT in a different location or extremity, the study should not be limited to the affected area. Serial studies may be needed if initial examination findings are negative but symptoms persist. Impedance plethysmography is a noninvasive test that helps detect disturbances in normal physiologic flow state through the venous system. Although venography is the most sensitive and specific test, its use has been limited because these less invasive tests have become available. A chest radiograph and V/Q scan should be obtained if shortness of breath or friction rub is present and the diagnosis of PE is considered. Coagulation studies should be obtained, particularly if there is a history of previous episodes.

After it is confirmed that the thrombophlebitis is indeed superficial, intervention is dictated by DVT risk factors and patient history. In the absence of risk factors and history of similar episodes, warm packs, compression hose, and NSAIDs can be used to treat superficial thrombophlebitis. Ambulation should be encouraged, because rest may promote stasis and enhance coagulation. In the presence of prior episodes, a history of DVT, decreased mobility, hypercoagulability, or extensive saphenous vein involvement, subcutaneous LMWH therapy should be initiated, with consideration for long-term warfarin use. The inflammation associated with superficial thrombophlebitis usually subsides over 2 weeks, with a firm cord remaining for a much longer period.

Acute DVT usually involves the veins of the lower extremities and pelvis. PE, a potentially fatal condition, is largely a sequela of DVT. Long-term sequelae of DVT include chronic venous insufficiency and venous ulceration.

Because the triad of venous stasis, vessel wall injury, and altered coagulation state is the primary mechanism underlying DVT (as it is with superficial thrombophlebitis), risk factors include prolonged rest, recent trauma, recent surgery (especially hip replacement), pregnancy, and recent childbirth. The hypercoagulation state associated with many malignancies presents considerable risk. The use of hormone-containing contraceptives and hormone therapy can increase the risk of DVT, particularly in cigarette smokers. Disorders of coagulation such as factor V Leiden, protein C and S deficiencies, and antithrombin III deficiencies have been recognized as a cause of DVT in younger, otherwise healthy adults.

Because the presentation of DVT varies, making the diagnosis from clinical presentation alone is problematic (Table 9–1). The minority of patients with suspected DVT have the diagnosis supported unless the Virchow triad of venous stasis, vessel wall injury, and coagulation abnormalities is present. With regard to risk as well as clinical presentation, Table 9–2 provides a guide for estimating clinical suspicion.

In order to establish the diagnosis and develop an appropriate plan of intervention, a thorough diagnostic evaluation is needed in patients suspected of having DVT. Contrast venography has the greatest sensitivity and specificity for the condition. However, because of cost and the invasive nature of the test, as well as the risk of allergy to the contrast medium, noninvasive tests are used more commonly. Duplex ultrasound is the most commonly used diagnostic technique in DVT. MRI is the diagnostic test of choice for suspected iliac vein or inferior vena caval thrombosis. In the second or third trimester of pregnancy, MRI is also more accurate than duplex ultrasound because the gravid uterus al-

TABLE 9–1

CLINICAL PRESENTATION OF DEEP VEIN
THROMBOPHLEBITIS (DVT)

Finding	Comment
Edema	Usually unilateral Most specific finding
Leg pain	Usually described as a tugging pain, heaviness, ache Present in ~50% of patients with DVT Degree of pain does not correlate well with extent of thrombus
Homan sign	Pain on dorsiflexion of the foot Present in about one third of patients with DVT and up to half without DVT
Pulmonary embolus signs and symptoms	Present in ~10% of patients with DVT
Warmth over area of thrombosis	Relatively rare
Venous distention and prominence of subcutaneous veins	Relatively uncommon
Fever	If present, typically mild
Tenderness	Found in about 75% of patients with DVT May also be found in many conditions other than DVT Degree of tenderness does not correlate well with extent of thrombus

Adapted from Schreiber, D. (2002). Deep Venous Thrombosis and Thrombophlebitis. Available at http://www.emedicine.com/emerg/topic 122.htm, accessed 5/22/03.

TABLE 9–2

WELLS CLINICAL PREDICTION GUIDE FOR DEEP VEIN
THROMBOPHLEBITIS

Clinical Parameter	Score
Active cancer (treatment ongoing, within 6 months, or palliative)	1
Paralysis or recent plaster immobilization	1
Recently bedridden for >3 days or major surgery <4 weeks earlier	1
Localized tenderness along the distribution of the deep venous system	1
Entire leg swelling	1
Calf swelling >3 cm in comparison with the asymptomatic leg	1
Pitting edema (greater in the symptomatic leg)	1
Collateral superficial veins (nonvaricose)	1
Alternative diagnosis (as likely or > that of DVT)	−2

Adapted from Anand S. S., Wells, P. S., Hunt, D., et al. (1998). Does this patient have deep vein thrombosis? JAMA 279:1094–1099.
Total of scores:
high probability : score ≥ 3;
moderate probability: score = 1 or 2;
low probability: score = 0.

ters Doppler venous flow characteristics. As for laboratory testing, levels of D-dimer, a fibrin degradation product, are elevated in DVT with high sensitivity but low specificity; similar results are found with recent surgery, trauma, myocardial infarction, pregnancy, and metastatic cancer. When findings are positive in DVT, the degree of D-dimer elevation is dependent on the size of the clot. A lower risk patient with a normal D-dimer level is unlikely to have DVT. A growing body of knowledge compels the NP to consider an underlying clotting disorder in the person with DVT, and testing for protein S, protein C, antithrombin III, factor V Leyden, prothrombin 20210A mutation, and antiphospholipid antibodies is appropriate.

Therapy for patients with DVT should be aimed at minimizing the risk of PE and extension of peripheral thrombus. Anticoagulation therapy with medications, usually first with heparin followed by warfarin, should be prescribed. These products are aimed at allowing natural fibrinolysis action and clot resolution to take place and minimize risk for clot extension; heparin and warfarin do not have intrinsic thrombolytic activity.

Because rapid anticoagulation is needed in DVT therapy, heparin is usually the initial treatment (Table 9–3). A naturally occurring acidic carbohydrate, heparin potentiates antithromboplastin III (a naturally occurring antithrombotic agent) and inhibits the activity of a number of coagulating factors. Its effect on thrombus formation is immediate, in contrast to warfarin (Coumadin), which usually requires 3 to 5 days of use before therapeutic effect is seen.

Heparin is available in the standard unfractionated form, with an average molecular weight of 15,000 d, as well as a low-molecular-weight form (LMWH), with a molecular weight of 4000 to 6500 d. Enoxaparin, dalteparin, and ardeparin are examples of LMWH. LMWH selectively enhances factor Xa and accelerates antithrombin III activity; because of limited bleeding risk, partial thromboplastin time monitoring is not required during its use. LMWH has certain additional advantages, including superior bioavailability, a

---

TABLE 9–3
INDICATIONS AND LENGTH OF WARFARIN TREATMENT

Condition	INR	Duration of therapy
Acute venous thrombosis		
• First episode	• 2–3	• 3–6 months
• High risk of recurrence	• 2–3	• Indefinitely
• W/antiphospholipid syndrome	• 3–4	• Lifelong
Prevention of systemic embolus		
• Tissue heart valves	• 2–3	• 3 months
• Valvular heart disease after thrombotic event	• 2–3	• Indefinitely
• Mechanical heart valve	• 2.5–3.5	• Indefinitely
• Acute myocardial infarction	• 2–3	• As deemed by clinical presentation
Atrial fibrillation		
• Chronic or intermittent	• 2–3	• Lifelong
• Cardioversion	• 2–3	• 3 weeks before and 4 weeks after conversion to sinus rhythm

Horton, J., and Bushwick, B. (1999). Warfarin therapy: Evolving strategies in anticoagulation. Am Family Phys. 59: 635–647.

longer half-life that allows for twice-a-day dosing, ease of calculating dosage, and limited antiplatelet effect. However, LMWH is more expensive than unfractionated heparin. Patients with an isolated calf vein DVT who are clinically stable with few risks for further embolic process and access to careful provider follow-up should be considered for initial outpatient treatment with self-administered injections of LMWH twice a day. In the absence of this scenario, inpatient admission and heparin anticoagulation are indicated.

Long-term warfarin therapy usually follows an initial heparin course. As a result of vitamin K antagonism, warfarin acts against coagulation factors II, VII, IX, and X. Warfarin is highly (99%) protein bound, primarily to albumin, and has a narrow therapeutic range. In order to avoid problems with warfarin therapy, patients must be well informed of the drug-to-drug and drug-to-food interactions (Table 9–4). Because cigarette smoking likely increases thrombotic risk while reducing warfarin's efficacy, developing a smoking cessation plan is important.

Prothrombin time is used as the measure of warfarin's efficacy and is reported as an INR. INR prolongation is seen in about 48 to 72

TABLE 9–4

WARFARIN: DRUG AND FOOD INTERACTIONS

Note: The concomitant use of warfarin with one of the following medications is not contraindicated. However, the prescriber and patient need to be aware of the impact of concurrent use on anticoagulation state.

Increased anticoagulant effect	Decreased anticoagulant effect	Variable effects
Alcohol (particularly with liver disease)	Barbiturates	Phenytoin
Amiodarone	Carbamazepine	Both increased and decreased
Cimetidine	Chlordiazepoxide	effects noted, as well as in-
Clofibrate	Cholestyramine	crease in phenytoin level.
Cotrimoxazole	Griseofulvin	
Erythromycin	Nafcillin	
Clarithromycin	Rifampin	
Fluconazole	Sucralfate	
Isoniazid	Dicloxacillin	
Metronidazole	Azathioprine	
Miconazole	Cyclosporine	
Omeprazole	Trazodone	
Phenylbutazone		
Piroxicam		
Propafenone		
Propranolol		
Acetaminophen (inconsistent)		
Ciprofloxacin		
Dextropropoxyphene disulfiram		
Itraconazole		
Quinidine		
Tamoxifen		
Tetracycline		
Influenza vaccine		

Tatro, D. (2001). Drug interaction facts. St. Louis: Facts and Comparisons.

hours after the first warfarin dose (Table 9–5). Warfarin anticoagulant therapy is usually prescribed for at least 3 to 6 months after the first DVT episode. Studies have supported low-intensity (INR = 1.5 to 2.0) warfarin anticoagulation long term to minimize thrombus risk even after a first DVT episode. With a second episode, abnormal clotting should be suspected and anticoagulant therapy lifelong. In the presence of a clotting disorder, such as factor V Leiden mutations, antiphospholipid antibodies, and the like, anticoagulation should be also be lifelong.

Approximately 2% to 10% of patients taking warfarin develop hemorrhage. This complication, however, is rarely seen in those with

---

TABLE 9–5

WARFARIN: INITIATION OF THERAPY AND LONG-TERM MANAGEMENT

- Warfarin's anticoagulation effect takes about 3–4 days of use to achieve. If immediate anticoagulation effect is needed, initiate heparin therapy while also starting warfarin 5–10 mg QD for 2 days, then reduce to 5 mg QD. Check INR daily; when at goal, discontinue heparin.
- If there is no need for immediate anticoagulation, warfarin should be initiated at 5 mg/d, anticipating therapeutic effect in about 4 days.
- If INR is not within goal during warfarin therapy, check for adherence to recommended therapy prior to adjusting dose as well as use of medications or foods that may interfere with warfarin effect.

INR goal = 2–3	Action
At desired range	Repeat INR at interval determined by duration of therapeutic INR and underlying condition • 4–6 weeks if stable condition and typically therapeutic INR • At least weekly when underlying condition can impact coagulation state (malignancy, clotting disorder, use of medications that can influence warfarin effect)
INR <2	• Increase weekly dose by 5–20% • Repeat INR 2–3 times/week until within desired range
INR 3–3.5	• Decrease weekly dose by 5–15% • Repeat INR 2–3 times/week until within desired range
INR 3.6–4	• Consider withholding 1 dose, decrease weekly dose by 10–15% • Repeat INR 2–3 times/week until within desired range
INR >4 without complications and no indication for rapid reversal of anticoagulation effect	• Consider withholding 1 dose, decrease weekly dose by 10–20% • Repeat INR 2–3 times/week until within desired range
INR >4 and need for rapid reversal of anticoagulant effect	Vitamin K 2.5–5 mg PO × 1–2 doses or 3 mg SC or slow IV
INR goal= 2.5–3.5	Action
At desired range	Repeat INR at interval determined by duration of therapeutic INR and underlying condition 4–6 weeks if stable. Repeat INR at interval determined by duration of therapeutic INR and underlying condition • 4–6 weeks if stable condition and typically therapeutic INR. • At least weekly when underlying condition can impact coagulation state (malignancy, clotting disorder, use of medications that can influence warfarin effect)
INR <2	• Increase weekly dose by 10–20% • Repeat INR 2–3 times/week until within desire range

INR goal = 2.5–3.5	Action
INR 2–2.4	• Increase weekly dose by 5–15% • Repeat INR 2–3 times/week until within desired range
INR 3.5–4.6	• Decrease weekly dose by 5–15% • Repeat INR 2–3 times/week until within desired range
INR 4.7–5.2	• Consider withholding 1 dose, decrease weekly dose by 10–20% • Repeat INR 2–3 times/week until within desired range
INR >5.2 without complications and no indication for rapid reversal of anticoagulation effect	• Withhold 1–2 doses, decrease weekly dose by 10–20% • Repeat INR 2–3 times/week until within desired range
INR >5.2 and/or need for rapid reversal of anticoagulant effect	Vitamin K 2.5 mg PO × 1–2 doses or 3 mg SC or slow IV

Horton and Bushwick (1999).

INRs of 2.0 to 3.0. In the presence of significant bleeding in patients taking warfarin, the drug should be discontinued and vitamin K should be given promptly. However, vitamin K has little effect on hemostasis for 24 hours afterward. If more prompt action is needed, such as in the case of hemorrhage or bleeding into an enclosed space, fresh-frozen plasma must be given. If anticoagulation therapy is continued after the bleeding crisis, response to warfarin may fluctuate, which necessitates close monitoring.

With a mortality rate as high as 20% to 40%, PE is a feared complication of DVT. However, the diagnosis is often missed because presentation is nonspecific. PE presentation usually includes dyspnea, pleuritic chest pain, and accentuation of the pulmonic component of S_2 heart sound; tachypnea (respiratory rate > 16 breaths per minute) is a nearly universal finding. DVT signs and symptoms may be noted, but their absence should not eliminate the consideration of a PE diagnosis. Hemoptysis, cyanosis, and change in level of consciousness are rarely encountered but are often considered to be part of the presentation.

In treating patients with PE, thrombolytic therapy may be used, followed by heparin and then warfarin therapy for a minimum of 3 to 6 months. If the patient is not a candidate for long-term anticoagulation therapy or if clotting occurs in spite of adequate anticoagulation therapy, a vena cava filter is often used to minimize the risk of future PE. Follow-up is recommended as needed to monitor INR and the underlying clinical condition.

DISCUSSION SOURCES

Feied, C., and Handler, J. (2002). Superficial Thrombophlebitis. Available at http://www.emedicine.com/ emerg/topic582.htm, accessed 8/8/04.

Hillman, R., and Ault, K. (2002). Normal hemostasis. In Hematology in Clinical Practice (3rd ed., pp. 301–307). New York: McGraw-Hill.

Hoffbrand, A., Pettit, J., and Moss, P. (2001). Thrombosis and antithrombotic therapy. In: Essential Hematology (4th ed., pp. 273–288). London: Blackwell Scientific.

Horton, J., and Bushwick, B. (1999). Warfarin therapy: Evolving strategies in anticoagulation. American Family Physician 59:635–647.

Pak, L., Messina, L., and Tierney, L. (2003). Blood vessels and lymphatics. In Tierney, L., McPhee, S., and Papadakis, M. (eds.). Current Diagnosis and Treatment (42nd ed., pp. 435–468). New York: Lange Medical Books/ McGraw-Hill.

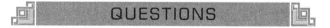

QUESTIONS

27. Which of the following is the most potent risk factor for lower extremity vascular occlusive disease?

A. hypertension
B. older age
C. cigarette smoking
D. leg injury

28. Clinical presentation of advanced lower-extremity vascular disease includes all of the following except:

    A. resting pain.
    B. absent posterior tibialis pulse.
    C. blanching of the foot with elevation.
    D. spider varicosities.

29. Drug therapy that may worsen symptoms in lower extremity arterial vascular disease includes:

    A. aspirin.
    B. cilostazol.
    C. pentoxifylline.
    D. propranolol.

30. Typically, the earliest sign of lower extremity venous insufficiency is:

    A. edema.
    B. altered pigmentation.
    C. skin atrophy.
    D. shiny skin.

31. Which of the following is the most appropriate topical antimicrobial therapy for patients with lower extremity venous stasis ulcer treatment?

    A. mupirocin
    B. bacitracin
    C. metronidazole
    D. polymyxin

32. Treatment options for venous stasis ulcers in the lower extremities include:

    A. cleansing with hydrogen peroxide.
    B. applying Burrow solution.
    C. prescribing oral corticosteroids.
    D. applying an occlusive hydroactive dressing.

33. Cilostazol (Pletal) should be used with great caution in the presence of which of the following diagnoses?

A. diabetes mellitus
B. congestive heart failure
C. hypertension
D. dyslipidemia

34. Clinical presentation of acute lower-extremity atherosclerotic arterial disease most likely includes:

    A. pain and paresthesia.
    B. pallor and pulselessness.
    C. poikilothermy.
    D. paralysis or loss of limb strength.

35. More common etiologies of acute lower-extremity atherosclerotic arterial disease include:

    A. arterial embolism with underlying atrial fibrillation.
    B. chronic venous insufficiency.
    C. extension of venous thrombosis.
    D. vessel trauma.

36. In comparison with standard arteriography, potential benefits of magnetic resonance angiography include:

    A. superior visualization of small vessel disease.
    B. the use of a relatively non-nephrotoxic contrast material.
    C. more accurate estimation of degree of stenosis.
    D. significantly less expense.

ANSWERS

| 27. C | 28. D | 29. D | 30. A | 31. C |
| 32. D | 33. B | 34. A | 35. A | 36. B |

DISCUSSION

Peripheral vascular disease is a term used to describe a group of conditions in which there is a reduction of blood flow to the extremities. Risk factors include diabetes mellitus, hypertension, and hyperlipidemia; tobacco use is the most potent risk factor. In the absence of these risk factors, peripheral vascular disease is rare except in advanced age; it is found in up to 10% of older adults.

In those with peripheral vascular disease, the venous, arterial, or lymphatic systems may be affected. Disease caused by atherosclerosis in the distal aorta or iliac, femoral, or popliteal arteries is the greatest clinical problem and is typically called lower extremity occlusive dis- ease. Presentation varies according to the area of vessel disease and dysfunction (Table 9–6). Atherosclerotic and calcific lesions usually cause occlusive disease of the aorta and its branches. Disease is often asymmetric because the distribution of obstructive lesions usually occurs in segments rather than continuously.

The diagnosis of lower extremity occlusive disease is made from clinical presentation and

TABLE 9–6

CLINICAL PRESENTATION OF LOWER EXTREMITY VASCULAR OCCLUSIVE DISEASE

Patient Presentation	*Clinical Significance*
Burning sensation or ache with walking	Usually indicates femoropopliteal arterial disease
Pain in calf, hip, or buttock with activity, relieved by rest	Classic report in intermittent claudication
Foot pain at rest	Blood flow to extremity ≤10% of normal; indicates profound disease and gangrene risk
Numbness, coldness, pain in extremity	More common than claudication report in the older adult
Absent posterior tibialis pulse	This pulse is always present in a healthy adult Dorsalis pedis pulse absent in about 5% of healthy adults
Nail thickening	Because numbness is often also a problem, meticulous nail hygiene while minimizing injury is needed Onychomycosis is often seen in PVD
Absent dorsalis pedis and tibial pulses	Proximal pulses may remain palpable
Blanching of the foot with elevation, poor capillary return, dependent rubor	≤10% of normal blood flow to extremity
Ache in anterior tibial muscles, foot, and metatarsal arch with activity	Most common with long-standing poorly controlled diabetes mellitus Can be confused with peripheral neuropathy
Sexual dysfunction	Most common in presence of smoking, hyperlipidemia, diabetes mellitus PVD contributes to its development but is likely one of a number of influencing factors

PVD, peripheral vascular disease.

select diagnostics. Gadolinium-enhanced magnetic resonance angiography and duplex ultrasonography help confirm the diagnosis and monitor disease progress. Angiography, although an invasive procedure, gives the best measure of the extent of the disease; the information gained from angiography is needed before the clinicians proceed with percutaneous treatment or surgery.

Because patients with lower extremity occlusive disease usually have other health problems, prevention and intervention measures such as aggressive risk factor reduction—including cessation of tobacco use and blood pressure, glucose, and lipid control—help improve overall well-being. In addition, the presence of concomitant disease such as cardiovascular or cerebrovascular disease may limit ability to exercise. Exercise such as walking helps to minimize symptoms and therefore should be encouraged; whereas the intervention was once thought to enhance collateral blood flow, the benefit is now recognized as being from increasing muscle anaerobic metabolism. Meticulous skin care is needed, and periodic podiatric care is recommended.

Pharmacotherapy for those with lower extremity occlusive disease often yields variable results. The use of pentoxifylline, a medication thought to reduce blood viscosity and improve blood flow by altering the ability of red blood cells to pass through diseased vessels, can be helpful in increasing exercise tolerance. Outcomes with pentoxifylline use are variable; patients without diabetes mellitus and milder symptoms appear to gain the most benefit. Cilostazol, a medication that impairs platelet aggregation and increases vasodilation, is often helpful but has limitations. Its use is contraindicated in heart failure and carries an approximately 20% rate of adverse effects, with headache, dizziness, and diarrhea. The use of these medications does not alter the course of the disease but, rather, reduces symptoms.

Although the use of vasodilators and anticoagulants appears not to alter the natural history of the disease, aspirin therapy is indicated, in part because of the increased risk of heart disease with the condition. Clopidogrel has been used in lower extremity occlusive disease therapy, particularly in patients who are aspirin allergic or intolerant or have an underlying hypercoagulable state; it prevents fibrinogen binding and may reduce the risk of thrombus formation. Warfarin therapy with a goal INR of 2.0 to 3.0 may be used for selected patients with high thrombus risk, particularly those who have undergone a vascular procedure.

Surgical evaluation for percutaneous or open procedures should be part of the care of patients with lower extremity occlusive disease; medical management of concomitant problems such as cardiovascular disease and diabetes mellitus needs to optimized preoperatively and surgical intervention for other forms of vascular disease also considered. Angioplasty and/or grafting procedures can help improve blood flow and minimize symptoms and complications.

Although lower extremity occlusive disease is characterized by a relatively predicable, slower progressive process, acute occlusion can occur. Caused by embolic, thrombotic, or traumatic events, acute limb ischemia usually presents with the so-called six Ps: pain, paresthesia (the two most common manifestations), pallor, pulselessness, poikilothermy (variation in limb temperature), and paralysis. When acute limb ischemia is caused by arterial embolism, the clot's origin is usually the heart with an underlying atrial fibrillation. When caused by arterial thrombosis, chronic arteriosclerotic occlusive disease is usually at the core of the problem. Prompt assessment is needed to support the diagnosis. Arteriography is usually considered the diagnostic "gold standard" but carries the risk of exposure to potentially nephrotoxic contrast material and ionizing radiation. Magnetic resonance angiography may replace diagnostic angiography because it is noninvasive, it does not require the use of ionizing radiation, and the contrast agent used is relatively non-nephrotoxic. Drawbacks include cost, limited availability, the limited depiction of small vessels, and the possible overestimation of the degree of stenosis. Treatment options for acute occlusive disease include endovascular therapies, surgical revascularization procedures, and thrombolytic and anticoagulant therapy.

Chronic venous insufficiency is a common sequela of DVT and leg trauma, although the absence of this history is noted in about 25% of patients. There is decreased venous return because of vessel damage, and lower extremity edema is usually the earliest sign. Symptoms usually include leg aching and itchiness. Over time, the edema becomes progressively worse; this results in the development of thin, shiny, atrophic skin, often with brown pigmentation. Subcutaneous tissue thickens and becomes fibrous.

The stage is set for stasis ulceration. Inflamed, red, pruritic patches usually precede the formation of an irregular ulceration with a clean base. Yellow eschar, which is occasionally found, necessitates débridement. After the ulcer base is clean, metronidazole gel should be applied to reduce bacterial growth and odor. An occlusive hydroactive dressing such as DuoDerm, followed by an Unna zinc paste boot, is applied and changed weekly. If healing does not ensue within a few weeks, the patient should be referred for surgical evaluation for possible skin grafts or for specialty wound care.

DISCUSSION SOURCES

Chahin, D. (2002). Lower-Extremity Atherosclerotic Arterial Disease. Available at http://www.emedicine.com/radio/topic895.htm, accessed May 21, 2003.

Pak, L., Messina, L., and Tierney, L. (2003). Blood vessels and lymphatics. In Tierney, L., McPhee, S., and Papadakis, M. (eds.). Current Diagnosis and Treatment (42nd ed., pp. 435–468). New York: Lange Medical Books/McGraw-Hill.

Scott, L. (2004). Peripheral vascular disorders. In Hektor Dunphy, L. Management Guidelines for Nurse Practitioners Working with Adults (2nd ed, pp 411–424). Philadelphia, F.A. Davis.

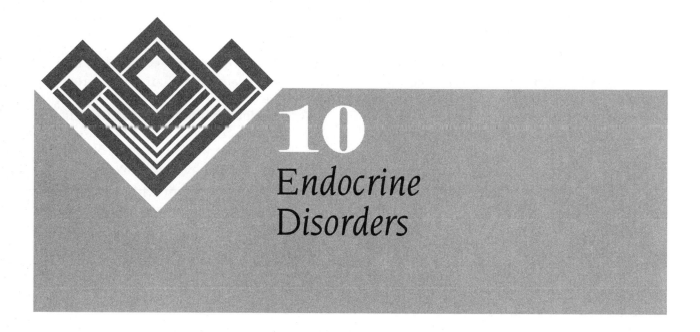

10

Endocrine Disorders

1. Which of the following characteristics applies to type 1 diabetes mellitus (DM)?

   A. Significant hyperglycemia and ketoacidosis result from lack of insulin.
   B. This condition is commonly diagnosed on routine examination or workup for other health problems.
   C. Initial response to oral sulfonylureas is usually favorable.
   D. Insulin resistance (IR) is a significant part of the disease.

2. Which of the following characteristics apply to type 2 DM?

   A. Major risk factors are heredity and obesity.
   B. Pear-shaped body type is commonly found.
   C. Exogenous insulin is needed for control of disease.
   D. Exercise increases IR.

3. You consider prescribing insulin G (Lantus) because of its:

   A. extended duration of action.
   B. rapid onset of action.
   C. ability to prevent diabetic end-organ damage.
   D. ability to preserve pancreatic function.

4. Lispro's (Humalog's) onset of action occurs in:

   A. less than 15 minutes.
   B. approximately 1 hour.
   C. 1 to 2 hours.
   D. 3 to 4 hours.

5. Which of the following medications should be used with caution in a person with suspected or known sulfa allergy?

   A. metformin
   B. glyburide
   C. Ultralente insulin
   D. NPH insulin

6. Metformin's (Glucophage's) mechanism of action is as:

   A. an insulin-production enhancer.
   B. a product virtually identical in action to the sulfonylureas.
   C. a drug that increases insulin action in the peripheral tissues and reduces hepatic glucose production.
   D. a facilitator of renal glucose excretion.

7. According to the American Diabetes Association (ADA) Clinical Practice Guidelines, testing for type 2 DM in asymptomatic, undiagnosed individuals older than 45 years should be conducted every ____.

   A. year
   B. 3 years
   C. 5 years
   D. 10 years

8. According to the ADA Clinical Practice Guidelines, testing for type 2 DM in asymptomatic, undiagnosed individuals younger than 45 years should be considered when there is:

   A. a family history of obesity.
   B. a personal history of high-density lipoprotein (HDL) less than 35 mg/dL.
   C. activity intolerance reported by the patient.
   D. poor response to efforts to maintain normal body mass index (BMI).

9. Criteria for the diagnosis of type 2 DM include:

   A. classic symptoms regardless of fasting plasma glucose measurement.
   B. plasma glucose level of 126 mg/dL as a random measurement.
   C. a 2-hour glucose measurement of 156 mg/dL after a 75-g anhydrous glucose load dissolved in water.
   D. a plasma glucose level of 126 mg/dL or higher after an 8-hour fast on more than one occasion.

10. Rosiglitazone's mechanism of action is as:

   A. an insulin-production enhancer.
   B. a reducer of pancreatic glucose output.
   C. an insulin sensitizer.
   D. a facilitator of renal glucose excretion.

11. Which of the following should be the goal measurement in treating a person with DM and hypertension?

   A. blood pressure of less than 130 mm Hg systolic and less than 80 mm Hg diastolic
   B. low-density lipoprotein (LDL) cholesterol level of less than 130 mg/dL
   C. triglyceride levels of 200 to 300 mg/dL
   D. HDL level of 35 to 40 mg/dL

12. In caring for a patient with DM, microalbuminuria measurement should be obtained:

   A. annually if urine protein is present.
   B. periodically in relationship to glycemia control.
   C. yearly if urinalysis is negative for protein.
   D. with each office visit related to DM.

13. The mechanism of action of the sulfonylureas is as:

   A. a catalyst of insulin receptor site activity.
   B. a product that enhances insulin release.
   C. a facilitator of renal glucose excretion.
   D. an agent that can reduce hepatic glucose production.

14. When caring for a patient with DM and hypertension, the nurse practitioner (NP) considers prescribing:

   A. furosemide.
   B. methyldopa.
   C. fosinopril.
   D. nifedipine.

15. Clinical presentation of type 1 DM usually includes all of the following except:

   A. report of recent weight gain.
   B. ketosis.
   C. thirst.
   D. polyphagia.

16. Which of the following should be periodically monitored with the use of a biguanide?

   A. creatine kinase (CK)
   B. alkaline phosphatase (ALP)

C. alanine aminotransferase (ALT)

D. creatinine (CR)

17. Which of the following should be periodically monitored with the use of a thiazolidinedione (TZD)?

A. CK

B. ALP

C. ALT

D. CR

18. All of the following are risks for lactic acidosis in metformin users except:

A. renal insufficiency.

B. dehydration.

C. radiographic contrast dye use.

D. chronic obstructive pulmonary disease.

19. Secondary causes of hyperglycemia include all of the following medications except:

A. niacin.

B. corticosteroids.

C. thiazide diuretics.

D. alpha blockers.

20. Hemoglobin A_{1C} provides information on glucose control over the past:

A. 21 to 47 days.

B. 48 to 63 days.

C. 64 to 90 days.

D. 90 to 120 days.

21. Which of the following is not true concerning the effects of exercise and IR?

A. Approximately 80% of the body's insulin-mediated glucose uptake takes place in skeletal muscle.

B. With regular aerobic exercise, IR is reduced by approximately 40%.

C. The IR-reducing effects of exercise persist for up to 48 hours after the activity.

D. Hyperglycemia can occur as a result of aerobic exercise.

22 to 25. With an 8:00 AM dose of the following drugs and inadequate dietary intake/excessive energy utilization, at approximately what time would hypoglycemia be most likely to occur?

22. Lispro _____

23. Regular insulin _____

24. Insulin N (NPH) _____

25. Insulin G (glargine, Lantus) _____

26. The meglitinide analogs are particularly helpful adjuncts in type 2 DM care to minimize risk of:

A. fasting hypoglycemia.

B. nocturnal hyperglycemia.

C. postprandial hyperglycemia.

D. postprandial hypoglycemia.

27. What is the most common adverse effect noted with alpha-glucosidase inhibitor use?

A. flatulence

B. hepatotoxicity

C. renal impairment

D. symptomatic hypoglycemia

28. Which of the following best describes the Somogyi effect?

A. Insulin-induced hypoglycemia triggers excess secretion of glucagon and cortisol, leading to hyperglycemia.

B. Early morning elevated blood glucose levels result in part from growth hormone and cortisol-triggering hepatic glucose release.

C. Late evening hyperglycemia is induced by inadequate insulin dose.

D. Episodes of postprandial hypoglycemia occur as a result of inadequate food intake.

29. Intervention in microalbuminuria for a person with DM includes:

A. improved glycemic control.

B. strict dyslipidemia control.

C. use of an angiotensin-converting enzyme inhibitor or angiotensin receptor blocker.

D. all of the above.

ANSWERS

1. A	2. A	3. A
4. A	5. B	6. C
7. B	8. B	9. D
10. C	11. A	12. C
13. B	14. C	15. A
16. D	17. C	18. D
19. D	20. D	21. D

22. Approximately 8:30–9:30 AM (with peak of insulin dose)
23. Approximately 10 AM to 11 AM (with peak of insulin dose)
24. Approximately 12 PM to 6 PM (with peak of insulin dose)
25. Because insulin G (glargine, Lantus) has no peak, an episode of hypoglycemia is unlikely. If hypoglycemia were to occur, the episode could be protracted if left untreated, because of the medication's protracted duration of activity.

26. C	27. A
28. A	29. D

DISCUSSION

Type 1 DM is a disease of insulin deficiency. This disease usually occurs in persons younger than 30 years, with symptomatic presentation often as the classic "polys": polydipsia, polyphagia, and polyuria. If type 1 DM is associated with ketoacidosis, DM presentation can be dramatic, with severe dehydration, abdominal pain, vomiting, and decreased level of consciousness. In any event, prompt intervention with appropriate insulin therapy is indicated.

Insulin resistance (IR) is a genetically predetermined condition that is central to the pathogenesis of type 2 DM. In IR, there is a reduced sensitivity in the tissues to insulin's action at a given concentration, which causes a subnormal effect on glucose metabolism. This results in hyperglycemia, which in turn stimulates pancreatic insulin production to reduce the blood glucose level. Euglycemia occurs, albeit in the presence of hyperinsulinemia. Elevated fasting insulin levels are noted to be an independent predictor for ischemic heart disease. When coupled with acquired or lifestyle characteristics that contribute to IR, such as obesity, physical inactivity, and high-carbohydrate (>60% total calories) diet, the body has greater difficulty maintaining a normal blood glucose level. Over time, usually after many years of IR, pancreatic beta cell deficiency usually occurs, resulting in impaired glucose tolerance, hyperglycemia, and the diagnosis of type 2 DM.

A number of conditions are seen in conjunction with IR. Increased IR is inversely related to decreased urinary uric acid clearance; this leads to a dramatic increase in the rate of gout. The majority of women with polycystic ovary syndrome are insulin resistant. Acanthosis nigricans, hyperpigmentation of the skin often in the neck and axilla, is also correlated with IR. This finding is most common in children and young adults with IR and DM risk.

Although the correlation of obesity with IR and DM type 2 is well established, not all body fat types and distribution are equally problematic. Some persons with IR and DM type 2 are of normal weight, whereas others with IR never develop hyperglycemia. However, obesity dramatically increases the risk of diabetes in the person with IR. "Apple-shaped" or central, abdominal obesity is made up of metabolically active fat and is associated with high insulin levels, IR, high mobilization rate of free fatty acids, and high insulin levels; the last trait is often associated with increased appetite. The genetic makeup that allows this to happen helped increase the likelihood of survival in times of famine. However, in these times of plentiful food, IR helps promote fat storage.

Patients with type 2 DM are most often asymptomatic at onset. As a result, the ADA recommends periodic fasting plasma glucose screening every 3 years in all adults, regardless of appearance of risk. Testing should be considered at a younger age or be carried out more frequently in individuals with the following type 2 DM risk factors:

- are overweight (BMI $\geq$ 25 kg/m^2)
- have a first-degree relative with diabetes
- are members of a high-risk ethnic population (e.g., African-American, Latino, Native American, Asian-American, Pacific Islander)
- have given birth to a baby weighing more than 9 lb or have been diagnosed with gestational diabetes
- are hypertensive
- have an HDL cholesterol level of $\Leftarrow$ 35 mg/dL (0.90 mmol/L) and/or a triglyceride level of $\Rightarrow$ 250 mg/dL (2.82 mmol/L)
- have other clinical conditions associated with IR (e.g., polycystic ovary syndrome, acanthosis nigricans, or glucose intolerance)

When a fasting plasma glucose threshold level of greater than 126 mg/dL after an 8-hour fast is used, this testing is 98% specific and 40% to 88% sensitive for type 2 DM. Typically, wide-scale screening done according to these guidelines yields a 6% true-positive rate. Additional ADA diagnostic criteria for type 2 DM include a casual (random) plasma glucose level greater than 200 mg/dL with classic diabetic symptoms and an oral glucose tolerance result of greater than 200 mg/dL at 2 hours. The ADA does not currently recommend the use of hemoglobin A_{1C} as a tool for diagnosing DM.

Therapeutic lifestyle changes are critically important for the person withDM. Tobacco use in any form should be discouraged. Because approximately 80% of the body's insulin-mediated glucose uptake takes place in muscle and is enhanced by physical activity, a regular program of aerobic exercise should be prescribed. Exercise reduces IR by approximately 40%, with the effects persisting for up to 48 hours after the activity, and aids in weight maintenance. For type 1 or type 2 DM, current ADA recommendations advise a diet of 300 mg or less of cholesterol per day, 8% to 9% or less of total dietary calories per day from saturated fat with similar proportions of polyunsaturated and monounsaturated fats, and 25 to 30 g of dietary fiber per day. Calories from protein should be no more than 10% to 20% of the daily total. Reinforcement of proper foot care and a clinical foot examination should be a part of every DM–related visit (Table 10–1).

Insulin therapy is indicated for all patients with type 1 DM and those with type 2 DM with insulinopenia. Insulins come in many forms, from shorter acting to long-acting forms with different onsets, peaks, and durations of action (Table 10–1). The NP needs to be aware of the characteristics of each insulin form and how they contribute to glycemic control. With insulin use, two conditions that can result in early morning hyperglycemia can occur. The Somogyi effect occurs when an insulin-

TABLE 10–1
INSULIN; ONSET, PEAK, AND DURATION OF ACTION

Type	Onset of Action	Peak	Duration of Action
Short-acting, rapid onset of action (Lispro, Humalog)	15 min	30–90 min	$<$=5 hr
Short-acting (Regular; Humulin R)	$^1/_2$–1 hr	2–3 hr	4–6 hr
Intermediate-acting (Humulin N, NPH)	2–4 hr	4–10 hr	14–18 hr
Long-acting (Humulin L, Lente)	3–4 hr	4–12 hr	16–20 hr
Extended-acting (Humulin U; Ultralente)	6–10 hr	None to minimal	20–30 hr
Insulin glargine (Lantus)	Hours	None	$>$ 24 hr

TABLE 10–2

MEDICATIONS COMMONLY USED TO TREAT TYPE 2 DM

Medication	Mechanism of action	Caution
Sulfonylurea (SU)	Insulin secretagogue	Sulfa allergy, renal dysfunction
Thiazolidinedione (TZD) (-glitazone suffix)	Insulin sensitizer	Periodically monitor ALT; hypoglycemia possible when used w/SU or insulin but not when used as solo agent
Biguanides (Metformin)	Insulin sensitizer	Monitor creatinine (Cr) lactic acidosis risk especially w/elevated Cr; hypoglycemia when used w/SU or insulin but not when used as solo agent. Potential GI side effects.
α-gulucosidase inhibitors	Delay intestinal carbohydrate absorption	Taken w/meals. Helpful in management of postprandial hyperglycemia. Potential GI side effects.
Meglitinides	Short-acting insulin secretagogue	Quick insulin burst, taken before meals, helpful in management of postprandial hyperglycemia

induced hypoglycemia triggers excess secretion of glucagon and cortisol; this in turns leads to hyperglycemia. Intervention is aimed at lowering the inappropriately high insulin dose, usually the dinnertime dose of intermediate-acting insulin. The dawn phenomenon is a result of reduced insulin sensitivity developing between 5:00 AM and 8:00 AM, caused by earlier spikes in growth hormone. The net result is cortisol release, which triggers hepatic glucose secretion and early morning hyperglycemia. The dawn phenomenon intervention includes splitting the evening intermediate insulin dose between dinner and bedtime. Alternative interventions include switching to a bedtime dose of insulin G or an insulin pump.

Sulfonylureas have been used for many years for the treatment of type 2 DM. These drugs help to control DM by stimulating insulin release from functioning beta cells and, to a lesser degree, help enhance insulin sensitivity. However, type 2 DM is a progressive disease, with about 5% to 20% patients per year failing therapy on sulfonylurea alone. As a result, multiple treatment modalities should be considered. The sulfonylureas have photosensitizing potential; patients should be advised to use sunscreen and sun-protective clothing. These medications also contain a sulfa molecule; they should be avoided or used with great caution by the person with sulfa allergy. Because of the sulfonylureas' action in enhancing insulin release, patients often note an increase in appetite and resultant weight gain after starting the medication (Table 10–2).

Metformin, a biguanide, increases muscle and adipose cell receptors' sensitivity to glucose. As a result, glucose uptake is more efficient and plasma glucose level is lowered. In addition, metformin suppresses hepatic glucose production and hepatic glycogen output. A modest weight loss, usually 3 to 5 kg, is often seen during the first months with the use of metformin, because there is a reduction of glucose absorption from the gastrointestinal tract. There is little hypoglycemia risk with the use of metformin alone, although this may be noted when it is used with a sulfonylurea or insulin.

The use of metformin can help improve lipid profile, decreasing LDL and triglyceride levels while increasing HDL. Metformin's major adverse effect is gastrointestinal upset, avoidable by increasing the dosage slowly. A rare but serious complication of metformin use is the development of lactic acidosis risk; this is highest in patients with complicating factors such as heart and liver disease, renal insufficiency, electrolyte imbalance, and the use of radiographic imaging contrast dyes. Because lactic acidosis risk is greatest in the person with renal insufficiency, serum creatinine levels should be periodically monitored. However, metformin is not an inherently renal toxic medication.

The TZDs, a class of medications whose names share the "-glitazone" suffix, are used in the treatment of DM. These products act by reducing IR and improving insulin sensitivity in muscle and adipose tissue. In addition, hepatic glucose output suppressed with TDZ use but somewhat less than with metformin use. Occasionally, modest weight loss and mild edema is reported with TZD use. There is little hypoglycemia risk when TZDs are used as monotherapy, but such risk is possible when TZDs are coupled with sulfonylurea or insulin use. These products have a positive lipid effect, decreasing triglyceride levels by approximately 15%, increasing HDL by about 7%, and decreasing LDL by about 10%. Periodic ALT monitoring is recommended in all patients on TZD therapy; the medication should be discontinued if ALT level reaches three times the upper limit of normal. The medication should not be started if ALT level is higher than 2.5 times the upper limit of normal at baseline.

Two classes of medications, the alpha-glucosidase inhibitors and the meglitinide analogs, are particularly helpful in managing postprandial glucose excursion These medications must be taken with meals and are indicated as part of overall therapy in type 2 DM. The alpha-glucosidase inhibitors are a family of drugs that include acarbose and miglitol and have a net effect of delaying intestinal absorption of carbohydrate, thus potentially preventing postprandial hyperglycemia. These drugs are poorly absorbed systemically and generally safe to use, with flatulence being the most common adverse effect. The meglitinide analogs such as repaglinide are structurally similar to glyburide, a sulfonylurea, but have a much more rapid onset of action and a very short half-life. These medications can be used at mealtime to provide a quick insulin burst, potentially preventing postprandial glucose increase.

DM is the leading cause of chronic renal failure. After the diagnosis of DM is made, periodic screening of renal function should be done. Often the serum creatinine measurement is used for this purpose. However, an increase in creatinine is not seen until at least 50% of the nephrons are not functioning. Thus, an elevated creatinine level is a late rather than early indicator of renal damage. A far more sensitive indicator of diabetic nephropathy is the presence of proteinuria, a harbinger of progressive renal failure. Urine protein consists of a number of forms, including the most abundant, albumin, as well as immunoglobulins, haptoglobin, and light chains. The standard dipstick test is sensitive to 100 to 150 mg/L of urine albumin, certainly an earlier marker of progressive renal failure than serum creatinine but still a later disease marker. However, the presence of a small amount of albumin (microalbumin, or >20 mg/L albumin, or >30 to 40 mg/day) is considered a predictor of glomerular dysfunction associated with diabetic nephropathy.

Microalbuminuria can precede development of DM by 10 years. With type 2 DM, the patient should be screened for microalbuminuria at onset of disease, with an annual recheck if results are normal. Collection of a first morning specimen is important because normal daily activity may cause a low level of protein spillage into the urine, creating a false-positive result. The diagnosis of microalbuminuria should be confirmed by obtaining at least two positive results from three collections in a 3- to 6-month period; results should be correlated with serum creatinine level. Intervention includes tightening of glycemic control, to hemoglobin A_{1C} of less than 7%, controlling elevated blood pressure (<130 mm Hg systolic and <80 mm Hg diastolic, per the Seventh Report of the Joint National Committee on the

Prevention, Detection, Evaluation, and Treatment of Hypertension guidelines); aggressive treatment of dyslipidemia; and the addition of an agent to preserve renal function by reducing efferent arteriolar pressure (angiotensin-converting enzyme inhibitors [drugs whose names have the "-pril" suffix], angiotensin receptor blockers [drugs whose names have the "-sartan" suffix], diltiazem, and/or verapamil).

Glycated hemoglobin, also know as hemoglobin A_1, increases in proportion to the amount of circulating glucose. The most abundant glycohemoglobin subtype of hemoglobin A_1 is A_{1C}, which constitutes about 4% to 6% of the body's total hemoglobin. Glycohemoglobin circulates as part of the red blood cell for about 120 days, the length of the red blood cell's life span. As a result, hemoglobin A_{1C} measurement provides a method for evaluating glucose control over time; it should be borne in mind that the measurement best reflects blood glucose trends over the preceding 4 to 6 weeks.

DISCUSSION SOURCES

American Diabetes Association Clinical Practice Recommendations (2004). Available at http://care.diabetesjournals.org/content/vol27/suppl_1, accessed 8/16/04.

Masharni, U., and Karam, J. (2003). Diabetes mellitus and hypoglycemia. In Tierney, L., McPhee, S., and Papadakis, M. (eds.). Current Medical Diagnosis and Treatment (42nd ed., pp. 1152–1198). New York: Lange Medical Books/McGraw-Hill.

Price, M., and Kent, D. (1999). Endocrine disorders: Diabetes mellitus. In Youngkin, E., Sawing, K., Kissinger, J., and Israel, D. (eds.). Pharmacotherapeutics: A Primary Care Clinical Guide (pp. 709–729). Stamford, CT: Appleton & Lange.

Thrush S., and McCaffrey, R. (2004). Endocrine and metabolic disorders. In Hektor Dunphy, L. Management Guidelines for Nurse Practitioners Working with Adults. Philadelphia, F.A. Davis.

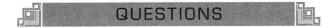

QUESTIONS

30. Risk factors for heat stroke include all of the following except:

A. obesity.

B. use of beta-adrenergic antagonists.

C. excessive activity.

D. use of a vasodilator.

31. Possible adverse outcomes from heat stroke include:

A. rhabdomyolysis.

B. anemia.

C. hypernatremia.

D. leukopenia.

32. Laboratory findings in heat stroke usually include:

A. elevated total creatine kinase level.

B. anemia.

C. metabolic alkalosis.

D. hypokalemia.

33. Intervention for patients with heat stroke includes:

A. total body ice packing.

B. rehydration.

C. fluid restriction.

D. potassium supplementation.

ANSWERS

30. D   **31.** A   **32.** A   **33.** B

DISCUSSION

Heat stroke is a life-threatening emergency caused by a failure of the body's thermoregulatory system, usually in response to extreme environmental and personal factors. Risk factors for heat stroke include the use of medications that alter adrenergic activity and possibly decrease cardiac output (negative inotropes), such as tricyclic antidepressants (drugs whose names have the "-triptyline" suffix), beta-adrenergic antagonists (beta blockers; drugs whose names have the "-lol" suffix), and vasoconstrictors such as decongestants. The use of these products negates the body's normal attempts to decrease core temperature, such as increasing cardiac output and cutaneous vasodilatation.

Assessment of a patient with heat stroke includes a complete evaluation of electrolytes, hematologic parameters, and liver function. Total creatine kinase level is typically elevated, owing to this enzyme's being released by skeletal muscle injured by muscle cramping and convulsion. Because of the release of this intracellular electrolyte with tissue damage, hyperkalemia is common. Heat stroke can lead to a transient polycythemia caused by volume constriction, hyponatremia with Na^+ level of less than 120 mEq/L, and stress-induced leukocytosis.

Intervention for a patient with heat stroke includes controlled cooling by the use of tepid sprays and fanning or by the application of cold packs to selected areas such as the axillae, neck, and groin. Rapid cooling by ice packing is discouraged because it may stimulate cutaneous vasoconstriction, inhibiting heat loss. Rehydration should be aggressive but with careful monitoring because of the risk of pulmonary edema from reduced cardiac output.

Optimally, a patient with heat stroke should be admitted to the hospital for at least 24 hours after stabilization because of the risk of late complications that includes one of the most feared complications: rhabdomyolysis, a condition of rapid muscle tissue destruction.

As the muscle breaks down, large amounts of myoglobin and other cellular products are released into circulation to be excreted by the kidney. As a result, about 50% of patients with rhabdomyolysis develop acute renal failure. In heat stroke, the presence of myoglobinuria is an early indicator of rhabdomyolysis. Typically, the patient also has complaints of muscle pain and weakness. Treatment of rhabdomyolysis is aimed at treating its potentially life-threatening consequences such as renal failure and profound hyperkalemia.

DISCUSSION SOURCES

Cohen, R., and Moelleken, B. (2003). Disorders due to physical agents. In Tierney, L., McPhee, S., and Papadakis, M. (eds.). Current Medical Diagnosis and Treatment (42nd ed., pp. 1536–1554). New York: Lange Medical Books/ McGraw-Hill.

Thrush S., and McCaffrey, R. (2004). Endocrine and metabolic disorders. In Hektor Dunphy, L. Management Guidelines for Nurse Practitioners Working with Adults. Philadelphia, F.A. Davis.

QUESTIONS

34. A 62-year-old woman has hypertension, a 100–pack-year history of cigarette smoking, and intermittent claudication. Triglyceride level is 280 mg/dL, HDL level is 38 mg/dL, and LDL level is 135 mg/dL. Which of the following represents the most appropriate pharmacologic intervention for this patient's lipid disorders?

   A. No further intervention is required.
   B. Multidrug therapy will likely be needed.
   C. A resin should be prescribed
   D. The use of ezetimibe will likely be sufficient to achieve dyslipidemia control.

35. You examine a 46-year-old smoker with hypertension. His lipid profile is as follows: HDL level is 48 mg/dL; LDL level is 192 mg/dL; and triglyceride level is 110 mg/dL. He had been on a low-cholesterol diet for 6 months when these tests were taken. Which of the following represents the best next step?

   A. No further intervention is required.
   B. A fibrate should be prescribed.
   C. A 3-hydroxy-3-methylglutaryl–coenzyme A (HMG-CoA) reductase inhibitor should be prescribed.
   D. A resin is the best choice of lipid-lowering agent for this patient.

36. You examine a 64-year-old man with hypertension and type 2 DM. Results are as follows: HDL level is 38 mg/dL; LDL level is 135 mg/dL; and triglyceride level is 180 mg/dL. His current medications include a sulfonylurea, TZD, biguanide, angiotensin-converting enzyme inhibitor, and thiazide diuretic, and he has acceptable glycemic and blood pressure control. He states, "I really watch the fats and sugars in my diet." Which of the following is the most appropriate advice?

A. No further intervention is needed.

B. His lipid profile should be repeated in 6 months.

C. Lipid-lowering drug therapy should be initiated.

D. The patient's dietary intervention appears adequate.

37. When providing care for a patient taking an HMG-CoA reductase inhibitor, periodic monitoring of which of the following is recommended?

A. potassium

B. aspartate aminotransferase

C. creatine kinase

D. blood urea nitrogen

38. When prescribing a fibrate, the NP expects to see the following changes in lipid profile:

A. marked decrease in LDL level

B. increase in HDL level

C. no effect on triglyceride level

D. increase in very-low-density lipoprotein (VLDL) level

39. When prescribing niacin, the NP expects to see the following changes in lipid profile:

A. marked decrease in LDL level

B. increase in HDL level

C. no effect on triglyceride level

D. increase in VLDL level

40. In prescribing niacin therapy for a patient with hyperlipidemia, the NP considers that:

A. postdose flushing is often reported.

B. hepatic monitoring is not warranted.

C. low-dose therapy is usually effective in raising LDL level.

D. drug-induced thrombocytopenia is a common problem.

41. With the use of ezetimibe (Zetia), the NP expects to see:

A. a marked increase in HDL cholesterol.

B. a reduction in LDL cholesterol.

C. a significant reduction in triglyceride levels.

D. increased rhabdomyolysis when the drug is used in conjunction with a HMG-CoA reductase inhibitor.

42. With ezetimibe (Zetia), which of the following should be periodically monitored?

A. ALP

B. LDH

C. CPK

D. No special laboratory monitoring is recommended.

43. With the use of a lipid-lowering resin, which of the following enzymes should be periodically monitored?

A. alkaline phosphatase

B. lactate dehydrogenase

C. aspartate aminotransferase

D. no particular monitoring is recommended

44. All of the following are risks for statin-induced myositis except:

A. advanced age.

B. use of a statin with a resin.

C. low body weight.

D. high statin dose.

45. According the recommendations of the National Cholesterol Education Program Adult Treatment Panel III guidelines, what is the average LDL reduction achieved with a change in diet as a single life-style modification?

A. less than 5%

B. 5% to 10%

C. 11% to 15%

D. 16% to 20% or more

46. You are seeing a patient who is taking atorvastatin and cholestyramine and provide the following advice:

A. "Take both medications together."

B. "You need to have extra blood tests while on this combination."

C. "Separate your cholestyramine from other medications by at least 2 hours."

D. "Make sure you take these medications on an empty stomach."

47. Which of the following medications is most effective against lipoprotein (a)?

A. HMG-CoA reductase inhibitors
B. niacin
C. bile acid sequestrants
D. fibrates

48. All of the following are common causes of secondary hypertriglyceridemia except:

A. hypothyroidism.
B. beta blocker use.
C. poorly controlled DM.
D. excessive alcohol use.

ANSWERS

34. B	**35.** C	**36.** C
37. B	**38.** B	**39.** B
40. A	**41.** B	**42.** D
43. D	**44.** B	**45.** B
46. C	**47.** B	**48.** B

DISCUSSION

Treatment of hyperlipidemia is an important part of cardiovascular and cerebrovascular risk reduction. Intensive therapeutic lifestyle changes should be the first line of therapy. Dietary advice includes, per ATP III Guidelines, lowering saturated fat and cholesterol intake to levels of previous American Heart Association Step II diet and adding dietary options to enhance LDL lowering, such as plant stanols and sterols, as well as increasing intake of viscous or soluble fiber. However, most adults achieve only a modest 5% to 10% reduction in LDL cholesterol with this as a single intervention. Weight management and a program of regular aerobic exercise should be prescribed for overall health. Dietary lipid improvement is often enhanced if coupled with exercise.

Pharmacologic intervention in hyperlipidemia will likely be needed in patients with considerable cardiovascular and cerebrovascular risk, including patients with DM, hypertension, and existing vascular disease. The choice of a lipid-lowering agent should be guided by the effect of the agent on the lipid profile, as well as the desired lipid levels (Tables 10–3, 10–4, and 10–5).

DISCUSSION SOURCES

Baron, R. (2003). Lipid abnormalities. In Tierney, L., McPhee, S., and Papadakis, M. (eds.). Current Medical Diagnosis and Treatment (42nd ed., pp. 1199–1211). New York: Lange Medical Books/McGraw-Hill.

Grundy, S., et al. Implications of recent clinical trials for the National Cholesterol Education Program Adult Treatment Panel III guidelines. Circulation 2004; 110:227–239.

National Heart, Lung, and Blood Institute (2002). Adult Treatment Panel III (ATP III) Guidelines National Cholesterol Education Program Adult Treatment Panel III Guidelines for Lipid Goals. Available at www.nhlbi.nih.gov/guidelines/cholesterol/index.htm, accessed 8/15/03.

Thrush, S., and McCaffrey, R. (2004). Endocrine and metabolic disorders. In Hektor Dunphy, L. Management Guidelines for Nurse Practitioners Working with Adults. Philadelphia, F.A. Davis.

QUESTIONS

49. The diagnosis of metabolic syndrome includes notation of:

A. abdominal obesity.
B. triglyceride levels higher than 150 mg/dL.
C. HDL cholesterol level of less than 40 mg/dL for men, less than 50 mg/dL for women.
D. all of the above.

50. Which of the following characteristics apply to metabolic syndrome?

A. IR is universally noted.
B. Lower body obesity is often noted.
C. Progress to type 2 DM occurs rapidly.
D. Increased peripheral vascular resistance is uncommon.

	TABLE 10-3	

EFFECT OF MEDICATIONS ON LIPID LEVELS

Medication	Effect	Comment
HMG CoA reductase inhibitor (statin)	↓LDL: 18–55% ↑HDL: 5–15% ↓TG: 7–30%	Small risk (<=1%) of hepatic enzyme rise with use. Check hepatic enzymes (esp. AST) prior to initiation, periodically post-initiation or dose adjustment as recommended in product information. Check CK at initiation to establish baseline. Ongoing CK evaluation in the absence of symptoms not warranted. Adverse effects: Rhabdomyolysis, myositis, rare but most often noted with higher statin dose, in combination with fibrate, in renal impairment, multiple comorbidities, low body weight, advanced age.
Resins (cholestyramine, colestipol, colesevelam)	↓LDL: 15–30% ↑HDL: 3–5%	Nonsystemic with no hepatic monitoring required. Minimal effect on TG with the exception of potential to increase TG if > 400 mg/dL. Adverse effects: GI distress, constipation, decreased absorption of other drugs if taken within 2 h of many medications.
Niacin	↑HDL: 15–35% ↓TG: 20–50% ↓LDL: 5–25%	Particularly effective against highly atherogenic lipoprotein (a) Adverse effect: Flushing (potentially minimized by taking aspirin 1 h prior to niacin dose), hyperglycemia, hyperuricemia, upper GI distress, hepatotoxicity Contraindications: Active liver disease, severe gout, peptic ulcer
Fibric acid derivatives Gemfibrozil (Lopid), fenofibrate (Tricor)	↑HDL: 10–20% ↓TG: 20–50% ↓LDL: 5–20% (with normal TG) May raise LDL-C (with high TG)	Adverse effects: Dyspepsia, gallstones, myopathy including rhabdomyolysis if taken with a statin. Contraindications: Severe renal or hepatic disease.
Ezetimibe (Zetia)	↓LDL-C: 15–20% ↑HDL-C: 3–5%	Minimal effect on TG. Most often prescribed with another lipid-lowering agent such as a statin to enhance LDL reduction. Adverse effects: Few due to limited systemic absorption.

Baron, 2003, Adult Treatment Panel III (ATP III) Guidelines National Cholesterol Education Program Adult Treatment Panel III Guidelines for Lipid Goals, available at www.nhlbi.nih.gov/guidelines/cholesterol/index.htm, accessed 10/4/04.

51. Which of the following characteristics is *not* descriptive of plasminogen activator inhibitor?

    A. increased levels noted in atherosclerotic lesion

    B. produced by the pancreas

    C. inhibits fibrin degradation by plasmin

    D. enhances clot formation

52. When counseling obese patients, the NP realizes that:

    A. a daily energy deficit of 500 to 1000 kcal/day leads to about a 1- to 2-lb weight loss per week.

    B. each pound of body fat represents approximately 6000 stored calories.

    C. exercise enhances IR.

    D. thyroid dysfunction is found in the majority of cases.

53. Which of the following presents the most problematic pattern of obesity?

TABLE 10–4

CAUSES OF SECONDARY HYPERLIPIDEMIA

Cause	Lipid Abnormality
Inactivity	↓ HDL
Alcohol abuse	↑ Triglycerides, ↑ HDL, ↑ LDL
Diabetes mellitus	↑ Triglycerides, ↓ HDL, ↑ TC
Hypothyroidism	↑ Triglycerides, ↑ TC
Higher-dose thiazide diuretics	↑ TC, ↑ LDL, ↑ triglycerides
Chronic renal insufficiency	↑ TC, ↑ triglycerides

HDL, high-density lipoprotein; LDL, low-density lipoprotein; TC, total cholesterol.

TABLE 10–5

RISK CATEGORIES THAT
MODIFY LDL-CHOLESTEROL
GOALS

Risk Categories	LDL Goal
CHD and CHD risk equivalents	<70–100 mg/dL
Multiple (2+) risk factors	<130 mg/dL
Zero to one risk factor	<160 mg/dL

From National Cholesterol Education Program Adult Treatment Panel III, (ATP III) guidelines. Available at www.nhlbi.nih.gov/ncep, accessed 10/4/04.
CHD, coronary heart disease; LDL, low-density lipoprotein.

    A. female fat distribution pattern
    B. male patient with BMI of less than 28.5
    C. female patient with BMI of 23 to 27
    D. male fat distribution pattern

54. Aerobic exercise can reduce IR for up to:

    A. 12 hours.
    B. 24 hours.
    C. 36 hours.
    D. 48 hours.

55. The TZDs have all of the following effects except:

    A. reduced IR.
    B. improved lipid levels.

    C. decreased intra-abdominal fat mass.
    D. increased blood pressure.

56. Metformin has all of the following effects except:

    A. improved insulin-mediated glucose uptake.
    B. modest weight loss with initial use.
    C. enhanced fibrinolysis.
    D. increased LDL cholesterol production.

57. Cardiovascular effects of hyperinsulinemia include:

    A. decreased renal sodium reabsorption.
    B. constricted circulating volume.
    C. greater responsiveness to angiotensin II.
    D. diminished sympathetic activation.

ANSWERS

49. D	**50.** A	**51.** B
52. A	**53.** D	**54.** D
55. D	**56.** D	**57.** C

DISCUSSION

Synonymous with a number of other names such as syndrome X, Reaven syndrome, the "deadly quarter," metabolic cardiovascular syndrome, atherothrombogenic syndrome, and cardiovascular dysmetabolic syndrome, the term metabolic syndrome is now most commonly used to describe a complex health problem that includes three or more of the following: obesity, blood pressure problems, dyslipidemia, and glucose intolerance. See Table 10–6. Metabolic syndrome arises from a number of causes, including predetermined genetic factors, such as IR, as well as acquired or lifestyle characteristics, such as obesity, physical inactivity, and high-carbohydrate (>60% of total calories) diets.

In IR, there is a reduced sensitivity in the tissues to insulin's action at a given concentration, which causes a subnormal effect on glucose metabolism. This results in hyperglycemia, which in turn stimulates pancreatic insulin production to reduce the blood glucose levels. Euglycemia occurs, albeit in the presence of hyperinsulinemia. High fasting insulin levels are noted to be an independent predictor for ischemic heart disease in men. Over time, usually many years, pancreatic beta cell deficiency usually occurs, resulting in impaired glucose tolerance and hyperglycemia.

Although present in nearly all persons with type 2 DM, IR is also found in a significant part of population who never develop clinically evident glucose intolerance. Also, although it is more common and severe as weight rises, some persons with IR are of normal weight. However, obesity dramatically increases the risk of diabetes in the person with IR.

TABLE 10–6
NATIONAL CHOLESTEROL
EDUCATION PROGRAM
(NCEP) ADULT TREATMENT
PANEL (ATP) III GUIDELINES
METABOLIC SYNDROME

⇒3 of the following:
- Abdominal obesity (Men >102 cm or 40 inches; women >88 cm or 35 inches)
- Triglycerides >150 mg/dL
- HDL cholesterol <40 mg/dL for men, <50 mg/dL for women
- BP >130/85 mm Hg
- Fasting glucose >110 mg/dL

A number of conditions are seen in conjunction with IR. Increased IR is inversely related to decreased urinary uric acid clearance; this leads to a dramatic increase in the rate of gout. The majority of women with polycystic ovary syndrome are insulin resistant; treatment with insulin-sensitizing medications can lead to a resumption of ovulation, return of fertility, and reduction in hirsutism. Acanthosis nigricans, hyperpigmentation of the skin often in the neck and axilla, is also correlated with IR. This finding is most common in children and young adults with IR and DM risk and should alert the NP to work aggressively with such patients on developing or maintaining a healthy lifestyle.

Although the correlation of obesity with IR and DM type 2 is well established, not all body fat types and distribution are equally problematic. "Apple-shaped" or central, abdominal obesity is made up of metabolically active fat and is associated with high insulin levels, IR, high mobilization rate of free fatty acids, and high insulin levels; the last trait is often associated with increased appetite. The genetic makeup that allows this to happen helped increase the likelihood of survival in times of famine. However, in these times of plentiful food, IR helps increase insulin levels and promote fat storage.

IR and its resulting metabolic syndrome are now recognized as contributing to a prothrombotic and proatherogenic state. Plasminogen activator inhibitor, produced by the liver and endothelial cells, inhibits fibrin degradation by plasmin and enhances clot formation; increased levels are found in atherosclerotic lesions. High levels of triglyceride-VLDL and oxidized LDL stimulate the production of plasminogen activator inhibitor. Plasminogen activator inhibitor levels are significantly correlated with increased body mass and high plasma insulin levels, whereas levels are reduced when endogenous insulin levels are reduced by exercise, weight loss, and/or insulin-sensitizing medications such as metformin and the TZDs.

Although the ADA guidelines for the diagnosis of diabetes includes a plasma glucose level higher than 126 mg/dL after an 8-hour fast, the clinician should bear in mind that most people without IR or glucose intolerance will have a fasting blood glucose level in the range of 70 to 90 mg/dL. Therefore, seeing a gradual increase in a patient's glucose level over the years should be considered an early warning sign of metabolic syndrome and future DM type 2.

Hypertension is usually seen in the person with IR. In contributing to the development of increased blood pressure, hyperinsulinemia leads to increased renal sodium reabsorption, which potentially expands circulating volume and increases vascular resistance. Additional cardiovascular affects include increased vascular smooth muscle proliferation, greater responsiveness to angiotensin II, and greater sympathetic activation. Endothelial dysfunction is correlated with decreased nitric oxide production and peripheral vasoconstriction in the muscle tissue, which can potentially increase blood pressure. IR also contributes significantly to dyslipidemia; the person with persistent hypertriglyceridemia is likely to be significantly insulin resistant.

One of the major goals of treating a person with metabolic syndrome is to work with the patient to minimize the core defect, IR. Cigarette smoking increases IR, as does inactivity and obesity. Conversely, most patients note an improvement in HDL cholesterol with smoking cessation and exercise. Also, the benefits of smoking cessation on lung and vascular health cannot be overstated. Because approximately 80% of the body's insulin-mediated glucose uptake takes place in muscle and is enhanced by physical activity, the positive effects of a program of regular aerobic exercise are significant. Exercise—as little as 20 to 30 minutes of brisk walking—reduces IR by approximately 40%, with the effects persisting for up to 48 hours after the activity. In addition, exercise aids in weight loss, reduces blood pressure, and improves lipid levels. Regular aerobic physical activity is one of most effective therapies to help decrease IR and prevent the development of DM.

Weight loss improves insulin sensitivity and lowers blood pressure; improvement is not related to the degree of weight loss. Eating frequent, high-fiber, small meals as well as foods with a low glycemic index and smaller serving sizes, should be encouraged. Dietary fat should be limited but not eliminated, with emphasis on decreasing saturated fats while using monounsaturated fat. A pound of fat contains approximately 3500 stored calories. Thus, a deficit of 500 to 1000 calories per day will lead to a 1- to 2-lb weight loss per week.

A number of medications are now available for the treatment of IR and DM. The TZDs (pioglitazone, rosiglitazone) help improve insulin sensitivity and metabolic parameters such as lipids and blood pressure, as well as decrease intra-abdominal fat mass. Metformin, a biguanide, improves insulin-mediated glucose uptake and metabolic parameters such as fibrinolysis. Although TZD use is usually associated with a modest weight gain, patients taking metformin usually have a modest weight loss. Insulin secretagogues such as a sulfonylurea or injectable insulin will likely be needed as pancreatic insulin production wanes. Dyslipidemia and hypertension must be aggressively treated to minimize risk of cardiovascular disease. Daily aspirin use is recommended to counteract the proinflammatory and prothrombotic effects of IR.

DISCUSSION SOURCES

Grundy, S., et al. Implications of recent clinical trials for the National Cholesterol Education Program Adult Treatment Panel III guidelines. Circulation 2004; 110:227–239.

National Heart, Lung, and Blood Institute (2002). Adult Treatment Panel III (ATP III) Guidelines National Cholesterol Education Program Adult Treatment Panel III Guidelines for Lipid Goals. Available at www.nhlbi.nih.gov/guidelines/cholesterol/index.htm, accessed 8/15/03.

Thrush, S., and McCaffrey, R. (2004). Endocrine and metabolic disorders. In Hektor Dunphy, L. Management Guidelines for Nurse Practitioners Working with Adults. Philadelphia, F.A. Davis.

58. Obesity is usually defined as having a BMI equal to or exceeding ____ kg/m².

A. 25
B. 30
C. 35
D. 40

59. An example of an appropriate question to poise to a person with obesity who is in the precontemplation stage is:

A. "How do you feel about your weight?"
B. "What are barriers you see to losing weight?"
C. "What is your personal goal for weight loss?"
D. "How do you envision my helping you meet your weight loss goal?"

60. An example of an appropriate question to poise to a person with obesity who is in the contemplation stage is:

A. "How do you feel about your weight?"
B. "What are barriers you see to losing weight?"
C. "What is your personal goal for weight loss?"
D. "How do you envision my helping you meet your weight loss goal?"

61. When advising a person who will be using orlistat as part of a weight loss program, the NP provides the following information about when to take the medication:

A. within an hour of each meal that contains fat
B. before any food with a high carbohydrate content
C. only in the morning, to avoid sleep disturbance
D. up to 3 hours after any meal, regardless of types of food eaten

62. The action of which of the following is believed to be responsible for satiety?

A. norepinephrine
B. epinephrine
C. dopamine
D. serotonin

63. Potential adverse effects of sibutramine use include:

A. bradycardia.
B. somnolence.
C. blood pressure increase.
D. diarrhea.

64. In the person with obesity, weight loss of ____% or more yields an immediate reduction in death rates from cardiovascular and cerebrovascular disease.

A. 5
B. 10
C. 15
D. 20

65. When counseling about bariatric surgery, the NP provides the following information:

A. Most people achieve ideal BMI postoperatively.
B. Nearly 50% of the weight loss occurs in the first few postoperative months.
C. The death rate directly attributable to surgery is about 10%.
D. Weight loss will continue for years postoperatively in most patients.

58. B	**59.** A	**60.** B
61. A	**62.** D	**63.** C
64. B	**65.** B	

Rates of obesity, usually defined as a BMI of 30 kg/m² or more (Table 10–7), in the United States are currently at record levels and are projected to double over the next 30 years. Although no specific endocrine disorder, including thyroid dysfunction, is usually found in obese individuals, the cause of obesity is likely a combination of environmental, gen-

TABLE 10–7
WORLD HEALTH ORGANIZATION CLASSIFICATION OF
OVERWEIGHT AND OBESITY

BMI (Kg/m^2)	WHO Classification	Popular description
<18.5	Underweight	Thin
18.5–24.9		Normal or acceptable
25–29.9	Grade 1 overweight	Overweight
30–39.9	Grade 2 overweight	Obesity
=>40	Grade 3 overweight	Morbid obesity

etic, and behavioral influences. Consequences of obesity include increased risk of all-cause morbidity and mortality, greater health care cost, lower workforce productivity, and increased workplace absentee rates and employer costs. Direct health care cost increases related to obesity are attributable largely to obesity-related disease, including coronary heart disease, DM, osteoarthritis, and dyslipidemia. Less tangible are issues of social and workplace discrimination.

Often, persons with obesity assume that only dramatic weight loss can produce healthy results. As little as a 10% body weight loss yields a nearly immediate improvement of death rates from heart disease and stroke. Clinical improvement in osteoarthritis and asthma symptoms is usually noted, as well as a reduction in sleep apnea symptoms.

The NP is well situated to help the person with obesity. For the person who desires weight loss, a first step is the discussion of achievable, reasonable goals. A first step can be to simply help the person halt weight gain or to lose as little as 5% to 10% of total body weight. Slow, steady weight loss usually leads to long-term health benefit and risk reduction. A pound of fat contains approximately 3500 stored calories. Thus, a deficit of 500 to 1000 calories per day will lead to a 1- to 2-lb weight loss per week.

A comprehensive approach to obesity treatment includes behavior modification and pharmacotherapy that lead to decreased food intake, and increased energy expenditure can lead to long-term success. Asking about readiness for change at every clinical visit can help facilitate success (Table 10–8).

Pharmacotherapy is an important tool in weight management. A number of antiobesity drugs are available. Orlistat is taken with meals and contributes to weight loss by reducing dietary fat absorption by approximately 30%. The fat passes undigested, and therefore weight loss is facilitated. The medication is taken three times daily with or within 1 hour of a meal. The most common adverse effect is gastrointestinal disturbance. Sibutramine (Meridia) acts in areas of the brain that control not only mood and sense of well-being but also appetite by influencing levels of norepinephrine, serotonin, and, to a lesser extent, dopamine that is available to neurons by interfering with the reabsorption of these substances (5-hydroxytryptamine [serotonin] facilitates satiety; norepinephrine and dopamine inhibit feeding). The result is diminished appetite and reduced food intake. Adverse effects include dry mouth, constipation, disturbed sleep, and mildly increased blood pressure; valvuloplasty, noted with dexfenfluramine use, has not been noted with sibutramine use. As with many other weight-loss medications, weight loss plateaus and then may slowly increase, particularly if lifestyle modification does not include increased activity and decreased caloric intake. Sympathomimetics such as dexamphetamine and

TABLE 10–8

FACILITATING CHANGE IN THE CARE OF THE PERSON WITH OBESITY

Stage	Questions to Ask	As the Provider, You Can:
Precontemplation (not interested in change)	How do you feel about your weight? How does your weight affect you? Are you considering/planning weight loss now? On a scale of 0–10, how ready are you to start a weight loss program?	Validate and acknowledge • This will take working together but can be done. Restate position, leave the door open • It's up to you to make the decision to lose weight. I cannot do this for you but am here to help you.
Contemplation (thinking about change)	What are the pros and cons of weight loss? Where are you on the scale of 0–10 as far as ready? What are barriers/supports you envision? How do you view me as helping?	Praise and validate • I am happy that you want to deal with this issue and feel ready to do so. Try to shift decisional balance • I am here to help you and point you in the direction of other sources of support. Arrange follow-up
Preparation for change	What is your usual food and activity pattern? What is your personal goal or weight loss? Health goal? Cosmetic goal?	Help set small behavioral goal related to diet, physical activity Assist in compiling food and activity diaries Begin to negotiate goal weight Identify support system Help set a date to start
Making change Maintaining change Dealing with relapse	How can I help? What is getting in your way? What is making this work?	Teach nutritional tactics to help control obesity • Learn energy values of different foods Monitor food consumption by keeping a food diary; reduce portion size Read and understand nutrition labels on foods • Learn new habits of food purchasing • Eliminate high-calorie foods from grocery list Limit fats and oils in cooking, recipes; high-calorie or "calorie-dense" foods Increase physical activity

From National Center for Chronic Disease Prevention and Health Promotion (2003). Overweight and Obesity. Available at www.cdc.gov/nccdphp/dnpa/obesity/index.htm, accessed 8/16/03.

phentermine work with norepinephrine and dopamine, reducing the appetite, with resulting reduction in food intake. Sleep disturbances and nervousness rank among the most adverse effects associated with the use of these medications.

Although there are a number of surgical options available for obesity intervention, gastric bypass is likely the most common. The ideal candidate for this bariatric surgical procedure is a person who is 100 lb or more above ideal body weight level, or with BMI => 40, or less with significant comorbidity, in whom behavioral and pharmacologic therapy has failed. A person considering bariatric surgery must have a realistic idea as to the anticipated outcome. The average weight loss is approximately 30% above ideal body weight; about half of the loss occurs in the first 3 months after surgery, with the loss proceeding more gradually until the patient reaches equilibrium about 12 or 15 months after surgery. About 75% of patients lose a great deal of weight without major complications and maintain this loss long term. About 20% have a significant problem after the surgery (e.g., reoperation, long hospital stay, insufficient weight loss, persistent nausea/vomiting), but most do well in the long term. About 5% have major unresolved problems over time, including, for some, death as a direct result of the surgery.

DISCUSSION SOURCE

National Center for Chronic Disease Prevention and Health Promotion (2003). Overweight and Obesity. Available at www.cdc.gov/nccdphp/dnpa/obesity/index.htm, accessed 8/16/03.

QUESTIONS

66. Risk factors for pancreatitis include all of the following except:

    A. hypothyroidism.
    B. hyperlipidemia.
    C. abdominal trauma.
    D. thiazide diuretic use.

67. A 28-year-old woman with a long-standing history of alcohol abuse presents with a 4-day history of a mid-abdominal ache that radiates through to the back, remains relatively constant, and has been accompanied by nausea and three episodes of vomiting. She has tried taking antacids without relief. Abdominal examination reveals slightly hyperactive bowel sounds with upper abdominal tenderness without localization or rebound. Her skin is cool and moist with a blood pressure of 90/72, pulse rate of 120, and respiratory rate of 24. The most likely diagnosis is:

    A. gastric ulcer.
    B. acute pancreatitis.
    C. acute alcohol poisoning.
    D. viral hepatitis.

68. Your next best action in caring for the patient in the previous question is to:

    A. refer her to the hospital for admission.
    B. attempt office hydration after administration of an analgesic agent.
    C. initiate cimetidine and antacid regimen.
    D. obtain serum electrolyte levels.

69. Which of the following is true when evaluating a patient with acute pancreatitis?

    A. Elevated amylase level is a highly accurate marker for the condition.
    B. Abdominal ultrasound assists with the diagnosis.
    C. Measuring serum lipase level along with amylase level increases diagnostic specificity.
    D. Hypocalcemia is common.

70. Presentation of pancreatic cancer includes:

    A. jaundice.
    B. polycythemia.
    C. hematuria.
    D. increased appetite.

71. Which of the following is the most reliable test for the detection of pancreatic cancer?

    A. elevated alkaline phosphate level
    B. magnetic resonance imaging
    C. abdominal ultrasound
    D. elevation of amylase level

ANSWERS

66. A	**67.** B	**68.** A
69. C	**70.** A	**71.** B

DISCUSSION

Acute pancreatitis, characterized by an acute or chronic inflammation of the organ, is a potentially life-threatening condition. The most common risks for pancreatitis include gallstones (45%) excessive alcohol use (35%), and elevated triglyceride levels and idiopathic causes (20% combined). Less common risk factors are use of opioids, steroids, and thiazide diuretics; viral infections; and abdominal trauma.

In a patient with pancreatitis, serum amylase level is typically elevated. However, because elevated amylase level may be found in a number of other conditions, concurrently measuring serum lipase level increases diagnostic specificity. Abdominal ultrasound may assist in diagnosing contributing gallbladder disease; it does not typically help with diagnosing pancreatitis because of limited views of the organ. Abdominal computed tomographic scan usually provides a diagnostic view of the inflamed pancreas.

Significant pain and volume constriction are common in patients with acute pancreatitis. Intervention includes parenteral hydration and analgesia, as well as gut rest. Treatment of the underlying cause, such as gallbladder disease or hypertriglyceridemia, or discontinuation of the causative agent, such as alcohol, corticosteroids, or thiazide diuretics, is also indicated. The clinical course of pancreatitis can range from a self-limiting condition to life-threatening illness. Ranson criteria are usually used in assessing pancreatitis severity. When three or more criteria are found on clinical presentation, a severe course can be predicted with significant risk for pancreatic necrosis.

Pancreatic cancer most commonly presents with abdominal pain, weight loss, anorexia, nausea, and vomiting. In addition, jaundice is often present but usually without the localized right upper quadrant abdominal tenderness seen in hepatic and biliary disorders such as cholecystitis and acute hepatitis. Pancreatic cancer is a condition with high mortality rates because presentation, unfortunately, usually occurs with late disease and the spread of the cancer.

Magnetic resonance imaging is helpful in identifying pancreatic cancer. The usefulness of abdominal ultrasound is somewhat limited by the presence of intestinal gas. Alkaline phosphatase and amylase levels may be mildly elevated in patients with pancreatic cancer, but these elevations are not specific for this disease (Table 10–9).

DISCUSSION SOURCES

Friedman, L. (2003). Liver, biliary tract, and pancreas. In Tierney, L., McPhee, S., and Papadakis, M. (eds.). Current Medical Diagnosis and Treatment (42nd ed., pp. 628–673). New York: Lange Medical Books/McGraw-Hill.

TABLE 10–9
LIPASE AND AMYLASE EVALUATION IN ACUTE PANCREATITIS

Amylase	Lipase

• In pancreatitis
• Appears 2–12 h after symptom onset
• Back to normal within 7 d of pancreatitis resolution
• Amylase level >1000 U/L
  • 80%= DX cholelithiasis
  • 6%= DX alcoholic pancreatitis
	• In pancreatitis
	• Appears 4–8 h after symptom onset
	• Peaks at 24 h, decreases 8–14 d of pancreatitis resolution

• Nonpancreatic amylase sources
  • Salivary glands
  • Ovarian cysts
  • Ovarian tumors
  • Tubo-ovarian abscess
  • Ruptured ectopic pregnancy
  • Lung cancer
	• Nonpancreatic reasons for elevated lipase
	  • Renal failure
	  • Perforated duodenal ulcer
	  • Bowel obstruction
	  • Bowel infarction

Thrush, S., and McCaffrey, R. (2004). Endocrine and metabolic disorders. In Hektor Dunphy, L. Management Guidelines for Nurse Practitioners Working with Adults. Philadelphia, F.A. Davis.

QUESTIONS

72. Increased thyroid disorder risk is found in individuals who are:

   A. obese.
   B. hypertensive.
   C. treated with corticosteroids.
   D. elderly.

73. Which of the following is most consistent with subclinical hypothyroidism?

   A. elevated free thyroxine (T_4) and thyroid-stimulating hormone (TSH) levels
   B. normal free T_4 and elevated TSH levels
   C. elevated TSH and low free T_4 levels
   D. low TSH and free T_4 levels

74. The most common cause of hypothyroidism is:

   A. primary pituitary failure.
   B. thyroid neoplasia.
   C. autoimmune thyroiditis.
   D. radioactive iodine exposure.

75. Which is most likely to be found in Graves disease?

   A. decreased free T_4 level
   B. decreased TSH level
   C. "cold spot" on thyroid scan
   D. solid lesion on thyroid ultrasound

76. Physical examination findings in patients with Graves disease include:

   A. muscle tenderness.
   B. coarse, dry skin.
   C. eyelid retraction.
   D. delayed relaxation phase of the patellar reflex.

77. The mechanism of action of radioactive iodine in the treatment of Graves disease is to:

   A. destroy the overactive thyroid tissue.
   B. reduce production of TSH.

   C. alter thyroid metabolic rate.
   D. relieve distress caused by increased thyroid size.

78. Which of the following is a helpful treatment option for relief of tremor seen with hyperthyroidism?

   A. propranolol
   B. diazepam
   C. carbamazepine
   D. verapamil

79. In prescribing T_4 therapy for the elderly patient, which of the following statements is true?

   A. Elderly persons require a rapid initiation of T_4 therapy.
   B. TSH should be checked about 2 days after dosage adjustment.
   C. The T_4 dose needed by elderly persons is 75% or less of that needed by younger adults.
   D. TSH should be suppressed to a nondetectable level.

80. Physical examination findings in hypothyroidism likely include:

   A. muscle tenderness.
   B. exophthalmos.
   C. smooth, silky skin.
   D. delayed relaxation phase of the deep tendon reflex.

81. In the report of a thyroid scan done on a 48-year-old woman with a thyroid mass, a "cold spot" is reported. This finding is most consistent with:

   A. autonomously functioning adenoma.
   B. Graves disease.
   C. Hashimoto disease.
   D. thyroid cyst.

82. Which of the following is likely to be found in the person with untreated hypothyroidism?

   A. hypokalemia
   B. hypernatremia
   C. hypertriglyceridemia
   D. microcytic anemia

83. The findings of a painless thyroid mass and TSH level of less than 0.1 IU/mL in a 35-year-old woman is most consistent with:

    A. autonomously functioning adenoma.
    B. Graves disease.
    C. Hashimoto disease.
    D. thyroid malignancy.

84. A fixed, painless thyroid mass accompanied by hoarseness and dysphagia should raise the suspicion of:

    A. autonomously functioning adenoma.
    B. Graves disease.
    C. Hashimoto disease.
    D. thyroid malignancy.

85. Which of the following is the most cost-effective method of distinguishing malignant from benign thyroid nodules preoperatively?

    A. ultrasound
    B. magnetic resonance imaging
    C. fine-needle aspiration biopsy
    D. radioactive iodine scan

86. Possible consequences of excessive levothyroxine use include:

    A. bone thinning.
    B. fatigue.
    C. renal impairment.
    D. constipation.

87. Optimally, at what interval should TSH be reassessed after a levothyroxine dosage is altered?

    A. 1–2 weeks
    B. 2–4 weeks
    C. 4–6 weeks
    D. 6–8 weeks

88. As part of an evaluation of a 3-cm, round, mobile thyroid mass, you obtain a thyroid ultrasound revealing a fluid-filled structure. The most likely diagnosis is:

    A. adenoma.
    B. thyroid cyst.

    C. multinodular goiter.
    D. vascular lesion.

89. Periodic monitoring for hypothyroidism is indicated in the presence of which of the following clinical conditions?

    A. digoxin use
    B. male gender
    C. Down syndrome
    D. alcoholism

90 to 106. Identify each of the following findings as associated with hyperthyroidism, hypothyroidism, or both.

_____ 90. heat intolerance
_____ 91. smooth, silky skin
_____ 92. thin nails that break with ease
_____ 93. frequent, low-volume, loose stools
_____ 94. chilling easily, cold intolerance
_____ 95. amenorrhea or low-volume menstrual flow
_____ 96. coarse, dry skin
_____ 97. menorrhagia
_____ 98. hyperreflexia with a characteristic "quick out–quick back" action
_____ 99. proximal muscle weakness
_____ 100. tachycardia with hypertension
_____ 101. hyporeflexia with a characteristic slow relaxation phase, the "hung-up" reflex
_____ 102. coarse hair with tendency to break
_____ 103. thick, dry nails
_____ 104. constipation
_____ 105. atypical presentation in the elderly person
_____ 106. change in mental status

ANSWERS

72. D	73. B	74. C	75. B
76. C	77. A	78. A	79. C
80. D	81. D	82. C	83. A
84. D	85. C	86. A	87. D
88. B	89. C		

90. Hyperthyroidism 91. Hyperthyroidism
92. Hyperthyroidism 93. Hyperthyroidism
94. Hypothyroidism 95. Hyperthyroidism
96. Hypothyroidism 97. Hypothyroidism
98. Hyperthyroidism 99. Hyperthyroidism
100. Hyperthyroidism 101. Hypothyroidism
102. Hyperthyroidism 103. Hypothyroidism
104. Hypothyroidism 105. Both
106. Both

DISCUSSION

Thyroid hormone is essential to normal body function because it assists cells in energy-releasing activities. When assessing a patient with thyroid dysfunction, look for signs of excessive energy release in hyperthyroidism or decreased energy release in hypothyroidism. This may present in the history and physical examination (Table 10–10).

Although thyroid disease probably exists in less than 7% of the population, it is important to maintain a high index of suspicion in those at particular risk. Risk factors and associated conditions include:

- Down syndrome: hypothyroidism
- the elderly: hypothyroidism or hyperthyroidism with a high propensity for atypical presentation in either situation
- use of certain medications causing an alteration in iodine metabolism (lithium, amiodarone): hypothyroidism
- female gender: hyperthyroidism or hy-

TABLE 10–10

COMPARISON OF HYPERTHYROIDISM WITH HYPOTHYROIDISM

	Hyperthyroidism	*Hypothyroidism*
Characteristics	Excessive energy release, rapid cell turnover	Reduced energy release, slow cell turnover
Causes	Graves disease, thyroiditis, metabolically active thyroid nodule	Post-thyroiditis (>90%), primary pituitary failure (rare)
Neurologic	Nervousness, irritability, memory problems	Lethargy, disinterest, memory problems
Weight	Weight loss (usually modest, present in ~50%)	Weight gain (usually 5–10 lb)
Environmental response	Heat intolerance	Chilling easily, cold intolerance
Skin	Smooth, silky skin	Coarse, dry skin
Hair	Fine hair with frequent loss	Thick, coarse hair with tendency to break
Nails	Thin nails that break with ease	Thick, dry nails
Gastrointestinal	Frequent, low-volume, loose stools	Constipation
Menstrual	Amenorrhea or low-volume menstrual flow	Menorrhagia
Reflexes	Hyperreflexia with a characteristic "quick out–quick back" action	Hyporeflexia with a characteristic slow relaxation phase, the "hung-up" reflex
Muscle strength	Proximal muscle weakness	No change
Cardiac	Tachycardia	Bradycardia in severe cases

pothyroidism; because most thyroid dysfunction is autoimmune in nature, it is more common in women than in men, as are the majority of autoimmune diseases

- postpartum period: a transient hypothyroidism is common, as is a transient thyroiditis
- personal and family history of autoimmune disease such as pernicious anemia, vitiligo, and type 1 DM: hyperthyroidism and hypothyroidism
- history of head and neck irradiation or surgery: hypothyroidism

Highly sensitive (89% to 95%) and specific (90% to 96%), the measurement of TSH is the most helpful thyroid test. TSH is produced by the anterior pituitary gland, with secretion stimulated by thyrotropin-releasing hormone through a negative feedback loop in response to amount of circulating thyroid hormone (T_4). Because only a small fraction of T_4 circulates free, with 99.7% bound to T_4-binding globulin or other plasma proteins, the unbound portion of T_4, or free T_4, is metabolically active. The measurement of free T_4 is the most helpful test to confirm an abnormal TSH level. Approximately 40% of T_4 is converted in periphery to triiodothyronine (T_3). In comparison with T_4, T_3 is likely four times more metabolically active.

The serum total T_4 level reflects the function of the thyroid gland. However, a number of factors can cause an increase or decrease in total T_4 that is not indicative of a change in metabolic status. These factors include a change in T_4-binding globulin, the principal carrier protein of T_3 and T_4. A metabolically insignificant increase in total T_4 is typically noted with the use of estrogen, tamoxifen, and opioids, as well as during pregnancy and acute-phase hepatitis. A metabolically insignificant decrease in total T_4 is often noted with the use of androgens and glucocorticoids, as well as in protein malnutrition and nephrotic syndrome. As a result, the clinical usefulness of total T_4 measurement is limited. The free T_4 index may be a more accurate measure for those with altered states of protein binding, such as with combined oral contraceptive use, pregnancy, and malnutrition.

The likelihood of normal free T_4 if TSH level is normal is in excess of 98%. In the small remainder, pituitary disorder is the likely cause. If the clinician suspects thyroid disorder, and TSH level is normal, it should be assumed that the hypothalamic-pituitary-thyroid axis is intact, with no further testing required. TSH level is increased in hypothyroidism; a 50% decrease in T_4 concentration can yield up to a 90-fold increase in TSH. Conversely, TSH level is decreased in hyperthyroidism. If TSH level is elevated, confirm hypothyroidism by obtaining a free T_4. If TSH is low or undetectable, confirm hyperthyroidism with a measurement of free T_4.

Because thyroid disease can produce low-level symptoms attributed to other conditions, especially stress, fatigue, and a variety of self-limiting illnesses, the issue of routine testing for thyroid disorder with TSH has been long debated. Clinical Preventive Services Guidelines advise that there is insufficient evidence to recommend for or against routine screening for thyroid disease, whereas the American College of Physicians recommends periodic screening in adults older than 50 years.

Chronic lymphocytic, or Hashimoto, thyroiditis is the most common inflammatory disease of the thyroid and the leading cause of hypothyroidism. This condition likely has a genetic predisposition as inherited dominant trait and is often linked with other autoimmune disorders such as systemic lupus erythematosus, pernicious anemia, rheumatoid arthritis, DM, and Sjögren syndrome. The condition is most often seen in women ages 30 to 50; clinical presentation may include a diffusely enlarged, firm thyroid with fine nodules, neck pain, and tightness. This Hashimoto goiter may regress over time; many have the first presentation of the condition in the hypothyroid state, which necessitates the use of T_4 replacement in the form of levothyroxine (Levothroid, Levoxyl, Synthroid).

Antimicrosomal thyroid antibodies, likely reflecting cell-mediated immunity, are found in nearly all patients with Hashimoto disease.

With an 8:1 female:male ratio, Graves disease is the most common form of thyrotoxicosis or hyperthyroidism. The age at onset is usually 20 to 40 years, and there is a significant correlation with autoimmune diseases such as pernicious anemia, myasthenia gravis, and DM. Clinical presentation of Graves disease includes diffuse thyroid enlargement, exophthalmos, nervousness, tachycardia, and heat intolerance. Thyroid scan reveals a large "hot" (metabolically active) gland with heterogeneous uptake. Graves disease treatment includes the use of antithyroid preparations such as methimazole, propylthiouracil, or radioactive iodine. Subsequent hypothyroidism is the norm, necessitating the use of levothyroxine.

Subclinical hypothyroidism is diagnosed from the presence of an elevated TSH level and a normal free T_4 level in the absence of symptoms. The estimated prevalence of this disorder is about 7% in women and 3% in men among community-dwelling individuals ages 60 to 89 years. There is an approximate 5% likelihood of development of overt hypothyroidism per year if these findings are noted with the presence of antithyroid antibodies. The management of patients with subclinical hypothyroidism is a matter of differing approaches; some authorities recommend levothyroxine therapy in the presence of antithyroid antibodies in comparison with a "watch and wait" approach, with periodic TSH and free T_4 testing every 6 months. However, when TSH level rises above 10 mU/L (normal range, 0.5 to 4 mU/L), even in the presence of a normal free T_4 level, a significant increase in LDL is often noted, and T_4 therapy should be initiated.

In the treatment of hypothyroidism, T_4 replacement is needed in the form of levothyroxine (Levothroid, Levoxyl, Synthroid). The anticipated dosage of thyroid replacement for the adult is 75 to 125 µg of levothyroxine, or about 1.6 µg/kg/day. For the elderly person, the anticipated dosage is 75% or less of the adult dosage. Because this drug has a long half-life, the effects of a dosage adjustment will not cause a change in TSH for approximately five to six drug half-lives, or about 6 to 8 weeks. Thyroid hormone requirements tend to remain stable over time. However, certain factors can influence thyroid hormone requirements. When levothyroxine is taken with iron, calcium, aluminum-containing antacids, or sucralfate, its absorption can be impaired; ingestion of these medications should be separated by a number of hours. When levothyroxine is taken with rifampin, phenytoin, carbamazepine, and phenobarbital, its metabolism can be increased.

The evaluation of a palpable thyroid nodule presents a challenge. In the absence of hyperthyroidism symptoms, the presentations of benign and malignant thyroid lesions are typically the same; the risk that any thyroid nodule is malignant is about 5%. A history of head or neck irradiation, localized pain, dysphonia, hemoptysis, regional lymphadenopathy, or a hard, fixed mass should raise suspicion. Initial testing for the person with a thyroid nodule should include obtaining a TSH measurement. A metabolically active or "hot" nodule has a low risk of malignancy and may cause a reduction in TSH production from the pituitary. A thyroid scan can identify areas of increased uptake. However, fine-needle aspiration biopsy is advised, regardless of TSH results, and is more helpful and cost effective in arriving at a definitive diagnosis than is ultrasound or thyroid scan. A properly performed fine-needle aspiration biopsy has a false-negative rate of less than 5% and a false-positive rate of about 1%.

DISCUSSION SOURCES

Danese, M., Powe, N. R., Sawin, C. T., and Ladenson, P. W. (1996). Screening for mild thyroid failure at the periodic health examination: A decision and cost-effectiveness analysis. Journal of the American Medical Association 276: 285–292.

Fitzgerald, P. (2003). Endocrinology. In Tierney, L., McPhee, S., and Papadakis, M. (eds.). Current Medical Diagnosis and Treatment (42nd ed., pp. 1067–1152). New York: Lange Medical Books/McGraw-Hill.

Thrush, S., and McCaffrey, R. (2004). Endocrine and metabolic disorders. In Hektor Dunphy, L. Management Guidelines for Nurse Practitioners Working with Adults. Philadelphia, F.A. Davis.

U.S. Preventive Services Task Force (2004) Screening for Thyroid Disease, available at http://www.ahrq.gov/clinic/uspstf/uspsthyr.htm, accessed 8/16/04.

Woeber, K. A. (1999). The year in review: The thyroid. Ann Intern Med 131:59–62.

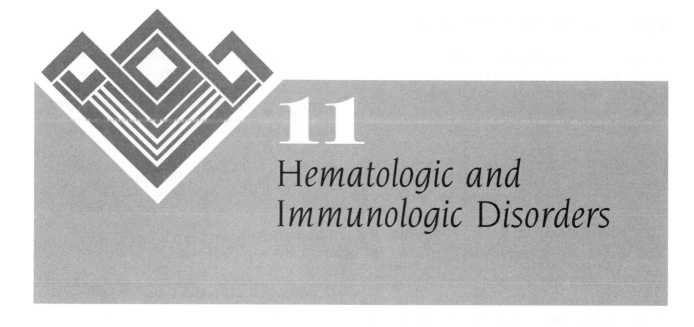

11

Hematologic and Immunologic Disorders

1. A 19-year-old man presents with sudden onset of edema of the lips and face, as well as a sensation of "throat tightness and shortness of breath," after a bee sting. Physical examination reveals inspiratory and expiratory wheezing. Blood pressure is 78/44; heart rate is 102 bpm; respiratory rate is 24. The most likely diagnosis is:

   A. urticaria.
   B. angioedema.
   C. anaphylaxis.
   D. reactive airway disease.

2. Your priority in caring for the patient in Question 1 is to:

   A. administer a rapidly acting antihistamine.
   B. ensure airway patency.
   C. initiate vasopressor therapy.
   D. increase circulating volume.

3. Which of the follow food-based allergies is likely to be found in adults and children?

   A. milk
   B. egg
   C. soy
   D. peanut

4. A person with latex allergy may also have a cross allergy to all of the following except:

   A. banana.
   B. avocado.
   C. kiwi.
   D. lettuce.

5. The first clinical manifestation of systemic anaphylaxis is usually:

   A. flushing.
   B. feeling of apprehension.
   C. urticaria.
   D. itch.

ANSWERS

1. C **2.** B **3.** D
4. D **5.** B

DISCUSSION

Anaphylaxis is an acute, life-threatening, systemic antibody-antigen reaction that is an example of a type I immune response or a hypersensitivity or allergic reaction. This type of reaction occurs after a person had been exposed to an allergen and has developed antibodies. Common allergens include insect venoms, latex, and select medications. Food allergens that occur more commonly in children but are often absent in adulthood include egg, soy, milk, and wheat. Shellfish, fish, tree nuts, and peanut allergies tend to manifest in childhood and persist throughout the lifespan.

The immunoglobulin E (IgE) antibodies that develop in response to allergen exposure occupy receptor sites on mast cells, causing a degradation of the mast cell and subsequent release of histamine, vasodilation, mucous gland stimulation, and tissue swelling. Type I hypersensitivity reactions are composed of two subgroups: atopy and anaphylaxis.

Atopy is a group of localized allergic reactions, including allergic rhinitis and eczema, that are bothersome but not life-threatening. Anaphylaxis, on the other hand, typically causes a systemic IgE–mediated reaction in response to exposure to an allergen. Anaphylaxis is characterized by widespread vasodilation, urticaria, angioedema, and bronchospasm, which create a life-threatening condition of airway obstruction coupled with circulatory collapse (Table 11–1). The first symptom is usually apprehension, followed by tingling sensation, palpitations, urticaria, and angioedema.

First-line treatment of anaphylaxis includes avoiding or discontinuing use of the offending agent. Simultaneously, maintaining airway patency is the greatest priority. Maintaining adequate circulation is also critical. Angioedema and urticaria are subcutaneous anaphylactic reactions that are not life-threatening unless tissue swelling impinges on the airway (Table 11–2)

DISCUSSION SOURCE

Kishiyama, J., and Adelman, D. (2003). Allergic and immunologic disorders. In Tierney, L., McPhee, S., and Papadakis, M. (eds.). Current Medical Diagnosis and Treatment (42nd ed., pp. 759–782). New York: Lange Medical Books/McGraw-Hill.

TABLE 11–1
CLINICAL PRESENTATION OF ANAPHYLAXIS

Most Common	Less Common
Apprehension	Upper airway edema
Tachycardia	Flush
Urticaria	Rhinitis
Angioedema	Headache
Dyspnea and wheezing	Substernal pain
Dizziness	Itch without rash
Syncope	
Hypotension	
GI symptoms	
Seizure	

From www.anaphylaxis.com, accessed 1/3/05.
GI, gastrointestinal.

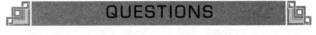

QUESTIONS

6. Worldwide, which of the following is the most common type of anemia?

   A. Pernicious anemia
   B. Folate deficiency anemia
   C. Anemia of chronic disease
   D. Iron deficiency anemia

7. The majority of the body's iron is obtained from:

   A. food sources.
   B. recycled iron content from aged red blood cells (RBCs).
   C. endoplasmic reticulum production.
   D. water supplies.

8. Which of the following is most consistent with iron-deficiency anemia?

   A. low mean corpuscular volume (MCV), normal mean corpuscular hemoglobin (MCH)
   B. low MCV, low MCH
   C. low MCV, elevated MCH
   D. normal MCV, normal MCH

9. One of the earliest laboratory markers in iron-deficiency anemia is:

   A. an increase in RBC distribution width.
   B. a reduced hemoglobin level.
   C. a low MCH level.
   D. an increased platelet count.

▬▬▬ **TABLE 11–2** ▬▬▬▬▬▬▬▬▬▬▬▬▬▬▬▬▬▬▬

MEDICATIONS USED IN THE TREATMENT OF ANAPHYLAXIS

Medications	Mechanism of action	Comments
Antihistamines	Antagonize H, receptor sites	First-generation products (diphenhydramine [Benadryl], chlorpheniramine [Chlor-Trimeton]) • Cross blood-brain barrier, causing sedation • Anticholinergic activity causes some drying of secretions Second-generation products (loratadine [Claritin], desloratadine [Clarinex], cetirizine [Zyrtec], fexofenadine [Allegra]) • Little transfer across blood-brain barrier; low rates of sedation • Less anticholinergic effect Prevents action of formed histamine, thus helpful in acute allergic reactions
Epinephrine	Alpha, beta$_1$, beta$_2$, agonist Potent vasoconstrictor, cardiac stimulant, bronchodilator	Initial therapy for anaphylaxis because of its multiple modes of reversing airway and circulatory dysfunction Anaphylaxis usually responds quickly to 0.3–0.5 mL SC of 1:1000 solution Use with caution in presence of cardiac disease
Decongestants (oral, topical via nasal spray)	Alpha agonist, vasoconstrictor	May cause increase in BP and heart rate when high-dose oral products are used Short-term use (<5 days) of nasal spray safe with few sequelae
Corticosteroids	Anti-inflammatory	Will not reverse airway obstruction or shock Can help limit recurrence, late-phase allergic response

BP, blood pressure; H$_1$, histamine 1; SC, subcutaneously.

10. A 48-year-old woman developed an iron-deficiency anemia after excessive perimenopausal bleeding, successfully treated by endometrial ablation. Her hematocrit (Hct) level is 25%, and she is taking iron therapy. At 5 days into therapy, you expect to find:

A. a correction of mean cell volume.
B. a 10% increase in Hct level.
C. brisk reticulocytosis.
D. a normal ferritin level.

11. A healthy 34-year-old man asks whether he should take an iron supplement. You respond that:

A. this is a prudent measure to ensure health.

B. iron-deficiency anemia is a common problem in men of his age.
C. this may cause iatrogenic iron overload.
D. excess iron is easily excreted.

12. Which of the following is the best advice on taking ferrous sulfate?

A. "Take with other medications to enhance adherence."
B. "Take on a full stomach."
C. "Take on an empty stomach to enhance absorption."
D. "Do not take with vitamin C."

13. A 40-year-old woman with pyelonephritis who is taking ciprofloxacin and is also being treated for iron-deficiency anemia

with ferrous sulfate asks about taking both medications. You advise that:

A. she should take the medications with a large glass of water.

B. an inactive drug compound may be formed if the two medications are taken together.

C. she may take the medications together to enhance adherence to therapy.

D. the ferrous sulfate may slow gastrointestinal motility and result in enhanced ciprofloxacin absorption.

14. One month into therapy for pernicious anemia, you wish to check the efficacy of the intervention. The best laboratory test is:

A. the Schilling test.

B. the hct level.

C. the reticulocyte count.

D. ferritin measurement.

15. A woman who is planning a pregnancy should increase her intake of which of the following to reduce the risk of neural tube defect?

A. iron

B. niacin

C. folic acid

D. vitamin C

16. Risk factors for folate-deficiency anemia include:

A. menorrhagia.

B. chronic ingestion of overcooked foods.

C. use of nonsteroidal anti-inflammatory drugs.

D. gastric atrophy.

17. Folate-deficiency anemia causes which of the following changes in the RBC indices?

A. microcytic, normochromic

B. normocytic, normochromic

C. microcytic, hypochromic

D. macrocytic, normochromic

18. Pernicious anemia is usually caused by:

A. dietary deficiency of vitamin B_{12}.

B. lack of production of intrinsic factor by the gastric mucosa.

C. RBC enzyme deficiency.

D. a combination of micronutrient deficiencies caused by malabsorption.

19. Pernicious anemia causes which of the following changes in the RBC indices?

A. microcytic, normochromic

B. normocytic, normochromic

C. microcytic, hypochromic

D. macrocytic, normochromic

20. Common physical examination findings in patients with pernicious anemia include:

A. hypoactive bowel sounds.

B. stocking-glove neuropathy.

C. thin, spoon-shaped nails.

D. retinal hemorrhages.

21. You examine a 47-year-old man with the following results on hemogram:

- Hemoglobin (Hg) = 15 g
- Hct = 45%
- MCV = 108 fL

The most likely diagnosis is:

A. pernicious anemia.

B. alcohol abuse.

C. thalassemia.

D. Fanconi disease.

22. You examine a 22-year-old woman of Asian ancestry. She is without complaint. Hemogram results are as follows: Hgb = 9.1 g (normal = 12 to 14 g); Hct = 28% (normal = 36% to 42%); RBC = 5 million (normal = 3.2 to 4.3 million); MCV = 68 fL (normal = 80 to 96 fL); RBC distribution width (RDW) = 13% (normal < 15%). The most likely diagnosis is:

A. iron-deficiency anemia.

B. Cooley anemia.

C. alpha-thalassemia minor.

D. hemoglobin Bart.

23. A 68-year-old man is usually healthy but presents with new onset of "huffing and puffing" with exercise. Physical examination reveals conjunctiva pallor and a

hemic murmur. Hgb = 7.6 g; MCV = 71 fL. The most likely problem is:

A. poor nutrition.
B. occult blood loss.
C. malabsorption.
D. microcytosis.

24. You examine a 57-year-old woman with rheumatoid arthritis and find the following results on hemogram:

- Hgb = 10.5 g
- Hct = 33%
- MCV = 88 fL

The most likely diagnosis is:
A. pernicious anemia.
B. anemia of chronic disease.
C. beta-thalassemia minor.
D. folate-deficiency anemia.

25. You examine a 27-year-old woman with menorrhagia and note the following results on hemogram:

- Hgb = 10.1 g
- Hct = 34%
- MCV = 72 fL.

Physical examination is likely to include:
A. conjunctiva pallor.
B. hemic murmur.
C. tachycardia.
D. no specific anemia-related findings.

26. Results of hemogram in anemia of chronic disease include:

A. microcytosis.
B. anisocytosis.
C. reticulocytopenia.
D. macrocytosis.

27. When prescribing erythropoietin supplementation, the nurse practitioner (NP) considers that:

A. the adrenal glands are its endogenous source.
B. it should be given with iron.
C. its use is an adjunct in treating thrombocytopenia.
D. with its use, the RBC lifespan is prolonged.

28. In the first weeks of pernicious anemia therapy with parenteral vitamin B_{12} in a 68-year-old woman, the patient should be carefully monitored for:

A. hypernatremia.
B. dehydration.
C. hypokalemia.
D. acidemia.

29. Which of the following conditions is unlikely to result in anemia of chronic disease?

A. rheumatoid arthritis
B. peripheral vascular disease
C. chronic renal insufficiency
D. chronic osteomyelitis.

ANSWERS

6. D	**7.** B	**8.** B	**9.** A
10. C	**11.** C	**12.** C	**13.** B
14. B	**15.** C	**16.** B	**17.** D
18. B	**19.** D	**20.** B	**21.** B
22. C	**23.** B	**24.** B	**25.** D
26. C	**27.** B	**28.** C	**29.** B

DISCUSSION

Anemia is defined as a decrease in the oxygen-carrying capability of the blood. It is not a disease but rather a sign of an underlying process. Anemia occurs only in the presence of a clinical insult severe enough to disturb the normal hematologic homeostatic mechanisms and exceed the body's ample hematologic reserves.

The clinical presentation of anemia is highly variable, and compensation is common because most anemias are usually gradual in onset. In addition, the oxyhemoglobin-dissociation curve is moved to the right as the hemoglobin level decreases, with the oxygen molecule given up more freely by the RBC. As a result, symptoms of anemia seldom present unless the hemoglobin level decreases to below 10 g/dL.

The health history may reveal clues as to the cause of the anemia (i.e., excessive menstrual flow, acute blood loss). Patients may have complaints of deep, sighing respiration with activity, often associated with a sensation of rapid, forceful heart rate. This is likely a reflection of the decreased oxygen-carrying capability of the blood and a corresponding compensatory mechanism. Fatigue and headache may also be present. In patients at risk for or who have coronary artery disease, angina may be reported.

The physical examination usually contributes little to the diagnosis of anemia unless anemia is severe. Pallor of the skin and mucous membranes is not a reliable indicator and is usually seen only when anemia is severe (hemoglobin < 8 g/dL). In elderly persons and in individuals with coronary artery disease, signs of congestive heart failure (i.e., distended neck veins, rales, tachycardia, right upper quadrant abdominal tenderness, hepatomegaly) may be seen with severe anemia. An early systolic murmur, also known as a hemic murmur, may be heard because of the increase of blood flow over the heart valves. Neurologic findings such as paresthesia, stocking-glove neuropathy, difficulty with balance, and, in extreme cases, confusion may be found in patients with vitamin B_{12} deficiency or folate-deficiency anemia.

In evaluating the hemograms of patients with anemia, the following questions should be answered in order to ascertain the origin of the anemia:

- What is the cell size? Is the RBC unusually small (microcytic or low MCV)? Because hemoglobin is a major contributor to cell size, microcytosis is usually seen in patients with anemia in whom hemoglobin synthesis is impaired, such as in those with iron-deficiency anemia and the thalassemias. In addition, because hemoglobin gives RBCs their characteristic red color, smallness and pallor go together. Thus, a microcytic cell can also be hypochromic (low mean hemoglobin concentration).
- Is the RBC unusually large (macrocytic)? Impaired RNA and DNA synthesis in young erythrocytes most commonly cause macrocytosis. Folic acid and vitamin B_{12} contribute significantly to this process. A lack of either or both of these micronutrients can cause a macrocytic anemia. Because hemoglobin synthesis is not the issue, macrocytic cells are usually of normal color (normochromic).

- Is the RBC of normal size (normocytic)? Generally in these anemias, there is no problem with RNA, DNA, or hemoglobin synthesis. Acute blood loss and anemia of chronic disease are examples of normocytic, normochromic anemia.

- What is the RDW? RDW is the degree of variation in RBC size. This may also be noted as anisocytosis on RBC morphologic study. RDW measurement is elevated when RBCs are of varying sizes, which implies that cells were synthesized under varying conditions. For example, in an iron-deficiency anemia, normal-sized cells produced before the iron depletion will continue to circulate until their 90- to 120-day lifespan ends. At the same time, the new, smaller, iron-deficient cells containing less hemoglobin are produced. Therefore, there will be wide variation in cell size and an increase in RDW. Because minor variation in cell size is normal, RDW is considered increased only when it is above 15%.

- What is the hemoglobin content (color) of the cell? The hemoglobin content of the cell is reflected in the MCH, reported as a percentage of the cell's volume. Because hemoglobin gives RBCs their characteristic red color, the suffix "-chromic" is used to describe the MCH. Thus, when a cell has a normal MCH, it is of normal color, or normochromic. When there is an impairment of hemoglobin synthesis, such as in iron-deficiency anemia or thalassemia, the cells are pale or hypochromic and the MCH is low. RBCs seldom are hyperchromic or contain excessive amounts of hemoglobin.

- What is the reticulocyte production index (RPI)?
The body's normal response to anemia is to

increase reticulocyte production in order to increase the hemoglobin level. Thus, an increase in the reticulocyte count, reticulocytosis, is an expected normal response to a drop in hemoglobin; if it is absent, suspect impaired marrow function or lack of erythropoietin stimulus. The RPI is an indicator of how rapidly new RBCs are produced and mature; the RPI is calculated as the reticulocyte percentage (corrected) divided by correction factor (Fig. 11–1). A RPI > 3 demonstrates adequate hematologic and bone marrow responses to the anemia, whereas a RPI < 2 indicates inadequate response.

Worldwide, iron deficiency is the most common reason for anemia. Because an estimated 8 years of poor iron intake are needed in adults before iron-deficiency anemia occurs, diet is rarely its origin. Rather, chronic blood loss causing a wasting of the RBCs' recyclable iron is the most common cause. Occult gastrointestinal blood loss, such as from an oozing gastritis or gastrointestinal malignancy, is a common reason, as is excessive menstrual flow.

Men and postmenopausal women require 1 mg of iron each day. During reproductive years, women require 1.5 to 3 mg/day of iron, in part because of the monthly loss of RBCs with the menses. In all these circumstances, these iron requirements are achievable with a well-balanced diet. One milliliter of packed RBCs contains 1 mg of iron, so even losses of 2 to 3 mL of blood through the gastrointestinal tract can lead to iron deficiency.

The laboratory diagnosis of iron-deficiency anemia is supported by the following findings:
- early disease: low to normal hemoglobin, low Hct, and low total RBC count; normocytic, possible hypochromic; RDW > 15%
- later disease: microcytic, hypochromic anemia with low RBC count and elevated RDW > 15%
- low serum iron level: reflecting iron concentration in circulation; may be falsely elevated as a result of recent high iron intake
- elevated total iron-binding capacity (TIBC): a measure of transferrin, a plasma protein that easily combines with iron; when more of transferrin is available for binding, the TIBC level increases, reflecting iron deficiency
- iron saturation less than 15%: calculated by dividing the serum iron level by the TIBC
- low serum ferritin level: the body's major iron storage protein
- absence of iron from bone marrow, if aspiration is done

In iron-deficiency anemia, the order of the laboratory markers is as follows:
- ferritin (decrease)
- iron in marrow (absent)
- serum iron (decrease)
- RDW (increase)
- TIBC (increase)
- hemoglobin (decrease)
- indices (decrease)

Therefore, a decrease in hemoglobin or RBC indices is a late rather than an early marker of disease. Therapy for patients with iron-deficiency anemia involves not only iron replacement but also treatment of the underlying cause. Drug interactions are common (Table 11–3).

Iron use without a distinct clinical indication, including the use of iron-fortified multiple vitamins, is not recommended because this may lead to an iatrogenic iron overload. Iron overload has been hypothesized to be a cardiovascular risk factor. A lower rate of car-

Correction factor table for calculating reticulocyte production index

Patient's hct (%)	Correction factor
40–45	1.0
35–39	1.5
25–34	2.0
15–25	2.5
<15	3.0

FIG. 11–1. Correction factor table for calculating reticulocyte production index.

TABLE 11–3

DRUG INTERACTIONS WITH ORAL IRON THERAPY

Drug	Effect	Comment
Antacids	Decreased iron absorption	Separate use by ≥2 hr
Caffeine	Decreased iron absorption	Separate use by ≥2 hr
Fluoroquinolones (ciprofloxacin, ofloxacin, levofloxacin, others)	Decreased fluoroquinolone effect	Avoid concurrent use
Levodopa	Decreased levodopa and iron effect	Separate medications by as much time as possible; increase levodopa dose as needed
Antihypertensives (ACE inhibitor, methyldopa)	Decreased antihypertensive effect	Separate medications by ≥2 hr, monitor BP Additional effect with IV iron: when ACE inhibitors are given concurrently, increased risk of systemic reaction to iron (fever, arthralgia, hypotension); concurrent use should be avoided
Tetracycline	Decreased tetracycline and iron effect	Do not use concurrently, or separate by ≥3–4 hr or use an enteric-coated iron product
Thyroid hormones	Decreased thyroxine effect	Take thyroid hormones ≥2 hr before or 4 hr after iron dose
Histamine 2 receptor antagonists	Decreased iron absorption	Minor interaction

Adapted from Tatro, 2004.
ACE, angiotensin-converting enzyme; BP, blood pressure; IV, intravenous.

diovascular disease has been noted in frequent blood donors with relatively low levels of stored iron in comparison with age controls. In addition, women's cardiovascular disease rates equal men's 5 to 10 years after menopause, a time when female and male ferritin levels are equal.

Reticulocytosis begins quickly after initiation of iron therapy, with the reticulocyte count peaking 7 to 10 days into therapy. Hemoglobin increases at a rate of 2 g/dL every 3 weeks in response to iron therapy and will likely take 2 months to correct. As a result, the following laboratory tests may be used to evaluate the resolution of iron-deficiency anemia: reticulocytes at 1 to 2 weeks to ensure marrow re-

sponse to iron therapy, hemoglobin at 6 weeks to 2 months to ensure anemia recovery, and ferritin at 2 months after measure of normal hemoglobin (or 4 months after initiation of iron therapy) to ensure documentation of replenished iron stores.

Folic acid (pteroylglutamic acid) is a water-soluble B complex vitamin found in abundance in peanuts, fruits, and vegetables. Through a complex reaction, folic acid is reduced to folate. Folate donates one carbon unit to oxidation at various levels, reactions vital to proper DNA synthesis. During times of accelerated tissue growth and repair, such as in childhood, pregnancy, recovery from serious illness, and recovery from hemolytic anemia, folic acid requirements increase from the baseline of twofold to fourfold. Folate deficiency causes a macrocytic, normochromic anemia.

The most common causes of folic acid-deficiency anemia are inadequate dietary intake, seen in elderly, alcoholic, and impoverished persons and in those with decreased ability to absorb folic acid, which occurs with malabsorption syndromes such as sprue and celiac disease. Folic acid deficiency can often be avoided with a healthy diet featuring folate-rich fruits and vegetables.

Folic acid transfers readily through the placenta to the fetus, with fetal levels usually higher than maternal levels; therefore, there is evidence that pregnancy is a maternal folate-depleting event. Repeated or multiple pregnancies, in particular, cause depletion of maternal folate stores. Folate deficiency during pregnancy can be largely avoided through the consistent use of prescriptive prenatal vitamins, each tablet usually containing 0.8 to 1.0 mg of folic acid. Over-the-counter prenatal vitamins contain significantly less of this micronutrient, usually about 0.4 mg per tablet. Supplementation should continue through lactation because approximately 0.5 mg/day of folic acid is transferred to breast milk. Accumulation of the vitamin in human milk takes precedence over maintaining maternal folate levels.

Maternal folic acid deficiency is a teratogenic state, particularly during neural tube formation. In order to reduce the rate of neural tube defects in their offspring, women planning a pregnancy should be advised to take additional amounts of folic acid, 0.4 mg/day, for 3 months before conception. This recommendation should be extended to all women capable of conception. Over-the-counter multivitamin or diet supplementation with vitamin-fortified foods can easily supply the recommended folate dose. If a woman has a history of giving birth to a child with a neural tube defect, the folic acid dose should be increased to 4 mg/day for 3 months before conception and continued at least through the first 12 weeks of pregnancy. If the pregnancy is unplanned or pre-conception counseling was not sought, initiating folic acid supplementation during the first 7 weeks of pregnancy appears to offer some neural tube protection. This can be supplied by a prescription prenatal vitamin supplement. However, if the pregnant woman cannot tolerate the prenatal vitamin supplement as a result of nausea, a common condition, she will likely be able to take folic acid alone without difficulty.

Recommended doses for folic acid replacement in adults range from 0.5 to 1 to 5 mg/day, the usual dose being 1 mg/day. The underlying cause of the folate deficiency must also be treated.

Reticulocytosis occurs rapidly, with a peak at 7 to 10 days into folic acid therapy. The Hct level increases by 4% to 5% per week and generally returns to normal within 1 month. Leukopenia and thrombocytopenia resolve within 2 to 3 days of therapy. A repeat hemogram in 1 to 2 months assists in the monitoring of therapeutic effect. Resolution of the related signs and symptoms generally follows the time frame needed for the resolution of the anemia.

Vitamin B_{12}, a member of the cobalamin family, is found in abundance in foods of animal origin and is essential to the development of the RBC. When vitamin B_{12} is ingested orally, it binds with intrinsic factor, a glycoprotein produced by the gastric parietal cells and transported systematically. Within the portal blood flow, the vitamin is attached to transcobalamin II, a polypeptide synthesized in the liver and ileum. Intrinsic factor is not absorbed, and the new compound is transported to the bone marrow and other sites, where it is available for use in RBC formation. Two additional glycoproteins, transcobalamin I and III, combine with vitamin B_{12} and are used in the formation of granulocytes. In synergy with folic acid, vitamin B_{12} plays a role essential to RBC DNA synthesis. When deficiencies of either of these micronutrients exist, DNA synthesis in the RBC is impaired, which leads to the distinct changes in the RBC and bone marrow.

Vitamin B_{12} therapy should be initiated when the diagnosis is made. Usually there is a brisk hematologic response, and the anemia is resolved within 2 months. Reversal of neurologic abnormalities is generally slower, but improvement is seen quickly.

Vitamin B_{12} is available generically and in oral and injectable forms. The parenteral form is preferred because of its excellent absorption. In oral form, vitamin B_{12} is erratically absorbed in the distal portion of the small intestine, which can potentially lead to treatment failure. The usual initial vitamin B_{12} dosage is 100 µg/day intramuscularly for the first week, then weekly for the first month, and then 100 µg monthly for the rest of the patient's life. Traditionally, doses as high as 1000 µg per injection have been used. However, a cyanocobalamin dose of more than 100 µg in a single injection exceeds the binding capacity of transcobalamin II; the excess is excreted via the kidney and wasted. Concomitant administration of folic acid and iron may help with hematologic recovery. Orally, a higher dose, 1000 µg/day, is needed. Vitamin B_{12} is also available in a nasal gel, usually used weekly at a dose of 500 µg. When the cause of the macrocytic anemia has not yet been established, a prudent course of action is to initially give parenteral vitamin B_{12} while giving folic acid, 1 to 2 mg/day. With this plan, no intervention time is lost. After the appropriate diagnosis is established, the correct vitamin supplement is continued; 1000 µg/day is needed; drug interactions should be noted (Table 11–4).

The hematologic response is generally rapid after therapy is begun. Reticulocytosis is brisk and peaks at 5 to 7 days. Hypokalemia, caused by serum-to-intracellular potassium shifts, is common if the anemia was particularly severe and is most likely seen with the peak of reticulocytosis. Monitoring serum potassium daily during the first week of therapy, especially in patients on diuretic therapy, at other risk of hypokalemia, or on digoxin, is important. If hypokalemia occurs, oral potassium replacement at 40 mEq/day is usually sufficient. Concomitant oral iron therapy is indicated if there is iron deficiency or low iron stores. Full hematologic recovery usually takes about 2 months.

Reversal of the signs and symptoms of vitamin B_{12} deficiency is generally rapid. A sense of improved well-being is usually reported within 24 hours of the onset of treatment. Neurologic changes, if present for less than 6 months, reverse quickly. However, neurologic reversal is likely not possible if these changes have been present for a protracted period.

Anemia is often noted in the person with select chronic health problems, such as acute and chronic inflammatory conditions (infection, arthritis), renal insufficiency, and hypothyroidism. In part, this condition, known as anemia of chronic disease, is caused by reduced erythropoietin response in the marrow, resulting in RBC hypoproliferation. Worldwide, anemia of chronic disease is second only to iron deficiency in occurrence. Bone marrow can be suppressed as a result of the use of certain drugs, such as large amounts of alcohol. Because normal RBC cell death occurs without

---

TABLE 11–4

ORAL VITAMIN B_{12} DRUG INTERACTIONS

Drug	Effect
Aminoglycosides	With concomitant use, decreased vitamin B_{12} absorption
Colchicine	With concomitant use, decreased vitamin B_{12} absorption
Potassium supplements	With concomitant use, decreased vitamin B_{12} absorption
Ascorbic acid	May destroy vitamin B_{12} if taken within 1 hr of vitamin B_{12} ingestion

Adapted from Rizack, M. (1998). Handbook of Adverse Drug Interactions. New Rochelle, NY: The Medical Letter.

the production of new RBC forms, anemia can occur. When glomerular filtration rate falls below 30 to 40 mL/minute, renal erythropoietin synthesis is reduced; a hypoproliferative normochromic, normocytic anemia develops, usually with hemoglobin level of 7 to 8 g/dL or higher. That is, as the kidney fails, erythropoietin production declines and anemia of chronic disease develops.

Recombinant human erythropoietin (epoetin alfa) is used in the treatment of anemias associated with end-stage renal disease, HIV, and cancer chemotherapy and of other forms of anemia of chronic disease. The drug can be administered parenterally (subcutaneously or intravenously) up to 3 times per week with an expected rise in Hct of approximately 4% over 2 weeks. Iron therapy is also needed unless iron overload is present. Patient symptoms, such as altered exercise capacity and sexual function, that are often attributed to renal disease are often attenuated if hemoglobin is corrected to 11 to 12 g/dL with the use of recombinant human erythropoietin (epoetin alfa).

DISCUSSION SOURCE

Fitzgerald, M. (2005). Hematologic disorders. In Youngkin, E., Sawin, K., Kissinger, J., and Israel, D. (eds.). Pharmacotherapeutics: A Primary Care Clinical Guideline (2nd ed). Saddle River, NJ: Prentice-Hall.

 QUESTIONS

30. Which of the following is most accurate about HIV testing?

    A. After office testing, results should be given over the phone.
    B. Most tests will detect HIV infection within 48 hours of virus acquisition.
    C. A positive enzyme-linked immunosorbent assay (ELISA) result is followed by a confirmatory Western blot for viral antigen.
    D. Most tests have a false-negative rate exceeding 10%.

31. A 28-year-old man with HIV has a CD4 count of 345 cells/μL. You realize that he is most likely at increased risk for:

    A. cytomegalovirus retinitis
    B. *Pneumocystis* pneumonia.
    C. staphylococcal skin infections.
    D. *Mycobacterium avium* complex infection.

32. Which of the following does not increase a woman's risk of contracting HIV infection from heterosexual vaginal intercourse?

    A. bacterial vaginosis
    B. male partner using a latex condom
    C. being postmenopausal
    D. use of a spermicide

33. When a pregnant woman passes the HIV virus on to her unborn child, it is known as what kind of transmission?

    A. vertical
    B. chorionic
    C. placental
    D. horizontal

34. A 38-year-old woman has advanced HIV disease. She presents with a chief complaint of a painless rash over her trunk. Examination reveals umbilicated vesicular-form lesions scattered over her thorax. This is most consistent with:

    A. herpes zoster.
    B. dermatitis herpetiformis.
    C. molluscum contagiosum.
    D. impetigo.

35. Which of the following represents the NP's most appropriate response to this patient's statement "I might as well just die now that I have HIV"?

    A. "You sound frightened."
    B. "What makes you say that?"
    C. "I am concerned about your health and safety."
    D. "We need more tests before your prognosis can be known."

36. The most common mode of HIV transmission worldwide is via:

A. male-to-male sexual contact.
B. heterosexual intercourse.
C. vertical transmission.
D. injection drug use with needle sharing.

ANSWERS

30. C   **31.** C   **32.** B
33. A   **34.** C
35. C   **36.** B

DISCUSSION

HIV infection is a systemic disease that causes a wide clinical spectrum of manifestations from asymptomatic state to fatal complications. Risk factors include close contact with blood and body fluids of a person with HIV, with heterosexual contact being the most common mode of transmission worldwide. The risk of contracting HIV from a single contaminated hollow-bore needle stick is about 1 in 250, considerably less than that of contracting hepatitis B from the same needle. In addition, the unborn child can become infected by vertical transmission from the mother. This risk is considerably reduced by the use of antiretroviral therapy during pregnancy. Postmenopausal women are at particular risk for infection through horizontal transmission from heterosexual vaginal intercourse because of the thinning of the vaginal mucosa associated with a low estrogen state. Male and female condom use and other barriers such as dental dams offer protection, although not elimination, of HIV transmission.

The presentation of HIV infection varies according to the point in the disease spectrum. Opportunistic infections are common as disease advances. In addition, infections that can occur in an immunocompetent person, such as staphylococcal skin infections, impetigo and molluscum contagiosum, can also occur in immunocompromised patients. Impetigo often presents initially as a vesicular-form lesion that is mildly itchy, followed by the formation of a honey-colored crust. Molluscum contagiosum usually presents as a painless vesicular-form lesion with an umbilicated center. However, the degree of severity is usually much worse for HIV-infected patients.

Unfortunately, prejudice against those who are infected with HIV exists. In addition, insurers and employers may make decisions on the basis of a person's perceived HIV risk. To this

---

TABLE 11-5
POINTS OF DISCUSSION
DURING HIV PRETEST
COUNSELING

HIV transmission and risk reduction opportunities

Natural history and clinical manifestations of HIV/AIDS

Risk of vertical transmission during pregnancy

Benefits of early diagnosis and treatment

Potential role for postexposure prophylaxis in select cases

History of prior HIV testing

Reason for current testing and expectations

Technical aspects (be aware of latest options)
• ELISA with confirmatory Western blot
• "Window period" between infection and seroconversion (≤6 weeks)

Testing options (home testing, anonymous, confidential)

Screening for STI; coinfections, including hepatitis A, B, C, D

Test obtained only with patient informed consent

Special testing consideration in the pregnant woman
• Universal testing strongly recommended
• Risk of vertical transmission
• Potential benefit of treatment to unborn child

From Clinician's Guide to HIV Counseling and Testing (2000). Boston: Massachusetts Department of Public Health, HIV/AIDS Bureau.
AIDS, acquired immunodeficiency syndrome; ELISA, enzyme-linked immunosorbent assay; HIV, human immunodeficiency virus; STI, sexually transmitted infection.

TABLE 11–6

POINTS OF DISCUSSION
DURING HIV POSTTEST
COUNSELING

Regardless of results
- Give in person only, not via mail or telephone call
- Review meaning of test
- Emphasize risk reduction
- Provide emotional support and assess need for immediate intervention
- Discuss community resources

With negative test
- Does not imply immunity from future infection
- Need for repeat testing for exposures occurring in "window" period

With positive test
- Review natural history of HIV/AIDS, benefits of treatment, and opportunistic infection (OI) prophylaxis
- Encourage partner counseling, entry into primary and HIV care
- If nonblood test, emphasize importance of confirming infection with serology or viral load testing
- Advise of potential discrimination based on disclosure and legal protections

Indeterminate test
- Discuss potential significance, including early seroconversion, cross-reacting antibodies
- Encourage return for repeat testing

From Clinician's Guide to HIV Counseling and Testing (2000). Boston: Massachusetts Department of Public Health, HIV/AIDS Bureau.
AIDS, acquired immunodeficiency syndrome; HIV, human immunodeficiency virus.

TABLE 11–7

ACUTE HIV INFECTION,
ACUTE RETROVIRAL
SYNDROME (ARS)

Onset: 2–4 weeks after exposure

Duration: ≤14 days

Common symptoms
- Fever (96%)
- Lymphadenopathy (74%)
- Maculopapular rash (70%)
- Pharyngitis (70%)
- Arthralgia/myalgia (54%)
- Night sweats (50%)

Diagnosis: Viral load, Western blot, P24 antigen

Treatment
- Three-drug regimen recommended with close follow-up and expert consultation
- No evidence that treatment during ARS will eradicate HIV

From Clinician's Guide to HIV Counseling and Testing (2000). Boston: Massachusetts Department of Public Health, HIV/AIDS Bureau.
HIV, human immunodeficiency virus.

end, an important part of primary care is counseling the patient about HIV testing. If testing is provided in a primary care office, held in a special manner during sampling and on the record, this usually qualifies as confidential testing. In this type of testing, the counselor or provider and the patient know one another's identity. The results are potentially traceable, which is helpful when the provider needs to find a patient who has not returned for results. However, insurers and others may be able to also trace the results, a potentially problematic situation. If testing is provided at an anonymous test site, the counselor does not know the patient's identity because a number or other designation is used. The result of this type of test is not traceable, and thus the patient's privacy is protected. However, the drawback is that the patient cannot be identified. Therefore, if the patient does not return for results, no follow-up care is possible. A number of home testing options and a growing number of office-based, rapid-result tests are available.

When counseling about HIV testing, inform patients that false-positive test results are rare and false-negative results are more common. This situation is caused by a "window period," the period from infection to development of antibodies. However, antibodies usually develop within 6 weeks of infection. Standard HIV testing includes an ELISA as a screening test. If the ELISA test result is positive, a confirming Western blot is obtained. A critically important part of care for patients infected with HIV is the ongoing support and counseling provided in the primary care relationship. As with other potentially life-threatening illnesses, patients display a range of emotions. However, NPs should maintain an objective stance and not attempt to assign feelings or badger the patient for additional information. Starting a counseling statement with "I" followed by a verb that conveys what you see or feel about a situation is very helpful when dealing with people in crisis. In the example given here, the patient states, "I might as well just die now that I am HIV positive." This may represent a suicidal statement. The NP must establish the safety status, as well as health status, of this person such as, "I am concerned about your health and safety," or "I am here to help you" (Tables 11–5, 11–6, 11–7).

Treatment of patients infected with HIV is a dynamic process with new therapies becoming available. As a result, it behooves NPs to be familiar with the latest testing options and therapies in order to afford the patient the best opportunity to achieve and maintain health.

DISCUSSION SOURCES

Hollander, H. (2003). Allergic and immunologic disorders. In Tierney, L. McPhee, S., and Papadakis, M. (eds.). Current Medical Diagnosis and Treatment (42nd ed., pp. 1272–1303). New York: Lange Medical Books/McGraw-Hill.

National Center for HIV, STD and TB Prevention, Divisions of HIV/AIDS Prevention (2004). Recommendations and Guidelines. Available at www.cdc.gov/hiv/pubs/guidelines.htm, accessed 8/15/04.

QUESTIONS

37. An 18-year-old woman presents with a chief complaint of a 3-day history of "sore throat and swollen glands." Her physical examination includes exudative pharyngitis, minimally tender anterior and posterior cervical lymphadenopathy, and maculopapular rash. Abdominal examination reveals right and left upper quadrant abdominal tenderness. Her most likely diagnosis is:

    A. group A beta-hemolytic streptococcal pharyngitis.
    B. infectious mononucleosis.
    C. rubella.
    D. scarlet fever.

38. Which of the following is most likely to be found in the laboratory data of a person with infectious mononucleosis?

    A. neutrophilia
    B. lymphocytosis with atypical lymphocytes
    C. presence of antinuclear antibody
    D. macrocytic anemia

39. You examine a 25-year-old man who has infectious mononucleosis with tonsillar hypertrophy, exudative pharyngitis, difficulty swallowing, and a patent airway. You prescribe the following:

    A. amoxicillin
    B. prednisone
    C. ibuprofen
    D. acyclovir

40. The rash associated with scarlet fever is usually described as:

    A. sandpaper-like.
    B. having lacelike borders.
    C. being limited to the trunk.
    D. starting with vesicular lesions.

41. What percentage of patients with Epstein-Barr virus mononucleosis have splenomegaly during the acute phase of the illness?

    A. at least 10%
    B. about 25%
    C. at least 50%
    D. nearly 100%

ANSWERS

37. B   **38.** B   **39.** B
40. A   **41.** C

DISCUSSION

Developing an accurate diagnosis of an acute febrile illness with associated rash and pharyngitis can be a daunting task. A few key points can help:

- Lymphadenopathy: Diffuse lymphadenopathy is most often seen in patients with diffuse infection, such as a systemic viral illness. When associated with a localized bacterial infection such as streptococcal pharyngitis, the affected lymph nodes are also localized (anterior cervical chain).

- Pharyngitis and associated symptoms: Systemic viral infection can cause pharyngitis but also involves other mucous membranes such as the conjunctiva and the oral and respiratory mucosa. These signs and symptoms are usually absent with a more localized infection such as "strep throat."

Infectious mononucleosis is an acute systemic viral illness usually caused by Epstein-Barr virus, a DNA herpesvirus that typically enters the body via oropharyngeal secretions and infects B lymphocytes. After an incubation period of 30 to 50 days, an intense T cell–mediated response develops and coincides with the onset of clinical illness. A 3- to 5-day prodrome of headache, malaise, myalgias, and anorexia is followed by acute symptoms that last about 5 to 15 days. The clinical presentation of acute infectious mononucleosis includes fatigue, exudative pharyngitis and tonsillar enlargement, fever, headache, and posterior cervical lymphadenopathy. Splenomegaly develops in more than 50% of patients and hepatomegaly in about 10%; these organs are also tender to palpation. Additional findings include jaundice, periorbital edema, soft palatal petechiae, generalized adenopathy, rubella-like rash, and a 30% incidence of concurrent streptococcal pharyngitis. Full recovery time is variable but is usually about 4 to 6 weeks.

Diagnostic testing for patients with infectious mononucleosis usually includes obtaining a heterophil antibody test (Monospot). However, this test is positive in only 60% of patients by the second week of illness and carries a false-negative rate of up to 15%. To further complicate this issue, acute infection with cytomegalovirus, adenovirus, *Toxoplasma gondii,* HIV, and other agents can cause an infectious mononucleosis–like illness with a risk of heterophil antibody cross-reactivity rate and a resulting infectious mononucleosis false-positive rate of 5% to 15%. Leukopenia with lymphocytosis is present. The presence of atypical lymphocytes is not unique to infectious mononucleosis and is commonly found in systemic viral infection (Table 11–8). Mild thrombocytopenia is seen in 50% of patients; 85% of infected individuals develop a twofold to threefold elevation in hepatic enzymes (aspartate and alanine aminotransferases) by the second and third weeks of the illness.

Treatment is usually supportive, with recovery slow but complete. However, there is a potential for obstruction and respiratory distress when enlarged tonsils and lymphoid tissue impinge on the upper airway. A corticosteroid such as prednisone, 40 to 60 mg/day for 3 days, is the treatment of choice. Neither the use of antiviral agents such as acyclovir nor routine prescribing of corticosteroid agents is indicated in uncomplicated infectious mononucleosis.

In the person who participates in contact or collision sports or other activities, the risk of splenic rupture, the most common cause of mortality and morbidity in patients with infectious mononucleosis, needs to be considered during both acute and convalescent stages. The risk for splenic rupture is greatest in the second and third weeks of illness, hence the mandate of at least 21 days without collision or contact sports. The risk of rupture is greatest in the enlarged spleen; the size of the normal spleen can be recalled by the "rules of odds": $1 \times 3 \times 5$ inches in size, weighing 7 oz (about 200 g), and lying between ribs 9 and 11. When the spleen is easily palpated, its size is usually increased by two or more times the norm. That said, the physical examination is a relatively insensitive measure of splenic size. Obtaining an ultrasound examination may be a prudent measure

TABLE 11-8

DIFFERENTIAL DIAGNOSIS OF ACUTE RASH-PRODUCING ILLNESS ASSOCIATED
WITH FEVER AND SORE THROAT

Clinical Condition With Causative Agent	Presentation	Comments
Roseola Agent: human herpesvirus-6 (HHV-6)	Discrete rosy-pink macular or maculopapular rash lasting hours to 3 days that follows a 3–7 day period of fever, often quite high	90% of cases seen in children younger than 2 years Febrile seizures in 10% of children affected Supportive treatment
Scarlet fever Agent: *Streptococcus pyogenes* (group A beta-hemolytic streptococci)	Scarlatinaform or sandpaper-like rash with exudative pharyngitis, fever, headache, and tender, localized anterior cervical lymphadenopathy	Rash may peel Treatment: identical to that for streptococcal pharyngitis
Rubella Agent: rubella virus	Mild symptoms; fever, sore throat, malaise, nasal discharge, diffuse maculopapular rash lasting about 3 days Posterior cervical and posturicular lymphadenopathy 5–10 days before onset of rash Arthralgia in about 25% (most common in women)	Incubation period about 14–21 days, with disease transmissible for ~1 week before onset of rash to ~2 weeks after rash appears Generally a mild, self-limiting illness Greatest risk is effect of virus on the unborn child, especially with first-trimester exposure (~80% rate of congenital rubella syndrome) Prevent by immunization
Measles Agent: rubeola virus	Usually acute presentation with fever, nasal discharge, cough, generalized lymphadenopathy, conjunctivitis (copious clear discharge), photophobia, Koplik spots (appear ~2 days before onset of rash as nearly pinpoint white lesions on mucous membranes, conjunctival folds) Pharyngitis is usually mild, without exudate Maculopapular rash onset 3–4 days after onset of symptoms, may coalesce to generalized erythema	Incubation period about 10–14 days, with disease transmissible for ~1 week before onset of rash to ~2–3 weeks after rash appears CNS and respiratory tract complications common Prevent by immunization Supportive treatment as well as intervention for complications
Hand, foot, and mouth disease Agent: Coxsackie virus A16	Fever, malaise, sore mouth, anorexia; 1–2 days later, lesions Also can cause conjunctivitis, pharyngitis Duration of disease 2–7 days	Transmission oral, fecal, or via droplet Highly contagious with incubation periods of 2–6 weeks Supportive treatment

Clinical Condition With Causative Agent	Presentation	Comments
Fifth disease Agent: human parvovirus-B19	3–4 days of mild flulike illness followed by 7–10 days of red rash that begins on face with slapped-cheek appearance, spreads to trunk and extremities Rash onset corresponds with disease immunity in patient Viremic and contagious before, but not after onset of rash	Droplet transmission Leukopenia common Risk of hydrops fetalis when contracted by women during pregnancy Supportive treatment
Infectious mononucleosis Agent: Epstein-Barr viruses (human herpesvirus-4)	Maculopapular rash in ~20%, rare petechial rash Fever, "shaggy" purple-white exudative pharyngitis, malaise, marked diffuse lymphadenopathy, hepatic and splenic tenderness and occasional enlargement Diagnostic testing: heterophil antibody test (Monospot) Leukopenia with lymphocytosis with atypical lymphocytes	Incubation period 20–50 days >90% will develop a rash if given amoxicillin or ampicillin Potential for respiratory distress when enlarged tonsils and lymphoid tissue impinge on the upper airway Corticosteroids may be helpful Avoid contact sports for at ≥1 month because of risk of splenic rupture
Acute HIV infection Agent: human immunodeficiency virus (HIV)	Maculopapular rash, fever, mild pharyngitis, ulcerating oral lesions, diarrhea, diffuse lymphadenopathy	Most likely to occur in response to infection with large viral load Consult with HIV specialist concerning initiation of antiretroviral therapy

CNS, central nervous system.

to ensure splenic regression before approving return to play. Recall, however, that all persons with infectious mononucleosis are at risk of splenic rupture, regardless of spleen size.

DISCUSSION SOURCE

MacKnight, J. M. (2002). Infectious mononucleosis: Ensuring a safe return to sport. The Physician and Sportsmedicine 30(1). Available at http://www.physsportsmed.com/issues/2002/01_02/macknight.htm, accessed 4/28/03.

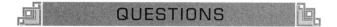

QUESTIONS

42. A 29-year-old woman has a sudden onset of right-sided facial asymmetry. She is unable to tightly close her right eyelid or frown or smile on the affected side. Her examination is otherwise unremarkable. This represents paralysis of cranial nerve:

   A. III.
   B. IV.
   C. VII.
   D. VIII.

43. From those listed below, which represents the most important diagnostic test for the patient in the previous question?

   A. complete blood cell count with white blood cell differential
   B. serum testing for *Borrelia burgdorferi* by ELISA
   C. computed tomographic scan of the head with contrast enhancement
   D. serum protein electrophoresis

44. Which of the following symptoms does a person with stage 1 Lyme disease have?

    A. peripheral neuropathic symptoms
    B. high-grade atrioventricular heart block
    C. Bell palsy
    D. single painless annular lesion

45. The preferred antimicrobials for the treatment of adults with Lyme disease include all of the following except:

    A. doxycycline.
    B. aminoglycoside.
    C. cephalosporin.
    D. penicillin.

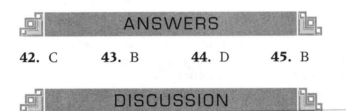

ANSWERS

42. C   **43.** B   **44.** D   **45.** B

DISCUSSION

Lyme disease is a multisystem infection caused by *B. burgdorferi*, a tick-transmitted spirochete. Although original reports of this disease, also known as Lyme borreliosis, were clustered through select areas of the United States, primarily in the Northeast and Mid-Atlantic states, it has now been diagnosed in every state. The origin of the disease's name comes from the town of Old Lyme, Connecticut, where it was first diagnosed after a community epidemic of rash and arthritis. Lyme disease is the most common vector-borne disease in the United States.

Overdiagnosis of Lyme disease is a problem, as is the issue of significant but understandable anxiety about any tick exposure. Infected ticks must feed on the human host for more than 24 hours in order to transmit the spirochete. In addition, not all ticks are infected, with rates varying from 15% to 65% in areas where Lyme disease is endemic.

Lyme disease is typically divided into three stages:

- Stage 1 (early localized disease): This is a mild flulike illness, typically with a single annular lesion with central clearing (erythema migrans). The lesion is rarely pruritic or painful. Signs and symptoms can resolve in 3 to 4 weeks without treatment.
- Stage 2 (early disseminated infection): Typically months later, the classic rash may reappear with multiple lesions, usually accompanied by arthralgias, myalgia, headache, and fatigue. Less commonly, cardiac manifestations such as heart block and neurologic findings such as acute facial nerve paralysis (Bell palsy) and aseptic meningitis may also be present. Individuals with Bell palsy should undergo careful examination and serologic testing for Lyme disease. Again, regression of symptoms can occur without treatment.
- Stage 3 (late persistent infection): Starting approximately 1 year after the initial infection, musculoskeletal signs and symptoms usually persist, ranging from joint pain with no objective findings to a frank arthritis with evidence of joint damage. Neuropsychiatric symptoms can appear, including memory problems, depression, and neuropathy.

Serum testing for *B. burgdorferi* by ELISA with a confirmatory Western blot assay for IgM antibodies help to support the clinical diagnosis of Lyme disease; IgM antibodies decline to low levels after 4 to 6 months of illness, whereas IgG is noted about 6 to 8 weeks after onset of symptoms and may persist at low levels in spite of successful treatment. Careful correlation of patient history and physical examination along with astute interpretation of laboratory diagnostics are critical, to prevent both overdiagnosing and underdiagnosing this condition.

Effective antimicrobials for Lyme disease treatment include doxycycline, cefuroxime axetil (Ceftin), and amoxicillin. Be aware of the latest recommendation for dosage as well as duration of treatment with these products.

Most adults with Lyme disease recover in a period of weeks with appropriate treatment, whereas some have a late relapse.

Prevention of Lyme disease includes avoiding areas with known or potential tick infestation, wearing long-sleeved shirts and pants, and using insect repellents. Inspecting the skin and clothing for ticks is also helpful.

DISCUSSION SOURCES

Centers for Disease Control and Prevention (2004). Lyme Disease. Available at www.cdc.gov/ncidod/dvbid/lyme/, accessed 8/16/04.

Jacobs, R. (2003). Infectious diseases: Spirochetal. In Tierney, L., McPhee, S., and Papadakis, M. (eds.). Current Medical Diagnosis and Treatment (42nd ed., pp. 1390–1410). New York: Lange Medical Books/McGraw-Hill.

12

Psychosocial Disorders

1. A 44-year-old man who admits to drinking a "few beers now and then" presents for examination. After obtaining a health history and performing a physical examination, you suspect he is a heavy alcohol user. Your next best action is to:

   A. obtain liver enzymes.
   B. administer the CAGE questionnaire.
   C. confront the patient with your observations.
   D. advise him about the hazards of excessive alcohol use.

2. During an office visit, a 38-year-old woman states, "I drink way too much but do not know what to do to stop." According to Prochaska's change framework, her statement is most consistent with a person at the stage of:

   A. precontemplation.
   B. contemplation.
   C. preparation.
   D. action.

3. Lorazepam is the preferred benzodiazepine for treating alcohol withdrawal symptoms when there is a concomitant history of:

   A. seizure disorder.
   B. folate-deficiency anemia.
   C. multiple substance abuse.
   D. hepatic disease.

4. Which of the following is the most helpful approach in the care of a patient with alcoholism?

   A. Tell the patient to stop drinking.
   B. Counsel the patient that alcohol abuse is a treatable disease.
   C. Inform the patient of the long-term health consequences of alcohol abuse.
   D. Refer the patient to Alcoholics Anonymous.

5. A 42-year-old man who has a long-standing history of alcohol abuse presents for primary care. He admits to drinking 12 to 16 beers daily for 10 years. He states, "I really do not feel like the booze is a problem. I get to work every day." Your most appropriate response is:

   A. "Work is usually the last thing to go in alcohol abuse."
   B. "Your family has suffered by your drinking."
   C. "I am concerned about your health and safety."
   D. "Alcoholics Anonymous can help you."

261

6. Which of the following agents offers effective control of tremor and tachycardia associated with alcohol withdrawal?

   A. phenobarbital
   B. propranolol
   C. verapamil
   D. naltrexone

7. Which of the following is most likely to be noted in a 45-year-old woman with laboratory evidence of chronic excessive alcohol ingestion?

   A. alanine aminotransferase (ALT) = 202 U/L (0 to 31 U/L), mean corpuscular volume (MCV) = 60 fL (80 to 96 fL)
   B. aspartate aminotransferase (AST) = 149 U/L (0 to 31 U/L), MCV = 81 fL (80 to 96 fL)
   C. ALT = 88 U/L (0 to 31 U/L), MCV = 140 fL (80 to 96 fL)
   D. AST = 80 U/L (0 to 31 U/L), MCV = 103 fL (80 to 96 fL)

ANSWERS

1. B	2. B	3. D
4. B	5. C	6. B
7. D		

DISCUSSION

Providing primary care for patients abusing alcohol presents a number of challenges because this is a complex disorder affecting family and social function and employment, as well as health. Often patients minimize the effect of alcohol abuse, pointing out that employment has not been affected. In reality, alcoholism is a progressive disease that usually affects family and personal relationships first, then health, and, much later, employment. The use of an effective screening tool for alcohol abuse such as the CAGE questionnaire (Box 12–1) is critical for disease detection. The National Institute on Alcohol Abuse and Alcoholism offers steps for alcohol screening and brief intervention (Fig. 12–1).

Counseling the patient and family about alcoholism as a lifelong but treatable disease is a helpful clinical approach. In addition, asking about current drinking habits and associated consequences for health with each visit is important. Consistently offering assistance in accessing treatment conveys the seriousness of this life-threatening condition. As with other health problems with a behavioral component, using statements beginning with "I" is important: "I continue to be very concerned about your health and safety when I hear that you are drinking every day."

In providing primary care, the nurse practitioner (NP) must maintain an attitude that, as with any substance abuse, the patient is capable of changing and achieving sobriety. Change occurs dynamically and often unpredictably. A commonly used change framework is based on

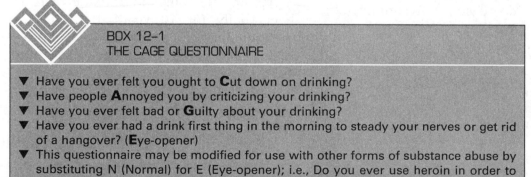

BOX 12–1
THE CAGE QUESTIONNAIRE

▼ Have you ever felt you ought to **C**ut down on drinking?
▼ Have people **A**nnoyed you by criticizing your drinking?
▼ Have you ever felt bad or **G**uilty about your drinking?
▼ Have you ever had a drink first thing in the morning to steady your nerves or get rid of a hangover? (**E**ye-opener)
▼ This questionnaire may be modified for use with other forms of substance abuse by substituting N (Normal) for E (Eye-opener); i.e., Do you ever use heroin in order to keep from getting sick or withdrawing?

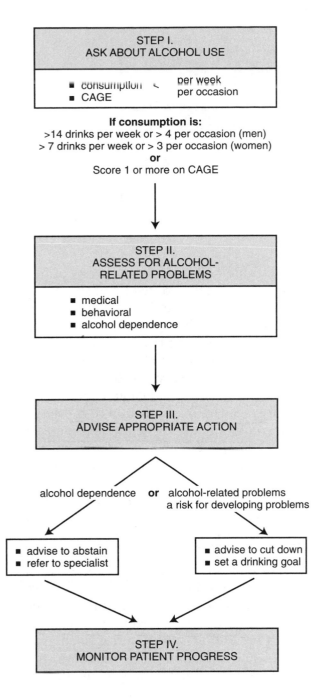

FIG. 12–1. Steps for alcohol screening and brief intervention. (From the National Institute on Alcohol Abuse and Alcoholism [1995]. The Physician's Guide to Helping Patients with Alcohol Problems [NIH Publication No. 95–3769]. Bethesda, MD: National Institutes of Health.)

the work of Prochaska, who noted five stages of preparation for change:

1. Precontemplation: The patient is not interested in change.
2. Contemplation: The patient is considering change and looking at its positive and negative aspects.
3. Preparation: The patient exhibits some change behaviors or thoughts but may feel that he or she does not have the tools to proceed.
4. Action: The patient is ready to go forth with change.
5. Maintenance/relapse: The patient learns to continue the change and to deal with backsliding.

As counselor, the NP provides a valuable role in continually "tapping" the patient with a message of concern about health and safety, thus possibly moving the patient from the precontemplation to the contemplation stage. After the patient is at this stage, presenting treatment options and support for change are critical parts of a NP's role.

In a patient who drinks more than one pint of hard liquor or six beers per day, alcohol withdrawal symptoms typically begin about 12 hours after the last drink. Peak symptoms are seen at 24 to 48 hours with abatement over the next few days. Abrupt withdrawal of alcohol use in the addicted person can lead to potentially life-threatening problems, with autonomic hyperactivity (i.e., agitation, hallucinations, disorientation) as well as seizures. Benzodiazepines are helpful in managing distressing symptoms as well as preventing seizures. Treatment of concurrent problems such as dehydration, malnutrition, and infection is also warranted. Inpatient detoxification is the safest treatment for high-risk individuals (Box 12–2).

A highly motivated patient with adequate support systems and a relatively low level of alcohol addiction may be a good candidate for outpatient detoxification. In this type of detoxification, the patient and support person con-

BOX 12–2
IN-PATIENT DETOXIFICATION CRITERIA

In-patient detoxification is the safest treatment in high-risk individuals, including those who have the following:

▼ Other acute illness, such as infection and cardiac disease.
▼ Severe alcohol-related symptoms prior to detoxification.
▼ Prior severe withdrawal characterized by delirium tremens or seizure.
▼ Coexisting mental health problems such as depression.

Saitz, Vaillant, Wolf (1998).

tract with the health care provider about a safe plan of detoxification. This includes daily office visits or contact, ongoing involvement in Alcoholics Anonymous, and counseling services as well as use of a limited supply of medications for managing withdrawal symptoms.

Benzodiazepines have long been used to treat alcohol withdrawal symptoms. Chlordiazepoxide (Librium) or diazepam (Valium), agents with a long half-life, are reasonable treatment options for a patient with adequate hepatic function, but lorazepam or similarly shorter acting benzodiazepines should be used in those with hepatic dysfunction. Providing a higher dosage of a long-acting benzodiazepine such as diazepam, 20 mg on day one, followed by a dosing schedule reduced by 5 mg daily, increased if symptoms are particularly severe, is often effective and is currently favored over fixed-dosage schedules. Carbamazepine offers an alternative to benzodiazepine use; antipsychotics play no role in managing alcohol withdrawal symptoms. Alpha-adrenergic agonists (e.g., clonidine) or beta-adrenergic antagonists (e.g., propranolol, atenolol) are helpful in managing the distressing physical manifestations of alcohol withdrawal such as tachycardia and tremors. Attention must be focused on treating alcohol-induced nutritional deficiencies, particularly with high-dose B vitamin supplementation, including thiamine, pyridoxine, and folic acid, as well as vitamin C.

Although it is tempting to rely on laboratory markers to make the diagnosis of alcoholism, few tests are helpful in reality. Tests of hepatic function are often ordered by health care providers who then have the problem of presenting the alcohol-abusing patient with a set of relatively normal test results. This may further reinforce the patient's denial or minimization of the effect excessive alcohol use has on health. All currently available hepatic tests indirectly measure liver function or capacity. The most commonly performed tests are measurements of hepatic enzymes, protein molecules acting as catalysts, and regulating metabolism within cells.

AST (formerly known as serum glutamic-oxaloacetic transaminase [SGOT]) is found in large quantities in hepatocytes. Small amounts are typically found in circulation for hepatic growth and repair. AST increases in response to hepatocyte injury, as may occur in alcohol abuse, the therapeutic use of HMG CoA reductase inhibitors (lipid-lowering drugs whose names have the "-statin" suffix, such as lovastatin), and acetaminophen overdose. AST is also found in skeletal muscle, myocardium, brain, and kidneys in smaller amounts; therefore, damage to these areas may also cause an AST increase. AST has a circulatory half-life of approximately 12 to 24 hours, and so levels increase in response to hepatic damage and clear quickly after damage ceases. AST elevation is generally found in only about 10% of problem drinkers. However, if AST is elevated with normal ALT and mild macrocytosis (MCV >100 fL, seen in about 30% to 60% of men who drink five or more drinks per day and in women at a threshold of three or more drinks per day), long-standing alcohol abuse is the likely cause.

ALT (formerly known as serum glutamate pyruvate transaminase [SGPT]) is more specific to the liver, having limited concentration in other organs. This enzyme has a longer half-life than AST, at 37 to 57 hours. Therefore, elevation persists longer after hepatic damage has ceased. The greatest elevation of this enzyme is likely seen in hepatitis caused by infection or inflammation. This enzyme is unlikely to increase in the presence of alcohol abuse.

When evaluating a patient with suspected substance abuse causing hepatic dysfunction, the NP must note both the degree of AST or ALT elevation and the AST/ALT ratio.

DISCUSSION SOURCES

Eisendrath, S., and Lichtmacher, J. (2003). Psychiatric disorders. In Tierney, L., McPhee, S., and Papadakis, M. (eds.). Current Diagnosis and Treatment (42nd ed., pp. 1006–1066). New York: Lange Medical Books/McGraw-Hill.

Landis, B.J., and Bryant, S. (1999). Mental health disorders. In Youngkin, E., Sawin, K., Kissinger, J., and Israel, D. (eds.). Pharmacotherapeutics: A Primary Care Clinical Guide (pp. 747–800). Stamford, CT: Appleton & Lange.

McQueen, K. (2004). Alcoholism. In Rakel, R. E., and Bope, E. T. (eds.). Conn's Current Therapy (pp. 1141–1145). Philadelphia: Elsevier.

National Institute on Alcohol and Alcoholism (1995). The Physicians' Guide to Helping Patients with Alcohol Problems (NIH Publication No. 95–3769). Rockville, MD: U.S. Department of Health and Human Services.

Saitz, R., Vaillant, G., and Wolf, D. (1998). Recognizing and treating patients with drinking problems. Patient Care 12:113–128.

QUESTIONS

8. When providing primary care for a middle-aged woman with a history of prescription benzodiazepine abuse, you consider that:

   A. she is unlikely to have a problem with misuse of other drugs or alcohol.
   B. rapid detoxification is the preferred method of treatment for this problem.
   C. there may be an underlying untreated psychiatric illness.
   D. she is at significant risk for drug-induced hepatitis.

9. Risk of benzodiazepine misuse can be minimized by use of:

   A. agents with a shorter half-life.
   B. the drug as an "as-needed" rescue medication for acute anxiety.
   C. more lipophilic products.
   D. products with longer duration of action.

10. While counseling an adolescent about the risks of marijuana use, the NP considers that:

    A. symptoms of physical and psychological dependency are rarely reported by regular users.
    B. chronic obstructive airway disease is often associated with its regular use.
    C. its use on a daily basis among teenagers is significantly less common than that of alcohol.
    D. driving ability is minimally impaired with its use.

11. When assessing a person with acute opiate withdrawal, you expect to find:

    A. constipation.
    B. hypertension.
    C. hypothermia.
    D. somnolence.

12. When providing care for a middle-aged man with acute cocaine intoxication, you inquire about:

    A. feelings of anxiety.
    B. poor sleeping patterns.
    C. chest pain.
    D. abdominal pain.

13. Use of flunitrazepam (Rohypnol) has been associated with:

A. agitation.
B. sexual assault.
C. increased appetite.
D. hallucination.

ANSWERS

8. C	**9.** D	**10.** B
11. B	**12.** C	**13.** B

DISCUSSION

The misuse and overuse of a variety of mood-altering products such as alcohol, opioids, cocaine, and amphetamines is often referred to as substance abuse. Substance abuse is a common problem, affecting 10% to 14% of primary care patients, with less than 10% being detected and appropriately treated. The Diagnostic and Statistical Manual of Mental Disorders, Fourth Edition (DSM-IV), describes substance abuse as a maladaptive pattern of use leading to clinically significant impairment or distress, manifested by one of more of the following, directly attributed to substance misuse within a 12-month period, with three or more of the following noted:

- tolerance, shown by either markedly increased intake of the substance (needed to achieve the same effect) or continued use of the same amount of the substance having markedly less effect
- withdrawal, shown by either substance's characteristic withdrawal syndrome or use of the substance (or one closely related) to avoid or relieve withdrawal symptoms
- the amount or duration of use often being greater than intended
- repeated attempts by the person to control or reduce substance use without success
- the person's spending much time using the substance, recovering from its effects, or trying to obtain it
- the person's reducing or abandoning important social, occupational, or recreational activities because of substance use

- the person's continuing to use the substance despite knowing that it has probably caused physical or psychological problems

When rendering primary care, remember that substance abuse commonly means misuse of multiple agents, including alcohol, prescription drugs, and illegal agents. Many substance abusers have an underlying psychiatric problem such as a mood disorder. Substance abuse, including alcoholism, may be a method of self-treatment in patients with an undetected or untreated psychiatric illness.

In comparison with men, women have higher rates of misuse of prescription medications, which is most likely caused by their more frequent use of the health care system. In addition, women are more likely to have disorders of mood, including anxiety and depression, and, consequently, have potential drugs of abuse such as benzodiazepines prescribed by the primary care provider. However, benzodiazepine abuse is likely less common than perceived by prescribers, who often fear that many patients receiving these anxiolytic agents will abuse or misuse the medications (Table 12–1). One issue that needs to be considered when benzodiazepines are prescribed is the issue of their abuse and misuse. Indeed, clinicians often hesitate to prescribe these highly effective agents because of fear of providing the patient with a potentially habituating drug with the possibility of needing increasing dosages. In reality, psychological dependence does occur on occasion, but careful prescribing can help avoid this.

Psychological dependence on benzodiazepines is usually associated with a rapid-onset agent, one that possibly produces a sensation of intoxication. In addition, dosing intervals that exceed duration of action of the drug produce alternating periods of drug effect and withdrawal. The perception of the difference is significant and possibly perceived as a buildup of unpleasant anxiety followed by a period of relief or rescue provided by the patient; the cycle is repeated with each drug dose. Interestingly, using a benzodiazepine as an "as-needed" product increases the likelihood of abuse

TABLE 12–1
ANXIOLYTICS

Anxiolytic	Pharmacokinetics	Indications	Onset of action	Comments
Buspirone (BuSpar)	Slow onset of action (> 7 days), lipophilic, T ½ of metabolite = 16 h.	Generalized anxiety syndrome, social phobia. May be used as adjunct in OCD, PTSD. Less effective in panic disorder, acute anxiety. Will not be helpful in alcohol withdrawal.	2–4 weeks for some relief of anxiety. 4–5 weeks for full therapeutic effect	5-HT1A receptor site agonist, not a benzodiazepine; not effective as a PRN or sleep aid drug. Minimal to no effect on performance, nonsedating. No tolerance withdrawal syndrome. No potentiation with alcohol. Little abuse potential. If anxiety is disabling, consider add short-term benzodiazepine while awaiting other agent's action.
Lorazepam (Ativan)	Plasma peak in 1–6 hours. About ½ as lipophilic as diazepam (Valium). No active metabolites T ½: 10–20 h.	Generalized anxiety syndrome, social phobia, adjunct in OCD, PTSD panic disorder. Helpful in acute anxiety, alcohol withdrawal.	Fairly slow onset of action. Sustained effect.	As with all benzodiazepines, abuse and habituation potential.
Oxazepam (Serax)	About ½ as lipophilic as diazepam. Slower onset of action. Plasma peak in 1–4 h. No active metabolites T ½: 5–15 h.	Generalized anxiety syndrome, social phobia, adjunct in OCD, PTSD panic disorder. Helpful in acute anxiety, alcohol withdrawal.	Slow onset of action. Relatively sustained effect.	As with all benzodiazepines, abuse and habituation potential. A good choice for anxious elders due to short elimination T½ and lack of active metabolites.
Alprazolam (Xanax)	Plasma peak in 1–2 h. About ½ as lipophilic as diazepam. Parent compound T ½: 12–15 h. Active metabolite ½ as active as parent compound.	Generalized anxiety syndrome, social phobia, adjunct in OCD, PTSD panic disorder. Helpful in acute anxiety, alcohol withdrawal.	Slow onset of action. Relatively sustained effect.	As with all benzodiazepines, abuse and habituation potential.

(continued)

TABLE 12–1
ANXIOLYTICS *(Continued)*

Anxiolytic	Pharmacokinetics	Indications	Onset of action	Comment
Clonazepam (Klonopin)	Plasma peak in 1–2 h. About ¼ as lipophilic as diazepam. No active metabolites T½: 18–50 h.	Generalized anxiety syndrome, social phobia, adjunct in OCD, PTSD panic disorder. Helpful in acute anxiety, alcohol withdrawal. Absence and petit mal seizures. Anxiety and panic.	Slow onset of action. Highly sustained effect.	As with all benzodiazepines, abuse and habituation potential. Protracted T½ may pose a problem when used in elders.
Diazepam (Valium)	Plasma peak in 0.5–2 h. Highly lipophilic. Three active metabolites with various T½. Desmethyldiazepam T½: 30–200 h. Oxazepam T½: 3–21 h. 3–hydroxydiazepam T½: 5–20 h.	Generalized anxiety syndrome, social phobia, adjunct in OCD, PTSD panic disorder. Helpful in acute anxiety, alcohol withdrawal. Anxiety, seizures. Musculoskeletal pain.	Rapid onset of action, relatively sustained effect	As with all benzodiazepines, abuse and habituation potential. Protracted T½ may pose a problem when used in elder.

Maxmen., N., Ward, N. (2002). Psychotropic Drugs: Fast Facts (3rd ed.). New York: WW Norton and Company.

because this heightens the patient's awareness of drug versus no-drug state. Psychological dependence on benzodiazepines can be avoided by using a slow-onset product with a long half-life, such as clonazepam. If using short-acting products, provide for an adequate number of doses per day. If they are used on an as-needed basis, advise a maximum number of available or prescribed doses per week, such as three to four times per week rather than once or twice a day. This may help avoid benzodiazepine tolerance, a situation in which the patient requires increasingly higher doses to reach therapeutic effect. Tolerance may lead to physical dependence.

Physical benzodiazepine dependence is a significant problem. When working with a patient to discontinue benzodiazepine use, consider reducing the dosage by 25% per week. Rapid withdrawal can lead to tremors, hallucinations, seizures, and a delirium tremens–like state. The onset of withdrawal symptoms occurs a few days after the last dose of a benzodiazepine with a shorter half-life (e.g., lorazepam) and to up to 3 weeks after the last dose of one with a longer half-life (e.g., clonazepam).

Benzodiazepines rarely cause hepatic or renal impairment. When taken alone in overdose, benzodiazepines have a rather favorable toxicity profile. However, sedation is enhanced when benzodiazepines are combined with alcohol and barbiturates, leading to a potentially life-threatening condition. Therefore, accidental and intentional fatalities often occur.

Opioid withdrawal shares many common characteristics with alcohol withdrawal. Hypertension, tachycardia, diarrhea, nausea, hyperthermia, restlessness, myalgia, lacrimation, and rhinorrhea are often reported. Although most distressing, the condition is not life-threatening and usually resolves within a few days. Clonidine, an alpha$_2$-adrenergic antagonist, helps minimize opioid withdrawal symptoms. As with any chemical dependence, long-term rehabilitation therapy is usually needed, necessitating a high level of patient desire for sobriety. The use of methadone, a long-acting opioid, may help curb the use of illegal drugs.

Marijuana has historically been considered a drug that has potential for psychological dependence but little potential for physical addiction. For teenagers in many communities, its daily use is more common than that of alcohol. However, the marijuana currently used is extremely potent because of its high tetrahydrocannabinol content. After a period of abstinence, physical withdrawal symptoms are often reported among daily marijuana users. Chronic marijuana use can lead to airway obstruction such as that found in heavy tobacco users. Driving and activities requiring concentration and/or physical skills such as operating a motor vehicle show significant impairment during marijuana intoxication.

Cocaine is a potent sympathomimetic. With its use, there are increases in heart rate and myocardial contractility, as well as generalized vasoconstriction, causing an increase in blood pressure. In addition, cocaine preferentially constricts the coronary and cerebral vessels, creating significant risk for cerebral ischemia and stroke, as well as myocardial ischemia and infarction. Inquiring about chest pain is prudent in caring for a patient with cocaine abuse.

Flunitrazepam (Rohypnol), also known as Ruffies or the date-rape drug, is a benzodiazepine. Particularly potent with a rapid onset of action, this product is not available for prescription use in North America. However, it is available and commonly used as a sleep aid in other countries. It has been misused, particularly on college campuses as a drug given to reduce sexual inhibition, usually given without the knowledge of the recipient. Flunitrazepam's use is often associated with amnesia. Thus, sexual assault can take place possibly without the victim's recalling the event.

DISCUSSION SOURCES

Eisendrath, S., and Lichtmacher, J. (2003). Psychiatric disorders. In Tierney, L., McPhee, S., and Papadakis, M. (eds.). Current Diagnosis and Treatment (42nd ed., pp. 1006–1066). New York: Lange Medical Books/McGraw-Hill.

Landis, B.J., and Bryant, S. (1999). Mental health disorders. In Youngkin, E., Sawin, K., Kissinger, J., and Israel, D. (eds.). Pharmacotherapeutics: A Primary Care Clinical Guide (pp. 747–800). Stamford, CT: Appleton & Lange.

Liebowitz, N. (2004). Anxiety disorders. In Rakel, R. E., and Bope, E. T. (eds.). Conn's Current Therapy (pp. 1151–1155). Philadelphia: Elsevier.

QUESTIONS

14. Which of the following is true concerning anorexia nervosa?

    A. It affects men and women equally.
    B. Onset is usually in the mid-20s for both men and women.
    C. Depression is often found concomitantly.
    D. Individuals with anorexia nervosa are aware of the extreme thinness associated with the disease.

15. Treatment for anorexia nervosa often includes:

    A. referral for parenteral nutrition evaluation.
    B. antidepressant therapy.
    C. use of psychostimulants.
    D. psychoanalysis.

16. Physical examination findings in patients with bulimia nervosa typically include:

    A. obesity.
    B. dental surface erosion.
    C. tachycardia.
    D. easily plucked hair.

17. Which of the following is most consistent with the diagnosis of bulimia nervosa?

    A. Patients with bulimia nervosa usually present asking for treatment.
    B. Periods of anorexia may occur.
    C. Hyperkalemia often results from laxative abuse.
    D. Most patients with bulimia nervosa are significantly obese.

18. All of the following pharmacologic interventions are used in the treatment of patients with bulimia nervosa except:

    A. fluoxetine (Prozac).
    B. desipramine (Norpramin).
    C. bupropion (Wellbutrin).
    D. paroxetine (Paxil).

19. Characteristics of binge eating disorder include all of the following except:

    A. lack of control over the amount and type of food eaten.
    B. behavior present for at least 6 months.
    C. marked distress, self-anger, shame, and frustration as a result of bingeing.
    D. purging activity.

20 to 24. Identify whether the following characteristics are noted in anorexia nervosa, bulimia nervosa, or in both disorders.

20. parotid gland enlargement

21. hypokalemia

22. lanugo

23. dental enamel erosion

24. dysrhythmias

ANSWERS

14. C   **15.** B   **16.** B
17. B   **18.** C   **19.** D
20. Bulimia nervosa; possible with anorexia nervosa if binge-purging type present
21. Bulimia nervosa; possible with anorexia nervosa if binge-purging type present
22. Anorexia nervosa

23. Bulimia nervosa; possible with anorexia nervosa if binge-purging type present
24. Both anorexia nervosa and bulimia nervosa

DISCUSSION

Anorexia nervosa is a potentially life-threatening disease. DSM-IV criteria for anorexia nervosa include:

- an inability or refusal to maintain body weight.
- 85% of normal weight for age and height.
- intense fear of gaining weight and becoming fat despite low body weight.
- a disturbance in perception of body weight and shape.

Denial of the seriousness of low body weight is often found in patients with anorexia nervosa. Often, despite extreme thinness, a patient with anorexia nervosa looks in the mirror and comments on the need to lose "just a few more pounds." Amenorrhea, common in patients with anorexia nervosa, contributes to establishing the diagnosis. The usual onset of anorexia nervosa in women is during the teens to early 20s, with ages 14 to 18 years being the most common; men present a few years later. This is an overwhelmingly female disease (90%), but affected members of either gender are often involved in an activity that has an emphasis on weight and shape. These activities, which include wrestling, modeling, dancing, gymnastics, and swimming, are occasionally called appearance as well as performance sports.

Persons with anorexia nervosa usually demonstrate one of two types of behavior. With the restricting type, a patient with anorexia nervosa severely limits food intake but does not use binge eating or purging. In the binge-purging type, a patient with anorexia nervosa has cycles of these behaviors.

Unlike bulimia nervosa, which is a secretive disease with relatively few findings, anorexia nervosa is usually easy to identify clinically. In addition to the marked reduction in weight, muscle wasting; abdominal distention with hepatomegaly; cheilosis; oral and gum disease; coarse, dry skin; and hypotension with bradycardia and hypothermia are common.

Treating anorexia nervosa usually includes cognitive-behavioral as well as pharmacologic therapy. In cognitive-behavioral therapy, the focus is on the disturbed eating and the patterns of thinking that help perpetuated the binge-purge cycle. For this therapy to be effective, a clinician who is expert in eating disorders should provide this form of treatment.

Pharmacologic therapy usually involves the use of antidepressants, which may have an effect because of the high rate of comorbid depression. All antidepressants can be used. The choice of a specific agent should be guided by the principles used in choosing therapy in the treatment of depression. Benzodiazepines are also sometimes used to reduce anxiety associated with eating. Cyproheptadine (Periactin) may be used before meals to enhance appetite and reduce anxiety.

Bulimia nervosa is more common in women and typically is present for many years before the patient presents for treatment or before the disorder is noted by a health care provider. Because this tends to be a secretive disease, few with bulimia nervosa present directly requesting intervention.

According to DSM-IV criteria, a patient with bulimia nervosa has episodes of binge eating characterized by eating excessive quantities of food in a discrete period, such as 2 hours. During this period, the patient feels a lack of control over the eating for both the amount and type of food ingested. In addition, there is a recurrent compensatory behavior used to prevent excessive weight gain from a binge, such as self-induced vomiting, excessive exercise, laxative or diuretic abuse, or fasting. Body weight and shape excessively influence self-worth.

Bulimia nervosa may be identified in the clinical setting by problems with erosion of the lingual surface of the upper teeth because of excessive exposure to gastric contents during induced vomiting, hypokalemia caused by laxative and diuretic use, and ipecac-induced cardiomyopathy. Body weight provides few clues because a patient is typically of average to slightly above-average weight.

Treatment of a patient with bulimia nervosa usually includes cognitive-behavioral as well as pharmacologic therapy. In cognitive-behavioral therapy, the focus is on the disturbed eating and the thinking patterns that help perpetuate the binge-purge cycle. For this therapy to be effective, a clinician who is expert in eating disorders should provide this form of treatment.

Pharmacologic therapy usually involves the use of antidepressants such as the selective serotonin reuptake inhibitors (SSRIs). This is usually highly successful in reducing both the frequency and amount of binges, in part because of their activity at the 5-HT 1A receptor site. All antidepressants can be used except for bupropion (Wellbutrin), which may induce further bingeing or seizures in patients with bulimia nervosa. The choice of a specific agent should be guided by the principles used in choosing depression therapy.

Binge eating disorder is characterized as a lack of control over the amount and type of food eaten, occurring two or more times per week for at least 6 months. The bingeing is accompanied by marked distress, self-anger, shame, and frustration as a result of the bingeing; there is no purging activity, and, as a result, the person with binge eating disorder is usually obese. As with all eating disorders, treatment requires an interdisciplinary approach with contributions from health care providers with expertise in this area.

DISCUSSION SOURCES

American Psychiatric Association (1994). Diagnostic and Statistical Manual of Mental Disorders, Fourth Edition (DSM-IV). Arlington, VA: American Psychiatric Publishing.

Eisendrath, S., and Lichtmacher, J. (2003). Psychiatric disorders. In Tierney, L., McPhee, S., and Papadakis, M. (eds.). Current Diagnosis and Treatment (42nd ed., pp. 1006–1066). New York: Lange Medical Books/McGraw-Hill.

Yager, J, (2004). Bulimia nervosa. In Rakel, R. E.,

and Bope, E. T. (eds.). Conn's Current Therapy (pp. 1155–1158). Philadelphia: Elsevier.

QUESTIONS

25. Which patient presentation is most consistent with the diagnosis of depression?

    A. recurrent diarrhea and cramping
    B. difficulty initiating sleep
    C. diminished cognitive ability
    D. consistent early morning wakening

26. Of the following in need of an antidepressant, who is the best candidate for fluoxetine (Prozac) therapy?

    A. an 80-year-old woman with depressed mood 1 year after the death of her husband
    B. a 45-year-old man with mild hepatic dysfunction
    C. a 28-year-old woman who occasionally "skips a dose" of her prescribed medication
    D. a 44-year-old woman with decreased appetite

27. In caring for the elderly, an NP considers that all of the following is true except:

    A. many older patients with dementia have a component of depression.
    B. dementia signs and symptoms usually evolve over months, but depression has a more rapid onset.
    C. with dementia, a patient is aware of difficulties with cognitive ability.
    D. treating concurrent depression may help improve symptoms of dementia.

28. Which of the following is most consistent with the diagnosis of dysthymia?

    A. a 23-year-old man with a 2-month episode of depressed mood after a job loss
    B. a 45-year-old woman with "jitteriness" and difficulty initiating sleep for the past 6 months
    C. a 38-year-old woman with fatigue and anhedonia for the past 2 years

    D. a 15-year-old boy with a school adjustment problem and weekend marijuana use for the past year

29. Drug treatment options for a patient with bipolar disorder often include all of the following except:

    A. fluoxetine (Prozac).
    B. lithium carbonate.
    C. risperidone (Risperdal).
    D. valproic acid (Depakote).

30. Which of the following drugs is likely to be the most dangerous when taken in overdose?

    A. a 4-week supply of fluoxetine
    B. a 2-week supply of nortriptyline
    C. a 3-week supply of nefazodone
    D. a 3-day supply of diazepam

31. One week into sertraline (Zoloft) therapy, a patient complains of a recurrent dull frontal headache that is relieved with acetaminophen. Which of the following is true in this situation?

    A. This is a common, transient side effect of SSRI therapy.
    B. She should discontinue the medication.
    C. Fluoxetine should be substituted.
    D. Desipramine should be added.

32. A patient has been taking fluoxetine for 1 week and complains of mild nausea and diarrhea. You advise that:

    A. this is a common, long-lasting side effect of SSRI therapy.
    B. he should discontinue the medication.
    C. another antidepressant should be substituted.
    D. he should be taking the medication with food.

33. Which of the following medications is most likely to cause sexual dysfunction?

    A. nefazodone (Serzone)
    B. fluoxetine (Prozac)
    C. nortriptyline (Pamelor)
    D. bupropion (Wellbutrin)

34. SSRI withdrawal syndrome is best characterized as:

A. bothersome but not life-threatening.
B. potentially life-threatening.
C. most often seen with agents that have a long half-life.
D. associated with seizure risk.

35. Which of the following is most consistent with the presentation of a patient with bipolar I disorder?

A. increased need for sleep
B. impulsive behavior
C. fatigue
D. anhedonia

36. According to the Agency for Health Care Policy and Research (AHCPR) treatment guidelines, pharmacologic intervention for patients with depression should:

A. generally be given for about 4 to 6 months.
B. continue for at least 6 months after remission is achieved.
C. be continued indefinitely with a first episode of depression.
D. be titrated to a lower dosage after symptom relief is achieved.

37. Depression often presents with all of the following except:

A. psychomotor retardation.
B. irritability.
C. palpitations.
D. increased feelings of guilt.

38. A 44-year-old man is taking an SSRI and complains of new onset of sexual dysfunction and difficulty achieving orgasm. You advise him that:

A. this is a transient side effect often seen in the first weeks of therapy.
B. switching to another SSRI will likely be helpful.
C. venlafaxine may offer a reasonable treatment alternative.
D. he should see a urologist for further evaluation.

39. Which of the following has the longest half-life?

A. fluoxetine
B. paroxetine
C. citalopram
D. sertraline

40. Patient presentation common to both anxiety and depression includes:

A. feelings of worthlessness.
B. psychomotor agitation.
C. dry mouth.
D. appetite disturbance.

41. Which of the following describes prescriptions for antidepressant medications written by primary care providers?

A. dosage too high
B. dosage too low
C. excessive length of therapy
D. appropriate length of therapy

ANSWERS

25. D	26. C	27. C
28. C	29. A	30. B
31. A	32. D	33. B
34. A	35. B	36. B
37. C	38. C	39. A
40. B	41. B	

DISCUSSION

Depression is a common health problem, with a minimum of 15% lifetime occurrence rate. DSM-IV criteria for depression include the presence of the particular symptoms and findings for at least 2 weeks, the person having had five or more of the following symptoms, which are a definite change from usual functioning. Either depressed mood or decreased interest or pleasure must be one of the five, with findings reported by the patient and/or noted by others.

• mood, often, with a marked diurnal variation in mood, with morning mood being more depressed than later in the day

- interests, with lack of interest or pleasure in activities normally or formerly found to be pleasurable
- eating, with a marked increase or decrease in appetite noted with corresponding change in weight
- sleep, with reports of excessive or insufficient amounts; reports of early morning wakening, such as 3:00 to 4:00 AM, with inability to fall back to sleep, are common
- motor activity, with reports of activity being agitated or retarded; agitated mood and irritability are commonly noted together
- fatigue, with report of lack of energy
- self-worth, with report of worthless or inappropriate guilt.
- concentration, with report of difficulty concentrating, trouble thinking clearly, and/or indecisiveness
- repeated thoughts about death (other than the fear of dying) or suicide (with or without a plan) or a suicide attempt

These symptoms cause clinically important distress or impair work, social, or personal functioning and cannot be attributed to another health condition.

Other symptoms of depression are often reported. Hypochondria is found in about 30% of patients; such patients are unable to process objective information that he or she has no health problems. Suicidal thoughts are often present, most often passive ideas without a plan. The patient often agrees with the statement "If I could just die in my sleep, it would be all right." As with anyone with suicidal ideation, a thorough safety evaluation should be completed.

Depression is sometimes mistaken for new-onset dementia. However, a patient with dementia typically has cognitive changes that are slowly progressive over months to years. The cognitive changes reported by patients with depression have usually evolved over a much shorter period, with the patient often accurately reporting what changes have occurred.

Anxiety is often reported by the depressed person and is an important differential diagnosis. However, in depressed patients, mood disturbance occurs first, followed in a number of weeks by the addition of anxiety-related symptoms. Consider depression rather than anxiety as the diagnosis if the patient reports feeling worse while taking benzodiazepines.

Psychomotor agitation with fidgeting and irritability is often found in patients with depression, especially in children and adolescents. In these age groups, this presentation is more likely than psychomotor retardation. This type of increased activity is also found in type A adults with depression.

Intervention for patients with depression includes a combination of support, counseling, and medication. Interpersonal therapy, including counseling and support, alone has a 40% to 60% efficacy with high relapse rates. As a single therapeutic modality, this is most effective for those with reactive depression. Combined therapy of pharmacologic intervention along with interpersonal therapy allow the patient to have effective therapy for what is now recognized as a biochemical disorder, while enabling the patient to acquire the cognitive skills that are helpful in dealing with what is often a chronic, relapsing condition.

Dysthymia is found in approximately 3% of the general population and is characterized by low-level daily depression with at least two of the previously identified depressive symptoms for at least 2 years in adults and 1 year in children. As with those who are depressed, patients with dysthymia respond well to a combination of interpersonal and pharmacologic interventions. In fact, a patient who reports a life-changing feeling with antidepressant use, often described as "feeling good to be alive for the first time," is likely dysthymic. The person's underlying personality emerges after being suppressed or altered by the debilitating effects of the low-level depression that characterizes dysthymia.

Depressed mood may follow a significant life stressor such as death of a loved one or loss of a job. If criteria for depression last longer than 3 months after the precipitating event, the diagnosis of major depression should be considered. Treatment for adjustment disorder with depressed mood lasting beyond 3 months is the same as that for major depression, in recognition that interpersonal therapy can be highly effective in assisting patients in dealing with loss.

Eighty percent of all antidepressant prescriptions are written by primary care providers; thus, the acquisition of skill in prescribing these helpful medications is crucial to practice. All prescription antidepressants are about equally effective if taken in therapeutic dosages for sufficient lengths of time. However, primary care providers tend to underdose antidepressants and prescribe the product for an insufficient length of therapy. The AHCPR offers guidelines for length of therapy (Box 12–3). Long-term antidepressant therapy should be considered when there is a high risk of depression relapse (Box 12–4).

When prescribing an antidepressant, encourage the patient to participate in psychotherapy to work on the skills building needed to help manage this usually long-term health problem. In particular, convey the message to the patient that the use of antidepressants can help facilitate therapy.

When choosing an antidepressant, the prescriber should ask the following questions:

- What has worked in the past? Unless now contraindicated, such medication should be the agent of choice.
- What has worked for relatives? Besides having heard positive comments about the medication from family members, certain medications appear to have greater activity at given serotonin receptor sites. Relatives often have similar serotonin receptor site activity and response to a given medication.
- What are the most bothersome signs and symptoms of the depression? Choose an antidepressant with activity against these or, at minimum, one that will not make these worse. For example, if insomnia and anxiety bother a depressed person, a highly energizing medication is a poor choice (Table 12–2).

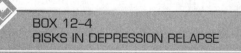

BOX 12–3
LENGTH OF PHARMACOLOGIC INTERVENTION IN
DEPRESSION PER AHCPR GUIDELINES

A minimum of 6–9 months therapy total:

▼ Acute-phase treatment to bring symptoms under control and into remission and lasts up to 3 months.
▼ Continue medication for a minimum of 6 months after depression remission achieved.
▼ Relapse highest in first 2 months after discontinuation of therapy .

With > 2 episodes, 80% relapse in 1 year without treatment:

▼ Consider maintenance therapy as with any chronic illness.

BOX 12–4
RISKS IN DEPRESSION RELAPSE

▼ Dysthymia preceding episode
▼ Poor recovery between episodes
▼ Current episode > 2 years
▼ Onset depression < age 20 years, > age 50 years
▼ Family history of depression
▼ Severe symptoms such as suicide and psychosis

TABLE 12–2
THE SELECTIVE SEROTONIN REUPTAKE INHIBITORS (SSRI)

SSRI	T½	Labeled indications	Adverse reaction profile	Comments
Paroxetine (Paxil)	T½ = 26 h. No active metabolites	Panic disorder, depression, obsessive compulsive disorder.	Rather sedating (HS dosing likely best). Some anticholinergic effect. More constipation (13%) than diarrhea (11%). Antihistamine-like activity may increase appetite.	Helpful in anxious depression. Elimination via renal and hepatic routes. Less problem with limited renal/hepatic function. Low mania induction in bipolar. With relatively short T½ and lack of active metabolites, helpful in the treatment of depression in elders. Due to short T½, a slow tapering dose when discontinuing medication is recommended to avoid significant withdrawal syndrome.
Fluvoxamine (Luvox)	T½ = 16 h. No active metabolites	Depression, panic disorder, obsessive compulsive disorder.	High rate of GI upset and sleep disturbance when compared with other SSRIs	Adverse effect profile can limit utility.
Sertraline (Zoloft)	T½ = 25–65 h. Metabolite T½ = 52–102 h.	Depression, panic disorder, obsessive compulsive disorder.	Equal numbers find it sedating and energizing. Low rate of nervousness, anorexia.	Take with food to enhance absorption
Citalopram (Celexa) Escitalopram (Lexapro)	Citalopram = racemic compound. T½ = 24–48 h for parent compound. Metabolite T½ = 2 days for one, 4 days for another. Escitalopram = single isomer of citalopram with shorter T½ = 33 h.	Depression	Equal numbers reporting somnolence and insomnia. Favorable GI profile. Low rates of agitation and anorexia.	Escitalopram 10 mg is therapeutically equivalent to citalopram 20–40 mg with a superior adverse effect profile.

SSRI	$T^{1/2}$	Labeled indications	Adverse reaction profile	Comments
Fluoxetine (Prozac)	$T^{1/2}$ = 24–72 h. Metabolite $T^{1/2}$ = 4–16 days.	Depression, obsessive compulsive disorder, bulimia nervosa.	Energizing, anorexia common	AM dosing recommended. Protracted $T^{1/2}$ may present problem in elders. Missed doses less of a problem due to protracted $T^{1/2}$. Weight loss common in early months of use but usually not sustained long-term.

Ward, N., Maxmen., N.(2002). Psychotropic Drugs: Fast Facts (3rd ed.). New York: WW Norton and Company.

When an antidepressant is chosen, the side-effect profile is critical. Often a given agent has a desirable side effect, such as sedation in a patient having difficulty with sleep or anxiety (Table 12–3). In addition, the drug's half-life influences the therapeutic choice, with shorter half-life products being desirable in elderly patients and in the presence of hepatic disease. The younger adult can benefit from the use of a longer half-life drug if this person skips a dose from time to time.

Another consideration in choosing an antidepressant is its toxicity when taken in overdose. The suicidal patient clearly needs hospitalization to ensure safety and appropriate treatment. However, as with many disease states, depression is a disease with episodes of improvement and deterioration. Therefore, the prescriber should consider the risk of an intentional overdose.

Taking a 2-week supply of a tricyclic antidepressant (TCA) in full therapeutic dose will likely be lethal, with significantly smaller amounts capable of causing seizures and dysrhythmias. In comparison, the SSRIs and atypical antidepressants have significantly better safety profiles when taken in overdose: usually more than a 2-month supply of a full therapeutic dose is needed to cause life-threatening effects (see Table 12–2).

Antidepressants generally work by causing an increase in availability of select neurotransmitters, such as serotonin, norepinephrine, and dopamine. This allows for greater activity at the neurotransmitter's respective receptor sites. Interestingly, there is evidence that interpersonal therapy also increases serotonin availability.

The SSRIs are a heterogenous group of drugs with a common mechanism of action, blocking reuptake of serotonin in the central nervous system and increasing amounts of scrotonin available to postsynaptic neuron. The end effect is that more serotonin is available for action at select receptors. Serotonin is active at a number of receptor sites (Table 12–4).

With all antidepressants, receptor site–induced effect is immediate when therapy is initiated. However, the length of onset of therapeutic action is usually a number of weeks. This length of onset is likely associated with time needed for change in receptor site activity.

When a patient who is depressed takes antidepressants and is undergoing a significant life stressor, such as family or marital discord or abuse, depressive symptoms usually subside as the medication takes effect. However, if the stressor continues, the antidepressant may appear to lose its initial effectiveness. Ongoing interpersonal therapy can be highly effective in augmenting pharmacologic treatment in such situations.

In early SSRI therapy, the patient often complains of drug-related side effects; these, which

TABLE 12–3

THE ATYPICAL, TRICYCLICS AND TETRACYCLIC ANTIDEPRESSANTS

Agent	T ½	Adverse reactions	Comments
Nefazodone (Serzone)	2–4 h	Low anxiety, insomnia rate. Excellent GI side-effect profile. Low-rate nausea, diarrhea. Problems with somnolence, dry mouth, dizziness. Take with food for slower absorption and less drowsiness. Excellent sexual function profile.	Inhibits neuron reuptake of serotonin and norepinephrine 5-HT2 antagonist. Antidepressant/anxiolytic agent. Good alternative for SSRI nonresponder or when SSRI sexual dysfunction an issue. Concerns about hepatotoxicity led FDA to add product warning.
Venlafaxine (Effexor)	T ½ = 3–5 h (4–24)	Stimulating in larger amounts. May need trazodone or other agent to help with sleep. Significant nausea with rapid onset of high dose. Dose-dependent increases in DBP. Average 5 mm Hg response.	SSRI-like effect only in low doses, with norepinephrine uptake blockade at medium to high doses, similar to TCA effect but with fewer adverse effects. Dopamine effect at very high doses, similar to bupropion. Withdrawal syndrome similar to SSRIs.
Bupropion (Wellbutrin)	T ½ = 9–14 h (3.9–24)	Few anticholinergic effects. Energizing. Possible increased libido, agitation (25%). Avoid with significant manifestation of anxiety, agitation, insomnia.	Possibly block reuptake of dopamine at the presynaptic neuron, especially in high doses, some increase in norepinephrine transmission. Dopamine receptor sites are likely stimulated in substance abuse, making bupropion a helpful antidepressant for the person with a history of substance abuse. Nonaddicting and nonintoxicating. Avoid use in presence of eating disorder or if anorexia is a major component of the depression. Weight loss often seen (28% >5 lb) after initiation of therapy. Do not give if history of or risk for seizure, closed head injury history, history of quiescent epilepsy. Seizure risk worsens if dose increased rapidly.
Mirtazapine (Remeron)	T ½ = 20–40 h	Potent H1 inhibitor, weight gain common. Major side effect is sedation that is worse in lower doses. Little sexual dysfunction or GI side effect.	Effect likely due to increase in central noradrenergic and serotonergic activity. Selectively stimulates 5HT1A while blocking 5HT2 and 5HT3. Higher doses more receptor-site selective and are associated with fewer side effects.

Agent	T $^1/_2$	Adverse reactions	Comments
Tricyclic antide-pressants (-ine suffix; includes nortriptyline {Pamelor-Active precursor of amitriptyline}, desipramine {Norpramin}, active metabolic of imipramine)	T $^1/_2$ = 24–32 h	Weight gain. Anticholinergic activity (blurred vision, dry mouth, memory loss, sweating, anxiety, postural hypotension, dizziness, and tachy-cardia). Constipation a problem but infrequent nausea. Little sexual dysfunc-tion.	Inexpensive, more effective than SSRI in more severe depression, likely due to its norepinephrine as well as serotonin activity More bothersome side-effect pro-file leads to high drop-out rate. Primary care providers seldom prescribe sufficient doses to relieve depression. Wean off over 2–4 weeks to avoid TCA withdrawal symptoms. Sleep disturbance, nightmares, GI upset, malaise, irritability.
Trazodone (Deseryl)	T $^1/_2$ = 5h (3–9 h)	Highly sedating, dizziness, favorable GI side-effect profile. Priapism risk found in 1 in 6000 males using drug. Patient should be in-formed to go to ED promptly for painful erection >30 minutes. Frequent issue in litigation.	Anxiolytic and antidepressant activity. 5-HT2 antagonist. Clinical use limited by marked sedation. Effective hypnotic with little AM drowsiness @ doses 25–100 mg taken 1 h before sleep. May use in low, frequent doses as benzodiazepine alternative for generalized anxiety. Risk of priapism when used in men.

Ward, N., Maxmen., N. (2002). Psychotropic Drugs: Fast Facts (3rd ed.). New York, NY: WW Norton and Company.

include headache, nausea, and diarrhea, re-solve within 2 to 6 weeks. Advising the patient that these are easily treatable and expected, but transient, problems helps avoid the prob-lem of self-discontinuation of this important therapeutic agent. The headache is usually frontal in location and resolves with acetamin-ophen. Using a nonsteroidal anti-inflamma-tory drug may contribute further to the gastrointestinal upset often found in the first weeks of SSRI use. Taking the medication with food can minimize nausea and diarrhea. Taking any medication with an antacid may limit the medication's effectiveness.

Use of SSRIs is often associated with sexual function problems. Decreased libido, anorgas-my, and erectile dysfunction are often reported. If this is a problem, switching the patient to an atypical antidepressant or TCA may be indi-cated, because the use of these products is much less often associated with sexual dys-function.

A withdrawal syndrome may be seen with SSRI use longer than 5 weeks when the prod-uct is rapidly discontinued. In SSRI withdrawal syndrome, there is a sudden change in the amount of serotonin available and an alter-ation in receptor site action. Its onset is related to the half-life of the drug, with five to seven half-lives before the drug clears fully. There-fore, symptoms occur more rapidly after SSRI discontinuation of a drug with a short half-life and may not occur at all after discontinuation of one with a protracted half-life (e.g., fluoxe-tine).

Symptoms of SSRI withdrawal syndrome include dizziness, paresthesia, anxiety, nausea, sleep disturbance, and insomnia. Although disturbing and uncomfortable, this syndrome, unlike benzodiazepine withdrawal, is not dan-

TABLE 12–4
SEROTONIN ACTIVITY

Serotonin receptor site	Activity when stimulated	Comments
5-HT1A	Antidepressant, antiobsessive-compulsive behavior, antipanic, antisocial phobia action, antibulimia effect.	Action at this site basis of most antidepressant, antipanic therapy. Reason that shyness often lifts with SSRI use.
5-HT1C, 5-HT2C	Influence CSF production, cerebral circulation. Regulation of sleep. Perception of pain. Cardiovascular function.	Reason tachycardia, dizziness, alteration of sleep patterns and change in pain perception occurs with SSRI use.
5-HT1D	Antimigraine activity	Triptan preparation works by stimulating this receptor site. TCA also works at this site and therefore helpful in preventing migraine headache.
5-HT2	Agitation, akathisia, anxiety, panic, insomnia, sexual dysfunction. Excessively upregulated in those with depression.	Receptor site highly stimulated in activating SSRI such as fluoxetine. Activity at this receptor site causes sexual dysfunction associated with SSRI use. Nefazodone (Serzone) and trazodone (Desyrel) antagonize action at this site and helpful in treatment of anxious depression and have a more favorable sexual function profile.
5-HT3	When stimulated, nausea, GI distress, diarrhea, headache.	Particularly stimulated with antidepressants with poor GI side-effect profile. Products such as ondansetron (Zofran) (a 5-HT3 antagonist) block activity at this site.

Maxmen, J., Ward, N. (2002). Psychotropic Drugs Fast (3rd edition). WW Norton and Company. New York.

gerous or life-threatening, generally resolving within days to a few weeks.

The TCAs are a group of helpful but often misunderstood and underused medications. The TCAs have a more problematic side-effect profile than do the SSRIs. In addition, they necessitate considerable prescriber skill and patient cooperation. These medications are likely superior to the SSRIs when depression is moderate to severe and characterized by emotional withdrawal, guilt, anorexia, and middle to late insomnia. In addition, they are effective in depressed patients who also have chronic pain, fibromyalgia, migraine, or the need for sedative or hypnotic agents. Choosing a TCA

(e.g., nortriptyline [Pamelor] or desipramine [Norpramin]) with less anticholinergic effect and slowly increasing the dosage helps enhance patient adherence.

If a patient with depression also has episodes of mania, bipolar I disorder is present. Bipolar disorders occur in approximately 1% of the general population. Characteristics of mania include the following for at least 1 week, or less; if hospitalized, the person's mood is persistently high, irritable, or expansive, coupled with three or more of these symptoms:
- grandiosity or exaggerated self-esteem
- reduced need for sleep
- increased talkativeness

- flight of ideas or racing thoughts
- easy distractibility
- psychomotor agitation or increased goal-directed activity (social, sexual, work, or school)
- poor judgment (as shown by spending sprees, sexual adventures, poor investments)

The severity of the symptoms is such that there is at least one of the following: material distress; impairment of work, social, or personal functioning; psychotic features; and the need for hospitalization to protect the person or others.

In bipolar I disorder, the patient usually presents with cycles of elevated or irritated mood lasting longer than 1 week. Bipolar I disorder is most common in women, with an onset around puberty. If a patient with depression has episodes of mania lasting less than 4 days with little social incapacitation, the diagnosis of bipolar II disorder is made. In patients with bipolar II disorder, the episodes of mania are relatively mild (hypomania) and may be rather productive, in contrast to the low point of depression.

Further descriptors of bipolar disease include rapid cycling and cyclothymic disorder. In rapid-cycle bipolar disorder, there are four or more hypomanic, manic, mixed, or major depressive episodes in a 1-year period. In cyclothymic disorder, the mood disorder has been present for at least 2 years with episodes of mania lasting less than 4 days, too brief to fit standard criteria of mania or hypomania. If a TCA is given to persons with bipolar disorder, approximately 15% develop mania. This may also happen when an energizing SSRI such as fluoxetine is given. Ongoing evaluation and treatment of the person with bipolar disorder require significant expertise; expert advice should be sought. Treatment usually includes the use of mood-stabilizing medications such as lithium carbonate, valproic acid, carbamazepine, and risperidone.

DISCUSSION SOURCES

Agency for Health Care Policy and Research (1993). Depression in Primary Care, Volume 2: Treatment of Major Depression. Washington, DC: U.S. Department of Health and Human Services.

American Psychiatric Association (1994). Diagnostic and Statistical Manual of Mental Disorders, Fourth Edition (DSM-IV). Arlington, VA: American Psychiatric Publishing.

Eisendrath, S., and Lichtmacher, J. (2003). Psychiatric disorders. In Tierney, L., McPhee, S., and Papadakis, M. (eds.). Current Diagnosis and Treatment (42nd ed., pp. 1006–1066). New York: Lange Medical Books/McGraw-Hill.

Landis, B. J., and Bryant, S. (1999). Mental health disorders. In Youngkin, E., Sawin, K., Kissinger, J., and Israel, D. (eds.). Pharmacotherapeutics: A Primary Care Clinical Guide (pp. 747–800). Stamford, CT: Appleton & Lange.

Maxmen, N., and Ward, N. (2002). Psychotropic Drugs: Fast Facts (3rd ed.). New York: W. W. Norton.

QUESTIONS

42. Which of the following is most consistent with the diagnosis of anxiety?

    A. nausea
    B. difficulty initiating sleep
    C. diminished cognitive ability
    D. consistent early morning wakening

43. When prescribing a benzodiazepine, the NP considers that:

    A. the drugs are virtually interchangeable, with similar durations of action and therapeutic effect.
    B. the onset of therapeutic effect is usually rapid.
    C. these drugs have a low abuse potential in substance abusers.
    D. elderly patients may use dosages similar to those needed by younger adults.

44. Buspirone (BuSpar) has:

    A. low abuse potential.
    B. significant antidepressant action.
    C. a withdrawal syndrome when discontinued, similar to the benzodiazepines.
    D. rapid onset of action.

45. A 24-year-old woman has a new onset of panic disorder. As part of her clinical presentation, you expect to find all of following except:

A. peak symptoms 10 minutes into the panic attack.
B. a history of agoraphobia.
C. a report of chest pain during panic attack.
D. a history of thought disorder.

46. As you develop the treatment plan in panic disorder, you consider prescribing:

A. carbamazepine (Tegretol).
B. risperidone (Risperdal).
C. paroxetine (Paxil).
D. bupropion (Wellbutrin).

47. Diagnostic criteria for generalized anxiety disorder includes all of the following except:

A. difficulty concentrating.
B. consistent early morning wakening.
C. apprehension.
D. irritability.

48. Which of the following is often reported by anxious patients?

A. constipation
B. muscle tension
C. hive-form rash
D. somnolence

49. According to the AHCPR treatment guidelines, pharmacologic intervention in anxiety should be:

A. generally given for about 4 to 6 months.
B. continued for at least 6 months after remission is achieved.
C. continued indefinitely with a first episode of anxiety.
D. titrated to a lower dosage after symptom relief is achieved.

50. The use of which of the following drugs often mimics generalized anxiety disorder?

A. sympathomimetics
B. benzodiazepines
C. anticholinergics
D. alpha beta antagonists

51. When prescribing a benzodiazepine, an NP should consider that:

A. the ingestion of as little as 3 to 4 days' therapeutic dose can be life-threatening.
B. the medication must be taken at the same hour every day.
C. concomitant use of alcohol should be avoided.
D. onset of therapeutic effect takes a number of days.

52. A middle-aged woman who has taken a therapeutic dosage of lorazepam for the past 6 years wishes to stop taking the medication. You advise her that:

A. she may discontinue the drug immediately if she thinks it no longer helps with her symptoms.
B. rapid withdrawal in this situation can lead to tremors and hallucinations.
C. she should taper down the dosage of the medication over the next week.
D. gastrointestinal upset is typically reported during the first week of benzodiazepine withdrawal.

53. Risk of benzodiazepine misuse is minimized by use of:

A. agents with a shorter half-life.
B. the drug as an as-needed rescue medication for acute anxiety.
C. more lipophilic products.
D. products with long durations of action.

54. Concomitant health problems found in a patient with panic disorder often include:

A. irritable bowel syndrome.
B. thought disorders.
C. hypothyroidism.
D. *Helicobacter pylori* colonization.

55. In providing primary care for a patient with post-traumatic stress disorder (PTSD), you consider that all of the following will likely be reported except:

A. agoraphobia.
B. feeling of detachment.
C. hyperarousal.
D. poor recall of the precipitating event.

56. Preferred pharmacologic treatment options for patients with PTSD include:

    A. methylphenidate (Ritalin).
    B. oxazepam (Serax).
    C. lithium carbonate.
    D. buspirone (BuSpar).

57. Which of the following medications is used to assist in treating irritability and impulsivity often found in patients with PTSD?

    A. carbamazepine
    B. trazodone
    C. kava kava
    D. diazepam

58. Which of the following is an over-the-counter herbal preparation used to relieve symptoms of depression?

    A. valerian root
    B. melatonin
    C. kava kava
    D. St. John's wort

59. Patients with treatment-resistant panic disorder may respond to the use of:

    A. imipramine.
    B. bupropion.
    C. clonidine.
    D. a monoamine oxidase inhibitor.

60 In treating a person with panic disorder using a SSRI, an NP should consider that there is:

    A. considerable abuse potential with these medications.
    B. no significant therapeutic advantage over the TCAs.
    C. reductions in number and severity of panic attacks.
    D. significant toxicity in overdose.

ANSWERS

42. B	**43.** B	**44.** A
45. D	**46.** C	**47.** B
48. B	**49.** B	**50.** A

51. C	**52.** B	**53.** D
54. A	**55.** D	**56.** D
57. A	**58.** D	**59.** D
60. C		

DISCUSSION

Anxiety is a normal human emotion that is an important part of fear response. It helps a patient focus on the issue at hand, such as anxiety associated with taking an important examination or making a presentation. Anxiety can also be protective, heightening senses when an individual encounters a dangerous situation. It should be a rational, expected emotion when present for appropriate reason and should dissipate with the cessation of the stressor. However, anxiety becomes problematic when it is exaggerated, is prolonged, or interferes with daily function.

Generalized anxiety disorder (GAD) is present in approximately 2% to 4% of the population. The typical age at onset is usually in the teens to young adult years; 15% have a first-degree relative with GAD. DSM-IV criteria for GAD include the following:

- excessive anxiety or worry, despite information to the contrary, present on most days for at least 6 months
- a report of difficulty controlling worry, with physical or mental distress causing impairment in social or occupational function
- these problems cannot be attributed to use of medications or alcohol, disease, or other conditions
- the above-mentioned criteria are associated with three or more of the following: muscle tension, restlessness, fatigue, difficulty concentrating, irritability, and difficulty initiating sleep

Anxiety often occurs in patients with depression, which makes the differentiation between these two common disorders problematic. However, a patient with depression that has an anxious component usually reports nervous feelings after the onset of depressed mood. Also in depression, the patient has feelings of worthlessness and the feeling that situations are hopeless; patients with anxiety often report feeling "worried sick" and helpless.

The cardinal presenting signs of anxiety disorder are related to the hypersympathetic state. Physical manifestations include tachycardia, hyperventilation, palpitations, tremors, and sweating. Therefore, in establishing the diagnosis of GAD, it is important to rule out a number of clinical conditions that can mimic the disorder, including thyroid toxicosis, alcohol withdrawal, or abuse of sympathomimetic drugs such as caffeine, amphetamines, and cocaine.

Treatment recommendations for pharmacologic intervention in anxiety disorders are similar to the AHCPR guidelines for depression. Treatment should begin with a 3-month trial period of working with the patient to find the correct medication and dose that help symptoms abate. Encourage the patient to participate in psychotherapy to work on skills building needed to help manage a long-term health problem. In particular, convey the message to the patient that the use of anxiolytic agents can help facilitate therapy. This acute-care phase should be followed with a 6- to 12-month maintenance period, although longer term therapy should be considered, especially if symptoms recur.

Choice of a therapeutic agent is guided by a number of factors, including asking about what has worked in the past and what has worked in the treatment of relatives with similar conditions.

Neurotransmitters implicated in anxiety include gamma-aminobutyric acid (GABA), the brain's major inhibitory chemical, and 5-hydroxytryptamine (5-HT), or serotonin. Norepinephrine, dopamine, and epinephrine likely play a role as well. Drug therapy for patients with anxiety disorders includes agents that enhance GABA function, such as the benzodiazepines, and products that enhance the availability of serotonin, such as the SSRIs.

The benzodiazepines' mechanism of action is as a mediator of GABA, enhancing its activity. Benzodiazepines are highly effective in the treatment of anxiety disorders. Because a number of benzodiazepines are available, choosing the appropriate agent may appear to be a daunting task. However, critical differences can be found in these agents. Some agents, such as diazepam (Valium), are more lipophilic, entering the brain more rapidly and igniting an effect promptly. Although this may appear to be a desired therapeutic effect for severely anxious patients, this rapid ignition can also be rather intoxicating. More hydrophilic benzodiazepines such as lorazepam produce reasonable therapeutic effect while having a slower onset of action and tend to be less intoxicating. In addition, with a highly lipophilic agent, excess is stored in body fat; this leaves a large repository for the drug and provides a longer half-life.

As with any drug, the half-life should be considered. Products such as diazepam and clonazepam with a long half-life give sustained effect without periods of withdrawal. With a shorter half-life, such as with oxazepam (Serax), therapeutic gaps can occur. However, the use of drugs with a shorter half-life and without active metabolites should be considered in treating elderly patients.

One issue that needs to be considered when benzodiazepines are prescribed is their abuse and misuse. Indeed, prescribers often hesitate to use these highly effective agents because of fear of providing the patient with a potentially habituating drug with the possibility of needing increasing doses. In reality, psychological dependence does occur on occasion, but careful prescribing can help avoid this.

Psychological benzodiazepine dependence is usually associated with a rapid-onset agent, which possibly produces a sensation of intoxication. In addition, dosing intervals that exceed the duration of action of the drug produce alternating periods of drug effect and withdrawal. The perception of the difference is significant and possibly perceived as a buildup of unpleasant anxiety followed by a period of relief or rescue provided by the patient; the cycle is repeated with each drug dose. Interestingly, using a benzodiazepine as an as-needed product increases the likelihood of abuse because this heightens the patient's awareness of drug versus no-drug state. Psychological benzodiazepine dependency can be avoided by using a slow-onset product that has a long half-life, such as clonazepam. If using short-acting products, provide for an adequate number of doses per day. If they are used on an as-needed basis, advise a maximum number of available or prescribed doses per week, such as three to four times per week rather than once or twice a day. Increasing tolerance to a high therapeutic dose, usually at a level two to four times the prescribed level, creates physical dependence on benzodiazepines.

When taken alone in overdose, benzodiazepines have a rather favorable toxicity profile. However, sedation is enhanced when benzodiazepines are combined with alcohol and barbiturates, leading to a potentially life-threatening condition. As a result, accidental and intentional fatalities often occur.

Physical benzodiazepine dependence is a significant problem. When working with the patient to discontinue benzodiazepine use, consider reducing the dosage by 25% per week. Rapid withdrawal can lead to tremors, hallucinations, seizures, and a delirium tremens–like state. Onset of withdrawal symptoms occurs a few days after the last dose of a benzodiazepine with a shorter half-life (e.g., lorazepam) to up to 3 weeks after the last dose of one with a longer half-life (e.g., clonazepam).

Panic disorder affects 2% to 4% of the general population. Average age at onset is 27 years; new onset is rare after age 45 years. There is a strong comorbidity with depression. The female:male ratio for panic disorder is approximately 1:1 if seen without agoraphobia. However, panic disorder with agoraphobia is decidedly more common in women than in men, by a ratio of 2:1. A strong family history of agoraphobia is often also reported.

DSM-IV criteria for panic disorder include a history of at least one attack followed by at least 1 month of worry about an additional attack, pondering implications of attacks, or significant change of behavior in relation to the attack.

The panic attack is central to panic disorder. This is a period of intense fear or discomfort developing abruptly and peaking within 10 minutes with at least four characteristic symptoms present. Panic attack symptoms include palpitations, tachycardia, sweating, trembling, shortness of breath, choking, chest pain, chills, nausea, dizziness, and a sensation of de-realization and depersonalization. Additional symptoms include fear of losing control or dying, paresthesia, and hot flashes. In addition to the characteristics mentioned, many individuals with panic disorder have problems with alcohol abuse, depression, dizziness, and chronic fatigue. Irritable bowel syndrome is often found in patients with panic disorder.

Because of the low abuse potential and favorable side effect profile, SSRIs have become the treatment of choice for persons with panic disorder. Their use helps decrease the number and severity of panic attacks and, to a lesser degree, phobia and anxiety related to the attacks. They are significantly more effective against panic disorders than are TCAs.

When using an SSRI for treating a patient with panic disorder, keep in mind that "start low, go slow" should guide therapy. Those with panic disorder usually do not tolerate a rapid induction or change in any therapy because of their heightened sympathetic state. Pick an agent with an early side-effect profile that the patient is likely to tolerate, such as a product that is less rather than more energizing with a lower rate of insomnia, nervousness, and akathisia, such as paroxetine (Paxil). Also realize that SSRI use may precipitate panic attacks with early use but prevent them after the full therapeutic effect is realized.

TCAs may also be used in treating patients with panic disorder. Because patients with panic disorder are sensitive to the sensation of tachycardia, choose a product with serotonergic rather than norepinephrine activity, such as clomipramine (Anafranil) or nortriptyline (Pamelor). As with SSRIs, start with a low dose and increase it slowly.

Monoamine oxidase inhibitors are the most potent drugs available for treating patients with panic disorder. Because of side effects and the need for dietary restriction while patients take the medications, their use is generally limited to patients with treatment-resistant panic disorder.

PTSD is an anxiety disorder that occurs after a significant single event such as a natural disaster, being the victim of a crime, or exposure to combat conditions. It may also be precipitated by recurrent trauma such as serving in combat, living in a war-torn area, or domestic abuse. Horror and helplessness are expected emotions in response to a traumatic life event for at least 1 month afterward. However, these emotions last significantly longer in patients with PTSD and are coupled with intrusive recall of the event, numbing of emotions, detachment, hyperarousal, and impaired social and occupational function.

Treatment of patients with PTSD requires an interdisciplinary approach of expert providers. Pharmacologic intervention often includes the use of an SSRI or a TCA. Benzodiazepines should be used with caution because substance abuse is a common co-condition in patients with PTSD. Buspirone (BuSpar), with its anxiolytic action and low abuse potential, provides a reasonable therapeutic option for the anxiety usually associated with this condition. Carbamazepine (Tegretol) and valproic acid (Depakote) have been used with some success in treating irritability, aggression, and impulsiveness. Clonidine and propranolol may be helpful in minimizing hyperarousal. Trazodone offers a nonaddicting option to enhance sleep.

Patients often choose to treat anxiety and depression with herbal products, which are available over the counter in unlimited supply. Although encouraging and facilitating patient self-care is an important part of the role of NPs, the use of herbal products should be approached with some caution. Herbal medications are considered nutritional supplements and are therefore not subject to the regulatory process common to prescription and over-the-counter medications. As a result, quality control in their production may be lacking, leading to inconsistent amounts of herbs per dose. In addition, when a patient takes an herb to treat symptoms of anxiety and depression, he or she is self-medicating a potentially life-threatening disease. Using herbs with prescription medications may lead to problems with drug interactions or additive effects, such as when St. John's wort is used concurrently with an SSRI. Both the NP and the patient need to be aware of the effects, efficacy, and side-effect profiles of these products (Table 12–5).

DISCUSSION SOURCES

American Psychiatric Association (1994). Diagnostic and Statistical Manual of Mental Disorders, Fourth Edition (DSM-IV). Arlington, VA: American Psychiatric Publishing.

Eisendrath, S., and Lichtmacher, J. (2003). Psychiatric disorders. In Tierney, L., McPhee, S., and Papadakis, M. (eds.). Current Diagnosis and Treatment (42nd ed., pp. 1006–1066). New York: Lange Medical Books/McGraw-Hill.

Landis, B. J., and Bryant, S. (1999). Mental health disorders. In Youngkin, E., Sawin, K., Kissinger, J., and Israel, D. (eds.). Pharmacotherapeutics: A Primary Care Clinical Guide (pp. 747–800). Stamford, CT: Appleton & Lange.

Maxmen, N., and Ward, N. (2002). Psychotropic Drugs: Fast Facts (3rd ed.). New York: W. W. Norton.

QUESTIONS

61. You note that a 25-year-old woman has bruises on her right shoulder. She states, "I fell up against the wall." The bruises appear finger-shaped. She denies that another person injured her. What is your best choice of statement in response to this?

    A. "Your bruises really look as if they were caused by someone grabbing you."

    B. "Was this really an accident?"

    C. "I notice the bruises are in the shape of a hand."

    D. "How did you fall?"

62. Which of the following is true concerning domestic violence?

================================ TABLE 12–5 ================================
OTC HERBAL PRODUCTS FOR ANXIETY AND DEPRESSION

Agent	Mechanism of action	Comments
St. John's wort	? Like MAOI/SSRI/TCA >10 active compounds	When compared with TCA: Less anticholinergic effect, weight gain, less efficacy in more severe depression. When compared with SSRI, similar potential for energizing such as fluoxetine, similar efficacy in mild to moderate depression with limited study. TID-QID dosing needed. 6–8 weeks prior to clinical effect. Little information on drug interactions; likely prudent to avoid concurrent use of SSRI, TCA, MAOI. Potentially photosensitizing, peripheral neuropathy in high doses.
Kava kava	Action at GABA receptors similar to benzodiazepines	Satisfactory response when compared with placebo, low-dose oxazepam (Serax). Sedating, can potentiate effects of alcohol. Cross-allergenic with pepper.
Valerian root	Action similar to benzodiazepines	5–10% with paradoxical stimulating effect. Available in a rather aromatic tea, but weaker, shorter duration of action. Less drug hangover than with benzodiazepines.

A. It is found largely among persons of lower socioeconomic status.

B. The person in an abusive relationship usually seeks help.

C. Routine screening is indicated during pregnancy.

D. A predictable cycle of violent activity followed by a period of calm is the norm.

63 to 67. The following questions should be answered true or false.

____ **63.** Access to a firearm by a male perpetrator is associated with increased risk of abuse of women in only lower socioeconomic income households.

____ **64.** The NP is in an ideal position to provide counseling to both members of a couple involved in domestic violence, particularly if both members of the couple are members of the NP's practice panel.

____ **65.** Women's violence against a male partner is likely to result in as serious an injury as is men's violence against women.

____ **66.** Interpersonal violence is uncommon in same-sex relationships.

____ **67.** Child abuse is present in about half of all homes in which partner mistreatment occurs.

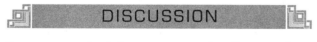

===================== ANSWERS =====================

61. C   **62.** C   **63.** False
64. False   **65.** False   **66.** False
67. True

===================== DISCUSSION =====================

Interpersonal violence among family members (i.e., domestic violence) is found in all socioeconomic and ethnic groups. However, because providers working with lower income and select ethnic groups usually are more vigilant about domestic violence, there is often an appearance that the abuse is more of a problem in certain groups.

Abuse can take a number of forms: psychological, financial, emotional, and physical. Acts of violence are typically thought to be against the victim but may include destruction of property, intimidation, and threats. A cycle of tension building, including criticism, yelling, and threats, followed by violence and then a quieter period of apologies and promises to change is often seen. However, this cycle usually accelerates over time, with the violence being less predictable. Love for the perpetrator, hope that things will change, and fear of the consequences of leaving the relationship help to keep the victim in the relationship. These considerations also usually prevent victims from coming forth and asking for help.

As with counseling and screening for other health problems, using objective statements beginning with "I" is helpful. When a patient denies that finger-shaped bruises are caused by intentional injury by another person, an NP can simply state what is seen. This reinforces the assessment of abuse and allows the patient to offer more information. In a situation in which a patient is verbally abused in your presence, reinforce your role as patient advocate by stating that the behavior is unacceptable in your presence. Some patients may fear that this can possibly precipitate another episode of abuse. However, this is unlikely.

Using the BATHE model is helpful in framing the problem and forming a therapeutic relationship and directing intervention. Developed by Stuart and Lieberman, this model provides a guide for gathering information while helping the patient reflect on the issues at hand. The components of the model are on page 377.

Interpersonal violence is likely as common in same-sex relationships as in opposite-sex relationships but not as well studied. Violent behavior by a woman against a male partner is unlikely to result in as serious an injury as is men's violence toward women. However, in all socioeconomic groups, access to a firearm by a male perpetrator is associated with increased risk of abuse toward women; indeed, this is also a risk for suicide. The NP is in an ideal position to direct the couple to the appropriate resources for help in domestic violence but should not attempt to provide this counseling, because of the complexity of this type of care. Individual treatment is the rule as long as the violent behavior continues. Child abuse is present in about half of all households in which there is partner abuse.

DISCUSSION SOURCES

American Psychiatric Association (1994). Diagnostic and Statistical Manual of Mental Disorders, Fourth Edition (DSM-IV). Arlington, VA: American Psychiatric Publishing.

Peace at Home, Inc. (1995). Domestic Violence: The Facts. Boston: Harvard Community Health Plan Foundation.

Stuart, M., and Lieberman, J. (2002). The 15-Minute Hour: Practical Therapeutic Intervention in Primary Care (3rd ed.). Philadelphia: Elsevier.

13

Female Reproductive and Genitourinary Systems

1. Which of the following is a contraindication to combined oral contraception (COC) use?

   A. mother with a history of breast cancer
   B. personal history of hepatitis A at age 10 years
   C. factor V Leiden mutation
   D. cigarette smoking

2. A 22-year-old woman taking a 35 µg ethinyl estradiol COC calls after forgetting to take her pills for 2 consecutive days. She is 2 weeks into the pack. You advise her to:

   A. Take two pills today and two pills tomorrow.
   B. Discard two pills and take two pills today.
   C. Discard the rest of the pack and start a new pack with the first day of her next menses.
   D. Continue taking the pills for the rest of the cycle but expect some breakthrough bleeding (BTB).

3. When counseling a woman about COC use, you advise that:

   A. long-term use is discouraged because the body needs a "rest" from birth control pills from time to time.
   B. fertility is often delayed for a number of months after their discontinuation.
   C. there is an increase in the rate of breast cancer after protracted use.
   D. premenstrual syndrome symptoms are often improved.

4. Noncontraceptive benefits of oral contraceptives include a decrease in all of the following except:

   A. iron-deficiency anemia.
   B. pelvic inflammatory disease (PID).
   C. cervicitis.
   D. ovarian cancer.

5. Which of the following women is the best candidate for progestin-only pill (POP) use?

   A. an 18-year-old woman who frequently forgets to take prescribed medications
   B. a 28-year-old woman with multiple sexual partners
   C. a 32-year-old woman who is breastfeeding a 3-week-old infant

D. a 26-year-old woman who wants to use the pill to help "regulate" her menstrual cycle

6. A 38-year-old nulliparous woman who smokes two and a half packs a day is in an "on-and-off" relationship. The woman presents seeking contraception. Which of the following represents the most appropriate method?

   A. copper-containing intrauterine device (IUD)
   B. oral contraceptive
   C. tubal ligation
   D. barrier method

7. Which of the following statements is true concerning vaginal diaphragm use?

   A. When in place, the woman is aware that the diaphragm fits snugly against the vaginal walls.
   B. It is a suitable form of contraception for women with recurrent urinary tract infection (UTI).
   C. After insertion, the cervix should be smoothly covered.
   D. The device should be removed within 2 hours of coitus to minimize the risk of infection.

8. All of the following are relative contraindications to the use of a copper-containing IUD except:

   A. valvular heart disease.
   B. multiple sexual partners.
   C. hypertension.
   D. lack of availability for follow-up care.

9. Which of the following is the most appropriate response to a 27-year-old woman who is taking phenytoin (Dilantin) for the treatment of a seizure disorder and is requesting hormonal contraception?

   A. "It is preferable for you to use a barrier method."
   B. "COC use is acceptable."
   C. "Depo-Provera (medroxyprogesterone acetate in a depot injection [DMPA])

will not interact with your seizure medication."
   D. "IUD use is contraindicated."

10. Which of the following is commonly found after 1 year of using DMPA (Depo-Provera)?

    A. weight gain
    B. hypermenorrhea
    C. acne
    D. rapid return of fertility when discontinued

The following questions should be answered by responding yes or no.
   According to the World Health Organization (WHO) guidelines, who is a COC candidate?

11. a 22-year-old who smokes one pack per day

12. a 29-year-old with PID

13. a 45-year-old with tension-type headache

14. a 32-year-old breast-feeding a 6-month-old infant

15. a 28-year-old with type 1 diabetes mellitus

According to the WHO guidelines, who is a candidate for a copper-containing IUD?

16. a 45-year-old with uterine fibroids

17. a 33-year-old who smokes two packs per day

18. a 25-year-old with seizure disorder

19. a 33-year-old with low-grade squamous intraepithelial lesions

20. As you prescribe COC containing the progestin drospirenone, you offer the following advice:

    A. "Always take this pill on a full stomach."
    B. "You should not use acetaminophen when using this birth control pill."
    C. "Avoid using potassium-containing salt substitutes."

D. "You may notice that premenstrual syndrome symptoms might become somewhat worse."

21. With genitourinary tract exposure to the spermicide nonoxynol-9, a woman is at increased risk for:

A. cervical stenosis.
B. UTI.
C. increased numbers of lactobacilli.
D. ovarian malignancy.

22. With the use of a levonorgestrel intrauterine system (Mirena), the following is normally noted:

A. endometrial hyperplasia
B. hypermenorrhea
C. increase in PID rates
D. reduction in menstrual flow

23. The reduction in free androgens noted in the woman taking oral contraceptives can yield an improvement in:

A. cycle control.
B. acne vulgaris.
C. breast tenderness.
D. rheumatoid arthritis.

24. In comparison with DMPA (Depo-Provera), the use of an estrogen-progestin injection such as Lunelle is usually associated with:

A. a monthly episode of vaginal bleeding.
B. less suppression of ovulation.
C. increased bone loss.
D. need for less frequent injections.

25. When can a woman safely conceive after discontinuing oral contraceptives?

A. immediately
B. after 1 to 2 months
C. after 3 to 4 months
D. after 5 to 6 months

26. When prescribing the contraceptive patch (Ortho Evra) or vaginal ring (NuvaRing), the nurse practitioner (NP) considers that:

A. these are progestin-only products.
B. candidates include women who have

difficulty remembering to take a daily pill.
C. there are significant drug interactions with both products.
D. contraceptive efficacy is less than that of COC.

ANSWERS

1. C	2. A	3. D
4. C	5. C	6. D
7. C	8. C	9. C
10. A	11. Yes	12. Yes
13. Yes	14. Yes	

15. Yes, in the absence of advanced vascular disease

16. No	17. Yes	18. Yes

19. Relatively contraindicated

20. C	21. B	22. D
23. B	24. A	25. A
26. B		

DISCUSSION

Despite the availability of numerous methods of highly reliable contraception, nearly one half of all pregnancies are unplanned. Rates of continued contraception use vary greatly according to the method. Helping a woman choose an effective and acceptable form of family planning is an important part of providing health care.

Available for more than three decades, COC has been used by millions of women. This highly reliable form of contraception usually results in 1 pregnancy per 1000 women with perfect use and 50 per 1000 with typical use.

Contraceptive effect is achieved through the action of the COC's progestin and estrogen components. Progestational effects help to inhibit ovulation by suppressing luteinizing hormone (LH), thickening endocervical mucus, and hampering implantation by endometrial atrophy. Through its estrogenic effects, ovulation is inhibited by suppression of follicle-stimulating hormone (FSH) and LH and by alteration of endometrial cellular structure.

When COC is discontinued, fertility usually returns promptly. Contrary to common belief, there is no need to delay conception after discontinuing COC; prolonged COC use is not associated with future infertility or other health problems.

Noncontraceptive benefits of COC include lower rates of benign breast tumors and dysmenorrhea. Menstrual volume is reduced by about 60%, resulting in decreased rates of iron deficiency anemia. Decreased rates of endometrial, ovarian, and breast cancers are particularly noted among long-term users (>5 years). Although COC is not protective against sexually transmitted infections (STIs), COC users have decreased frequency of PID, which results from thickened endocervical mucus; this results in a lower rate of future ectopic pregnancy. Decreased rates of acne, hirsutism, and ovarian cyst; reduction in premenstrual syndrome; and improvement in rheumatoid arthritis symptoms are also noted among COC users.

The highest dropout rates with COC and POP use are in the first 3 months of use. The most frequently mentioned reasons are BTB and inconvenience of use. Although BTB is bothersome, it is not harmful and does not indicate lesser contraceptive benefit. BTB can be minimized by taking the COC or POP within the same 4-hour period every day. Cigarette smoking, a relative contraindication to COC use, increases the likelihood of BTB and should therefore be discouraged. The BTB rate rises dramatically when pills are missed. Advice about what to do in the event of missed pills is an important part of providing contraceptive care (Fig. 13–1).

Nausea with COC and hormone therapy (HT) is often reported. This is usually a transient problem noted in the first months of use and can be minimized by taking the medication with food or at bedtime. If vomiting occurs within 2 hours of taking COC, the dose should be retaken.

COC can interact with a limited number of drugs. However, interaction is noted with a number of antiepileptic drugs (AEDs), including phenytoin, carbamazepine, phenobarbital, and primidone, potentially causing a reduction

With use of 30–35 μg ethinyl estradiol pills
- Missed 1 or 2 active pills
  - Take active pill as soon as possible and then continue taking pills daily, one each day.
  - No additional contraceptive protection

- Missed ⇒ 3 active pills or if she starts a pack 3 or more days late
  - Take an active (hormonal) pill as soon as possible and then continue taking pills daily, one each day.
  - Use condoms or abstain from sex until she has taken active pills for 7 days in a row.

With use of 20 μg or less ethinyl estradiol pills
- Missed 1 active pill
  - Take active pill as soon as possible and then continue taking pills daily, one each day.
  - No additional contraceptive protection

- Missed ⇒ 2 active pills or if she starts a pack 2 or more days late
  - Take active (hormonal) pill as soon as possible and then continue taking pills daily, one each day.
  - Use condoms or abstain from sex until she has taken active (hormonal) pills for 7 days in a row.

Source: www.who.int/reproductive-health/publications/spr_2/index.html, accessed 11.4.04.

FIG. 13–1. Missed combined oral contraceptive pill advice.

in therapeutic levels of these important medications. The BTB rate is greater in women using COC and AEDs partly because of more rapid metabolism of estrogen. A woman with a seizure disorder who wishes to use hormonal contraception will likely have a reduction appear to in frequency and severity of seizures while using DMPA (Depo-Provera), inasmuch as progestin use has long been noted to be protective against seizures. In addition, DMPA does not appear to interact with AEDs. Levonorgestrel implants may have the same effect. Use of barrier methods, IUDs, or levonorgestrel-containing intrauterine systems does not interfere with AEDs and has no effect on seizure threshold.

The progestins used in most COCs are testosterone derivatives. Drospirenone, found in the COC Yasmin is an analog of an aldosterone antagonist and therefore has potassium-sparing qualities. Thus, drospirenone should be used with caution in hepatic or renal dysfunction or with concomitant use of an angiotensin receptor blocker, angiotensin-converting enzyme inhibitor, salt substitute, or potassium-sparing diuretics. A potential benefit of a drospirenone-containing COC is improvement in premenstrual syndrome symptoms.

Although not consistently suppressing ovulation, POP likely provides contraception through thickening of endocervical mucus, as well as through the alteration of the endometrium. POP use offers certain advantages and disadvantages in comparison with COC. With failure rates of 1% to 4%, POP is a less effective contraceptive than COC. The nausea rate with its use is significantly lower than with COC use, owing to the lack of estrogen. POPs are taken daily, a schedule many women find more convenient than the typically 3-weeks-on, 1-week-off schedule with COCs. However, POP must be used daily for maximum efficacy. For lactating women who wish to use an oral hormonal contraceptive, POP use is highly effective and does not alter the quality or quantity of breast milk. One significant disadvantage with POP use is bleeding irregularity, ranging from prolonged flow to amenorrhea.

The contraceptive patch (OrthoEvra) and contraceptive intravaginal ring (NuvaRing) contain estrogen and progestin as a birth control method via a non-oral form. Both of these methods have the advantage of infrequent dosing, with a new patch needed once a week and a new ring every 3 weeks. With proper use, contraceptive efficacy is similar to that of COC. Adverse effects and contraindications to patch and ring use are similar to those of COC. Women who dislike or forget to take a daily pill often welcome the opportunity to use the patch or ring (Table 13–1).

DMPA (Depo-Provera), given every 90 days, is a highly reliable form of contraception (99.7% efficacy). DMPA is best suited for women who do not wish a pregnancy for at least 18 months, because resumption of fertility is frequently delayed by 6 to 12 months. When the injection is given within the first few days of menses, the contraceptive effect is immediate. When it is started 5 days after the onset of menses, it is prudent to use a backup method for 1 week. Depo-Provera may be started immediately postpartum if the woman is not breast-feeding and initiated 3 to 6 weeks postpartum if she is breast-feeding. Earlier use may diminish quantity but not quality of breast milk.

Irregular bleeding, a common problem during the first few months of DMPA injection use, can be minimized by the use of a prostaglandin inhibitor such as ibuprofen, 400 mg TID, or naproxen sodium, 375 to 540 mg BID, for 3 to 5 days. Estrogen supplements, such as a 0.1-mg estrogen patch used for 7 to 10 days, may also be helpful. After 1 year of use, 30% to 50% of women have amenorrhea. According to observation from limited study, bone density may be reduced in women using DMPA. However, this is unlikely to be a long-term problem. Calcium supplementation should be recommended, at 1000 to 1500 mg/day.

Some women like to have an injectable form of contraception but are bothered by the lack of regular menstrual bleeding. An estrogen-progestin injection (Lunelle) given monthly offers similar contraceptive efficacy in comparison with medroxyprogesterone (MPA) injection but a short and fairly predictable episode of monthly vaginal bleeding.

Standard IUDs such as the copper-containing ParaGard T are an effective form of contraception with a failure rate of 0.5% to 2.9%. Their mechanism of contraceptive action is not entirely understood, but it is unlikely that these are abortifacients. Although there may be an increase in menstrual bleeding and upper reproductive tract infection with their use, and because of a number of absolute and relative contraindications (Fig. 13–2), IUDs are, unfortunately, not widely used. Mirena is a levonorgestrel-containing intrauterine system of drug delivery, producing marked endometrial

atrophy. As a result, about 50% of Mirena users are amenorrheic at the end of 1 year of use. Thickened endocervical mucus is also noted, which limits the ascent of infection into the upper reproductive tract and minimizes PID risk. This is a particularly helpful method of contraception for the woman with menorrhagia.

The diaphragm, a barrier method of contraception, is placed in the vagina before intercourse. This device, which has an effectiveness rate of 80% to 95%, should be used in conjunction with a spermicide and removed no sooner than 6 hours after coitus. When properly fitted and in the appropriate position, the woman and partner should be unaware of the

---

TABLE 13–1

WORLD HEALTH ORGANIZATION PRECAUTIONS FOR THE USE OF ORAL CONTRACEPTIVE PILLS

Category 4 Refrain from use	Category 3 Exercise caution	Category 2 Advantages outweigh risk	Category 1 No restriction
• Venous thromboembolism • CHD, CVA • Structural heart disease • Breast cancer • Pregnancy • Lactation (<6 wk pp) • Acute hepatitis • Hepatic adenoma • HA w/ focal neuro symptoms • Major surgery with prolonged mobilization • Age > 35, smoking => 20 cigs/day • HTN (>160/>100 or w/ vascular disease) • Known thrombotic mutations (Factor V Leiden, prothrombin mutations, protein S, C, or antithrombin deficiency)	• Postpartum < 21 d • Lactation (6 wk – 5 mo) • Undiagnosed vaginal bleeding • Age => 35 and smoking < 20 cigs/day • Hx breast cancer but no recurrence in p 5 years • Interacting drugs • Gallbladder disease	• Severe HA w/ OC use • DM • Major surgery w/o immobilization • Sickle cell disease • HTN w/ BP 140/100-159/109 • Undx breast mass • Cervical cancer • Age > 50 • Non adherence factors • Fm hx lipid disorders • Fm hx premature MI • BMI => 30	• Postpartum => 21 d • Post TAB, SAB • GDM hx • Varicose veins • Mild HA • PID, STD hx • HIV • Benign breast disease • Fm hx breast, cervical, ovarian cancer • Cervical ectropion • Uterine fibroids • Past hx ectopic pregnancy • Obesity • Thyroid disease • Depression • Uterine fibroids • Minor surgery without mobilization • Menorrhagia • Irregular menses

http://www.who.int/reproductive-health/, accessed 11.4.04.

diaphragm's presence. If either partner can feel the diaphragm, it is either the wrong size or not properly inserted. Because a diaphragm should always be used with a spermicide, a woman with a history of recurrent UTI is not an ideal candidate for diaphragm use. Although the thought behind this long-held advice is that the diaphragm increases UTI risk as a result of potential pressure on the woman's lower urinary tract, the risk more likely arises from the concurrent use of a spermicide. The woman who is exposed to the spermicide nonoxynol-9, either through vaginal use or with a male partner who uses condoms with this spermicide, is at increased risk of UTI. The proposed mechanism of this risk is the spermicide's antibacterial effect, which is to reduce lactobacilli, a normal component of the periurethral flora. Lactobacilli produce hydrogen peroxide and lactic acid, providing the periurethral area and vagina with a pH that inhibits bacterial growth and blocks potential sites of attachment, as well as being toxic to uropathogens.

DISCUSSION SOURCES

Brown, K. (2004). Management Guidelines for Nurse Practitioners Working with Women (2nd ed.) (pp. 153–173). Philadelphia: F. A. Davis.

Kennedy-Malone, L., Fletcher, K., and Plank, L. (2004). Management Guidelines for Nurse Practitioners Working with Older Adults (2nd Ed.). Philadelphia: F. A. Davis.

QUESTIONS

27. An 18-year-old woman requests emergency contraception after having unprotected intercourse approximately 18 hours ago. Today is day 12 of her normally 27- to 29-day menstrual cycle. You advise her that:

    A. emergency contraception use reduces the risk of pregnancy by approximately 33%.

    B. all forms of emergency contraception must be used within 12 hours after intercourse.

    C. the likelihood of conception is minimal.

    D. taking oral contraceptive hormones in multiple doses is an effective emergency contraceptive option.

28. Which of the following is likely not among the proposed mechanisms of action of COC when used for emergency contraception?

    A. It inhibits ovulation
    B. It is an abortifacient
    C. It slows sperm transport
    D. It slows ovum transport

29. A 24-year-old woman who requests emergency contraception with COC wants to know its effects if pregnancy does occur. You respond that there is the risk of increased rate of:

    A. spontaneous abortion.
    B. birth defects.
    C. placental abruption.
    D. none of the above.

30. A woman who has used hormonal emergency contraception should be advised that if she does not have a normal menstrual period within _____ weeks, a pregnancy test should be obtained.

    A. 1
    B. 1 to 2
    C. 2 to 3
    D. 3 to 4

ANSWERS

27. D   28. B   29. D
30. D

DISCUSSION

As previously mentioned, nearly one half of all pregnancies are unplanned. Emergency contraception, used after coitus to minimize the risk of unintended pregnancy when a contraceptive method fails or is not used, is an effective method of minimizing the number of

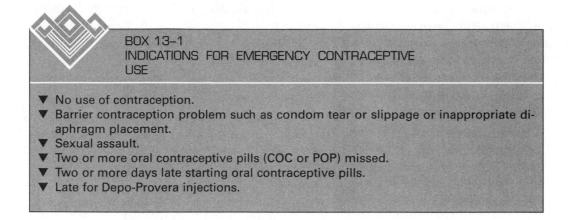

unintended pregnancies (Box 13–1). An estimated 800,000 annual pregnancy terminations could be avoided if knowledge of and access to emergency contraception were widely available.

A number of methods are available, including the use of COCs, POPs, and copper-containing IUDs. Emergency contraception with oral hormonal agents is highly effective, reducing the risk of pregnancy by 75% or more, according to the following model: If 100 fertile women have unprotected heterosexual intercourse in the second to third weeks of their cycles, eight typically become pregnant. Two or fewer typically become pregnant when using emergency contraception. Its mechanism of action is not clearly established, but it may help reduce pregnancy risk by multiple methods, including inhibiting or delaying ovulation or impairing ovum or sperm transport. Emergency contraception is unlikely to prevent pregnancy by preventing implantation of a fertilized ovum, because the resulting minor endometrial changes would likely not be sufficient to prevent implantation. Oral hormonal emergency contraception use will not interrupt an established pregnancy or increase risk of early pregnancy loss. In pregnancy that does occur, use of emergency contraception does not appear to be teratogenic. A theoretical but not observed risk of ectopic pregnancy exists due to its slowed tubal motility.

A copper-containing IUD such as the ParaGard T 380A can be inserted within 5 days after intercourse as a form of emergency contraception. Because of the risk of upper reproductive tract infections, its use is contraindicated in the presence of an STI. IUD insertion also provides a hormone-free emergency contraception option, as well as ongoing contraception.

Menstrual bleeding should be expected within 3 to 4 weeks of using emergency con-

Patient factors in CU-IUD use	
Appropriate candidates	**Contraindications**
• Stable, mutually monogamous relationship • Parous (preferred) • Not candidate for OCP	• Pregnancy • Undiagnosed uterine bleeding • Abnormal pap (relative) • Abnormal uterine shape (fibroids, septum, others) • Allergy to IUD components • Increased risk of infection • Immune system compromise (relative)

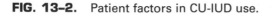

http://www.who.int/reproductive-health/, accessed 11.4.04.

FIG. 13–2. Patient factors in CU-IUD use.

traception. If none occurs, a pregnancy test should be done.

DISCUSSION SOURCES

Brown, K. (2004). Management Guidelines for Nurse Practitioners Working with Women (2nd ed.). Philadelphia: F.A. Davis.

Dickey, R. (2002). Managing Contraceptive Pill Patients (11th ed.) Dallas: EMIS.

QUESTIONS

31. In advising a woman about menopause, you offer the following information:

    A. The average age at last menstrual period for a North American woman is 47 to 48 years.
    B. Hot flashes and night sweats occur in about 80% of women.
    C. Women with surgical menopause usually have milder symptoms.
    D. FSH and LH levels are suppressed.

32. Findings in estrogen deficiency (atrophic) vaginitis include:

    A. a malodorous vaginal discharge.
    B. an increased number of lactobacilli.
    C. a reduced number of white blood cells.
    D. a pH greater than 5.

33. A 53-year-old woman who is taking HT with conjugated equine estrogen (CEE), 0.625 mg/day, with MPA, 2.5 mg, has bothersome atrophic vaginitis symptoms. You advise that:

    A. her oral estrogen dose should be increased.
    B. topical estrogen may be helpful.
    C. the MPA component should be discontinued.
    D. baking soda douche should be used.

34. Relative contraindications to postmenopausal HT include all of the following except:

    A. unexplained vaginal bleeding.
    B. seizure disorder.

C. dyslipidemia.
D. migraine headache.

35. Absolute contraindications to postmenopausal HT include:

    A. endometrial cancer.
    B. seizure disorder.
    C. dyslipidemia.
    D. migraine headache.

36. In advising a perimenopausal woman about HT, you consider that it may:

    A. reduce the risk of venous thrombotic events.
    B. significantly lower serum triglyceride levels.
    C. worsen hypertension in most women.
    D. preserve bone density.

37. Postmenopausal HT may cause:

    A. a reduction in the rate of cardiovascular disease.
    B. an increase in the rate of rheumatoid arthritis.
    C. a reduction in the frequency of spinal and hip fractures.
    D. a disturbance in sleep patterns.

38. The progestin component of HT is given to:

    A. counteract the negative lipid effects of estrogen.
    B. minimize endometrial hyperplasia.
    C. help with vaginal atrophy symptoms.
    D. prolong ovarian activity.

39. Concerning selective estrogen receptor modulator (SERM) therapy such as raloxifene (Evista), which of the following is correct?

    A. Concurrent progestin opposition is needed.
    B. Hot flashes are reduced in frequency and severity.
    C. Its use is contraindicated when a woman has a history of breast cancer.
    D. Osteoporosis risk is reduced with its use.

40. During perimenopause, which of the following is likely to be noted?

A. Symptoms are most likely in the week before the onset of the menses.
B. The length of the perimenopausal period is predictable.
C. Symptoms are less severe in women who smoke.
D. Hot flashes are uncommon.

41. Which of the following is likely to be noted with short-term (<1- to 2-year) hormone replacement therapy (HRT) use in a post-menopausal woman?

A. reduction in dementia risk
B. significant increase in breast cancer risk
C. minimized menopausal symptoms
D. increase in cardiovascular risk

42. Which body area has the greatest concentration of estrogen receptors?

A. vulva
B. vascular bed
C. heart
D. brain

43. Reported effects of black cohosh use include:

A. hirsutism.
B. insomnia.
C. decreased frequency and severity of hot flashes.
D. resolution of urogenital atrophy symptoms.

44. Adding an androgen to HT may be well suited for the woman with:

A. late-onset menopause.
B. severe hot flashes in spite of maximized estrogen therapy.
C. low osteoporosis risk.
D. alopecia.

45. The typical HT regimen contains _____ of the estrogen dose of COC.

A. one-eighth
B. one-fourth
C. half
D. three-fourths

46. When reviewing the action of black cohosh during perimenopause, the NP considers that it likely:

A. binds to estrogen receptors.
B. lowers FSH levels.
C. increases LH levels.
D. increased prolactin levels.

47. Which of the following statements is true?

A. Many over-the-counter progesterone creams contain sterols that the human body is unable to use.
B. All progesterones are easily absorbed via the skin.
C. Soy is an example of a phytoprogesterone.
D. Progesterones, whether synthetic or plant-based, should not be used by a woman who has undergone a hysterectomy.

ANSWERS

31. B	32. D	33. B
34. A	35. A	36. D
37. C	38. B	39. D
40. A	41. C	42. A
43. C	44. B	45. B
46. A	47. A	

DISCUSSION

Menopause marks a transition in a woman's reproductive life and the cessation of the menses. Perimenopause is the time surrounding menopause; its onset is marked by the beginning symptoms of menopause and ends with the cessation of menses. The average age at menopause, marked by the last menstrual period, is 50 to 51 years, with a woman living up to one third of her life after this time. Perimenopause is the period of time leading to menopause and usually starts at around ages 40 to 45 years, earlier in cigarette smokers. The woman may note hot flashes or flushes during the week before the onset of the menses, a time when hormonal shifts are most dramatic.

Estrogen receptors are found in greatest concentration in the vulva, vagina, urethra, and trigone of the bladder. As a result, urogenital atrophy symptoms caused by estrogen deficiency are a common menopausal problem. These receptors are found in lower concentrations in the vascular bed, heart, brain, bones, and eyes.

With menopause, LH and FSH levels increase dramatically as the pituitary gland sends out an abundance of these substances in an attempt to induce ovulation, with the ovaries failing to respond. Levels of estrogen forms (estradiol, estrogen) are reduced, as are androgens (testosterone, progesterone, androsterone, dehydroepiandrosterone [DHEA], and DHEA sulfate). Hot flashes, in part induced by the LH surge, occur in about 80% of women going through menopause, from mildly bothersome to debilitating. In comparison with naturally occurring menopause, women with surgical menopause usually have more severe symptoms because hormonal shifts are more rapid and dramatic.

Vasomotor symptoms can be debilitating, causing disturbed sleep, avoidance of social situations in which a hot flash occurs, and numerous other problems. HT is likely the most effective therapy to attenuate the frequency and severity of hot flashes. When given during the first years after menopause at the equivalent of CEE, 0.325 to 0.625 mg/day, an anticipated reduction of hot flashes by 50% to 75% is expected. Using higher estrogen doses causes sex hormone–binding globulin levels to increase. This can result in a hypoandrogenic state as free androgens become bound and become inactive.

On occasion, a woman with significant vasomotor symptoms does not or cannot use HT for relief. Low-dose antidepressant therapy can afford a 50% greater reduction in the frequency and severity of hot flashes. Examples of options include venlafaxine (Effexor), 37.5 mg QD; sertraline (Zoloft), 25 to 50 mg; and paroxetine (Paxil), 10 to 20 mg.

Phytoestrogens are chemical substances similar to estrogen, particularly estradiol, that are found in more than 300 plants, including apples, carrots, coffee, potatoes, yams, soy products, flax seed, ginseng, bean sprouts, red clover sprouts, sunflower seeds, rye, wheat, sesame seeds, linseed, black cohosh, and bourbon. These are active substances that bind to estrogen receptor sites and have a mild estrogenic effect, as well as some antiestrogenic activity in some areas, by binding to and blocking sites in the breast, colon, and rectum. Black cohosh is an herb that has long been used as a menopausal remedy. Its actions are estrogenic and help to suppress LH but not FSH, increase serotonin levels, and enhance sleep. An example of a food containing phytoprogesterones is wild yams. These are often compounded into creams that are poorly absorbed with low bioavailability. Micronization may help with absorption. Some creams sold as phytoestrogens actually contain herbal precursors such as sarsasapogenin and diosgenin, sterols that cannot be used by the body. Certain vitamin and mineral supplements can be helpful in the management of menopausal symptoms. Vitamin E, 800 IU/day, reduces the number and frequency of hot flashes. Vitamin B_6, 25 mg/day, is recommended to improve mood in women with premenstrual dysphoria.

In the woman who continues to menstruate but is having significant perimenopausal symptoms, low-dose oral contraceptives can be helpful for symptom relief as well as for cycle regulation. Oral contraceptives contain approximately three to four times the estrogen dose of usual-dose HT. Because the woman taking oral contraceptives cyclically will continue to have monthly vaginal bleeding, the question often arises as to how to know when menopause occurs. If the woman is of an appropriate age (45 years or older) and has symptoms such as hot flashes during placebo week, she may be in menopause. Checking levels of estradiol, LH/FSH on day 7 of the pill-free interval can help confirm this; a FSH:LH ratio of 1 or higher with an estradiol level less than 25 pg/mL usually indicates menopause.

After menopause, androgen levels also decrease, leading to loss of lean muscle mass, attenuated libido, and additional bone loss. Androgen supplementation can be helpful in the woman with postmenopausal low libido and in those with continued hot flashes in spite of maximized estrogen dosage, a particularly common problem in the younger woman who has undergone surgical menopause. An estrogen-androgen supplement such as CEE, 0.625 mg, with methyltestosterone, 1.25 mg (Estratest H.S.), can be used for these purposes. The prescriber and the patient need to be aware of the risks of estrogen supplementation, as well as those of specific androgens, such as acne and hirsutism (common) and alopecia, vocal changes, and clitoral enlargement (less common).

Estrogen deficiency is a potent risk factor in the development of osteoporosis, which is most common in postmenopausal woman. By age 80, the average woman has lost greater than 30% of her premenopausal bone density. When taken with calcium supplements, postmenopausal HT can help reduce the risk of postmenopausal fracture by as much as 50% by minimizing further bone loss. However, because of the greater observed rate of venous thrombotic events and invasive breast cancer with short- and long-term HT use, and the availability of other medications to treat bone thinning such as the bisphosphonates and salmon calcitonin (Miacalcin), HT should not be used solely for this purpose.

Because the vaginal introitus remains colonized with protective flora when HT is used, there are lower rates of urogenital atrophy and UTIs. However, some women using HT may continue to need topical estrogen in the form of a vaginal cream, tablet, or estrogen-impregnated ring (Estring) to help minimize urogenital atrophy symptoms.

Endometrial cancer risk with unopposed estrogen use is considerable, with the rate of 4 to 5 per 1000 users per year, a 5-year risk of 2%, and a 10-year risk of 4%. There has been an observed increase risk of breast cancer with HT use. HT use in women with a history of breast cancer has been considered contraindicated; recent studies may contradict this (Table 13–2).

Estrogen typically acts at target-particular sites found in the breast, brain, reproductive tract, and cardiovascular system. As a result, postmenopausal estrogen use acts on body systems in which its effects are positive, such as enhanced endothelial function and reduced risk of certain types of dementia. In addition, it acts in areas in which its effects are not desirable, such as by increasing breast and endometrial cancer risk with unopposed estrogen use.

Estrogen deficiency, or atrophic, vaginitis is a noninfectious disease that affects postmenopausal women. During the process, there is a rise in vaginal pH (>5), thinning of vaginal tissue, and loss of vaginal lubrication. Urinary frequency and burning without UTI are often reported. On physical examination, the vaginal tissue appears fragile and vaginal rugae are lost.

Intervention for atrophic vaginitis includes using lubricants during sexual activity to minimize tissue trauma. Avoiding tight-fitting clothing and wearing cotton underwear can be helpful. Topical estrogen in the form of a cream

---

TABLE 13–2

CONTRAINDICATIONS TO POSTMENOPAUSAL ESTROGEN THERAPY

Absolute contraindication
- Unexplained vaginal bleeding
- Acute liver disease
- Chronic impaired liver function
- Thrombotic disease
- Endometrial cancer
- Neuro-opthalmologic vascular disease
- Breast cancer (controversial)

Relative contraindication
- Seizure disorder
- Dyslipidemia
- Migraine headache
- Thrombophlebitis
- Gallbladder disease

Jones, N., and Judd, H. (2002). Menopause and postmenopause. In DeCherney, A. H., and Nathan, L. (eds.). Current Obstetric and Gynecologic Diagnosis and Treatment (9th ed., pp. 1018–1040). New York: Lange Medical Books/McGraw-Hill.

or obtained through the use of an estrogen-impregnated intravaginal ring or tablet can also be used and is highly effective. However, many women who use oral HT continue to have symptoms of atrophic vaginitis; the addition of topical estrogen can be helpful. Increasing the dosage of oral estrogen is seldom helpful and likely increases HT adverse effects.

Tamoxifen is a SERM that locks out estrogen's effects on the breasts. It is useful both as the primary prevention of breast cancer in high-risk women and as a means of lowering breast cancer recurrence. Because endometrial sites are not antagonized, there is a small increase in endometrial cancer rate when tamoxifen is used. Evaluation of unexplained vaginal bleeding is critical during tamoxifen use.

Raloxifene (Evista) is a SERM with activity in the cardiovascular system and the bone but little to no activity in breast, uterine, or brain tissue. Raloxifene's cardiac effects occur in part because of a change in vessel response, as well as its ability to lower total cholesterol and fibrinogen levels. In addition, it is helpful in preventing osteoporosis because of its ability to preserve bone density. Because it lacks breast tissue effect, raloxifene may emerge as a reasonable treatment option for cardiovascular and bone protection in postmenopausal women with a history of or at high risk for breast cancer. Hot flashes are among the most commonly reported side effect with raloxifene use, with few reports of the breast tenderness and bloating often noted with estrogen therapy.

DISCUSSION SOURCES

Brown, K. (2004). Management Guidelines for Nurse Practitioners Working with Women (2nd ed). Philadelphia: F. A. Davis.

Jones, N., and Judd, H. (2002). Menopause and postmenopause. In DeCherney, A. H., and Nathan, L. (eds.). Current Obstetric and Gynecologic Diagnosis and Treatment (9th ed., pp. 1018–1040). New York: Lange Medical Books/McGraw-Hill.

Kennedy-Malone, L., Fletcher, K., and Plank, L. (2004). Management Guidelines for Nurse Practitioners Working with Older Adults (2nd ed.). Philadelphia: F.A. Davis.

QUESTIONS

48. Patients with urge incontinence often report urine loss:

    A. with exercise.
    B. at night.
    C. associated with a strong sensation of needing to void.
    D. as dribbling after voiding.

49. Patients with urethral stricture often report urine loss:

    A. with exercise.
    B. during the day.
    C. associated with urgency.
    D. as dribbling after voiding.

50. Patients with stress incontinence often report urine loss:

    A. with lifting.
    B. at night.
    C. associated with a strong sensation of needing to void.
    D. as dribbling after voiding.

51. Factors that contribute to stress incontinence include:

    A. detrusor overactivity.
    B. pelvic floor weakness.
    C. urethral stricture.
    D. UTI.

52. Factors that contribute to urge incontinence include:

    A. detrusor overactivity.
    B. pelvic floor weakness.
    C. urethral stricture.
    D. UTI.

53. Pharmacologic intervention for patients with urge incontinence includes:

    A. doxazosin (Cardura).
    B. terodiline (Detrol).
    C. finasteride (Proscar).
    D. pseudoephedrine.

54. Behavioral intervention for patients with stress incontinence includes:

A. establishing a voiding schedule.
B. gentle bladder-stretching exercises.
C. Kegel exercises.
D. restricting fluid intake.

55. Which form of urinary incontinence (UI) is most common in elderly persons?

A. stress
B. urge
C. iatrogenic
D. overflow

ANSWERS

48. C	**49.** D	**50.** A
51. B	**52.** A	**53.** B
54. C	**55.** B	

DISCUSSION

UI is the involuntary loss of urine in sufficient amounts to be a problem. This condition is often thought by many women to be a normal part of aging. In reality, numerous treatment options are available after the cause of UI is established (Table 13–3). In all cases, urinalysis and urine culture and sensitivity should be obtained. If UTI is present, treatment with the appropriate antimicrobial is indicated.

Urge incontinence is the most common form of UI in elderly persons. Behavioral therapy, including a voiding schedule and gentle bladder stretching, are helpful. Pharmacologic intervention is indicated in conjunction with behavioral therapy (Table 13–4). Terodiline is a selective muscarinic receptor antagonist that blocks bladder receptors and limits bladder contraction. Helpful in the treatment of urge incontinence, its use is associated with a decrease in the numbers of micturations and of incontinent episodes, along with an increase in voiding volume. Oxybutynin is a nonselective muscarinic receptor antagonist that blocks both receptors in the bladder and oral cavity, with activity similar to that of terodiline; adverse effects include dry mouth and constipation.

DISCUSSION SOURCES

Brown, K. (2004). Management Guidelines for Nurse Practitioners Working with Women (2nd ed). Philadelphia: F. A. Davis.

Kennedy-Malone, L., Fletcher, K. and Plank, L. (2004). Management Guidelines for Nurse Practitioners Working with Older Adults (2nd ed.). Philadelphia: F.A. Davis.

Stoller, M., and Carrol, P. (2003). Urology. In Tierney, L., McPhee, S., and Papadakis, M. (eds.). Current Medical Diagnosis and Treatment (42nd ed., pp. 903–945). New York: Lange Medical Books/McGraw-Hill.

QUESTIONS

56. Which of the following is not a normal finding in a woman during the reproductive years?

A. vaginal pH of 4.5 or less
B. lactobacillus as the predominant vaginal organism
C. thick, white vaginal secretions during the luteal phase
D. vaginal epithelial cells with adherent bacteria

57. Which of the following findings is most consistent with vaginal discharge during ovulation?

A. dry and sticky
B. milky and mucoid
C. stringy and clear
D. tenacious and odorless

58. Physical examination of a 19-year-old woman with a 3-day history of vaginal itch reveals moderate perineal excoriation; vaginal erythema; and a white, clumping discharge. Expected microscopic examination findings include:

A. a pH higher than 6.0.
B. an increased number of lactobacilli.
C. hyphae.
D. an abundance of white blood cells.

59. Women with bacterial vaginosis typically present with:

TABLE 13–3

CLINICAL ISSUES IN URINARY INCONTINENCE

Type of urinary incontinence	Etiology and population most often affected	Clinical presentation	Treatment options
Urge incontinence	Detrusor overactivity causing uninhibited bladder contractions. Most common form of incontinence in elders.	Strong sensation of needing to empty the bladder that cannot be suppressed, often coupled with involuntary loss of urine.	Avoiding stimulants, gentle bladder stretching by increasing voiding interval by 15–30 minutes after establishing a half-hour voiding schedule. Add agent to reduce bladder contraction; tolterodine (Detrol) or oxybutynin (Ditropan)
Stress incontinence	Weakness of pelvic floor and urethral muscles. Most common form of incontinence in women; rare in men.	Loss of urine with activity that causes increase in intra-abdominal pressure such as coughing, sneezing, exercise.	Kegel exercises, support to the area through the use of a vaginal tampon, urethral stents, injections, and pessary use. Topical and systemic estrogen if associated with postmenopausal urogenital atrophic changes. Phenylpropanolamine (alpha-adrenergic agonist). Surgical intervention can be helpful in 75%–80%.
Urethral obstruction	Obstruction of bladder outflow through urethral obstruction (prostatic, stricture, tumor) resulting in urinary retention with overflow and detrusor instability. Most commonly found in older men.	Dribbling post-void coupled with urge incontinence on presentation.	Treatment of urethral obstruction.
Transient incontinence	Associated with acute event such as delirium, UTI, medication use, restricted activity.	Presentation consistent with underlying process.	Treatment of underlying process, discontinuation of offending medication.

A. vulvitis.
B. pruritus.
C. dysuria.
D. malodorous discharge.

60. Treatment of vulvovaginitis caused by *Candida albicans* includes:

A. metronidazole gel.
B. clotrimazole cream.
C. hydrocortisone ointment.
D. clindamycin cream.

61. A 24-year-old woman presents with a 1-week history of thin, green-yellow vaginal

━━━━ **TABLE 13–4** ━━━━━━━━━━━━━━━━━━━━━━━━━━━━━━

SELECT MEDICATIONS AND THEIR EFFECT ON URINARY CONTINENCE

Type of medication	Effect on urinary continence
Diuretics	Increase in volume and frequency of voiding.
Drugs with anticholinergic activity such as first-generation antihistamines, tricyclic antidepressants, antipsychotics	Urinary retention, overflow incontinence, alteration in sensorium, fecal impaction.
Opioids	Urinary retention, overflow, alteration in sensorium, fecal impaction.
Alcohol	Increase in volume, frequency, and urgency of voiding alteration in sensorium.
Sedatives, hypnotics, benzodiazepines	Alteration in sensorium, reduced mobility.
Alpha-adrenergic antagonists (prazosin, doxazosin, terazosin)	Relaxing internal urethral sphincter. This may be a desired effect in the man with BPH.

discharge with perivaginal irritation. Physical examination findings include vaginal erythema with petechial hemorrhages on the cervix, numerous white blood cells, and motile organisms on microscopic examination. These findings most likely represent:

A. motile sperm with irritative vaginitis.
B. trichomoniasis.
C. bacterial vaginosis.
D. condyloma acuminatum.

62. The preferred treatment option for trichomoniasis is:

A. metronidazole.
B. clindamycin.
C. acyclovir.
D. azithromycin.

63. Treatment options for bacterial vaginosis include all of the following except:

A. oral metronidazole.
B. clindamycin cream.
C. oral clindamycin.
D. azithromycin.

64. A 30-year-old woman presents without symptoms but states that her male partner has dysuria without penile discharge. Examination reveals a friable cervix cov-

ered with thick yellow discharge. This description is most consistent with an infection caused by:

A. *Chlamydia trachomatis.*
B. *Neisseria gonorrhoeae.*
C. human papillomavirus (HPV).
D. *Trichomonas vaginalis.*

65. Which of the following is active against *N. gonorrhoeae?*

A. cefixime
B. metronidazole
C. ketoconazole
D. amoxicillin

66. Which of the following is active against *C. trachomatis?*

A. amoxicillin
B. metronidazole
C. azithromycin
D. ceftriaxone

67. Which of the following is true of gonococcal infection?

A. The risk of transmission from an infected woman to a male sexual partner is about 80%.

B. Most men have asymptomatic infection.

C. The incubation period is about 2 to 3 weeks.

D. The organism rarely produces beta-lactamase.

68. Complications of gonococcal and chlamydial genitourinary infection in women include all of the following except:

A. PID.
B. tubal scarring.
C. pyelonephritis.
D. peritonitis.

69. What percentage of sexually active adults has human herpesvirus 2 (HHV-2) (herpes simplex type 2) antibodies?

A. 5
B. 15
C. 25
D. 35

70. All of the following are likely reported in the woman with an initial episode of genital HHV-2 infection except:

A. painful ulcer.
B. inguinal lymphadenopathy.
C. thin vaginal discharge.
D. pustular lesions.

71. Treatment options for HHV-2 genital infection include:

A. ribavirin.
B. indinavir.
C. famciclovir.
D. cyclosporine.

ANSWERS

56. D	**57.** C	**58.** C
59. D	**60.** B	**61.** B
62. A	**63.** D	**64.** A
65. A	**66.** C	**67.** B
68. C	**69.** C	**70.** D
71. C		

DISCUSSION

Vulvovaginitis is one of the most common gynecologic problems. Treatment is guided by presentation and causative organism (Table 13–5). Chlamydial infection is one of the most common STIs, affecting primarily adolescents and adults younger than 25 years. The causative organism, *C. trachomatis* immunotype D-K, is an obligate intracellular parasite closely related to gram-negative bacteria. This infection causes cervicitis in the majority of infected women. About are half have urethral infection, and one-third have endometrial involvement. Despite this, many women are asymptomatic, but mucopurulent vaginal discharge, dysuria, dyspareunia, and postcoital bleeding may be reported.

Clinical presentation of *C. trachomatis* genitourinary infection in women typically includes the presence of mucopurulent discharge, often adherent to a friable cervix. Cervical motion and adnexal tenderness may be present when there is endometrial involvement. Diagnostic testing includes DNA probe endocervical testing or urinalysis for ligase chain reaction.

Treatment options for *C. trachomatis* infection include antibiotics that act against intracellular organisms. These include doxycycline, erythromycin, and azithromycin. Azithromycin is given in a highly efficacious, well-tolerated, single-dose oral therapy.

Gonorrhea, caused by the gram-negative diplococcus *N. gonorrhoeae*, is one of the most common STIs. It has a short incubation period, of 1 to 5 days, and is likely to cause infection in approximately 20% of men who have sexual contact with infected women and approximately 80% of women who have sexual contact with infected men.

The majority of men with gonococcal infection have no symptoms. In women, presentation typically includes dysuria with a milky to purulent, occasionally blood-tinged, vaginal discharge. With anal-insertive sex, rectal infection leading to proctitis is often seen. Because the organism frequently produces

TABLE 13–5

GUIDELINES FOR ASSESSMENT AND TREATMENT OF GENITOURINARY
INFECTION

Conditions	Causative organism	Clinical presentation	Treatment options
Bacterial vaginosis	Overgrowth of anaerobes including *Gardnerella* species and *Mycoplasma hominis.*	Increased volume of vaginal secretions; thin, gray, homogeneous discharge; burning; pruritus. On microscopic exam: vaginal pH>4.5, clue cells, positive whiff test, few WBCs.	***Preferred per CDC STD guidelines*** Metronidazole 500 mg BID × 7 d *or* Metronidazole gel 0.75%, 1 applicator (5 g) intravaginally QD × 5 d *or* Clindamycin cream 2%, 1 applicator (5g) intravaginally at HS × 7 d. ***Alternative regimens*** Metronidazole 2 g as single dose *or* Clindamycin 300 mg BID × 7 d *or* Clindamycin ovules 100 g intravaginally at bedtime × 3 d
Candidiasis	*Candida albicans, Candida glabrata, Candida tropicalis*	Itching, burning, thick white to yellow adherent, curd-like discharge, vulvovaginal excoriation, erythema, excoriation. On microscopic exam: Hyphae, pseudohyphae, pH <5, few WBCs.	Miconazole Butoconazole Terconazole Tioconazole Fluconazole
Chancroid	*H. ducreyi*	Painless genital ulcer	Azithromycin 1 g orally in a single dose, *or* ceftriaxone 250 mg intramuscularly (IM) in a single dose, *or* ciprofloxacin 500 mg orally twice a day for 3 days, *or* erythromycin base 500 mg orally three times a day for 7 days.
Human herpes virus (Herpes simplex)	Human herpes virus-2 (HHV-2) (also known as herpes simplex, type 2); rarely by HHV-1 (also known as herpes simplex, type 1)	Painful ulcerated lesions, lymphadenopathy, thin vaginal discharge if lesion located at vagina or introitus	For initial infection: Acyclovir 400 mg PO TID × 7–10 days or acyclovir 200 mg 51D × 7–10 days or famciclovir 250 mg PO TID × 7–10 days or valacyclovir 1 g PO BID × 7–10 days. For episodic recurrent infection: Acyclovir 400 mg PO TID × 5 days *or* famciclovir 125 mg PO BID × 5 days *or* valacyclovir 1 g PO QD × 5 days *or* valacyclovir 500 mg PO BID × 5 days. For suppression of recurrent infection: Acyclovir 400 mg PO BID *or* famciclovir 250 mg PO BID *or* valacyclovir 1g PO QD *or* valacyclovir 500 mg–1 g PO for extended period.

Conditions	Causative organism	Clinical presentation	Treatment options
Lymphogranuloma venereum	Invasive serovar L1, L2, L3 of *C. trachomatis*	Vesicular or ulcerative lesion on the external genitalia with inguinal lymphadenitis or buboes.	Doxycycline 100 mg PO BID × 21 days *or* erythromycin 500 mg QID × 21 days.
Nongonococcal urethritis and cervicitis (adult or adolescent women, not pregnant)	*C. trachomatis*	Cervicitis, irritative voiding symptoms, occasional mucopurulent discharge.	Recommended therapy: Azithromycin 1 g PO as a single dose *or* doxycycline 100 mg PO BID × 7 days. Alternative therapy: Erythromycin 500 mg PO QID × 7 days *or* ofloxacin 300 mg BID × 7 days *or* levofloxacin 500 mg QD × 7 d.
Gonococcal urethritis and vaginitis (adult or adolescent women, not pregnant)	*N. gonorrhoeae*	Irritative voiding symptoms, occasional purulent discharge.	Recommended therapy: Single-dose therapy for uncomplicated infection. Cefixime 400 mg PO, ceftriaxone 125 mg IM *or* ciprofloxacin 500 mg *or* ofloxacin 400 mg *or* levofloxacin 250 mg. Concurrently treat with azithromycin 1 g as a single dose *or* doxycycline 100 mg BID × 7 days if chlamydial infection has not been ruled out. Alternative therapy: Spectinomycin 2 g IM as a single dose.
Pelvic inflammatory disease	*N. gonorrhoeae, C. trachomatis, E. coli, Mycoplasma* and *Ureaplasma* species, others	Irritative voiding symptoms, fever.	Recommended therapy: Regimen A: ofloxacin 400 mg PO BID *or* levofloxacin 500 mg PO QD with or without metronidazole 500 mg PO BID × 14 days. Regimen B: Ceftriaxone 250 mg IM as a single dose plus doxycycline 100 mg BID × 14 days with or without metronidazole 500 mg BID × 14 days.
Trichomoniasis	*T. vaginalis*	Dysuria, itching, vulvovaginal irritation, dyspareunia, yellow-green vaginal discharge, cervical petechial hemorrhages ("strawberry spots") in about 30%. On microscopic exam: motile organisms and WBCs	Recommended therapy: Metronidazole 2 g as a one-time dose. Alternative therapy: Metronidazole 500 mg PO BID × 7 days.

(continued)

TABLE 13–5

GUIDELINES FOR ASSESSMENT AND TREATMENT OF GENITOURINARY
INFECTION *(continued)*

Conditions	Causative organism	Clinical presentation	Treatment options
Genital warts (Condyloma acuminata)	Human papilloma virus	Verruca-form lesions or may be subclinical or unrecognized	Recommended therapy: Patient applied therapy: Podofilox 0.5% solution *or* imiquimod 5% cream. Provider applied therapy: Liquid nitrogen or cryoprobe, trichloroacetic acid, podophyllin resin, or surgical removal.

Center for Disease Control and Prevention (2002). 2002 Guidelines for Treatment of Sexually Transmitted Disease. Available at http://www.cdc.gov./STD/treatment/, accessed 9/28/03.

beta-lactamase, the choice of a therapeutic agent should include agents with beta-lactamase stability, such as select fluoroquinolones, ceftriaxone, and cefixime.

Genital herpes is a result of infection with a HHV. Most often, HHV-2 is the causative organism; HHV-1, the virus form that causes cold sores, is rarely implicated. However, HHV-2 can infect the perioral area. The clinical presentation usually includes a painful ulcerated genital lesion, often accompanied by inguinal lymphadenopathy. If lesions involve the vagina or its introitus, a thin, sometimes profuse discharge accompanies the infection. Treatment with an antiviral such as acyclovir, famciclovir, or valacyclovir for acute infection, recurrence, and/or suppression is highly effective.

As with all STIs, a critical part of care is the discussion of preventive strategies, including condom use and limiting the number of sexual partners. NPs should offer and encourage testing for other STIs, including human immunodeficiency virus (HIV).

DISCUSSION SOURCES

Brown, K. (2004). Management Guidelines for Nurse Practitioners Working with Women (2nd ed). Philadelphia: F.A. Davis.

Centers for Disease Control and Prevention (2002). 2002 Guidelines for Treatment of Sexually Transmitted Disease. Available at http://www.cdc. gov/STI/treatment/, accessed 9/28/03.

Chambers, H. (2003). Infectious disease: Bacterial and chlamydial. In Tierney, L., McPhee, S., and Papadakis, M. (eds.). Current Medical Diagnosis and Treatment (42nd ed., pp. 1346–1389). New York: Lange Medical Books/McGraw-Hill.

QUESTIONS

72. Women with PID typically present with all of the following except:

    A. dysuria.
    B. leukopenia.
    C. cervical motion tenderness.
    D. diffuse abdomen pain.

73. The most likely causative pathogen in a 26-year-old woman with PID is:

    A. *Escherichia coli.*
    B. Enterobacteriaceae species.
    C. *C. trachomatis.*
    D. *Pseudomonas* species.

74. Which of the following is a treatment option for a 30-year-old woman with PID and severe penicillin allergy?

    A. ofloxacin with metronidazole
    B. amoxicillin with gentamicin
    C. cefixime with vancomycin
    D. clindamycin with azithromycin

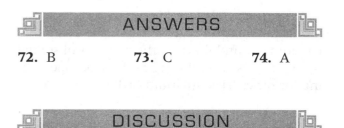

ANSWERS

72. B   **73.** C   **74.** A

DISCUSSION

PID is an infectious disease consisting of endometritis, salpingitis, and oophoritis. It is caused by a variety of pathogens, including *C. trachomatis, N. gonorrhoeae, H. influenzae, Streptococcus* species, select anaerobes, *Mycoplasma* species, and *Ureaplasma* species; approximately 60% of infections are acquired through sexual transmission. Clinical presentation includes lower abdominal pain, abnormal vaginal discharge, dyspareunia, fever, gastrointestinal upset, and abnormal vaginal bleeding. An adnexal mass may be palpable when tubo-ovarian abscess is present. Supporting laboratory findings may include elevated erythrocyte sedimentation rate or C-reactive protein level, as well as leukocytosis with neutrophilia. Although diagnosis can usually be made from clinical findings, transvaginal ultrasound may demonstrate tubal thickening with or without free pelvic fluid or tubo-ovarian abscess.

Treatment options differ according to patient presentation. When a woman with PID is severely ill, is pregnant, or has tubo-ovarian abscess, hospitalization for hydration and parenteral antibiotic therapy is indicated. In most situations, outpatient therapy with oral or parenteral antibiotics is sufficient. Ceftriaxone, 250 mg intramuscularly as a one-time dose, followed by doxycycline, 100 mg BID for 2 weeks, is likely the most commonly used treatment regimen and is highly effective. Ofloxacin, 400 mg BID, with metronidazole, 500 mg BID, for 2 weeks offers an effective oral treatment option that is a reasonable alternative in the presence of severe penicillin allergy.

As with all STIs, a critical part of care is the discussion of preventive strategies, including condom use and limiting the number of sexual partners. NPs should offer and encourage testing for other STIs, including HIV.

DISCUSSION SOURCES

Centers for Disease Control and Prevention (2002). 2002 Guidelines for Treatment of Sexually Transmitted Disease. Available at http://www.cdc.gov/STI/treatment/, accessed 1/2/04.

Chambers, H. (2003). Infectious disease: Bacterial and chlamydial. In Tierney, L., McPhee, S., and Papadakis, M. (eds.). Current Medical Diagnosis and Treatment (42nd ed., pp. 1346–1389). New York: Lange Medical Books/McGraw-Hill.

QUESTIONS

75. Sequelae of genital condyloma acuminatum can include:

   A. cervical carcinoma.
   B. PID.
   C. vaginal fistula.
   D. Reiter syndrome.

76. Which of the following best describes the lesions associated with condyloma acuminatum?

   A. verruciform
   B. plaquelike
   C. vesicular form
   D. bullous

77. Treatment options for patients with condyloma acuminatum include:

   A. imiquimod (Aldara).
   B. azithromycin.
   C. acyclovir.
   D. metronidazole.

78. Which HPV types are most likely to cause condyloma acuminatum?

   A. 1, 2, and 3
   B. 6 and 11
   C. 16 and 18
   D. 22 and 24

79. Which HPV types are most often associated with cervical cancer?

   A. 1, 2, and 3
   B. 6 and 11
   C. 16 and 18
   D. 22 and 24

80. What percentage of anogenital and cervical cancers can be attributed to HPV infection?

   A. less than 30
   B. 30 to 50
   C. 50 to 8
   D. 95 or higher

81. Which of the following describes the mechanism of action of imiquimod (Aldara)?

   A. keratolytic
   B. immune modulator
   C. cryogenic
   D. cytolytic

ANSWERS

75. A	**76.** A	**77.** A
78. B	**79.** C	**80.** D
81. B		

DISCUSSION

Condyloma acuminatum is a verruciform lesion seen in genital warts and is an STI. The causative agent is HPV, and infection with multiple HPV types is usually seen with genital infection. Anal, penile, and cervical carcinomas can be consequences of HPV infection. However, not all HPV types are correlated with malignancy. HPV types with high malignancy risks include types 16, 18, 31, 33, 35, 39, and 45, whereas low malignancy risks are seen with infection with types 6, 11, 40, 42, 43, 44, 54, 61, 70, 72, and 81. HPV types 6 and 11 most often cause genital warts. About 50% of patients have a spontaneous regression of warts without intervention. Treatment options include podofilox, imiquimod, trichloroacetic acid, or cryotherapy. Prescribing patient-administered therapies such as imiquimod (Aldara) or podofilox saves the cost and inconvenience of office visits. Surgical intervention is typically reserved for complicated, recalcitrant lesions (see Table 7–1).

As with all STIs, a critical part of care is the discussion of preventive strategies, including condom use and limiting the number of sexual partners. NPs should offer and encourage testing for other STIs, including HIV.

DISCUSSION SOURCES

Centers for Disease Control and Prevention (2002). 2002 Guidelines for Treatment of Sexually Transmitted Disease. Available at http://www.cdc.gov/STI/treatment/, accessed 1/2/04.

Chambers, H. (2003). Infectious disease: Bacterial and chlamydial. In Tierney, L., McPhee, S., and Papadakis, M. (eds.). Current Medical Diagnosis and Treatment (42nd ed., pp. 1346–1389). New York: Lange Medical Books/McGraw-IIill.

QUESTIONS

82. How long after contact does the onset of clinical manifestations of syphilis typically occur?

   A. less than 1 week
   B. 1 to 3 weeks
   C. 2 to 4 weeks
   D. 4 to 6 weeks

83. Which of the following is not representative of the presentation of primary syphilis?

   A. painless ulcer
   B. palpable inguinal nodes
   C. flulike symptoms
   D. spontaneously healing lesion

84. Which of the following is not representative of the presentation of secondary syphilis?

   A. generalized rash
   B. chancre
   C. arthralgia
   D. lymphadenopathy

85. Which of the following is found in tertiary syphilis?

   A. arthralgia
   B. lymphadenopathy

    C. macropapular lesions involving the palms and soles

    D. gumma

86. Syphilis is most contagious during which of the following?

    A. before onset of signs and symptoms

    B. at the primary stage

    C. at the secondary stage

    D. at the tertiary stage

87. First-line treatment options for syphilis include:

    A. penicillin.

    B. ciprofloxacin.

    C. erythromycin.

    D. ceftriaxone.

ANSWERS

82. C	**83.** C	**84.** B
85. D	**86.** C	**87.** A

DISCUSSION

Caused by the spirochete *Treponema pallidum*, syphilis is a complex, multiorgan disease. Sexual contact is the usual route of transmission. The initial lesion forms about 2 to 4 weeks after contact; contagion is greatest during the secondary stage. Treatment is guided by the stage of disease and clinical manifestations.

As with all STIs, a critical part of care is discussion of prevention strategies, including condom use and limiting the number of sexual partners. Offer and encourage testing for other STIs, including HIV.

DISCUSSION SOURCES

Centers for Disease Control and Prevention (2002). 2002 Guidelines for Treatment of Sexually Transmitted Disease. Available at http://www.cdc.gov/STI/treatment/, accessed 1/2/04.

Jacobs, R. (2003). Infectious diseases: Spirochetal. In Tierney, L., McPhee, S., and Papadakis, M. (eds.). Current Medical Diagnosis and Treatment (42nd ed., pp. 1390–1410). New York: Lange Medical Books/McGraw-Hill.

14

Pediatrics

QUESTIONS

1. Which of the following is appropriate advice to give to a mother who is breast-feeding her 10-day-old infant?

   A. "Your milk will come in today."
   B. "To minimize breast tenderness, the baby should not be kept on each breast for more than 5 to 10 minutes."
   C. "A pacifier should be offered between feedings."
   D. "The baby's urine should be light or colorless."

2. Which of the following is appropriate advice to give to a mother who is breast-feeding her 12-hour-old infant?

   A. "You will likely have enough milk to feed the baby within a few hours of birth."
   B. "The baby may need to be awakened to be fed."
   C. "Supplemental feeding is needed unless the baby has at least four wet diapers in the first day of life."
   D. "A seedy yellow stool is anticipated."

3. In comparison with the use of infant formula, advantages of breast-feeding include all of the following except:

   A. lower incidence of diarrheal illness.
   B. greater weight gain in the first few weeks of life.
   C. reduced risk of allergic disorders.
   D. a lower occurrence of constipation.

4. At 3 weeks of age, the average-weight formula-fed infant should be expected to take:

   A. 2 to 3 oz every 2 to 3 hours.
   B. 2 to 3 oz every 3 to 4 hours.
   C. 3 to 4 oz every 2 to 3 hours.
   D. 3 to 4 oz every 3 to 4 hours.

5. Solid foods are best introduced no earlier than:

   A. 1 to 3 months.
   B. 3 to 5 months.
   C. 4 to 6 months.
   D. 6 to 8 months.

6. Nursing infants generally maximally receive about which percentage of the maternal dose of a drug?

A. 1
B. 3
C. 5
D. 10

7. Most drugs pass into breast milk through:

A. active transport.
B. facilitated transfer.
C. simple diffusion.
D. creation of a pH gradient.

8. In order to remove a drug from breast milk through "pump and dump," the process must be continued for:

A. two infant feeding cycles.
B. approximately 8 hours.
C. three to five half-lives of drug.
D. a period of time that is highly unpredictable.

9. When counseling a breast-feeding woman about alcohol use during lactation, you describe the following:

A. It enhances the let-down reflex.
B. Because of its high molecular weight, relatively little alcohol is passed into breast milk.
C. Maternal alcohol use causes a reduction in the amount of milk ingested by the infant.
D. Infant intoxication may be seen with as little as one to two maternal drinks.

10. A 23-year-old woman is breast-feeding her newborn. She wishes to use hormonal contraception. Which of the following represents the best regimen?

A. combined oral contraception initiated at 2 weeks
B. progesterone-only oral contraception initiated at 3 weeks
C. medroxyprogesterone acetate (Depo-Provera) given day 1 postpartum
D. all forms are contraindicated during lactation

11. The anticipated average daily weight gain during the first 3 months of life is approximately:

A. 15 g.
B. 20 g.
C. 25 g.
D. 30 g.

12. The average required caloric intake in an infant from age 0 to 3 months is usually:

A. 40 to 60 kcal/kg/day.
B. 60 to 80 kcal/kg/day.
C. 80 to 100 kcal/kg/day.
D. 100 to 120 kcal/kg/day.

ANSWERS

1. D   2. B   3. B   4. A   5. C   6. A
7. C   8. C   9. C   10. B   11. D   12. D

DISCUSSION

Breast-feeding provides the ideal form of nutrition during infancy. In the United States, nearly 60% of all infants are breast-fed at birth, with only about 25% continuing by 6 months. Nurse practitioners (NPs) can help influence successful breast-feeding.

The content of commercially prepared formula available in the developed world continues to be improved to be closer in composition to breast milk. However, infant formula continues to lack critically important components. Breast milk contains immunoactive factors that help protect infants against infectious disease and may reduce the frequency of allergic disorders. Nutritionally, formula lacks a number of micronutrients found in breast milk. If a baby is formula-fed, the parents and caregivers should be encouraged to hold the child during feeding in order to have the interaction inherent in breast-feeding.

Frequency, amount, and type of feedings are often questions asked during well-child visits. Counseling should be offered to help ensure optimal nutrition (Box 14–1 and Table 14–1).

If a nursing mother becomes ill or has a chronic health problem, she is often erroneously encouraged to discontinue breast-feeding on the basis of the incorrect assumption by the

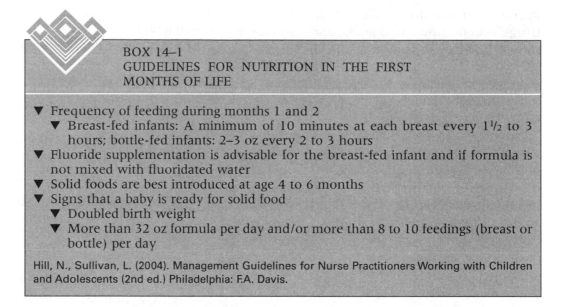

BOX 14–1
GUIDELINES FOR NUTRITION IN THE FIRST
MONTHS OF LIFE

▼ Frequency of feeding during months 1 and 2
  ▼ Breast-fed infants: A minimum of 10 minutes at each breast every 1½ to 3 hours; bottle-fed infants: 2–3 oz every 2 to 3 hours
▼ Fluoride supplementation is advisable for the breast-fed infant and if formula is not mixed with fluoridated water
▼ Solid foods are best introduced at age 4 to 6 months
▼ Signs that a baby is ready for solid food
  ▼ Doubled birth weight
  ▼ More than 32 oz formula per day and/or more than 8 to 10 feedings (breast or bottle) per day

Hill, N., Sullivan, L. (2004). Management Guidelines for Nurse Practitioners Working with Children and Adolescents (2nd ed.) Philadelphia: F.A. Davis.

TABLE 14–1
ANTICIPATED WEIGHT GAIN AND CALORIC
REQUIREMENTS IN THE FIRST THREE YEARS OF LIFE

Age	Anticipated Average Weight Gain per Day (in grams)	Required Kilocalorie per kilogram per Day
0–3 months	26–31	100–120 kcal
3–6 months	17–18	105–115 kcal
6–9 months	12–13	100–105 kcal
9–12 months	9	100–105 kcal
1–3 years	7–9	100 kcal

health care provider that most medications are not safe to use. In fact, most medications can be used during lactation, but the benefit of improved maternal health should be balanced against the risk of exposing an infant to medication.

Postpartum contraception is usually an important concern of new mothers. Some women may opt not to breast-feed, fearing an inability to access reliable hormonal contraception while lactating. In fact, a number of options are available, including the use of the progestin-only pill (POP) and medroxyprogesterone acetate. For lactating women who wish to use an oral hormonal contraceptive, POP is

highly effective and does not alter the quality or quantity of breast milk. One significant disadvantage of POP use is bleeding irregularity, ranging from prolonged flow to amenorrhea. Medroxyprogesterone acetate in a depot injection (Depo-Provera) given every 90 days is a highly reliable form of contraception, at 99.7% efficacy. Depo-Provera use may be started immediately postpartum if the woman is not breast-feeding and started at 3 to 6 weeks postpartum if she is breast-feeding. Earlier use may diminish the quantity but not quality of breast milk.

Nearly all breast-feeding mothers use some type of medication (most often analgesic agents such as nonsteroidal anti-inflammatory drugs, acetaminophen, opioids, and antibiotics) in the first 2 weeks after giving birth. About 25% need to use medication intermittently to manage episodic disease. Such medication usually includes analgesics, antihistamines, decongestants, and antibiotics.

About 5% of breast-feeding women have a chronic health problem necessitating daily use of a medication; the most common chronically used are for treating asthma, mental health problems, seizure disorder, and hypertension. Nursing infants usually get about 1%, often less, of the maternal dose, and only a small number of drugs are contraindicated.

The "pump-and-dump" procedure is a less-than-helpful way to reduce drug levels in a mother's milk because it creates an area of lower drug concentration in the empty breast. This enables the drug to diffuse from the area of high concentration (maternal serum) to the area of low concentration (breast milk). If the mother takes a medication that may be problematic for the nursing infant, pumping while discarding the milk needs to continue for three to five half-lives of the medication.

Alcohol has a low molecular weight and is highly lipid soluble; both of these characteristics allow it to have easy passage into breast milk. Even in small amounts, alcohol ingestion by a nursing mother can cause a smaller amount of milk produced and reduction in the let-down reflex, as well as less rhythmic and frequent sucking by the infant. This results in a smaller volume of milk ingested. Cigarette smoking is similarly problematic. Nicotine, a highly lipid-soluble substance with a low molecular weight, passes easily into breast milk. Maternal cigarette smoking may reduce milk supply, as well as expose an infant to passive smoke. Infant crankiness, diarrhea, tachycardia, and vomiting have been reported with high maternal nicotine intake.

DISCUSSION SOURCES

Hale, T. (2004). Medications and Mothers' Milk (14th ed.). Amarillo, TX: Pharmasoft Medical Publishers.

Hill, N., and Sullivan, L. (2004). Management Guidelines for Pediatric Nurse Practitioners Working with Children and Adolescents, 2nd ed. (pp. 3–28). Philadelphia: F. A. Davis.

QUESTIONS

13. Which of the following is most consistent with a normal developmental examination for a 3-month-old full-term infant?

    A. sitting briefly with support
    B. experimenting with sound
    C. rolling over
    D. having a social smile

14. Which of the following is most consistent with a normal developmental examination for a thriving 5-month-old infant born at 32 weeks' gestation?

    A. sitting briefly with support
    B. experimenting with sound
    C. rolling over
    D. performing hand-to-hand transfers

15. A healthy baby between the ages of 3 to 5 months should be able to:

    A. recognize parents.
    B. bring hands together.
    C. reach with one hand.
    D. feed self biscuit.

16. A healthy baby between the ages of 9 to 11 months is expected to:

    A. roll back to stomach.
    B. imitate "bye-bye."
    C. play peek-a-boo.
    D. hand toy on request.

17. The typical 2-year-old child is able to:

    A. speak in phrases of two or more words.
    B. throw a ball.
    C. scribble spontaneously.
    D. ride a tricycle.

18. At which age will a child likely start to imitate housework?

A. 15 months
B. 18 months
C. 24 months
D. 30 months

19. A healthy 3-year-old child is expected to:

A. give his or her first and last names.
B. use pronouns.
C. kick a ball.
D. name a best friend.

20. A healthy 6–7-month-old infant is able to:

A. roll back to stomach.
B. feed self cracker.
C. reach for object.
D. crawl on abdomen.

21. You examine a healthy 9-month-old infant from a full-term pregnancy and expect to find that he or she:

A. sits without support.
B. cruises.
C. has the ability to recognize his or her own name.
D. imitates a razzing noise.

22. A healthy 3-year-old child is in your office for well-child care. You expect this child to be able to:

A. name three colors.
B. alternate feet when climbing stairs.
C. speak in two-word phrases.
D. tie shoelaces.

23. Which of the following would not be found in newborns?

A. best vision at a range of 8 to 12 inches
B. presence of red reflex
C. light-sensitive eyes
D. lack of defensive blink

24. Which of the following do you expect to find in an examination of a 2-week-old infant?

A. a visual preference for the human face
B. a preference for low-pitched voices
C. indifference to the cry of other neonates
D. poorly developed sense of smell

25. Which of the following is the most appropriate response in the developmental examination of the average 5-year-old child?

A. the ability to name a best friend
B. giving gender appropriately
C. naming an intended career
D. hopping on one foot

ANSWERS

13. B	14. B	15. B
16. C	17. A	18. A
19. A	20. A	21. C
22. B	23. D	24. A
25. A		

DISCUSSION

Performing a developmental assessment is one of the most important parts of providing pediatric primary care. Besides providing a marker for evaluating the child, the assessment also affords an important learning tool for the parents. Pointing out milestones to be achieved in the near future and their impact on safety can help the family prepare appropriately (Table 14–2).

DISCUSSION SOURCE

Health Plan of New York Practice Management Tools, available at http://www.hipusa.com/Providers/ny/products_services/PediatricAnticipatoryGuidelines.pdf, accessed 1/1/05.

QUESTIONS

26. At which of the following ages in an infant's life is parental anticipatory guidance about teething most helpful?

A. 1 to 2 months
B. 2 to 4 months
C. 4 to 6 months
D. 8 to 10 months

27. At which of the following ages in a young child's life is parental anticipatory guid-

TABLE 14–2

ANTICIPATED EARLY CHILDHOOD DEVELOPMENTAL MILESTONES

Age	Able to Be Observed During Office Visit	Reported by Parent or Caregiver
Newborn	• Moves all extremities • Spontaneous stepping • Reacts to sound by blinking, turning • Responds to cries of other neonates • Well-developed sense of smell • Preference for higher-pitched voices Reflexes • Tonic neck • Palmar grasp • Babinski response • Rooting awake and asleep • Sucking	• Able to be calmed by feeding, cudding • Reinforces presence of developmental tasks seen in examination room
1–2 months	• Lifts head • Holds head erect • Regards face • Follows objects through visual field • Moro reflex fading	• Spontaneous smile • Recognizes parents
3–5 months	• Grasps cube • Reaches for objects • Brings objects to mouth • Raspberry sound • Sits with support	• Laughs • Recognizes food by sight • Rolls back to side
6–8 months	• Sits briefly without support • Scoops small object with rake grip; some thumb use • Hand-to-hand transfers • Imitates "bye-bye"	• Rolls back to stomach • Recognizes "no"
9–11 months	• Stands alone • Imitates peek-a-boo and pat-a-cake • Picks up small object with thumb and index finger	• Cruises • Follows simple command, such as "Come here."
12–15 months	• Walks solo • "Mama," "Dada" specific • Neat pincher grasp • Places cube in cup • Hands over objects on request • Builds tower of two bricks	• Says one to two words • Indicates wants by pointing • Scribbles spontaneously
15–20 months	• Points to several body parts • Throws a ball • Seats self in chair	• Uses a spoon with little spilling • Walks up and down steps with help • Understands two-step commands • Feeds self • Carries and hugs doll
24 months	• Speaks in phrases of two words or more • Kicks ball on request • Jumps with both feet • Uses pronouns • Developing handedness	• Runs • Copies vertical and horizontal lines • Has 50-word vocabulary • Washes and dries hands • Parallel play

Age	Able to Be Observed During Office Visit	Reported by Parent or Caregiver
30 months	• Walks backward • Hops on one foot • Copies circle	• Gives first and last names • Uses plurals
36 months	• Holds crayons with fingers • Nearly all speech intelligible to people not in daily contact with child • Three-word sentences	• Walks down stairs alternating steps • Rides tricycle • Copies circles • Dresses with supervision
3–4 years	• Responds to command to place object in, on, or under a table • Knows gender • Draws circle when one is shown	• Takes off jacket and shoes • Washes and dries face • Cooperative play • Speech includes plurals, personal pronouns, verbs • Skips
4–5 years	• Runs and turns while maintaining balance • Stands on one foot for at least 10 seconds • Counts to four • Draws a person without torso • Copies (1) by imitation • Verbalizes activities to do when cold, hungry, tired	• Buttons clothes • Dresses self (not including tying shoelaces) • Can play without adult input for about 30 minutes
5–6 years	• Catches ball • Knows age • Knows right from left hand • Draws person with six to eight parts, including torso • Identifies best friend • Likes teacher	• Able to complete simple chores • Understands concept of 10 items; likely counts higher by rote • Has sense of gender
6–7 years	• Copies a triangle shape • Draws person with at least 12 parts • Prints name • Reads multiple single-syllable words	• Ties shoelaces • Counts to 30 or beyond • Able to differentiate morning from later in day • Generally plays well with peers • No significant behavioral problems in school • Can name intended career
7–8 years	• Copies a diamond shape • Reads simple sentences • Draws person with at least 16 parts	• Ties shoes • Knows day of the week
8–9 years	• Able to give response to question such as what to do if an object is accidentally broken	• Able to add, subtract, borrow, carry • Understands concept of working as a team
9–10 years	• Knows month, day, year • Gives months of the year in sequence	• Able to multiply and do complex subtraction • Has increased reading fluency
10–12 years	• Beginning of pubertal changes for many girls	• Able to perform simple division • Has complex reading skills • May have interest in opposite sex

ance about temper tantrums most helpful?

A. 8 to 10 months
B. 10 to 12 months
C. 12 to 14 months
D. 14 to 16 months

28. At which of the following ages in a young child's life is parental anticipatory guidance about using "time out" as a discipline method most helpful?

A. 18 months
B. 24 months
C. 30 months
D. 36 months

29. At which of the following ages in a young child's life is parental anticipatory guidance about protection from falls most helpful?

A. at birth
B. 2 months
C. 4 months
D. 6 months

30. At which of the following ages in a young child's life is parental anticipatory guidance about toilet training readiness most helpful?

A. 12 months
B. 15 months
C. 18 months
D. 24 months

31. At which of the following ages in a young child's life is parental anticipatory guidance about infant sleep position most helpful?

A. birth
B. 2 weeks
C. 2 months
D. 4 months

ANSWERS

26. C	**27.** B	**28.** B
29. A	**30.** C	**31.** A

DISCUSSION

Providing health advice to the growing family is a critical part of an NP's role. During anticipatory guidance counseling, an NP should review the normal developmental landmarks that the child is expected to reach in the near future, coupled with advice about how parents can cope with, adapt to, and avoid problems with these changes. This guidance is tailored to meet the needs of the family but typically follows a developmental framework.

DISCUSSION SOURCE

Hill, N., and Sullivan, L. (2004). Management Guidelines for Nurse Practitioners Working with Children and Adolescents (2nd ed). Philadelphia: F.A. Davis.

QUESTIONS

32. When considering a person's risk for measles, mumps, and rubella, the NP considers the following:

A. Children should have two doses of the measles, mumps, and rubella (MMR) vaccine before the sixth birthday.
B. Considerable mortality and morbidity occur with all three diseases.
C. Most cases in the United States occur in infants.
D. The use of the vaccine is often associated with protracted arthralgia.

33. Which of the following is true about the MMR vaccine?

A. It contains live virus.
B. Its use is contraindicated in persons with a history of egg allergy.
C. Revaccination of an immune person is associated with risk of allergic reaction.
D. One dose is recommended for young adults who have not been previously immunized.

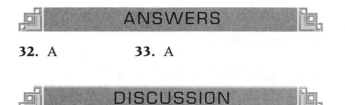

ANSWERS

32. A   **33.** A

DISCUSSION

The MMR vaccine is a live, attenuated vaccine. The recommended schedule for early childhood immunization is two doses of MMR vaccine given between 12 and 15 months and between 4 and 6 years (Fig. 14–1). Two immunizations 1 month apart are recommended for older children who were not immunized earlier in life. As with other immunizations, giving additional doses to those with an unclear immunization history is safe.

Rubella, also known as German measles, typically causes a relatively mild, 3- to 5-day illness with little risk of complication for the person infected. However, when rubella is contracted during pregnancy, the effects on the fetus can be devastating. Immunizing the entire population against rubella protects unborn children from the risk of congenital rubella syndrome. Measles can cause severe illness with serious sequelae, including encephalitis and pneumonia; sequelae of mumps include orchitis.

In the past, a history of egg allergy was considered a contraindication to receiving the MMR vaccine. However, use of the vaccine in such cases now appears safe, but a 90-minute observation period after vaccination is recommended. The MMR vaccine is safe to use during lactation, but its use in pregnant women is discouraged because of the possible risk of their developing congenital rubella syndrome from the live virus contained in the vaccine. However, this is likely more a theoretical than an actual risk. The MMR vaccine is well tolerated, with rare reports of mild, transient adverse reaction such as rash and sore throat. Systemic reaction to the MMR vaccine is rare.

DISCUSSION SOURCES

Centers for Disease Control and Prevention (2003). Recommended Childhood Immunization Schedule—United States, 2004. Available at http: cispimmunize.org/pro/pro_main.html, accessed 1/5/05.

Centers for Disease Control and Prevention (2004). Vaccine Preventable Disease: Measles. Available at http://www.cdc.gov/nip/diseases/child-vpd. htm#measles, accessed 1/1/05.

Centers for Disease Control and Prevention (2004). Vaccine Preventable Disease: Mumps. Available at http://www.cdc.gov/nip/diseases/child-vpd. htm#mumps, accessed 1/1/05.

Centers for Disease Control and Prevention (2004). Vaccine Preventable Disease: Rubella. Available at http://www.cdc.gov/nip/diseases/child-vpd. htm#rubella, accessed 1/1/05.

QUESTIONS

34. When advising parents about injectable influenza immunization, the NP considers the following about the vaccine:

   A. It may be given to at-risk infants older than 6 months.

   B. Its use is limited to children older than 2 years.

   C. It contains live virus.

   D. Its use is not recommended for members of households of high-risk patients.

35. A 7-year-old child with type 1 diabetes mellitus is about to receive injectable influenza vaccine. His parents and he should be advised that:

   A. The vaccine is more than 90% effective in preventing influenza.

   B. The vaccine's use is contraindicated during antibiotic therapy.

   C. Localized immunization reactions are fairly common.

   D. A short, intense, flulike syndrome typically occurs after immunization.

36. When giving influenza vaccine to a 7-year-old who has not received this immunization in the past, the NP considers that:

   A. two doses 4 weeks or more apart should be given.

Recommended Childhood and Adolescent Immunization Schedule
United States · July–December 2004

Vaccine ▼ / Age ▶	Birth	1 mo	2 mo	4 mo	6 mo	12 mo	15 mo	18 mo	24 mo	4–6 y	11–12 y	13–18 y
Hepatitis B[1]	HepB #1	only if mother HBsAg (-)	HepB #2			HepB #3					HepB series	
Diphtheria, Tetanus, Pertussis[2]			DTaP	DTaP	DTaP		DTaP			DTaP	Td	Td
Haemophilus influenzae Type b[3]			Hib	Hib	Hib	Hib						
Inactivated Poliovirus			IPV	IPV		IPV				IPV		
Measles, Mumps, Rubella[4]						MMR #1				MMR #2	MMR #2	
Varicella[5]						Varicella					Varicella	
Pneumococcal[6]			PCV	PCV	PCV	PCV			PCV		PPV	
Influenza[7]						Influenza (Yearly)				Influenza (Yearly)		
Hepatitis A[8]											Hepatitis A Series	

Range of Recommended Ages · Catch-up Immunization · Preadolescent Assessment

Vaccines below red line are for selected populations

Indicates age groups that warrant special effort to administer those vaccines not previously given.

This schedule indicates the recommended ages for routine administration of currently licensed childhood vaccines, as of April 1, 2004, for children through age 18 years. Any dose not given at the recommended age should be given at any subsequent visit when indicated and feasible. Indicates age groups that warrant special effort to administer those vaccines not previously given. Additional vaccines may be licensed and recommended during the year. Licensed combination vaccines may be used whenever any components of the combination are indicated and the vaccine's other components are not contraindicated. Providers should consult the manufacturers' package inserts for detailed recommendations. Clinically significant adverse events that follow immunization should be reported to the Vaccine Adverse Event Reporting System (VAERS). Guidance about how to obtain and complete a VAERS form can be found on the Internet: www.vaers.org or by calling 800-822-7967.

1. Hepatitis B (HepB) vaccine. All infants should receive the first dose of hepatitis B vaccine soon after birth and before hospital discharge; the first dose may also be given by age 2 months if the infant's mother is hepatitis B surface antigen (HBsAg) negative. Only monovalent HepB can be used for the birth dose. Monovalent or combination vaccine containing HepB may be used to complete the series. Four doses of vaccine may be administered when a birth dose is given. The second dose should be given at least 4 weeks after the first dose, except for combination vaccines which cannot be administered before age 6 weeks. The third dose should be given at least 16 weeks after the first dose and at least 8 weeks after the second dose. The last dose in the vaccination series (third or fourth dose) should not be administered before age 24 weeks.

Infants born to HBsAg-positive mothers should receive HepB and 0.5 mL of Hepatitis B Immune Globulin (HBIG) within 12 hours of birth at separate sites. The second dose is recommended at age 1–2 months. The last dose in the immunization series should not be administered before age 24 weeks. These infants should be tested for HBsAg and antibody to HBsAg (anti-HBs) at age 9–15 months.

Infants born to mothers whose HBsAg status is unknown should receive the first dose of the HepB series within 12 hours of birth. Maternal blood should be drawn as soon as possible to determine the mother's HBsAg status; if the HBsAg test is positive, the infant should receive HBIG as soon as possible (no later than age 1 week). The second dose is recommended at age 1–2 months. The last dose in the immunization series should not be administered before age 24 weeks.

2. Diphtheria and tetanus toxoids and acellular pertussis (DTaP) vaccine. The fourth dose of DTaP may be administered as early as age 12 months, provided 6 months have elapsed since the third dose and the child is unlikely to return at age 15–18 months. The final dose in the series should be given at age ≥4 years. Tetanus and diphtheria toxoids (Td) is recommended at age 11–12 years if at least 5 years have elapsed since the last dose of tetanus and diphtheria toxoid-containing vaccine. Subsequent routine Td boosters are recommended every 10 years.

3. Haemophilus influenzae type b (Hib) conjugate vaccine. Three Hib conjugate vaccines are licensed for infant use. If PRP-OMP (PedvaxHIB or ComVax [Merck]) is administered at ages 2 and 4 months, a dose at age 6 months is not required. DTaP/Hib combination products should not be used for primary immunization in infants at ages 2, 4 or 6 months but can be used as boosters following any Hib vaccine. The final dose in the series should be given at age ≥12 months.

4. Measles, mumps, and rubella vaccine (MMR). The second dose of MMR is recommended routinely at age 4–6 years but may be administered during any visit, provided at least 4 weeks have elapsed since the first dose and both doses are administered beginning at or after age 12 months. Those who have not previously received the second dose should complete the schedule by the visit at age 11–12 years.

5. Varicella vaccine. Varicella vaccine is recommended at any visit at or after age 12 months for susceptible children (i.e., those who lack a reliable history of chickenpox). Susceptible persons age ≥13 years should receive 2 doses, given at least 4 weeks apart.

6. Pneumococcal vaccine. The heptavalent pneumococcal conjugate vaccine (PCV) is recommended for all children age 2–23 months. It is also recommended for certain children age 24–59 months. The final dose in the series should be given at age >12 months. Pneumococcal polysaccharide vaccine (PPV) is recommended in addition to PCV for certain high-risk groups. See MMWR 2000;49(RR-9):1-35.

7. Influenza vaccine. Influenza vaccine is recommended annually for children aged ≥6 months with certain risk factors (including but not limited to asthma, cardiac disease, sickle cell disease, HIV, and diabetes), healthcare workers, and other persons (including household members) in close contact with persons in groups at high risk (see MMWR 2004;53;[RR-6]:1-40) and can be administered to all others wishing to obtain immunity. In addition, healthy children aged 6–23 months and close contacts of healthy children aged 0–23 months are recommended to receive influenza vaccine, because children in this age group are at substantially increased risk for influenza-related hospitalizations. For healthy persons aged 5–49 years, the intranasally administered live, attenuated influenza vaccine (LAIV) is an acceptable alternative to the intramuscular trivalent inactivated influenza vaccine (TIV). See MMWR 2004;53;[RR-6]:1-40. Children receiving TIV should be administered a dosage appropriate for their age (0.25 mL if 6–35 months or 0.5 mL if ≥3 years). Children aged ≤8 years who are receiving influenza vaccine for the first time should receive 2 doses (separated by at least 4 weeks for TIV and at least 6 weeks for LAIV).

8. Hepatitis A vaccine. Hepatitis A vaccine is recommended for children and adolescents in selected states and regions and for certain high-risk groups; consult your local public health authority. Children and adolescents in these states, regions, and high-risk groups who have not been immunized against hepatitis A can begin the hepatitis A immunization series during any visit. The 2 doses in the series should be administered at least 6 months apart. See MMWR 1999;48(RR-12):1-37.

For additional information about vaccines, including precautions and contraindications for immunization and vaccine shortages, please visit the National Immunization Program Web site at www.cdc.gov/nip/ or call the National Immunization Information Hotline at 800-232-2522 (English) or 800-232-0233 (Spanish).

Approved by the Advisory Committee on Immunization Practices (www.cdc.gov/nip/acip), the American Academy of Pediatrics (www.aap.org), and the American Academy of Family Physicians (www.aafp.org).

FIG. 14–1. Immunizations.

B. a single dose is adequate.

C. children in this age group have the highest rate of influenza-related hospitalization.

D. the vaccine should not be given to a child with shellfish allergy.

37. With regard to influenza prevention in well children, the NP considers that:

A. children ages 6 to 23 months have an increased risk of influenza-related hospitalization.

B. a full adult dose of influenza vaccine should be given starting at age 4 years.

C. the use of the influenza vaccine in well children is discouraged.

D. widespread use of the vaccine will likely increase risk of eczema.

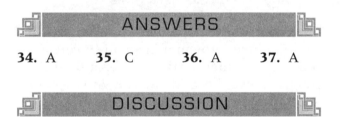

ANSWERS

34. A   35. C   36. A   37. A

DISCUSSION

Influenza is a viral illness that typically causes many days of incapacitation and suffering as well as the risk of death. Immunization is about 70% to 80% effective in preventing influenza A and B and reducing the severity of the disease.

Having a mild illness or taking an antibiotic is not a contraindication to any immunization, including influenza. The injectable vaccine does not contain live virus and is not shed; therefore, there is no risk of shedding an infectious agent to household contacts. Injectable influenza vaccine is recommended for household members of high-risk patients in order to avoid transmission of infection.

The nasal-spray flu vaccine, also known as attenuated influenza vaccine (LAIV), differs from the injectable influenza vaccine or "flu shot" because it contains weakened live influenza viruses instead of killed viruses and is administered by nasal spray instead of injection. The nasal-spray flu vaccine contains three different influenza viruses that are sufficiently weakened as to be incapable of causing disease but that have sufficient strength to stimulate a protective immune response. The viruses in the LAIV are cold-adapted and temperature-sensitive. As a result, the viruses can grow in the nose and throat but not in the lower respiratory tract where the temperature is higher. LAIV is currently approved for use in healthy people between the ages of 5 and 49 years. Individuals who should not receive LAIV include patients less than 5 years or more than 50 years of age; those with a medical condition that places them at high risk for complications from influenza, including those with chronic heart or lung disease, such as asthma or reactive airways disease, diabetes or kidney failure, immunosuppression; children or adolescents on chronic aspirin therapy; people with a history of Guillain-Barré syndrome; pregnant women, and people with a history of allergy to any of the components of LAIV or to eggs. In addition, there is a slight risk of transmission of the vaccine viruses and subsequent illness to close contacts. Adverse effects include nasal irritation and discharge, muscle aches, sore throat, and fever.

The optimal time to receive influenza vaccine is usually in October or November, about a month prior to the anticipated onset of the flu season. When a child younger than 8 years of age receives influenza vaccine for the first time, two doses => 4 weeks apart should be given. Annual influenza vaccine is recommended for children => 6 months of age with chronic health problems. In addition, because of their increased risk of hospitalization if influenza disease is contracted, all children age 6 to 12 months should receive immunization against influenza.

DISCUSSION SOURCES

Centers for Disease Control and Prevention, Preventing Influenza (2004). Available at http://www.cdc.gov/flu/protect/preventing.htm, accessed 1/2/05.

Centers for Disease Control and Prevention, Q & A: The Nasal-Spray Flu Vaccine (Live Attenuated

Influenza Vaccine [LAIV]). Available at http://www.cdc.gov/flu/about/qa/nasalspray.htm, accessed 1/2/05.

QUESTIONS

38. Which of the following is true about the hepatitis B virus (HBV) vaccine?

   A. It contains live HBV.
   B. Children should have hepatitis B surface antibody (HBsAb) (anti-HBs) titers drawn after three doses of vaccine.
   C. Hepatitis B immunization should be offered to all children, with the series completed by the child's 12th birthday.
   D. Serologic testing for hepatitis B surface antigen (HBsAg) should be checked before HBV vaccination is initiated in children.

39. You are making rounds in the nursery and examine the neonate of a mother who is HBsAg-positive. Your most appropriate action is to:

   A. administer hepatitis B immune globulin (HBIG).
   B. isolate the child.
   C. administer hepatitis B immunization.
   D. give hepatitis B immunization and HBIG.

40. Hepatitis B vaccine should not be given to the child with a history of anaphylactic reaction to:

   A. egg.
   B. baker's yeast.
   C. neomycin.
   D. streptomycin.

41. Infants who have been infected perinatally with HBV have an estimated ___% lifetime chance of developing hepatocellular carcinoma or cirrhosis.

   A. 10
   B. 25
   C. 50
   D. 75

42. When advising a patient about immunization with the nasal spray flu vaccine, the nurse practitioner (NP) considers the following:

   A. Its use is acceptable during pregnancy.
   B. Its use is limited to children younger than age 6 years.
   C. It contains live virus
   D. It is recommended for household members of high-risk patients.

ANSWERS

38. C   **39.** D   **40.** B
41. B   **42.** C

DISCUSSION

A small, double-stranded DNA virus that contains the inner protein of hepatitis B core antigen and an outer surface of hepatitis surface antigen causes hepatitis B. The virus is transmitted through exchange of body fluids. Hepatitis B infection can be prevented by limiting exposure to blood and body fluids, as well as through immunization. Recombinant hepatitis B vaccine, which does not contain live virus, is well tolerated but is contraindicated in the person who has a history of anaphylactic reaction to baker's yeast. Children should be immunized in early childhood, preferably in the first year of life. The well-child visit at age 11 to 12 years offers an opportunity to update hepatitis B and other immunizations before adolescence.

Infants who have been infected perinatally with HBV have an estimated 25% lifetime chance of developing hepatocellular carcinoma or cirrhosis. As a result, all pregnant women should undergo screening for HBsAg at the first prenatal visit, regardless of HBV vaccine history. The HBV vaccine is not 100% effective, and a woman may have carried HbsAg since before pregnancy. During the first 24 hours of life, a neonate born to a mother with HBsAg should receive HBV as well as HBIG in order to minimize the risk of perinatal transmission and subsequent development of chronic hepatitis B.

About 90% to 95% of those who receive the vaccine develop HBsAb after three doses, which implies protection from the virus. Therefore, routine testing for the presence of HBsAb after immunization is not generally recommended.

Administration of HBIG after exposure with a repeat dose in 1 month is about 75% effective in protecting from hepatitis B after percutaneous, sexual, or mucosal exposure to HBV. With postexposure HBIG, HBV vaccine series should be started.

DISCUSSION SOURCE

Centers for Disease Control and Prevention (2004). Vaccine Preventable Disease: Hepatitis B. Available at http://www.cdc.gov/nip/menus/diseases. htm#hepb, accessed 1/1/05.

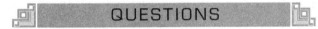

QUESTIONS

43. Which of the following is correct about the varicella vaccine?

   A. It contains killed varicella-zoster virus (VZV).
   B. A short febrile illness is common during the first days after vaccination.
   C. Children should have a varicella titer drawn before receiving the vaccine.
   D. Mild cases of chickenpox have been reported in immunized patients.

44. Expected outcomes with the use of varicella vaccine include a reduction in the rate of all of the following except:

   A. shingles.
   B. Reye syndrome.
   C. aspirin allergy.
   D. invasive varicella.

45. A parent asks about varicella-zoster immune globulin, and you reply that it is a:

   A. synthetic product that is well tolerated.

   B. pooled blood product that has been known to transmit infectious disease.
   C. blood product obtained from a single donor.
   D. pooled blood product with an excellent safety profile.

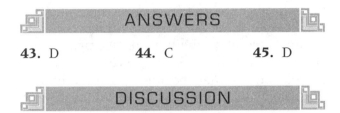

ANSWERS

43. D   **44.** C   **45.** D

DISCUSSION

The VZV causes the highly contagious, systemic disease commonly known as chickenpox. Varicella infection usually confers lifetime immunity. However, reinfection may be seen in immunocompromised patients. More often, reexposure causes an increase in antibody titers without causing disease.

The VZV can lie dormant in sensory nerve ganglion. Later reactivation causes shingles, a painful, vesicular-form rash in a dermatomal pattern. About 15% of those who have had chickenpox develop shingles at least once during their lifetime. Shingles rates are markedly reduced in people who have received varicella vaccine in comparison with those who have had chickenpox.

A patient-reported history of varicella is considered a valid measurement of immunity, with 97% to 99% of persons having serologic evidence of immunity. Among older children and adults with an unclear or negative varicella history, the majority are also seropositive. Confirming varicella immunity through varicella titers, even in the presence of a positive varicella history, should be done in health care workers because of their risk of exposure and potential transmission of the disease.

The varicella vaccine contains attenuated virus. The vaccine is administered in a single dose after the first birthday. Older children (age 13 years and older) and adults with no history of varicella infection or previous immunization should receive two immunizations 4 to 8 weeks apart. In particular, health care workers, family contacts of immunocompromised patients, and day care workers without evidence of varicella immunity should be targeted for varicella vaccine. In addition, adults who are in environments with high risk of varicella transmission (e.g., college dormitories, military barracks, long-term care facilities) should receive the immunization if there is no evidence of varicella immunity.

The vaccine is highly protective against severe, invasive varicella. However, mild forms of chickenpox may be reported after immunization. Varicella immune globulin, as with all forms of immune globulin (IG), provides temporary, passive immunity to infection. IG is a pooled blood product with an excellent safety profile. Although the majority of cases are seen in children younger than age 18 years, the greatest varicella mortality is found in persons ages 30 to 49 years.

DISCUSSION SOURCE

Centers for Disease Control and Prevention (2004). Vaccine Preventable Disease: Varicella. Available at http://www.cdc.gov/nip/diseases/child-vpd.htm#varicella, accessed 1/2/05.

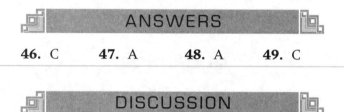

QUESTIONS

46. An 11-year-old child presents with no documented primary tetanus immunization series. Which of the following represents the immunization needed?

    A. three doses of diphtheria, tetanus, and acellular pertussis vaccine 2 months apart
    B. tetanus immune globulin now and two doses of tetanus-diphtheria (Td) 1 month apart
    C. Td now, with repeat doses in 1 and 6 months
    D. Td as a single dose

47. Problems after tetanus immunization typically include:

    A. localized reaction at site of injection.
    B. myalgia and malaise.
    C. low-grade fever.
    D. diffuse rash.

48. Which wound presents the greatest risk for tetanus infection?

    A. a puncture wound obtained while playing in a garden
    B. a laceration obtained from a knife used to trim raw beef
    C. a human bite
    D. an abrasion obtained by falling on a sidewalk

49. Infection with *Corynebacterium diphtheriae* usually causes:

    A. a diffuse rash.
    B. meningitis.
    C. pseudomembranous pharyngitis.
    D. a gastroenteritis-like illness.

ANSWERS

46. C   47. A   48. A   49. C

DISCUSSION

Tetanus infection is caused by *Clostridium tetani*, an anaerobic, gram-positive, spore-forming rod. This organism, which is found in soil, particularly if it contains manure, enters the body through a contaminated wound and causes a life-threatening systemic disease characterized by painful muscle weakness and spasm ("lockjaw"). Diphtheria, the "d" part of the Td vaccine, is caused by *C. diphtheriae*, a gram-negative bacillus. This disease is typically transmitted person to person or through contaminated liquids such as milk. Diphtheria is characterized by severe respiratory tract infection, including the appearance of pseudomembranous pharyngitis.

Tetanus and diphtheria are uncommon infections because of widespread immunization. A primary series of three Td or diphtheria, tetanus, and acellular pertussis vaccine injections sets the stage for long-term immunity. A booster Td dose every 10 years is recommended, but protection is likely for up to 20 to 30 years after a primary series. Using Td rather than tetanus toxoid for the primary series and booster doses in adults assists in keeping diphtheria immunity as well. At the time of wound-producing injury, tetanus immune globulin affords temporary protection for individuals who have not received tetanus immunization.

Tetanus and diphtheria immunizations are well tolerated and produce few adverse reactions. A short-term, localized area of redness and warmth is quite common and is not predictive of future problems with tetanus immunization.

DISCUSSION SOURCES

Centers for Disease Control and Prevention (2004). Vaccine Preventable Disease: Diphtheria, Available at http://www.cdc.gov/nip/diseases/child-vpd. htm#diptheria, accessed 1/2/05.

Centers for Disease Control and Prevention (2004). Vaccine Preventable Disease: Tetanus. Available at http://www.cdc.gov/nip/diseases/child-vpd. htm#tetanus, accessed 1/2/05.

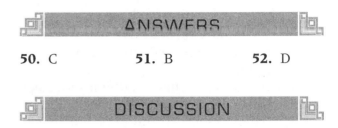

QUESTIONS

50. Which of the following is the primary source of hepatitis A infection?

   A. blood products
   B. shellfish
   C. contaminated drinking water
   D. intimate person-to-person contact

51. When answering questions about hepatitis A vaccine, you consider that it:

   A. contains live virus.
   B. should be given to children living in select high-risk states.
   C. frequently causes systemic post-immunization reaction.
   D. is 100% protective after a single injection.

52. Usual treatment options for a child with hepatitis A include:

   A. alpha-interferon.
   B. ribavirin.

   C. acyclovir.
   D. supportive care.

ANSWERS

50. C   **51.** B   **52.** D

DISCUSSION

Hepatitis A infection is caused by HAV (hepatitis A virus), a small RNA virus. Transmitted primarily by fecally contaminated drinking water and food supplies, hepatitis A is typically a self-limited infection with a very low mortality rate that responds well to supportive care. Although raw shellfish growing in contaminated water can be problematic, fecally contaminated water supplies are the most common source of infection. In developing countries with limited pure water, the majority of the children contract this disease by age 5 years. In North America, adults ages 20 to 39 years account for nearly 50% of the reported cases; children are more often affected than adults.

Children who live in select states and regions with increased HAV infection prevalence and select high-risk groups should be immunized against HAV. The local public health department should be consulted for further advice. Two doses of vaccine are recommended to ensure a greater immune response. Hepatitis A vaccine, which does not contain live virus, is usually well tolerated without systemic reaction.

DISCUSSION SOURCES

Centers for Disease Control and Prevention (2004). Vaccine Preventable Disease: Hepatitis A. Available at http://www.cdc.gov/nip/diseases/child-vpd.htm#hepa, accessed 1/2/05.

Friedman, L. (2003). Liver, biliary tract and pancreas. In Tierney, L., McPhee, S., and Papadakis, M. (eds.). Current Diagnosis and Treatment (42nd ed., pp. 628–673). New York: Appleton Medical Books/McGraw-Hill.

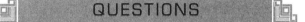

QUESTIONS

53. Which of the following is true about oral poliovirus vaccine (OPV)?

   A. It contains killed virus.
   B. It is the preferred method of immunization.
   C. Two doses should be administered by a child's fourth birthday.
   D. After administration of OPV, poliovirus may be shed from the stool.

54. Which of the following is true about inactivated poliovirus vaccine (IPV)?

   A. It contains live virus.
   B. It is the preferred method of immunization.
   C. Two doses should be administered by a child's fourth birthday
   D. After administration of IPV, poliovirus may be shed from the stool.

55. Which of the following is the route of transmission of the poliovirus?

   A. fecal-oral
   B. droplet
   C. blood and body fluids
   D. skin-to-skin contact

ANSWERS

53. D   **54.** B   **55.** A

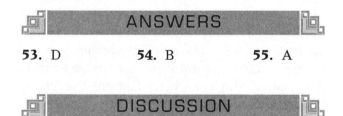

DISCUSSION

Polioviruses are highly contagious and capable of causing paralytic, life-threatening infection. The infection is transmitted fecally-orally. Rates of infection among household contacts may be as high as 96%. However, since 1994, North and South America have been declared free of indigenous poliomyelitis, largely because of the efficacy of the OPV. This live-virus vaccine is given orally, with a small amount of the poliovirus shed through the stool. This shedding presents household members with

possible exposure to poliovirus. Virtually all recent cases of paralytic poliomyelitis found in the United States were vaccine-associated (vaccine-associated paralytic poliomyelitis [VAPP]). Use IPV instead of OPV, as recommended. Because of VAPP risk, OPV is no longer used in the United States.

DISCUSSION SOURCE

Centers for Disease Control and Prevention (2004). Vaccine Preventable Disease: Polio. Available at http://www.cdc.gov/nip/diseases/child-vpd.htm#polio, accessed 1/2/05.

QUESTIONS

56. Which of the following is most likely to have lead (Pb) poisoning?

   A. a developmentally disabled 5-year-old child who lives in a 15-year-old house in poor repair
   B. an infant who lives in a 5-year-old home with copper plumbing
   C. a toddler who lives in a 65-year-old home
   D. a preschooler who lives nears an electric generating plant

57. You are devising a program to screen preschoolers for Pb poisoning. The most sensitive component of this campaign is:

   A. environmental history.
   B. physical examination.
   C. hematocrit level.
   D. hemoglobin level.

58. Patients with plumbism present with which kind of anemia?

   A. macrocytic, hyperchromic
   B. normocytic, normochromic
   C. hemolytic
   D. microcytic, hypochromic

59. Which of the following is the recommended screening for a child with significant risk of Pb poisoning?

   A. start at age 3 months; repeat every 3 months

B. start at age 6 months; repeat every 6 months
C. start at age 1 year; repeat every year
D. start at age 2 years; repeat annually

60. Intervention for a child with a Pb between 10 and 20 μg/dL usually includes all of the following except:

   A. removal from the Pb source.
   B. iron supplementation.
   C. chelation therapy.
   D. encouraging a diet high in vitamin C.

61. Intervention for a child with a Pb of 40 to 50 μg/dL usually includes:

   A. chelation.
   B. calcium supplementation.
   C. exchange transfusion.
   D. iron depletion.

ANSWERS

56. C	**57.** A	**58.** D
59. B	**60.** C	**61.** A

DISCUSSION

Pb poisoning, or plumbism, remains a significant public health problem. This is a reportable disease found in more than 2 million children and adults in the United States and is caused by exposure to Pb in the environment. Ingested Pb inactivates heme synthesis by inhibiting the insertion of iron into the protoporphyrin ring. This leads to the development of a microcytic, hypochromic anemia; basophilic stippling is often noted on red blood cell morphology. In addition, Pb is significantly toxic to the solid organs, bones, and the nervous system.

The major source of Pb poisoning in children is Pb-based paint. This paint has not been available in the United States for more than 25 years. However, unless deleading procedures have occurred, the majority of homes built before 1957 contain Pb-based paint. A diet low in calcium, iron, zinc, magnesium, and copper, as well as high in fat, typical for children living in poverty, enhances oral Pb absorption.

For Pb poisoning to occur, there must be an intersection between the environmental hazard and the child. In older homes, the point of greatest risk is the window because the windowsills and putty have high Pb concentration. Because toddlers are the ideal height to reach windowsills and are often drawn to open windows, the age of greatest risk is 2 to 3 years. Summer is the season of greatest risk. Children can acquire Pb through two sources: inhaled paint powder and ingested paint chips. Inhalation of paint dust is a potent Pb source for infants and for children with Pb levels below 45 μg/dL, although toddlers and children with Pb levels of more than 45 μg/dL are typically poisoned by also eating paint chips.

Besides paint, other Pb hazards may be encountered. Pb-glazed pottery used to store and serve acidic beverages, soft water delivered by Pb-lined pipes, Pb-soldered vessels used for cooking, and fumes from burnt casings of batteries can contribute to Pb burden. In addition, soil around the base of the home may contain Pb-based paint, and soil around highways often contains Pb residual from automotive fuel. Certain folk medicines from the Middle East and Mexico may contain Pb.

Clinical manifestation of Pb poisoning is usually not apparent until a child's Pb level is markedly elevated. Because most children have low-level, chronic Pb exposure with few or no symptoms, periodic screening of all children is recommended. Primary prevention of Pb poisoning should be the goal, with the goal of reducing risk for all children. After Pb risk is identified, removing the child or limiting exposure is vital. Most children with Pb levels of 10 to 35 μg/dL are typically treated with removal from the source, with improved nutrition, and with iron therapy. With Pb levels of 36 to 50 μg/dL, chelation with an agent such as succimer along with the previously listed interventions is indicated. With Pb levels of more than 51 μg/dL, hospital admission with expert evaluation is likely the most prudent course to avoid serious problems (including encephalopathy) associated with markedly elevated Pb levels.

DISCUSSION SOURCE

Centers for Disease Control and Prevention (2004). Lead: Topic Home. Available at http://www.cdc.gov/lead/, accessed 1/2/05.

QUESTIONS

62. The most likely causative organism of bronchiolitis is:

    A. *Haemophilus influenzae.*
    B. parainfluenza virus.
    C. respiratory syncytial virus.
    D. Coxsackie virus.

63. One of the most prominent clinical features of bronchiolitis is:

    A. fever.
    B. vomiting.
    C. wheezing.
    D. conjunctival inflammation.

64. In the majority of children with bronchiolitis, intervention includes:

    A. aerosolized ribavirin therapy.
    B. supportive care.
    C. oral theophylline therapy.
    D. ibuprofen therapy.

65. Long-term sequelae of bronchiolitis may include:

    A. recurrent airway reactivity.
    B. dilated terminal airways.
    C. hypoxemia.
    D. bronchopulmonary dysplasia.

ANSWERS

62. C   **63.** C   **64.** B   **65.** A

DISCUSSION

Bronchiolitis is a common illness in early childhood; its peak incidence is in children younger than 2 years. The most likely causative organism is respiratory syncytial virus; it is less often caused by parainfluenza and influenza virus and adenovirus. In most children, bronchiolitis runs a course of 2 to 3 weeks of mild upper respiratory symptoms with expiratory wheezing; supportive therapy is usually sufficient. In infants younger than 3 months and in children with chronic health problems, hypoxemia and hypercapnia are more common, necessitating hospital admission, hydration, and oxygenation. The use of corticosteroids and bronchodilators remains controversial. Long-term sequelae of bronchiolitis often include recurrent airway reactivity.

DISCUSSION SOURCE

Larsen, G., Accurso, F., Deterding, R., et al. (2003). Respiratory tract and mediastinum. In Hay, W., Hayward, A., Levin, M., and Sondheimer, J. (eds.). Current Pediatric Diagnosis and Treatment (16th ed., pp. 492–545.). New York: McGraw-Hill.

QUESTIONS

66. You examine a newborn with a capillary hemangioma on her thigh. You advise her parents that this lesion:

    A. will likely increase in size over the first year of life.
    B. should be treated to avoid malignancy.
    C. usually resolves within the first months of life.
    D. may develop a superimposed lichenification.

67. You examine a 2-month-old infant with a port-wine lesion over her right cheek. You advise the parents that this lesion:

    A. needs to be surgically excised.
    B. grows proportionally with the child.
    C. becomes lighter over time.
    D. may become malignant.

68. A 10-day-old child presents with multiple raised lesions resembling flea bites over the trunk and nape of the neck. The infant

is nursing well and has no fever or exposure to animals. This may represent:

A. erythema neonatorum toxicum.
B. milia.
C. neonatal acne.
D. staphylococcal skin infection.

69. An Asian couple comes in with their 4-week-old infant, who has blue-black macules scattered over the buttocks. These most likely represent:

A. mottling.
B. mongolian spots.
C. ecchymosis.
D. hemangioma.

70. The most important aspect of skin care for patients with eczema is:

A. frequent bathing with antibacterial soap.
B. consistent use of medium- to high-potency topical steroids.
C. application of lubricants.
D. treatment of dermatophytes.

71. One of the more common sites for eczema in infants is the:

A. dorsum of the hand.
B. face.
C. neck.
D. flexor surfaces.

ANSWERS

66. A	**67.** B	**68.** A
69. B	**70.** C	**71.** B

DISCUSSION

A number of dermatologic conditions are found in early infancy. Parents understandably have concerns about these lesions. A thorough knowledge of the more common conditions is an important part of the NP's role.

Capillary hemangioma is a congenital vascular malformation. Such lesions become evident shortly after birth and grow rapidly in the first year, then plateau in size, and eventually regress. About 90% are gone by age 9, usually leaving bluish vascularity over the area. If the lesion is large or involves a vital organ such as the eye, treatment may be indicated. This can include the use of corticosteroids, lasers, or alpha-interferon injection.

A port-wine stain is a flat hemangioma with a stable course. These lesions have a predilection for appearing on the face and are usually present at birth. Port-wine stains tend to deepen in color as time goes on and grow proportionally with the child. Although not malignant, the lesions are often disfiguring and can be minimized or eliminated through the use of laser therapy.

Milia are typically white pinpoint papular lesions caused by sebaceous hyperplasia. The usual distribution is over the nose, cheeks, and other areas with an abundance of sebaceous glands. The cause is likely the maternal androgenic effect on the sebaceous glands. Benign in nature, milia resolve without special therapy by 4 weeks to 6 months of life.

Erythema toxicum neonatorum is a benign rash of unknown etiology that occurs in about 50% of full-term infants. Usually beginning in the first 10 days of life, the lesions look like flea bites and are widely distributed; the palms and soles are spared. The lesions usually fade by 5 to 7 days after eruption without specific treatment.

Mongolian spots occur in about 90% of children of African and Asian ancestries and in fewer than 10% of those of European ancestry. The distribution is usually over the lower back and buttocks but can occur over a wider area. Caused by an accumulation of melanocytes, these are benign lesions that typically fade by age 7 without special therapy.

Acne neonatorum consists of open and closed comedones and pustules over the forehead and cheeks, similar to the adolescent version of the condition. The etiology is likely the effect of maternal androgens on the infant's skin. It usually resolves in about 4 to 8 weeks but may persist up to age 1 year. Low-dose benzoyl peroxide may be used.

Eczema or atopic dermatitis is one manifestation of a type I hypersensitivity reaction. This type of reaction is caused when immunoglobulin E antibodies occupy receptor sites on mast cells, causing a degradation of the mast cells and subsequent release of histamine, vasodilatation, mucous gland stimulation, and tissue swelling. Type I hypersensitivity reactions comprise two subgroups: atopy and anaphylaxis.

Within the atopy subgroup are a number of common clinical conditions such as allergic rhinitis, atopic dermatitis, allergic gastroenteropathy, and allergy-based asthma. Atopic diseases have a strong familial component and tend to cause localized rather than systemic reactions. Individuals with atopic disease are often able to identify allergy-inducing agents. Treatment for atopic disease of eczema includes avoidance of offending agents and minimizing skin dryness by limiting soap and water exposure, as well as consistent use of lubricants. The NP should explain to the patient that the skin tends to be sensitive and needs to be treated with some care. When flares occur, the skin eruption is largely caused by histamine release. Antihistamines and corticosteroids should be used to control eczema flares. With an acute flare of eczema or with contact dermatitis, an intermediate- to high-potency topical corticosteroid is likely needed to control acute symptoms. After this is achieved, the lowest potency topical corticosteroid that yields the desired effect should be used.

DISCUSSION SOURCES

Hill, N., and Sullivan, L. (2004). Management Guidelines for Nurse Practitioners Working with Children and Adolescents (2d ed.) Philadelphia: F.A. Davis.

Morelli, J., and Weston, W. (2003). Skin. In Hay, W.,Hayward, A., Levin, M., and Sondheimer, J. (eds.). Current Pediatric Diagnosis and Treatment (16th ed., pp. 400–419). New York: McGraw-Hill.

QUESTIONS

72. Which of the following is the most prudent first-line treatment choice for a toddler with acute otitis media (AOM) who requires antimicrobial therapy?

A. ceftibuten
B. amoxicillin
C. cefuroxime
D. azithromycin

73. The majority of AOM is caused by:

A. select gram-positive and -negative bacteria.
B. gram-negative bacteria and pathogenic viruses.
C. rhinovirus and *Staphylococcus aureus*.
D. predominately beta-lactamase–producing organisms.

74. Which of the following represents the best choice of clinical agents for a child who has severe type 1 penicillin allergy who requires antimicrobial therapy?

A. ciprofloxacin
B. clarithromycin.
C. amoxicillin
D. cefixime

75. Which of the following does not represent a risk factor for recurrent AOM in younger children?

A. pacifier use after age 10 months
B. history of first episode of AOM before age 3 months
C. exposure to second-hand smoke
D. penicillin allergy

76. Which of the following antimicrobial agents affords the most effective activity against *S. pneumoniae*?

A. ciprofloxacin
B. cefixime
C. trimethoprim-sulfamethoxazole (TMP-SMX)
D. cefuroxime

77. A 3-year-old boy with AOM continues to have otalgia and fever >39° C after 3 days of amoxicillin 80 mg/kg/d with clavulanate. Which of the following is recommended?

A. watch and wait while using analgesics
B. azithromycin

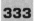

C. clindamycin
D. ceftriaxone

78. Which of the following is most consistent with the diagnosis of AOM?

A. ear pulling in the infant
B. tympanic membrane (TM) retraction
C. TM immobility to insufflation
D. anterior cervical lymphadenopathy

79. Which of the following is absent in otitis media with effusion (OME)?

A. fluid in the middle ear
B. otalgia
C. fever
D. itch

80. Treatment of OME usually includes:

A. symptomatic treatment.
B. antimicrobial therapy.
C. an antihistamine.
D. a mucolytic.

81. Clindamycin is most effective against:

A. *S. pneumoniae.*
B. *H. influenzae.*
C. *M. catarrhalis.*
D. Adenovirus.

82. Charecteristics of *Morexella catarrhalis* include:

A. high rate of beta-lactamase production.
B. antimicrobial resistance due to altered protein binding sites.
C. being often found in middle ear exudate on recurrent otitis media.
D. gram-positive organism.

83. Characteristics of *H. influenzae* include:

A. rare beta-lactamase production.
B. antimicrobial resistance due to altered protein binding sites.
C. organism most commonly isolated from mucoid middle ear effusion.
D. gram-positive organism.

84. Characteristics of *S. pneumoniae* include:

A. beta-lactamase production common.
B. antimicrobial resistance due to altered protein binding sites.
C. organism most commonly isolated from mucoid middle ear effusion.
D. gram-negative organism.

ANSWERS

72. B	73. A	74. B
75. D	76. D	77. D
78. C	79. C	80. A
81. A	82. A	83. C
84. B		

DISCUSSION

In children, AOM is among the most frequent diagnoses noted in office visits in children younger than age 15 years. *Streptococcus pneumoniae, Haemophilus influenzae, Moraxella catarrhalis,* and a variety of viruses contribute to the infectious and inflammatory processes of the middle ear. Nearly two thirds of all children have at least one episode by their second birthday; one third have more than three episodes.

The eustachian tubes provide drainage of middle ear secretions as well as protection of the middle ear from pharyngeal secretions and bacterial contaminates. As a result, conditions that cause eustachian tube dysfunction (ETD) or eustachian tube obstruction (ETO), such as allergic rhinitis, upper respiratory infection (URI), and craniofacial abnormalities, encourage status of secretions and allow aspiration of pharyngeal flora into the middle ear, resulting in acute otitis media (AOM). Passive cigarette smoke exposure, feeding in a supine position, and pacifier use beyond age 10 months likely also predispose a child to AOM due to ETD or ETO. As children in day care typically have more URIs, attendance at group child care is a risk factor as well as for nasopharyngeal carriage of bacteria implicated in AOM. Bottle feeding is a risk factor for AOM, with rates significantly lower among infants who were breast-fed for the first 6 to 12 months of life; boys and children of Native American ancestry

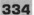

are also at increased risk. Additional interventions to reduce AOM risk, such as immunization against influenza, has been advocated by some sources. The pneumococcal conjugate vaccine is effective in reducing risk of invasive pneumococcal disease and, to a lesser degree, in minimizing AOM risk.

S. pneumoniae causes 40% to 50% of AOM; it is the least likely of the three major causative bacteria to resolve without antimicrobial intervention while causing the most significant symptoms. This organism has recently exhibited resistance to a number of antibiotic agents, including amoxicillin, cephalosporins, and the macrolides. The mechanism of resistance is an alteration of intracellular protein-binding sites, which can typically be overcome by using higher doses of amoxicillin and select cephalosporins.

H. influenzae and *M. catarrhalis* are gram-negative organisms capable of producing beta-lactamase. Although these two organisms have relatively high rates of spontaneous resolution (50% and 90%, respectively), without antimicrobial intervention, *H. influenzae* is the organism most commonly isolated from mucoid and serious middle ear effusion. Beta-lactamase production by organisms probably contributes less to AOM treatment failure than to prescribing an inadequate dosing of amoxicillin needed to eradicate drug-resistant *S. pneumoniae* (DRSP). Respiratory syncytial virus is commonly isolated from the middle ear fluid in children with AOM. Other common viral agents include human rhinovirus and coronavirus. AOM caused by these viral agents usually resolves in 7 to 10 days with supportive care alone.

Appropriate assessment is critical to arriving at the diagnosis of AOM. Ear pulling in preverbal children may be noted but is not considered diagnostic for the condition. The TM may be retracted or bulging and is typically reddened with loss of translucency and mobility on insufflation. With recovery, TM mobility returns in about 1 to 2 weeks, but middle ear effusion typically persists for 4 to 6 weeks, often up to 3 months. The components of AOM include objective findings such as a bulging, erythematous TM with limited or absent mobility and distinct otalgia with discomfort clearly referable to the ear(s) that results in interference with or precludes normal activity or sleep. Additional components include an air-fluid level behind the TM and otorrhea.

AOM is a common clinical problem. Bearing this in mind, the American Academy of Pediatrics (AAP) has developed treatment recommendations focused on the care of the child age 2 months through 12 years with AOM. These recommendations apply only to the otherwise healthy child without underlying conditions that may alter the natural course of AOM, including anatomic abnormalities such as cleft palate; genetic conditions such as Down syndrome, immunodeficiencies, presence of cochlear implants, and children with a clinical recurrence of AOM within 30 days or AOM with underlying chronic otitis media with effusion (OME).

According to the AAP recommendations, the management of AOM should include an assessment of pain. If pain is present, the clinician should recommend treatment to reduce pain.

One important point made in the AAP AOM treatment guidelines is that "watch and wait" can be an appropriate approach to treating AOM. Placebo-controlled trials of AOM over the past 30 years have shown consistently that most children do well, without adverse sequelae, even without antibacterial therapy. As a result, observation without use of antibacterial agents in a child with uncomplicated AOM is

TABLE 14–3	
DEFINITIONS OF OTITIS MEDIA TERMS	
Acute otitis media	The presence of fluid in the middle ear in association with local or systemic illness including otalgia, otorrhea, fever
Otitis media with effusion	The presence of fluid in the middle ear in the absence of signs or symptoms of acute infection

an option for selected children based on diagnostic certainty, age, illness severity, and assurance of follow-up. For example, consider the care of a child => 2 years of age presenting with AOM and nonsevere illness (mild otalgia and fever <39°C in the past 24 hours) or severe illness (moderate to severe otalgia or fever => 39°C) with an uncertain AOM diagnosis. A period of 48 to 72 hours of symptomatic treatment only without antimicrobial therapy is a viable option provided that follow-up can be ensured and antibacterial agents started if symptoms persist or worsen. Amoxicillin remains the first-line antimicrobial for the treatment of AOM in children with less severe illness. Given the wide therapeutic index of this medication and the prevalence of drugresistant *S. pneumoniae*, 80–90 mg/kg/d is the recommended dose. Amoxicillin/clavulanate (Augmentin), again with the 80–90 mg/kg/d recommended dose, is recommended as first-line therapy for the child with AOM and severe illness or in the case of treatment failure with amoxicillin.

Children younger than 3 months of age should be routinely seen in 1 to 2 days due to increased risk of treatment failure. In the child older than 3 months, otalgia, fever, and other symptoms that persist beyond 3 days of therapy may indicate treatment failure, and repeat evaluation is in order. If the child appears to be recovering, follow-up at 4 to 8 weeks is often advised, in part to evaluate for OME. OME is also called serous otitis media; it is defined as the presence of fluid in the middle ear in the absence of signs or symptoms of acute infection. With OME, 80% of children will clear the middle ear by 8 weeks. If OME persists beyond 8 weeks, the presence of communication problems and other symptoms dictate the need for further evaluation and treatment. Routine re-treatment with an antimicrobial is not indicated for OME. When a child is seen at follow-up, measures to reduce AOM risk should be reviewed and reinforced.

DISCUSSION SOURCES

Dowell, S., Butler, J. Giebink, S., Jacobs, M., Jernigan, D., Musher, D. Rakowsky, A., Schwartz, B. and the Drug-resistant *Streptococcus pneumoniae* Therapeutic Working Group (1999). Acute otitis media: Management and surveillance in an era of pneumococcal resistance. A report from the Drug-Resistance *Streptococcus pneumoniae* Therapeutic Working Group. Pediatric Infectious Disease Journal. 18:1–9.

Hill, N., and Sullivan, L. (2004). Management Guidelines for Nurse Practitioners Working with Children and Adolescents (2nd ed.) Philadelphia: F.A. Davis.

Subcommittee on Management of Acute Otitis Media (2004). Diagnosis and Management of Acute Otitis Media, Pediatrics, 113: 1451–1465, available at www.aap.org, accessed 1/2/05.

QUESTIONS

85. Which of the following is most likely to be part of the clinical presentation of urinary tract infection (UTI) in the 20-month-old child?

    A. urinary frequency and urgency
    B. fever
    C. suprapubic tenderness
    D. nausea and vomiting

86. Which of the following is the most common UTI organism in the child?

    A. *Pseudomonas aeruginosa*
    B. *Escherichia coli*
    C. *Klebsiella pneumoniae*
    D. *Proteus mirabilis*

87. All of the following uropathogens are capable of reducing urinary nitrates to nitrites except:

    A. *E. coli.*
    B. *Proteus* species.
    C. *K. pneumoniae.*
    D. *Staphylococcus saprophyticus.*

88. Which of the following is considered the ideal method for obtaining a urine sample for culture and sensitivity in a 1 to 1½ year-old girl with suspected UTI?

    A. suprapubic aspiration
    B. transurethral bladder catheterization
    C. bag collection
    D. diaper sample

89. When choosing an antimicrobial agent for the treatment of UTI in the febrile child, the NP considers that:

    A. gram-positive organisms are the most likely cause of infection.
    B. a parenteral aminoglycoside is the preferred treatment choice.
    C. the use of an oral third-generation cephalosporin is acceptable if gastrointestinal function is intact.
    D. TMP-SMX use is contraindicated.

90. When evaluating the urinalysis of a 10-month-old with UTI, the NP considers that:

    A. leukocytes will consistently be noted.
    B. proteinuria is usually absent.
    C. urobilinogen can be present.
    D. up to 20% of urinalyses will be normal.

91. In children ages 2 months to 2 years with UTI, antimicrobial therapy should be prescribed for:

    A. 3 to 5 days.
    B. 5 to 10 days.
    C. 7 to 14 days.
    D. 14 to 21 days.

92. The preferred urinary tract imaging study for a 22-month-old girl with first-time UTI is:

    A. renal ultrasound.
    B. renal scan.
    C. cytogram.
    D. none unless a second UTI occurs.

93. The urinary tract abnormality most often associated with UTI in the younger child is:

    A. bladder neck stricture.
    B. ureteral stenosis.
    C. renal scarring.
    D. vesicoureteral reflux.

ANSWERS

85. B	**86.** B	**87.** D
88. A	**89.** C	**90.** D
91. C	**92.** C	**93.** D

DISCUSSION

Although often thought of as a problem primarily of women, UTIs do occur in early childhood. Rates in girls younger than 1 year are around 6.5% and at 1 to 2 years are 8.1%. The rates are lower in boys: 3.3% at ages younger than 1 year and 1.9% at 1 to 2 years. Uncircumcised boys have a rate of UTI up to 20 times higher than that in circumcised boys, but this difference decreases dramatically once normal penile growth loosens the foreskin, usually occurring by the time the child is 1 to 2 years old.

The clinical presentation of UTI in children can be without the classic symptoms such as frequency, dysuria, or flank pain. In younger children, UTI often presents as irritability, lethargy, and fever with no obvious focal infectious source. Older children may present with abdominal pain and/or unexplained fever. UTI should be considered in infants and young children 2 months to 2 years of age with unexplained fever, particularly in boys younger than 6 months and girls younger than 2 years who have a temperature of 39° C (102.2° F) or higher.

A urinalysis should be obtained in a child with unexplained fever or symptoms that suggest a UTI; however, the urinalysis may be negative in up to 20% of cases. Any of the following findings are suggestive, although not diagnostic, of UTI: positive leukocyte esterase, positive nitrite, more than five white blood cells (WBCs) per high-power field in spun specimen, and bacteria present in unspun Gram-stained specimen. A septic evaluation should also be initiated if clinical presentation warrants.

The method of obtaining a urinalysis in the younger child has been long debated. Clearly, suprapubic bladder aspiration yields the specimen that is least likely to be contaminated; for the parent and child, this method can be fraught with fear and requires special provider skill. Next best is transurethral bladder catheterization. Less acceptable is a urine specimen collection via bag, because of the high rate of skin and fecal contamination.

UTIs in children can be associated with anatomic abnormalities, with vesicoureteral reflux the most commonly associated problem. Reflux nephropathy causes scarring and is a risk factor for renal failure but is largely avoidable with early reflux recognition and proper treatment. Little difference is usually found in the clinical presentation and laboratory findings of cystitis or pyelonephritis in the febrile child, and determining whether a UTI is limited to the lower urinary tract or involves the soft tissue of the kidney is not clinically significant. The management of the child with UTI is dictated by the clinical severity of the illness, rather than by the specific site of infection in the urinary tract. As a result, a single documented UTI in a child must be taken seriously.

If the infant or young child 2 months to 2 years of age with suspected UTI is assessed as toxic, dehydrated, or unable to retain oral intake, hospitalization should be considered. Initial antimicrobial therapy should be administered parenterally, usually with a second- or third-generation cephalosporin. An aminoglycoside is a second-line choice and may be used if there is a history of severe penicillin allergy. For the child who is well hydrated and able to take an antimicrobial and fluids orally, home-based care is reasonable. An oral second- or third-generation cephalosporin is a reasonable initial therapy; there is a small risk of treatment failure with the use of TMP-SMX. In children ages 2 months to 2 years, a 7- to 14-day antimicrobial course should be prescribed, with at least 7 days of therapy for older children. If the child responds to therapy, antimicrobial prophylaxis with an oral cephalosporin or TMP-SMX should be continued until imaging and urologic evaluations are complete.

Urinary tract abnormality is a major risk factor for pediatric UTI, with vesicoureteral reflux noted in 30% to 50% of cases. Reflux increases the risk of ascending infection, which leads to pyelonephritis and renal scarring. Therefore, urinary tract imaging should be considered for all children with UTI, particularly if this occurs before toilet training. Renal ultrasound is an easily obtained, noninvasive test, but when used as the sole study, reflux will often be missed. The preferred test for vesicoureteral reflux is the cystogram. A renal scan is the best study for detecting renal scarring, a finding present only after infection, but will miss reflux, and might therefore identify patients at particular risk for reflux. If reflux or other urinary tract abnormality is noted on imaging, antimicrobial prophylaxis should continue until the abnormality is corrected.

DISCUSSION SOURCES

Desai, S. (2004). Clinician's Guide to Laboratory Medicine (3rd ed.). Hudson, OH: Lexi-Comp.

Practice parameter: The diagnosis, treatment, and evaluation of the initial urinary tract infection in febrile infants and young children. American Academy of Pediatrics Committee on Quality Improvement. Subcommittee on Urinary Tract Infection (1999). Pediatrics 103:843–852.

QUESTIONS

94. You examine a 10-year-old boy with suspected streptococcal pharyngitis. His mother asks if he can get a "shot of penicillin." You consider the following when counseling her about the use of IM penicillin:

   A. There is nearly a 100% cure rate in strep pharyngitis when IM penicillin is used.

   B. Treatment failure rates with IM penicillin approach 20%.

   C. The risk of severe allergic reaction with IM products is similar to that of oral preparations.

   D. Injectable penicillin has a superior spectrum of antimicrobial coverage in comparison with the oral form of the drug.

95. You examine a 15-year-old child presenting with a 1-day history of sore throat, low-grade fever, maculopapular rash, and cervical and occipital lymphadenopathy. The most likely diagnosis is:

A. scarlet fever.
B. roseola.
C. rubella.
D. rubeola.

96. A 4-year-old child presents with fever, exudative pharyngitis, anterior cervical lymphadenopathy, and a fine, raised, pink rash. The most likely diagnosis is:

   A. scarlet fever.
   B. roseola.
   C. rubella.
   D. rubeola.

97. An 18-year-old woman has a chief complaint of "a sore throat and swollen glands" for the past 3 days. Her physical examination reveals exudative pharyngitis, minimally tender anterior and posterior cervical lymphadenopathy, and maculopapular rash. Abdominal examination reveals right and left upper quadrant abdominal tenderness. The most likely diagnosis is:

   A. group A beta-hemolytic streptococcal pharyngitis.
   B. infectious mononucleosis.
   C. rubella.
   D. scarlet fever.

98. Which of the following is most likely to be found in the laboratory data of a child who has infectious mononucleosis?

   A. neutrophilia
   B. lymphocytosis with atypical lymphocytes
   C. positive antinuclear antibody
   D. macrocytic anemia

99. You examine a 15-year-old boy who has infectious mononucleosis with marked tonsillar hypertrophy, exudative pharyngitis, difficulty swallowing, and a patent airway. You prescribe the following:

   A. amoxicillin
   B. prednisone
   C. ibuprofen
   D. acyclovir

100. A 2-year-old girl presents with pustular, ulcerating lesions on the hands and feet, as well as oral ulcers. The child is cranky, well hydrated, and afebrile. The most likely diagnosis is:

   A. hand-foot-and-mouth disease.
   B. aphthous stomatitis.
   C. herpetic gingivostomatitis.
   D. Vincent angina.

101. A 6-year-old boy presents with a 1-day history of fiery red, maculopapular facial rash concentrated on the cheeks. He has had mild headache and myalgia for the past week. The most likely diagnosis is:

   A. erythema infectiosum.
   B. roseola.
   C. rubella.
   D. scarlet fever.

ANSWERS

94. B	95. C	96. A
97. B	98. B	99. B
100. A	101. A	

DISCUSSION

Developing an accurate diagnosis of an acute febrile illness with associated rash or skin lesion can be a daunting task. Knowledge of the infectious agent, its incubation period, its mode of transmission, and its common clinical presentation can be helpful. See the following table on pages 339–340.

QUESTIONS

102. Which of the following best describes asthma?

   A. intermittent airway inflammation with occasional bronchospasm
   B. a disease of bronchospasm leading to airway inflammation
   C. chronic airway inflammation with superimposed bronchospasm
   D. relatively fixed airway constriction

Clinical condition with causative agent	Presentation	Comments
Roseola Agent: Human herpesvirus 6 (HHV-6)	Discrete rosy-pink macular or maculopapular rash, lasting hours to 3 days, that follows a 3–7 day period of fever, often quite high	90% of cases seen in children <2 years. Febrile seizures in up to 10% of children affected. Treatment: supportive
Scarlet fever Agent: *S. pyogenes* (group A beta hemolytic streptococci)	Scarlatina form or sandpaper-like rash with exudative pharyngitis, fever, headache, tender, localized anterior cervical lymphadenopathy	Rash may peel during treatment. Treatment: identical to *S. pyogenes* pharyngitis ("strep throat")
Rubella Agent: Rubella virus	Mild symptoms; fever, sore throat, malaise, nasal discharge, diffuse maculopapular rash lasting about 3 days. Posterior cervical and postauricular lymphadenopathy 5–10 days prior to onset of rash. Arthralgia in about 25% (most common in women)	Incubation period about 14–21 days with disease transmissible for ~1 week prior to onset of rash to ~2 weeks after rash appears. Generally a mild self-limiting illness. Greatest risk is effect of virus on the unborn child, especially with 1st trimester exposure (~80% rate congenital rubella syndrome). Treatment is supportive. Prevent with immunization.
Measles Agent: Rubeola virus	Usually acute presentation with fever, nasal discharge, cough, generalized lymphadenopathy, conjunctivitis (copious clear discharge), photophobia, and maculopapular rash. Onset 3–4 days after onset of symptoms may coalesce to generalized erythema. Koplik spots found in about half, appearing ~2 days prior to onset of rash as nearly pinpoint white lesions on mucous membranes, conjunctival folds, clear about 3 days after rash erupts. Pharyngitis is usually mild without exudate.	Incubation period about 10–14 days with disease transmissible for ~1 week prior to onset of rash to ~2–3 weeks after rash appears. CNS and respiratory tract complications common. Treatment is supportive with intervention as needed for complications. Prevent by immunization.
Hand, foot, and mouth disease. Agent: Coxsackie virus A16	Fever, malaise, sore mouth, anorexia. 1–2 days later are lesions. Also can cause conjunctivitis, pharyngitis. Duration of disease 2–7 days.	Transmission via oral, fecal, or droplet. Highly contagious, with incubation periods of 2–6 weeks. Treatment is supportive.
Fifth disease Agent: Human parvovirus B19	3–4 days of mild flu-like illness followed by 7–10 days of red rash that begins on face, with slapped cheek appearance; spreads to trunk and extremities. Rash onset corresponds with disease immunity with patient. Viremic and contagious prior but not after onset of rash.	Droplet transmission. Leukopenia common. Risk of hydrops fetalis when contracted by woman during pregnancy. Treatment is supportive.

(continued)

Clinical condition with causative agent	Presentation	Comments
Infectious mononucleosis (IM) Agent: Epstein-Barr viruses (human herpesvirus-4 or HHV-4)	Rash: Maculopapular rash in ~20%, rare petechial rash. Fever, "shaggy" purple-white exudative pharyngitis, malaise, marked diffuse lymphadenopathy, hepatic and splenic tenderness and occasional enlargement. Diagnostic testing: heterophil antibody test (monospot). Leukopenia with lymphocytosis with atypical lymphocytes.	Incubation period 20–50 days. >90% will develop a rash if given amoxicillin or ampicillin. Potential for respiratory distress when enlarged tonsils and lymphoid tissue impinge on the upper airway; corticosteroids may be helpful if upper airway compromised or severe dysphagia. Avoid contact sports for at =>1 month due to risk of splenic rupture. Treatment is otherwise supportive.
Acute HIV infection Agent: Human immunodeficiency virus	Maculopapular rash, fever, mild pharyngitis, ulcerating oral lesions, diarrhea, diffuse lymphadenopathy.	Most likely to occur in response to infection with large viral load. Consult with HIV specialist concerning initiation of antiretroviral therapy.

103. A 5-year-old boy has a 3-year history of moderate persistent asthma that is normally well controlled with budesonide via nebulizer twice a day and the use of albuterol once or twice a week as needed for wheezing. Three days ago, he developed a sore throat, clear nasal discharge, and a dry cough. In the past 24 hours, he has had intermittent wheezing, necessitating the use of albuterol, two puffs every 3 hours, with partial relief. Your next most appropriate action is to obtain:

A. a chest radiograph.
B. an oxygen saturation measurement.
C. a peak expiratory flow (PEF) measurement.
D. a sputum smear for WBCs.

104. You examine a 4-year-old girl who has an acute asthma flare. She is using budesonide and albuterol as directed and continues to have difficulty with coughing and wheezing. Her PEF is 55% of predicted with fair effort. Respiratory rate is within 50% of upper limits of normal for her age. Her medication regimen should be adjusted to include:

A. theophylline.
B. salmeterol (Serevent).
C. prednisolone.
D. montelukast (Singulair).

105. Which of the following is not consistent with the diagnosis of asthma?

A. a troublesome nocturnal cough
B. cough or wheeze after exercise
C. morning sputum production
D. colds "go to the chest" or take more than 10 days to clear

106. Celeste is a 9-year-old with moderate intermittent asthma. She is not using a prescribed inhaled corticosteroid but is using albuterol PRN to relieve her cough and wheeze. According to her mother, she currently uses about six albuterol doses per day. You respond that:

A. albuterol use may continue.
B. excessive albuterol use is a risk factor for asthma death.
C. she should also use salmeterol (Serevent) to reduce her albuterol use.
D. theophylline should be added to her treatment plan.

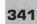

107. In the treatment of asthma, leukotriene modifiers should be used as:

    A. long-acting bronchodilators.
    B. inflammatory inhibitors.
    C. rescue drugs.
    D. intervention in acute inflammation.

108. According to the National Asthma Education and Prevention Program Expert Panel Report 2 (NAEPP EPR-2) guidelines, which of the following is not a risk factor for asthma death?

    A. hospitalization or an emergency department visit for asthma in the past month
    B. current use of systemic corticosteroids or recent withdrawal from systemic corticosteroids
    C. difficulty perceiving airflow obstruction or its severity
    D. rural residence

109. A middle-school student presents, asking for a letter stating that he should not participate in gym class because he has asthma. The most appropriate response is to:

    A. write the note, because gym class participation may trigger an asthma flare.
    B. excuse him from outdoor activities only in order to avoid pollen exposure.
    C. remind him that with appropriate asthma care, he should be capable of participating in gym class.
    D. excuse him from indoor activities only in order to avoid dust mite exposure.

110. After inhaled corticosteroid or leukotriene modifier therapy is initiated, clinical effects will be seen:

    A. immediately.
    B. within the first week.
    C. in about 1 to 2 weeks.
    D. in about 1 to 2 months.

111. In comparison with albuterol, levalbuterol (Xopenex):

    A. has a different mechanism of action.
    B. has the ability to provide greater bronchodilatation with a lower dose.
    C. has an anti-inflammatory effect similar to that of an inhaled corticosteroid.
    D. is contraindicated for use in children.

112. In caring for the child with an acute asthma flare, the NP considers that, according to the NAEPP EPR-2 guidelines, antibiotic use is recommended:

    A. routinely.
    B. with evidence of infection.
    C. when asthma flares are frequent.
    D. with sputum production.

ANSWERS

102. C	**103.** C	**104.** C
105. C	**106.** B	**107.** B
108. D	**109.** C	**110.** C
111. B	**112.** B	

DISCUSSION

Asthma is a chronic airway inflammatory disease involving an increase in bronchial hyper-responsiveness with superimposed bronchospasm and a resulting decrease in the ratio of forced expiratory volume in 1 second to forced vital capacity. Although the condition ranks second after allergic rhinitis as the most common chronic respiratory disease in North America, many persons with asthma continue to be undiagnosed and therefore untreated (see Table 5–1).

The goals of asthma care according to the NAEPP EPR-2 are presented as follows, with a brief explanation of the rationale for each objective:

- minimal or, ideally, no chronic symptoms such as cough and wheeze, including nocturnal symptoms

    Asthma symptoms typically follow a circadian rhythm, in which bronchospasm is worse during the night sleep hours. Therefore, a marker of effective airway inflammation control is minimal nocturnal symptoms. With young children, parents often report awakening to the child's repeated cough while the child continues to sleep. Conversely, asthma flares are often harder to control during the nighttime hours.

- no emergency room or emergency visits

  When airway inflammatory control is poor, children with asthma typically use emergency services for treatment of frequent acute flares. With appropriate asthma family teaching to help with management of acute and chronic airway inflammation and its resulting symptoms, emergency visits can be minimized or eliminated.

- minimal (ideally no) use of PRN short-acting beta$_2$ agonist (certainly two or fewer uses of beta$_2$ agonist per week)

  Asthma is a disease of airway inflammation with superimposed bronchospasm. The need for short-acting beta$_2$ agonist use as a rescue drug should be viewed as failure to provide adequate airway inflammatory control. Excessive beta$_2$ agonist use is a risk factor for asthma death (see the following table on pages 343–344)

- no limitations on activities, including physical activity

  When airway inflammation is inadequate, asthma symptoms such as cough or wheeze can accompany or immediately follow physical activity. The child with well-controlled asthma should be able and encouraged to participate in fitness and leisure activities.

- PEF circadian variation of less than 20%

  The body's normal circadian rhythm provides a variation of awakening to late evening PEF of 10% to 15%. With asthma, this variation increases to more than 15%, reflecting the nocturnal bronchospasm that is a part of the disease. Usually the child younger than 4 to 5 will have some difficulty with obtaining a peak flow.

- (near) normal PEF

  With asthma treatment that focuses on the prevention of airway inflammation and bronchospasm, the PEF can be normal or near normal.

- no or minimal side effects while optimal medications are given

  Because of the wide range of asthma medications currently available, the NP, patient, and family can work together to find a lifestyle and treatment regimen that provides optimal care with minimal to few adverse medication effects.

The backbone of therapy for mild persistent, moderate persistent, or severe persistent asthma is the use of an inflammatory controller drug such as an inhaled corticosteroid, mast cell stabilizers such as nedocromil or cromolyn, and leukotriene modifiers such as montelukast or zafirlukast. Although all these products afford anti-inflammatory capability, the inhaled corticosteroids have proved to be the most effective in preventing airway inflammation and are recognized as the preferred asthma controller drug. Rescue medications that relieve acute superimposed bronchospasm include short-acting beta$_2$ agonists, such as albuterol, levalbuterol, and pirbuterol. In comparison with albuterol and pirbuterol, some of levalbuterol's therapeutic advantages include greater bronchodilatation with fewer side effects and at a lower dosage. Long-acting beta$_2$ agonists such as salmeterol and formoterol provide bronchospasm protection. In moderate or severe persistent asthma, adding a long-acting beta$_2$ agonist to the inhaled corticosteroid is more effective in achieving symptom control than is increasing the inhaled corticosteroid dosage. Adding a leukotriene modifier to an inhaled corticosteroid or doubling the dosage of the inhaled corticosteroid also improves asthma outcome, but the evidence is not as substantial as that for adding a long-acting beta$_2$ agonist. It is important to remember that the clinical effects of the inhaled corticosteroid and leukotriene modifier take at least 1 to 2 weeks to be seen. Theophylline remains helpful in preventing

Medication	Mechanism of action	Indication	Comment
Inhaled corticosteroids	Inhibit eosinophilic action and other inflammatory mediators, potentate effects of beta-2 agonists	Controller drug, prevention of inflammation	Need consistent use to be helpful
Mast cell stabilizer Cromolyn sodium (Intal), nedocromil (Tilade)	Halts degradation of mast cells and release of histamine and other inflammatory mediators (mast cell stabilizer)	Controller drug, prevention of inflammation	• Need consistent use to be helpful • Less clinical effect when compared with inhaled corticosteroids
Leukotriene modifier (LTM) Leukotriene antagonists (LTRA) (montelukast [Singulair], zafirlukast[Accolate])	Inhibits action of inflammatory mediator, leukotriene, by blocking select receptor sites	Controller drug, prevention of inflammation	Likely less effective than inhaled corticosteroids. Particularly effective add-on medication when disease control inadequate with inhaled corticosteroid, when asthma complicated by allergic rhinitis
Oral corticosteroids	Inhibit eosinophilic action and other inflammatory mediators	Treatment of acute inflammation such as in asthma flare	• Indicated in treatment of acute asthma flare to reduce inflammation • In higher dose and with longer therapy (>2 weeks), adrenal suppression may occur • No taper needed if use is short-term (<10 days) and at lower dose • Potential for causing gastropathy, particularly gastric ulcer and gastritis
Beta-2 agonist Albuterol (Ventolin, Proventil), pirbuterol (Maxair), levalbuterol (Xopenex)	Bronchodilation via stimulation of B_2 receptor site	Rescue drugs for treatment of acute bronchospasm	• Onset of action = 15 minutes • Duration of action = 4–6 hours

(continued)

Medication	Mechanism of action	Indication	Comment
Long-acting beta-2 agonists (Salmeterol (Serevent), formoterol (Foradil)	Beta-2 agonist; bronchodilation via stimulation of B_2 receptor site	Prevention of bronchospasm	Salmeterol • Onset of action = 1 hour • Duration of action = 12 hours • Indicated for prevention rather than treatment of bronchospasm • Patient should also have short-acting beta-2 agonist as rescue drug Formoterol • Onset of action = 15–30 hours • Duration of action = 12 hours • Indicated for prevention rather than treatment of bronchospasm • Patient should also have short-acting beta-2 agonist as rescue drug
Anticholinergics (Ipratropium bromide [Atrovent] Tiotropium bromide [Spiriva])	Anticholinergic and muscarinic antagonist, yielding bronchodilatation	Treatment and prevention of bronchospasm	• Onset of action =>1 h Best used to avoid rather than treat the bronchospasm associated with COPD and asthma • Well tolerated
Theophylline	Mild bronchodilator, helps with diaphragmatic contraction	Prevention of bronchospasm, mild anti-inflammatory	• Narrow therapeutic index drug with numerous drug interactions. • Monitor carefully for toxicity by checking drug levels and clinical presentation.

bronchospasm; as a narrow therapeutic index medication, the theophylline dose must be closely titrated and monitored with serial serum drug levels, which significantly limit the drug's usefulness.

When acute asthma flare is present with increased symptoms and, if measured, PEF is less than 50% to 80% of predicted, rapidly acting higher potency anti-inflammatory therapy with an oral corticosteroid is needed. Adding more bronchodilators, such as theophylline and salmeterol, does not reverse the cause of the bronchospasm, which is significant airway inflammation. The leukotriene modifiers are helpful in preventing, but not acutely treating, inflammation (see Table 5–4).

Because this is a lower airway disease, the person with asthma has more of a problem with expiration, or getting air out, than with inspiration, or getting air in. This leads to findings characteristic of air trapping such as decreased PEF rate, prolonged expiratory phase, thoracic hyperresonance on percussion, and hyperinflation is seen on chest radiographs.

Oxygen desaturation is a late finding in an acute asthma flare.

DISCUSSION SOURCES

Hill, N., and Sullivan, L. (2004). Management Guidelines for Nurse Practitioners Working with Children and Adolescents (2nd ed.) Philadelphia: F. A. Davis.

Larsen, G., Accurso, F., Deterding, R., et al. (2003). Respiratory tract and mediastinum. In Hay, W., Hayward, A., Levin, M., and Sondheimer, J. (eds.). Current Pediatric Diagnosis and Treatment (16th ed., pp. 492–545). New York: McGraw-Hill.

National Asthma Education and Prevention Program, Expert Panel Report 2: Guidelines for the Diagnosis and Management of Asthma. Available at http://www.nhlbi.nih.gov/guide-lines/asthma/, accessed 1/5/05.

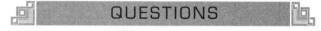

QUESTIONS

113. Which of the following advice should you give to a breast-feeding mother whose infant has gastroenteritis?

   A. Discontinue breast-feeding.
   B. Give the infant oral rehydration solution.
   C. Continue breast-feeding.
   D. Supplement with flat ginger ale.

114. Which of the following is the advice you should give to the parents of a toddler with gastroenteritis?

   A. Try sips of cola.
   B. Give the child sips of an oral rehydration solution.
   C. Give the child sips of Gatorade.
   D. Try sips of apple juice.

115. The onset of symptoms of food poisoning caused by *Staphylococcus* species is typically how many hours after the ingestion of the offending substance?

   A. 0.5 to 1
   B. 1 to 4
   C. 4 to 8
   D. 8 to 12

116. The onset of symptoms in food poisoning caused by *Salmonella* species is typically how many hours after the ingestion of the offending substance?

   A. 2 to 8
   B. 8 to 12
   C. 12 to more than 24
   D. 24 to 36

117. In order to obtain the most accurate hydration status in a child with acute gastroenteritis, a NP should ask about:

   A. the time of last urination.
   B. thirst.
   C. quantity of liquids taken.
   D. number of episodes of vomiting and diarrhea.

118. What percentage of body weight is typically lost in a child with moderate dehydration?

   A. 2 to 3
   B. 3 to 5
   C. 6 to 10
   D. 11 to 15

119. Clinical features of shigellosis include all of the following except:

   A. bloody diarrhea.
   B. high fever.
   C. malaise.
   D. vomiting.

ANSWERS

113. C	**114.** B	**115.** B
116. C	**117.** A	**118.** C
119. D		

DISCUSSION

Acute gastroenteritis is a common episodic disease of childhood. Usually viral in nature, the child presents with vomiting and diarrhea of short duration that typically are free of blood and pus. In addition, the child usually does not have a fever. Usually there is a history of contacts with children or adults who have similar symptoms. The duration of illness is usually short (less than 4 days with no sequelae). One of the most important parts of the assessment of a child with acute gastroenteritis is determining hydration status. Asking about the last urination provides a helpful way of evaluating this. If the child has voided within the previous few hours, the degree of dehydration is minimal. A number of other clinical parameters are helpful in assessing for dehydration (Table 14–4). Although mild dehydration can usually be managed with frequent small-volume feedings of oral rehydration solutions such as Pedialyte, a child with moderate to severe dehydration likely needs parenteral fluids. Sports drinks such as Gatorade and soda are not appropriate for rehydration solution. The use of antidiarrheal agents is usually discouraged because of the risk of increasing the severity of illness if a toxin-producing bacteria is the causative agent.

Warning signs during acute gastroenteritis include fever coupled with bloody or pus-filled stools. If these are present, consider a bacterial source of infection such as shigellosis. Stool culture should be obtained and appropriate antimicrobial therapy initiated.

Improperly handled food is a common source of gastrointestinal infection. Knowledge of the timing of the onset of symptoms is helpful when attempting to discern the offending organism. Most food poisoning episodes are short and self-limiting, resolving over a few hours to days without special intervention.

DISCUSSION SOURCES

Hill, N., and Sullivan, L. (2004). Management Guidelines for Nurse Practitioners Working with Children and Adolescents (2nd ed.). Philadelphia: F.A. Davis.

Sondheimer, J. (2003). Gastrointestinal tract. In Hay, W., Hayward, A., Levin, M., and Sondheimer, J. (eds.). Current Pediatric Diagnosis and Treatment (16th ed., pp. 614–646). New York: McGraw-Hill.

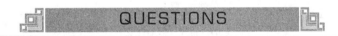

QUESTIONS

120. The most common reason for precocious puberty in girls is:

    A. ovarian tumor.
    B. adrenal tumor.

TABLE 14–4

CLINICAL PRESENTATION OF PATIENTS WITH DEHYDRATION

Clinical Presentation	Mild Dehydration	Moderate Dehydration	Severe Dehydration
Skin turgor	Normal	Slightly to moderately decreased	Markedly decreased with tenting possible
Capillary refill	2 sec	2–4 sec	>4 sec
Tears	Normal to slightly decreased	Slightly decreased	Markedly decreased to absent
Pulse	Normal	Slightly increased	Tachycardia
Blood pressure	Normal	Normal	Low
Mucous membranes	Normal to slightly dry	Dry	Parched
Urine output	Mildly decreased	Decreased	Anuria

Reference: Ford, D. (2003). Fluid, electrolyte and acid-base therapy. In Hay, W., Hayward, A., Levin, M., & Sondheimer, J. *Current Pediatric Diagnosis and Treatment* (16th ed.) St. Louis: McGraw-Hill/Appleton & Lange.

C. exogenous estrogen.

D. early onset of normal puberty.

121. The most common reason for precocious puberty in boys is:

   A. testicular tumor.
   B. a number of relatively uncommon health problems.
   C. exogenous testosterone.
   D. early onset of normal puberty.

122. Which of the following is noted in the child with premature thelarche?

   A. breast enlargement
   B. accelerated linear growth
   C. pubic hair
   D. body odor

123. Which of the following is noted in the child with premature adrenarche?

   A. breast enlargement
   B. accelerated linear growth
   C. pubic hair
   D. menstruation

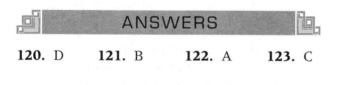

ANSWERS

120. D   **121.** B   **122.** A   **123.** C

DISCUSSION

Precocious puberty in girls has long been defined as the onset of secondary sexual characteristics before the eighth birthday. More recent study reveals that there may be a group of girls who have the onset of slowly developing secondary sexual characteristics between ages 6 and 8 years as a benign variant. As a result, the most common reason for precocious puberty in girls is early onset of normal puberty. However, a subset of girls, particularly those with pubertal changes noted before the sixth birthday, often have significant health problems such as ovarian or adrenal tumors.

Expert evaluation and referral are indicated. Evaluation typically includes measuring bone age, level of follicle-stimulating hormone, and level of luteinizing hormone and abdominal ultrasound. Treatment depends on the cause. In the absence of an adrenal or ovarian tumor, counseling about the nature of the process of early puberty should be discussed with the child and family. Because girls typically achieve nearly all of their adult height 1 year after the first menstrual period, a girl achieving menarche at a premature age may have short stature. If the child and family wish to attempt to halt the onset of puberty, a gonadotropin-releasing hormone analog may be given by injection to counteract the effects of endogenous hormones. The long-term effect of this therapy on fertility is not known.

Premature thelarche is a relatively common, benign process in which breast enlargement is noted in female toddlers. It is present unilaterally or bilaterally, and there are no other signs of puberty, including accelerated linear growth. Reassurance and ongoing monitoring are the typical course of treatment. In premature adrenarche, a parent usually reports that the child between ages 5 and 6 years has body odor, pubic hair, and, rarely, axillary hair. There are no other signs of puberty, including accelerated linear growth. Reassurance and ongoing monitoring constitute the typical course of treatment.

In boys, precocious puberty is defined as the onset of secondary sexual characteristics before the ninth birthday. Overall, this condition is less common in boys than in girls and is less likely to be a benign normal variation. Gonadal and adrenal tumors, as well as a number of genetically based diseases, are the most likely causes. Prompt referral to expert care is indicated.

DISCUSSION SOURCE

Kappy, M., Steelman, R., Teaver, S., and Zeiter, P. (2003). Endocrine disorders. In Hay, W., Groothuis, J., Hayward, A., and Levin, M. (eds.).

Current Pediatric Diagnosis and Treatment (16th ed., pp. 937–976). New York: McGraw-Hill.

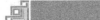

QUESTIONS

124. An innocent murmur has which of the following characteristics?

    A. It occurs late in systole.

    B. It has a localized area of auscultation.

    C. It becomes softer when the patient moves from the supine to standing position.

    D. It frequently obliterates the second heart sound (S_2).

125. The murmur of atrial septal defect is usually:

    A. found in children with symptoms of cardiac disease.

    B. first found on a 2- to 6-month well-child examination.

    C. found with mitral valve prolapse.

    D. presystolic in timing.

126. A Still murmur:

    A. is heard in the presence of cardiac pathology.

    B. has a humming or vibratory quality.

    C. is a reason for denying sports participation clearance.

    D. has the ability to become louder when the patient is standing.

ANSWERS

124. C   **125.** B   **126.** B

DISCUSSION

The ability to appropriately assess children with a heart murmur is an important part of the role of an NP. Knowledge of the most common murmurs, clinical presentation, and impact on a child's health is critical to appropriate assessment. It is also necessary to be able to determine the need for specialty referral (Table 14–5).

QUESTIONS

127. When assessing a febrile child, the NP considers that:

    A. any degree of temperature elevation is harmful.

    B. nuchal rigidity is usually not found in early childhood meningitis.

    C. fever-related seizures usually occur at the peak of the temperature.

    D. most children with temperatures of 101° to 104° F have a potentially serious bacterial infection.

128. Which of the following is *not* seen during body temperature increase found in fever?

    A. lower rate of viral replication

    B. toxic effect on select bacteria

    C. negative effect on *S. pneumoniae* growth

    D. increased rate of atypical pneumonia pathogen replication

129. When providing care for the febrile child, the NP bears in mind that all of the following are true except that:

    A. the use of antipyretics has been associated with prolonged illness.

    B. antipyretics shorten the course of viral and bacterial illness.

    C. fever increases metabolic demand.

    D. in the pregnant woman, increased body temperature is a potential first-trimester teratogen.

130. Concerning the use of antipyretics in the febrile young child, which of the following is true?

    A. A child with a serious bacterial infection will not have fever reduction with an antipyretic.

    B. The degree of temperature reduction in response to antipyretic therapy is not predictive of presence or absence of bacteremia.

    C. In comparison with ibuprofen, aceta-

TABLE 14–5

DIFFERENTIAL DIAGNOSIS OF COMMON HEART MURMURS IN CHILDREN

When evaluating a child with cardiac murmur:

- Ask about the major symptoms of heart disease: chest pain, congestive heart failure symptoms, palpitations, syncope, activity intolerance, and poor growth and development.
- The bell of the stethoscope is most helpful for auscultating lower-pitched sounds, and the diaphragm is better for those with higher pitch.
- Systolic murmurs are graded on a 1 to 6 scale, from barely audible to audible with stethoscope off the chest. Diastolic murmurs are usually graded on the same scale but abbreviated to grades 1 to 4 because these murmurs will not be loud enough to reach grades 5 and 6.
- A critical part of the evaluation of a child with a heart murmur is the decision to offer antimicrobial prophylaxis. No prophylaxis is needed with benign murmurs. Please refer to the American Heart Association's Guidelines for the latest advice.

Murmur	Important Cardiac Examination Findings	Additional Findings	Comments
Newborn	Gr 1–2/6 early systolic, vibratory, heard best at LLSB with little radiation Pulses intact, otherwise well neonate	Subsides or disappears when pressure applied to abdomen	Heard in first few days of life; disappears in 2–3 weeks Benign condition
Still's (vibratory innocent murmur)	Gr 1–3/6 early systolic ejection, musical or vibratory, short, often buzzing, heard best midway between apex and LLSB	Softens or disappears when sitting, standing, or with Valsalva maneuver Louder when supine or with fever or tachycardia	Usual onset age 2–6 years; may persist through adolescence Benign condition
Hemic	Gr 1–2/6 systolic ejection, high-pitched, heard best in pulmonic and aortic areas	Heard only in the presence of increased cardiac output, such as fever, anemia, stress	Disappears when underlying condition resolves Usually seen without cardiac disease Most often heard in children and younger adults with thin chest walls
Venous hum	Gr 1–2/6 continuous musical hum heard best at the URSB and ULSB and the lower neck	Disappears in supine position, when jugular vein is compressed Common after age 3 years	Believed to be produced by turbulence in the subclavian and jugular veins Benign condition
Pulmonary outflow ejection murmur	Gr 1–2/6 soft, short, systolic ejection murmur, heard best at LLSB, usually localized.	Softens or disappears when sitting, standing, or with Valsalva maneuver Louder when supine	Heard throughout childhood Benign condition but has qualities similar to murmurs caused by pathologic condition such as ASD, COA, PS

Murmur	Important Cardiac Examination Findings	Additional Findings	Comments
Patent ductus arteriosus	Gr 2–4/6 continuous murmur heard best at ULSB and left infraclavicular area	In premature newborns, seen with active precordium. In older children, with full pulses	Normal ductus closure occurs by day 4 of life Often isolated finding but may be seen with COA, VSD Accounts for +/− 12% of all congenital heart disease Twice as common in females In preterm infants < 1500 g, rate as high as 20%–60%
Atrial septal defect	Gr 1–3/6 systolic ejection murmur heard best at the ULSB with widely split fixed S_2	Accompanying mid-diastolic murmur heard at the fourth ICS LSB commonly caused by increased flow across tricuspid valve	Two times as common in females Child may be entirely well or present with CHF Often missed in the first few months of life or even entire childhood Watch for children with easy fatigability Cyanosis rare
Ventricular septal defect	Gr 2–5/6 regurgitant systolic murmur heard best at LLSB Occasionally holosystolic, usually localized	Thrill may be present as well as a loud P_2 with large left-to-right shunt	Usually without cyanosis Children with small- to moderate-sized left-to-right shunt without pulmonary hypertension likely to have minimal symptoms Larger shunts may result in CHF with onset in infancy
Aortic stenosis	Gr 2–5/6 systolic ejection murmur heard best in ULSB or a second RICS, possibly with paradoxically split S_2	Ejection click at apex, third LICS, second RICS Radiation or thrill to the carotid arteries	More common in males than females In children, usually caused by unicuspid (if noted in infancy) or bicuspid (if noted in childhood) valve Mild exercise intolerance common
Coarctation of the aorta (COA)	Gr 1–5/6 systolic ejection murmur heard best at the ULSB and left interscapular area (on back)	Weak or absent femoral pulses, hypertension in arms	Often seen with AS, MR Presence of dorsalis pedis pulse in child essentially rules out this condition
Mitral valve prolapse	Gr 1–3/6 midsystolic click followed by a late systolic murmur heard best at the apex	Murmur heard earlier in systole and often louder with standing or squatting	Often with pectus excavatum, straight back (>85%)
Pulmonic valve stenosis	Gr 2–5/6 heard best at ULSB, ejection click at second LICS	Radiates to the back S2 may be widely split	No symptoms with mild to moderate disease Usually a fusion of valvular cusps

References: Park, M. (2002). *Pediatric Cardiology for Practitioners, 4th ed.* St. Louis: Mosby-Yearbook.

minophen is more effective in reducing higher fevers.

   D. Ibuprofen should not be used if the child is also taking a macrolide.

131. When evaluating the child who has bacterial meningitis, the NP expects to find cerebrospinal fluid (CSF) results of:

   A. low protein.
   B. predominance of lymphocytes.
   C. glucose at about 30% of serum levels.
   D. low opening pressure.

132. When evaluating the child who has aseptic or viral meningitis, the NP expects to find CSF results of:

   A. low protein.
   B. predominance of lymphocytes.
   C. glucose at about 30% of serum levels.
   D. low opening pressure.

133. Sepsis is defined as the:

   A. clinical manifestation of systemic infection.
   B. presence of bacteria in the blood.
   C. circulation of pathogens.
   D. allergenic response to infection.

134. Gina is 2-year-old who presents with a 3-day history of fever, crankiness, and congested cough. Her respiratory rate is more than 50% of the upper limits of normal for age. Tubular breath sounds are noted at the right lung base. Skin turgor is within normal limits, and she is wearing a wet diaper. She is alert, is age-appropriately resisting the examination, and engages in eye contact. Temperature is 101° F. Gina's diagnostic evaluation should include:

   A. chest x-ray.
   B. urine culture and sensitivity measurement.
   C. lumbar puncture.
   D. sputum culture

135. As part of the evaluation in a febrile 3-year-old boy, the following WBC count with differential is obtained:

WBCs = 22,100/mm^3
Neutrophils = 75% (normal = 40% to 70%) with toxic granulation
Bands = 15% (normal = 0% to 4%)
Lymphocytcs = 4% (normal = 30% to 40%)
These results increase the likelihood that the cause of this child's infection is:
   A. viral.
   B. parasitic.
   C. fungal.
   D. bacterial.

136. As part of the evaluation in a febrile 18-month-old girl, the following WBC count with differential is obtained:

WBCs = 6100/mm^3
Neutrophils = 35% (normal = 40% to 70%)
Bands = 3% (normal = 0% to 4%)
Lymphocytes = 52% (normal = 30% to 40%)
Reactive lymphocytes = 10%
These results increase the likelihood that the cause of this child's infection is:
   A. viral.
   B. parasitic.
   C. fungal.
   D. bacterial.

137. Which of the following is the most appropriate way of reducing fever and discomfort in a child with varicella?

   A. ibuprofen
   B. aspirin
   C. acetaminophen
   D. alcohol rub

138. Which of the following is the most effective way of reducing fever in an 18-month-old with a temperature of 103.5° F and AOM?

   A. ibuprofen
   B. aspirin
   C. acetaminophen
   D. cool water bath

139. Which of the following medications can be given at the onset of a febrile illness to minimize the risk of recurrence in a child with a history of febrile seizure?

A. ibuprofen
B. phenytoin
C. phenobarbital
D. diazepam

ANSWERS

127. B	**128.** D	**129.** B
130. B	**131.** C	**132.** B
133. A	**134.** A	**135.** D
136. A	**137.** C	**138.** A
139. D		

DISCUSSION

Most young children with an acute febrile illness do not have a serious bacterial infection and recover fully without sequelae. However, about 4% to 6% of febrile young children with no obvious source of infection may suffer serious sequelae or death. As a result, the evaluation and treatment of the febrile child is an important part of providing pediatric primary care.

Fever is a complex physiologic reaction that occurs when exogenous pyrogens (microorganisms and their products, drugs, incompatible blood products) are introduced to the body. This triggers the production of endogenous pyrogens (polypeptides produced by host cells such as monocytes, macrophages; interleukin-1α, interleukin-1α, interferon-α, interferon-β, tumor necrosis factor) that in turn increase prostaglandin synthesis. Prostaglandins activate thermoregulatory neurons and alter the hypothalamic set point. Vasomotor center reactions increase heat conservation and heat production.

Although parents and health care providers usually treat fever with antipyretics and other options, an increase in body temperature has benefits. During fever, viral replication rate is reduced. Increased body temperature is toxic to encapsulated bacteria, particularly *S. pneumoniae*. In both animal models and clinical trials in humans, the presence of fever has been associated with improvement in the morbidity and mortality associated with infectious diseases. The use of antipyretics has also been associated with prolonged illness. Conversely, the child with fever is often uncomfortable and cranky, which reinforces the perception that this is a condition that warrants treatment. Fever also increases metabolic demands, a potential problem in the child or adult with a chronic health problem; in pregnancy, fever is potentially teratogenic in the first trimester and increases metabolic demands throughout pregnancy. Fear of febrile seizure also contributes to the propensity to aggressively treat fever, with the thought that if the body temperature is reduced, seizure risk is reduced. In reality, a simple febrile seizure is most likely to occur as fever rises rather than at its peak. A familial tendency has been noted with febrile seizure, but the condition is not predictive of the development of epilepsy. A simple febrile seizure is a benign and common event in children between the ages of 6 months and 5 years; a child who has had one seizure is at increased risk for a recurrence. Although there are effective therapies, which need to be daily, that reduce risk and could prevent the occurrence of additional simple febrile seizures, including phenobarbital and phenytoin (Dilantin), the potential adverse effects of these therapies outweigh the potential benefit in this self-limiting, though frightening, condition. In situations in which parental anxiety about febrile seizures is severe, intermittent oral diazepam (Valium) at the onset of febrile illness may be effective in preventing recurrence. Antipyretics, although they may improve the comfort of the child, will not prevent febrile seizures.

In the first 2 years of life, most children average four to six acute febrile episodes per year, with health care sought in about two thirds of cases. Of these younger children with temperatures lower than 39° C (102.2° F), 80% to 90% have a viral or obvious bacterial source, and 10% to 20% have no obvious source for fever and therefore risk for occult bacteremia and subsequent serious bacterial illness. The most common causes of fever in young children are viruses and bacteria, with fungi, parasites, neoplasms, collagen vascular disease, and factitious disease being important but less common. Before pneumococcal conjugate vaccine (PCV7 [Prevnar]) was available, *S. pneumoniae* was implicated in approximately 90% of cases of occult bacteremia in febrile infants and young children. This vaccine provides activity against the seven most common pneumococcal serotypes implicated in invasive pneumococcal disease and dramatically reduces but does not eliminate the risk of invasive pneumococcal disease.

In the previously well, nontoxic febrile child 3 months to 3 years of age without identifiable source of fever and temperature lower than 39° C, the evaluation for source of fever should start with a careful history and physical examination. If the child is alert and has a nontoxic appearance, no tests or antibiotics are needed. The child's caregivers should be advised about the use of antipyretics, increased fluid intake, and signs of deteriorating condition. Follow-up in 48 hours is prudent if fever persists, sooner if the child's condition worsens.

Advising the child's caregivers about the appropriate choice and use of antipyretics is an important part of providing care for the child with non–life-threatening illness and fever. As previously mentioned, fever plays an important role in controlling infection. If the child with fever appears fairly comfortable, no treatment is needed. Indeed, even the cranky child will usually not be harmed and may be helped by allowing the fever to run its course. If the child is uncomfortable with fever, common-sense measures include dressing the child lightly and increasing fluid intake. A cooling bath should not be used, because shivering, which would drive up body temperature, usually follows this. The choice of an antipyretic is dictated by a number of factors. These include the length of time for onset of action of this product (ideally, less than half an hour) and its duration of action (ideally, 4 to 8 hours), with no or few major reported adverse effects. Ibuprofen and acetaminophen are the most commonly prescribed antipyretics, both with

onset of action within half of the dose. Acetaminophen's duration of action is about 4 hours, whereas ibuprofen's is around 6 hours. Acetaminophen's antipyretic potential is equal to that of ibuprofen for lower grade fevers (<102.5° F); with fever above this level, ibuprofen has greater antipyretic potential. Acetaminophen has an excellent gastrointestinal adverse event profile but can be hepatotoxic with excessive use and high dose. Ibuprofen is usually well tolerated but does have the potential to cause gastric ulcer, albeit with long-term high-dose use. Aspirin should not be prescribed to a child with a febrile illness because of its association with Reye syndrome. Ibuprofen should not be prescribed for varicella because its use is implicated in necrotizing fasciitis.

The young child with high fever (=>40.9° C [105.6° F]) is three times more likely to be bacteremic than is the child with a temperature of 39° C or less. The degree of temperature reduction in response to antipyretic therapy is not predictive of presence or absence of bacteremia. In one major study, among infants with bacteremia but without meningitis, differences from nonbacteremic children were detected in clinical appearance before fever reduction but not after defervescence. All children with meningitis appeared seriously ill before and after defervescence.

When sepsis is suspected, a septic workup should be initiated (Table 14–6). Empirical antimicrobial therapy with ceftriaxone, 50 mg/kg IM every 24 hours, with supportive care is prudent, pending the outcome of evaluation. The child can be managed in the home if the child is intact neurologically, if hydration can be maintained via the oral route, if the caregiver is willing and able to provide the needed close attention to the child, and if follow-up and emergency care are easily accessible.

A total WBC count with differential is obtained as part of the evaluation of the child with suspected sepsis. The most typical WBC pattern found in severe bacterial infection is the "left shift." A "left shift" is usually seen in the presence of severe bacterial infection, such

TABLE 14–6
FEVER IN THE YOUNG
INFANT

- CBC with manual WBC differential
  - Identify viral versus bacterial shifts, general leukocytic response
- Blood culture
  - Potentially identifying causative organism in sepsis
- Urinalysis (UA) and urine culture via transurethral catheter or suprapubic tap
  - Rule in or out UTI, pyelonephritis
- Particularly important in child < 2 years
- LP for CSF analysis and culture
  - Rule in or out meningitis
- Particularly important if alterations in neurological examination
- Chest x-ray (CXR)
  - Particularly if dyspnea, tachypnea, decreased breath sounds, WBC>20,000 mm3
- Stool culture, fecal WBC count
  - Particularly if diarrhea

as appendicitis and pneumonia. The following is typically noted:

- Leukocytosis: An elevation in the total WBC count
- Neutrophilia: An elevation in the number of neutrophils in circulation, defined as more than 10,000 neutrophils/mm^3. Neutrophils are also known as polys or segs, both referring to the polymorph shape of the segment nucleus of this WBC.
- Bandemia: An elevation in the number of bands or young neutrophils in circulation. Usually, fewer than 4% of the total WBCs in circulation are bands. When this percentage is exceeded and the absolute band counts exceed 500/mm^3, bandemia is present. This indicates that the body has called up as many mature neutrophils that were available in storage pool and is now accessing less mature forms. This further reinforces the seriousness of the infection.
- Toxic granulation: often reported on WBC morphologic study.

There are other neutrophil forms that do not belong in circulation even with severe infection. These include myelocytes and metamyelocytes, immature neutrophil forms that are typically found in granulopoiesis pool. The presence of these cells in the circulation is an ominous marker for life-threatening bacterial infection.

In viral infection, the total WBC count can be elevated but is often normal or slightly depressed (leukopenia). Lymphocytes, the leukocytes most active in viral infection, predominate. Atypical or reactive lymphocytes are often reported on WBC morphology.

To eliminate or support the diagnosis of meningitis, lumbar puncture with CSF evaluation should be part of the evaluation of the febrile younger child who has an altered neurologic examination. Pleocytosis, defined as a CSF WBC count of more than 5 cells/mm^3, is an expected finding in meningitis caused by bacterial, viral, tubercular, fungal, or protozoan infection. An elevated CSF opening pressure is also a nearly universal finding. Typical CSF response in bacterial meningitis includes a median WBC count of 1200 cells/mm^3 with 90% to 95% neutrophils; additional findings are a reduction in CSF glucose below the normal level of about 60% of the plasma level and an elevated CSF protein level. CSF results in viral or aseptic meningitis include normal glucose level, normal to slightly elevated protein level, and lymphocytosis. Further testing to ascertain the causative organism is warranted.

Treatment of the child with meningitis includes supportive care and the use of the appropriate anti-infective agent. Acyclovir is an option in aseptic meningitis, pending identification of the offending virus. Ceftriaxone with vancomycin is usually the treatment of choice in suspect bacterial meningitis, pending bacterial sensitivity results. Treatment of other forms of sepsis in the younger child is dependent on its cause.

DISCUSSION SOURCES

Baraff L.J., Bass J.W., Fleisher G.R., et al. (1993): Practice guideline for the management of infants and children 0 to 36 months of age with fever without source. Pediatrics 92:1–12.

Egland, A. (2004). Fever in the young child, available at http://www.emedicine.com/ped/topic 2698.htm, accessed 1/1/05.

Hill, N., and Sullivan, L. (2004). Management Guidelines for Nurse Practitioners Working with Children and Adolescents (2nd ed.) Philadephia: F.A. Davis.

QUESTIONS

140. When treating a 3-year-old well child with community-acquired pneumonia (CAP), the NP realizes that the most likely causative pathogen is:

  A. *Mycoplasma pneumoniae.*
  B. a respiratory virus.
  C. *H. influenzae.*
  D. *S. pneumoniae.*

141. Which of the following is the most appropriate antimicrobial for treatment of CAP in a 2-year-old?

  A. azithromycin
  B. doxycycline
  C. TMP-SMX
  D. levofloxacin

142. Which of the following is most likely to be noted in the 3-year-old with CAP?

  A. complaint of pleuritic chest pain
  B. sputum production
  C. report of dyspnea
  D. tachypnea

143. What percentage of children will have an episode of pneumonia by age 5?

  A. less than 10%
  B. about 10%
  C. about 20%
  D. about 30%

144. Which of the following antimicrobials provides effective activity against atypical pathogens?

  A. amoxicillin
  B. cefprozil
  C. ceftriaxone
  D. clarithromycin

ANSWERS

140. B	**141.** A	**142.** D
143. C	**144.** D	

DISCUSSION

Pneumonia remains the most common cause of death from infectious disease and the sixth leading cause of overall mortality in the United States. Although pneumonia is often considered to be a disease primarily of older adults and the chronically ill, about 20% of children will develop pneumonia by age 5 years. Most often caused by bacteria or viruses, pneumonia is an acute lower respiratory tract infection involving lung parenchyma, interstitial tissues, and alveolar spaces. The term community-acquired pneumonia is used to describe the onset of the disease in the child who resides within the community, not in a nursing home or other care facility, with no recent (within 2 weeks) hospitalization.

The majority of children with pneumonia present with cough. However, tachypnea is the most sensitive, though not specific, finding. In particular, the diagnosis of lower respiratory tract disease should be considered with a respiratory rate exceeding 50 breaths/minute in children younger than 1 year and a rate exceeding 40 breaths/minute in children older than 1 year. Pulse oximetry is also informative but less so than respiratory rate. In comparison with an adult with pneumonia, the child is less likely to complain of dyspnea, produce sputum, or report pleuritic chest pain. Diagnostic evaluation of the child with CAP usually includes a chest x-ray; further evaluation for invasive disease (sepsis) should be dictated by clinical presentation.

Although a number of organisms are implicated in CAP in children, relatively few are seen with frequency. Respiratory viruses are the causes in the majority; *S. pneumoniae* and the atypical pathogens are also implicated. As with adults with CAP, sputum specimens are usually unobtainable or unreliable in the child with CAP.

Successful community-based care of the child with CAP requires a number of factors. The child must have intact gastrointestinal function and be able to take and tolerate oral medications, as well as adequate amounts of fluids. A competent caregiver must be available. Also, the child should be able to return for follow-up examination and evaluation.

As with CAP treatment in the adult, CAP antimicrobial therapy in children is chosen empirically. In adequate dosages, amoxicillin or a cephalosporin provides activity against *S. pneumoniae* but is ineffective against the atypical pathogens. A macrolide such as azithromycin or clarithromycin provides activity against *S. pneumoniae* and the atypical pathogens. Although the tetracyclines are used in treating CAP in the adult, these medications should not be prescribed to children because of the risk of tooth staining. Because the majority of childhood CAP is viral in origin, watchful waiting can also be used, whereby the child is not placed on an antimicrobial regimen but rather is observed to see whether the illness improves over a few days.

NPs are ideally positioned to help minimize risk for pneumonia through immunization and hygienic measures. Nearly two thirds of all fatal pneumonia is caused by *S. pneumoniae*, the pneumococcal organism. Pneumococcal conjugate vaccine is recommended for all children, starting in infancy. The use of influenza vaccine can help minimize the risk of post-influenza pneumonia. Ensuring adequate ventilation, reinforcing cough hygiene, and proper hand washing can help minimize pneumonia risk.

DISCUSSION SOURCES

Larsen, G., Accurso, F., Deterding, R., et al. (2003). Respiratory tract and mediastinum. In Hay, W., Hayward, A., Levin, M., and Sondheimer, J. (eds.). Current Pediatric Diagnosis and Treatment (16th ed., pp. 492–545). New York: McGraw-Hill.
Wubbel, L., Muniz, L., Ahmed, A., et al. (1999). Etiology and treatment of community-acquired pneumonia in ambulatory children. Pediatric Infectious Disease Journal 18:98–104.

QUESTIONS

145. Sam is a 4-year-old boy who presents with a 1-week history of intermittent fever, rash, and "watery red eyes." Clinical presentation is of an alert child who is cooperative with examination but irritable, with temperature of 37° C, pulse rate of 132, and respiratory rate of 38. Physical examination findings include nasal crusting; dry, erythematous, cracked lips; red, enlarged tonsils without exudate; and elevated tongue papillae. The diagnosis of Kawasaki disease is being considered. Additional findings will likely include:

   A. vesicular-form rash.
   B. exudative conjunctivitis.
   C. peeling hands.
   D. occipital lymphadenopathy.

146. Laboratory findings in Kawasaki disease include all of the following except:

   A. sterile pyuria.
   B. elevated liver enzyme levels.
   C. blood cultures positive for offending bacterial pathogen.
   D. elevated erythrocyte sedimentation rate.

147. Long-term consequences of Kawasaki disease include:

   A. renal insufficiency.
   B. coronary artery obstruction.
   C. hepatic failure.
   D. hypothyroidism.

148. The cause of Kawasaki disease is:

   A. fungal.
   B. viral.
   C. bacterial.
   D. unknown.

149. An important part of the treatment of Kawasaki disease includes:

A. antibiotics.
B. antivirals.
C. immune globulin.
D. antifungals.

ANSWERS

145. C	**146.** C	**147.** B
148. D	**149.** C	

DISCUSSION

Kawasaki disease, also known as Kawasaki syndrome, is self-limited vasculitis of unknown etiology. Clinical presentation includes fever, skin rash, mucocutaneous lesion, myocarditis (early disease stage), and the development of coronary artery aneurysms (later disease stage) (Table 14–7).

Occurring primarily in the late winter and spring at 3-year intervals, Kawasaki disease now surpasses rheumatic fever as the leading cause of acquired heart disease in the United States among children younger than 5. The development of coronary artery aneurysms can lead to coronary artery obstruction, myocarditis, congestive heart failure, pericarditis, mitral or aortic insufficiency, and dysrhythmias. Risk of aneurysm is increased in patients who have fever for more than 16 days, have recurrence of fever after an afebrile period of at least 48 hours, are male, are younger than 1 year, and have cardiomegaly at the time of diagnosis.

Although no specific laboratory test for Kawasaki disease exists, the presence of certain laboratory findings can support the diagnosis when coupled with clinical presentation. In the acute stage (days 1 to 11), leukocytosis with a left shift and elevated erythrocyte sedimentation rate are found, both neither sensitive nor specific for the condition. Blood and urine cultures fail to identify an offending organism. In the subacute stage (days 11 to 21), the platelet count is often markedly elevated, with a measurement of more than $1,000,000/mm^3$ being common. These values begin to normalize during the convalescent stage (days 21 to 60) but may not reach baseline values for up to 8 weeks.

During the acute stage of Kawasaki disease or if the diagnosis is in question, an echocardiogram should be obtained. The study should be repeated in the second or third week of disease and repeated 1 month after laboratory tests have resolved. Treatment of Kawasaki disease includes the use of immune globulin and aspirin. Confirmation of the diagnosis and treatment will likely involve consultation with a specialist in this disease. Long-term prognosis is generally related to the degree of permanent cardiac involvement.

TABLE 14–7

DIAGNOSTIC CRITERIA FOR KAWASAKI DISEASE

- Fever =>5 days in duration usually abrupt in onset, symptoms with no response to antibiotic therapy, if given, usually with irritability out of proportion to the degree of fever or other signs
- In addition to fever of at least 5 days' duration, => 4 of the following should be present:
  - Changes in extremities (erythema, edema, desquamation), usually with discomfort so that child may refuse to bear weight
  - Desquamation of the fingers and toes begins in the periungual region, may also involve the palms and soles, usually noted at 1–2 weeks after onset of fever
  - Bilateral, nonexudative conjunctivitis
  - Polymorphous rash
  - Cervical lymphadenopathy
  - Changes in lips and oral cavity (pharyngeal edema, dry/fissured or swollen lips, strawberry tongue)

(NB: If fever is present with fewer than four of the above symptoms the diagnosis is established with echocardiogram to evaluate the coronary arteries to either support or exclude the disease)

DISCUSSION SOURCE

Scheinfeld, N., and Silverberg, N. (2004). Kawasaki Disease, available at http://www.emedicine.com/ped/topic1236.htm, accessed 1/1/05.

15
Childbearing

QUESTIONS

Match the stage of pregnancy with the appropriate term

_____**1.** Fertilization ovum

_____**2.** Up to 2 weeks postconception

_____**3.** To 8–12 weeks

_____**4.** 13 weeks to term

  A. Embryo
  B. Fetus
  C. Blastocyst
  D. Zygote

ANSWERS

1. D   **2.** C   **3.** A
4. B

QUESTIONS

Match uterine size with stage of pregnancy.

_____**5.** Nongravid

_____**6.** 8 weeks

_____**7.** 10 weeks

_____**8.** 12 weeks

_____**9.** 16 weeks

_____**10.** 20 weeks

  A. Size of a baseball
  B. Size of a softball or grapefruit
  C. Size of a large lemon
  D. Size of a tennis ball or orange
  E. Uterine fundus at umbilicus
  F. Uterine fundus halfway between symphysis pubis and umbilicus

ANSWERS

5. C   **6.** D   **7.** A
8. B   **9.** F   **10.** E

QUESTIONS

11. Approximately _____ percent of fetuses are in the vertex position by the 36th week of pregnancy.

  A. 30
  B. 50
  C. 75
  D. 95

12. Recommended weight gain during pregnancy for a woman with a normal BMI is:

A. 15–20 lbs.
B. 20–30 lbs.
C. 25–35 lbs.
D. 35–45 lbs.

13. For a healthy woman with a normal prepregnancy BMI, daily caloric requirements during pregnancy are typical baseline caloric needs plus _____ kcal.

A. 100
B. 300
C. 600
D. 1000

14. For a healthy woman with a normal prepregnancy BMI, daily caloric requirements during lactation are typical baseline caloric needs plus _____ kcal.

A. 250
B. 500
C. 750
D. 1000

15. Recommended calcium intake for a woman during pregnancy is _____ mg of elemental calcium per day.

A. 500–750
B. 750–1000
C. 1000–1200
D. 1200–1500

16. Increased folic acid intake prior to conception will likely reduce the risk of which of the following birth defects?

A. Cleft palate
B. Ventricular septal defect
C. Club foot
D. Open neural tube defect

17. Maternal iron requirements are greatest during what part of pregnancy?

A. First trimester
B. Second and third trimesters
C. Equal throughout pregnancy
D. Preconception

18. The most common form of acquired anemia during pregnancy is:

A. iron deficiency.
B. folate deficiency.
C. vitamin B_{12} deficiency.
D. hypoproliferative.

19. Concerning the use of maternal alcohol during pregnancy, which of the following is most accurate?

A. Although potentially problematic, maternal alcohol intake does not increase the risk of miscarriage.
B. Fetal exposure risk is greatest in the third trimester.
C. No level or time of exposure is considered safe.
D. Fetal alcohol syndrome risk is noted only if exposure has been throughout the pregnancy.

20. Pica (ingestion of nonfood substances) during pregnancy should be considered:

A. a harmless practice common in certain ethnic groups.
B. only problematic if more nutritional food sources are left out of the diet and are replaced by the nonfood substance.
C. a way of providing select micronutrients not usually found in food products.
D. potentially dangerous due in part to contaminants in the nonfood substance.

21. Examples of neural tube defect include all of the following except:

A. Anencephaly.
B. Spina bifida.
C. Encephalocele.
D. Omphalocele.

ANSWERS

11. D	**12.** C	**13.** B
14. B	**15.** D	**16.** D
17. B	**18.** A	**19.** C
20. D	**21.** D	

DISCUSSION

The NP must have knowledge of nutritional requirements during pregnancy in order to provide appropriate counseling. Folic acid deficiency is a teratogenic state, leading to an increased risk of neural tube defect (NTD) and other defects in the developing pregnancy. NTDs are some of the most common serious fetal malformations in the United States, second only to cardiac defects, with an incidence of 1.2 NTDs for every 1000 births. Examples of NTDs include anencephaly, spina bifida, and encephalocele. Correcting folic acid deficiency prior to pregnancy by increased dietary and supplement intake dramatically reduces this risk, and continuing this measure throughout pregnancy minimizes the mother's risk of developing folate-deficiency anemia. If a woman has carried a pregnancy with an NTD or there is a family history of NTD, recommended folic acid intake increases to 4 mg per day 1 month prior to pregnancy and during the first 3 months of gestation. Most prescription prenatal multivitamins contain 1 mg of folic acid.

Increased calcium intake is important to the development of bone and teeth; the required amount can usually be met by ensuring 3–4 servings of high-quality dairy products per day. Examples of a single dairy serving include 8 ounces of milk, 1 ounce of cheese, 1 cup of yogurt, or 1 cup of calcium-fortified juice. Although dietary source calcium is best, supplementation is sometimes required if a woman is lactose intolerant or is otherwise unable to meet these goals. Maternal iron requirements increase in the second and third trimester of pregnancy, in part due to the fetus's need to build iron stores. Iron deficiency is the most common form of anemia during pregnancy, with most being due to the woman entering pregnancy iron deficient rather than developing this problem because of increased iron requirements. Pregnancy-related iron requirements, given in terms of elemental iron, are as follows: in the absence of iron deficiency, 30 mg/d; with iron deficiency or in a multiple-gestation pregnancy, 60 to 100 mg/d; and with iron deficiency anemia, 200 mg/d. A 325-mg ferrous sulfate tablet contains 65 mg of elemental iron, whereas most prescription prenatal vitamins contain 30 to 65 mg.

Fetal alcohol syndrome has most often been noted in the offspring of women who drank heavily throughout pregnancy. More common are babies, whose mothers drink lightly or moderately, who are born with lesser degrees of alcohol-related problems. Given that fetal alcohol syndrome is the leading preventable cause of mental retardation and is absolutely preventable by avoiding alcohol consumption throughout pregnancy, no level of maternal alcohol intake during pregnancy is deemed safe. Maternal alcohol intake also increases the risk of miscarriage. Less is known about fetal risks due to exposure to other recreational drugs, such as marijuana, a substance often considered more benign and "natural" than alcohol. However, a safe level of maternal ingestion during pregnancy for this and other intoxicating substances has not been established, and abstinence should be encouraged.

Pica is the ingestion of nonfood substances, such as clay, cornstarch, laundry starch, dry milk of magnesia, paraffin, coffee grounds, or ice. Although usually noted to be more common in select ethnic groups, pica is noted in all socioeconomic groups. Certain pica habits, such as sucking on ice chips, are likely harmless and likely do little to replace more nutritional substances. Most other pica forms contain potential risk because nonfood substances are taken in preferably over more nutritious food sources. With the ingestion of clay, starches, and paraffin, there are risks of constipation, bowel obstruction, and nutritional deficiency. In particular, many common pica substances can be contaminated with heavy metals, such as lead or mercury and other industrial pollutants that are particularly toxic to the mother and the developing fetus. The issue of pica should be raised with all pregnant women. Some women believe that pica is normal or are encouraged to eat substances like clay by well-meaning friends and family members as a way of relieving tension. Advice should be given recognizing this but informing the woman about the potential risks of pica.

DISCUSSION SOURCES

Brown, K.P. (2004) Antenatal care. In: Management Guidelines for Nurse Practitioners Working with Women (2nd ed., pp. 177–223). Philadelphia: F.A. Davis.

March of Dimes: During Your Pregnancy: Your Healthy Diet. Available at www.modimes.org, accessed 3/10/04.

QUESTIONS

Identify the following changes in a normal pregnancy as true (normal, anticipated finding) or false (not associated with normal pregnancy).

_____ **22.** Blood volume increases by 40 to 50 percent, peaking at week 32.

_____ **23.** Drop in diastolic blood pressure most notable during second trimester.

_____ **24.** S_1 heart sound becomes louder.

_____ **25.** Physiologic systolic ejection murmur is usually evident.

_____ **26.** Dilatation of renal collecting system.

_____ **27.** Physiologic glucosuria and proteinuria common.

_____ **28.** Decrease in transverse thoracic diameter and diaphragmatic contraction.

_____ **29.** Lower esophageal sphincter more relaxed.

_____ **30.** Increased intestinal motility.

_____ **31.** Gallbladder doubles in size.

_____ **32.** Insulin levels increase by two- to tenfold over prepregnancy levels.

_____ **33.** Fasting plasma glucose increases slightly.

_____ **34.** Thyroid decreases in size.

ANSWERS

22. True	**23.** True	**24.** True
25. True	**26.** True	**27.** True
28. False	**29.** True	**30.** False
31. True	**32.** True	**33.** False
34. False		

DISCUSSION

A woman's body changes dramatically throughout pregnancy. Knowledge of these normative physiologic changes in pregnancy is crucial to providing safe and competent prenatal care. See Table 15–1.

DISCUSSION SOURCES

Brown, K.P. (2004) Antenatal care. In: Management Guidelines for Nurse Practitioners Working with Women (2nd ed., pp 177–223). Philadelphia: F.A. Davis.

QUESTIONS

35. The recommended frequency of prenatal visits in weeks 28–32 of pregnancy is every:

  A. 1 week
  B. 2 weeks
  C. 3 weeks
  D. 4 weeks

36. Testing for sexually transmitted infection should be initially obtained:

  A. As early as possible in pregnancy
  B. During the second trimester
  C. During the third trimester
  D. As close to anticipated date of birth as possible

37. The "triple screen" should be obtained at about weeks _____ of pregnancy.

  A. 6–10
  B. 11–15
  C. 16–20
  D. 21–25

TABLE 15–1

PHYSIOLOGIC CHANGES DURING PREGNANCY

Body Area	Physiologic Adaptation During Pregnancy
Uterus	Increases from approximately 10-mL capacity and 70-g weight prepregnancy to 5000-mL capacity and 1100-g weight at term. The uterine isthmus becomes soft and compressible (Hegar's sign)
Cervix	Color and texture change, becoming cyanotic (Chadwick's sign) and less firm (Goodell's sign)
Skin	Striae (stretch marks) in about 50%, melasma (pregnancy mask), linea nigra (hyperpigmented line on abdomen) appears or darkens as melanocytes are stimulated
Breast	Nipples, areolae darken and increase in size. Venous congestion noted. Breast tissue becomes more nodular due to proliferation of lactiferous glands.
Blood	Blood volume increases by 40%–50%, peaking at week 32. Red blood cell production increases by 33% but results in a dilutional physiologic anemia of pregnancy.
Cardiovascular	Decrease in systolic blood pressure throughout pregnancy, with drop in diastolic blood pressure most notable during second trimester. Cardiac output dependent on maternal position, with a noted decrease if in supine position due to reduced venous return caused by vena cava compression to an increase of 30%–50% with lateral recumbent position. S_1 heart sound becomes louder, physiologic systolic ejection murmur usually evident. Heart is displaced, resulting in a left-axis deviation.
Renal	Increased renal blood flow, glomerular filtration rate (GFR), and dilatation of renal collecting system. Physiologic glucosuria and proteinuria occur due in part to increase in GFR and a resulting inability of the renal tubules to reabsorb glucose and protein.
Respiratory	Due in part to increased abdominal content, there are increases in transverse thoracic diameter and diaphragmatic contraction and the costal angle widens. Tidal volume increases with reduced residual volume in later pregnancy.
Digestive	Lower esophageal sphincter more relaxed while corresponding pressures increase, resulting in increased esophageal reflux. Decreased stomach and intestinal motility, allowing for greater nutrient absorption but increased risk for constipation. (Increased progesterone levels influence the aforementioned changes.) Gallbladder doubles in size, with more dilute bile and less soluble cholesterol, increasing risk of stones.
Metabolic/endocrine	Insulin levels increase by 2- to 10-fold over prepregnancy levels. Fasting plasma glucose drops slightly. Thyroid and pituitary increase in size. Maternal weight changes account for weight gain in the first half of pregnancy, whereas the components of the pregnancy account for the majority of weight gain in the later half.

Brown, K.P. (2004) Antenatal care. In: Management Guidelines for Nurse Practitioners Working with Women (2nd ed., pp 177–223). Philadelphia: F.A. Davis Company.

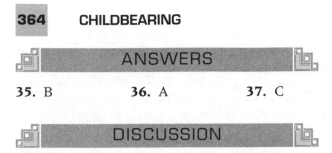

ANSWERS

35. B   **36.** A   **37.** C

DISCUSSION

There are a number of recommendations on the frequency of prenatal care and associated laboratory and other testing. It is important to remember that these are simply guidelines for the care that is needed for the well woman with a low physiologic and psychosocial risk pregnancy. More frequent visits and testing are often indicated, but a minimum of 8–10 visits should be scheduled. Additional testing is often indicated, such as screening for genetically based conditions risk (e.g., cystic fibrosis or Tay-Sachs disease) (Tables 15–2 through 15–5).

TABLE 15–2
NATIONAL ACADEMY OF SCIENCE RECOMMENDED WEIGHT GAIN DURING PREGNANCY

Prepregnancy BMI	Recommended Gain
<19.8	28–40 lb
19.8–26	25–35 lb
26–29	15–25 lb
>29	15+ lb

TABLE 15–3
FREQUENCY OF PRENATAL VISITS

Time in Pregnancy	Frequency of Visits
Up to 28 weeks	Q 4 weeks
28–36 weeks	Q 2 weeks
≥ 36 weeks	Q week

Modified from AAFP Guidelines. Available at www.AAFP.org

TABLE 15–4
PRENATAL CARE: FIRST VISIT, EARLY IN PREGNANCY

Pap smear	CBC
Rubella titer	Blood type, antibody screen
VDRL/RPR, HIV	GC/chlamydia
PPD	Hg electrophoresis (consider w/African, Asian ancestry)
HBsAg	UA, urine C & S

Modified from AAFP Guidelines. Available at www.AAFP.org

DISCUSSION SOURCE

Brown, K.P. (2004) Antenatal care. In: Management Guidelines for Nurse Practitioners Working with Women (2nd ed., pp 177–223). Philadelphia: F.A. Davis.

QUESTIONS

38. The rate of spontaneous fetal loss related to amniocentesis averages about 1 in _____ procedures

    A. 50
    B. 100
    C. 200
    D. 300

39. All of the following can cause an elevated maternal alpha-fetoprotein (AFP) except:

    A. underestimated gestational age.
    B. open neural tube defect.
    C. meningomyelocele.
    D. Down syndrome.

40. Edwards syndrome is the clinical manifestation of trisomy____.

    A. 13
    B. 15
    C. 18
    D. 21

41. In Edwards syndrome, which of the following is true?

TABLE 15–5

PRENATAL CARE LATER IN
PREGNANCY

Time	Test
16–20 weeks	Triple marker/screen ultrasound
24–28 weeks	1-hr glucose load If Rh negative, type and screen
28–32 weeks	Hg STI testing as indicated (VDRL, HIV, HBsAg, GC, chlamydia) RhoGAM as indicated
32–36 weeks	Fetal presentation Kick count (fetal movements ≥4 in 1 hr; ≥10 in 2 hr)
35–37 weeks	Group B streptococcus culture (rectal and vaginal)
40–42 weeks	Vaginal examination to assess cervical ripeness, fetal station (optional)
41+ weeks	Nonstress test, biophysical profile

Modified from AAFP Guidelines. Available at
www.AAFP.org

    A. More common than Down syndrome.
    B. Most affected infants die during the
        first year of life.
    C. Unlikely to cause developmental dis-
        ability.
    D. Associated with elevated AFP.

42. In Down syndrome, which of the following is true?

    A. Most babies affected with Down syn-
        drome are born to women older than
        age 35 years.
    B. Noted in about 1 in 10,000 live births.
    C. Associated with decreased maternal
        serum AFP.
    D. Antenatal serum analysis is sufficient
        to make the diagnosis.

43. Down syndrome is the clinical manifestation of trisomy ___.

    A. 13
    B. 15

    C. 18
    D. 21

44. Components of the antenatal screening
test known as the "triple screen" include
all of the following except:

    A. AFP.
    B. hCG.
    C. unconjugated estriol.
    D. progesterone.

ANSWERS

38. C	**39.** D	**40.** C
41. B	**42.** C	**43.** D
44. D		

DISCUSSION

The issue of prenatal screening and diagnostic
procedures is an important clinical issue, although one that often carries a component of
confusion, emotional charge, and disagree-
ment among providers and patients. One point
of confusion is the difference between screening and diagnostic tests. Commonly offered
prenatal tests include maternal serum analysis
for AFP, human chorionic gonadotropin (hCG)
and unconjugated estriol levels, also known as
the triple screen. When the amounts of these
substances are analyzed, increased risk of open
NTDs, trisomy 21 (Down syndrome), and trisomy 18 (Edwards syndrome) can be detected.
However, an abnormal triple screen result is
not diagnostic of any condition, and further
testing is required. Down syndrome results in
mental retardation and increased risk of cardiac and gastrointestinal malformation and
early-onset Alzheimer disease. The risk of
Down syndrome is approximately 1 in 1000
live births, with this number increasing to 1 in
270 in women 35 to 40 years of age and 1 in
100 in women older than 40 years. As maternal age is a well-known risk factor for Down
syndrome and other genetically based congenital anomalies, women who are 35 years or
older at the time of delivery should be offered

the opportunity for prenatal diagnosis with amniocentesis or chorionic villus sampling. It is important to remember that approximately 75 percent of all babies with Down syndrome are born to mothers younger than age 35. This is in part due to the fact that women in this age group are more likely to give birth than older women, and they undergo a lower rate of antenatal diagnostics, such as amniocentesis.

Edwards syndrome is much less common, occurring in 1 in every 6000 births, and is associated with low birth weight, mental retardation, and cranial, cardiac and renal malformations. The complexity and severity of these problems are such that most affected infants will die within the first year of life.

NTDs are second only to cardiac defects in frequency, with an incidence of 1.2 for every 1000 births. Examples of open NTD, such as meningomyelocele, anencephaly, or spina bifida; all carry risk of significant disability and the potential for shortened life span.

Alpha-fetoprotein is synthesized in the yolk sac, gastrointestinal tract, and liver of the fetus. Maternal levels can be elevated for a number of reasons, including open neural tube defect, such as meningomyelocele, anencephaly, or spina bifida, fetal nephrosis, cystic hygroma, fetal gastrointestinal obstruction, omphalocele, intrauterine growth restriction, multiple fetuses, or fetal demise. Underestimated gestational age can also lead to a misinterpreted test, given that maternal AFP is higher in earlier pregnancy. The placenta from precursors provided by the fetal adrenal glands and the liver produces unconjugated estriol; maternal levels are decreased in trisomy 21 and trisomy 18. hCG is produced by trophoblast shortly after implantation into the uterine wall, with levels increasing rapidly in the first 8 weeks of pregnancy, then steadily decreasing until week 20, when levels plateau. An increased hCG level appears to be the most sensitive marker for detecting trisomy 21, whereas a low hCG level is associated with trisomy 18. The hCG levels are typically normal in the presence of NTDs.

Interpreting the results of a triple screen requires knowledge of a number of factors, including the risk of false-positive and false-negative results, the significance of the results, and the woman's individual risk of having an affected pregnancy. In addition, all antenatal testing must be offered to a woman in a manner that allows her to make an informed decision to have or decline the test. Part of informed consent includes the information that the triple screen is simply that, a screening test that identifies higher-risk situations but is not diagnostic for the condition. With abnormal results, further testing is indicated, and results that are within normal limits do not ensure that no problem will occur with the pregnancy but do indicate that the risk is minimized.

As previously mentioned, if a triple screen yields abnormal results, further testing is indicated. For the detection of a genetic abnormality, such as trisomy 18 or 21, the most commonly used test is amniocentesis, a procedure that carries a rate of spontaneous fetal loss of about one in every 200 procedures. If a woman chooses not to have invasive testing, noninvasive follow-up evaluation after abnormal triple screen includes a level 2 ultrasound, a high-resolution study that can reveal fetal abnormalities such as an open NTD or increased nuchal folds and other anomalies often found in Down syndrome. Again, ultrasound can assist with diagnosis but does not take the place of genetically based studies.

DISCUSSION SOURCES

Brown, K.P. (2004) Antenatal care. In: Management Guidelines for Nurse Practitioners Working with Women (2nd ed., pp 177–223). Philadelphia: F.A. Davis.

Graves, C., Miller, K., and Sellers, A. (2002). Maternal Serum Triple Analyte Screening in Pregnancy. American Family Physician. Available at www.aafp.org/afp, accessed 3/10/04.

QUESTIONS

45. Medications most commonly pass through the placenta via:

A. facilitated transport.
B. passive diffusion.

C. capillary pump action.

D. mechanical carrier state.

46. A drug with demonstrated safety for use in pregnancy is risk category:

A. A

B. B

C. C

D. D

47. A drug demonstrated to cause teratogenic effects in human study but with benefit potentially outweighing risk of use in a life-threatening situation is assigned risk category:

A. A

B. B

C. C

D. D

48. An example of a medication that is pregnancy risk category D when used in the third trimester of pregnancy is:

A. Misoprostol

B. Captopril

C. Cefuroxime

D. regular insulin

49. A drug demonstrated to cause teratogenic effects in animal studies but not in human studies is available and is assigned risk category:

A. A

B. B

C. C

D. D

50. When treating a woman with a urinary tract infection who is 38 weeks pregnant, the NP prescribes:

A. TMP-SMX

B. Nitrofurantoin

C. Ciprofloxacin

D. Amoxicillin with clavulanate

51. According to Hale's Lactation Risk Category, a medication in which there is no controlled study on its use during lactation or controlled study shows minimal, non–life-threatening risk is listed as category:

A. L2

B. L3

C. L4

D. L5

52. According to Hale's Lactation Risk Category, a medication in which there is evidence of risk with its use in lactation but may be used if there is a maternal life-threatening situation is listed as category:

A. L2

B. L3

C. L4

D. L5

53. In the pregnant woman with asthma, in what part of her pregnancy do symptoms and bronchospasm worsen?

A. 6–14 weeks

B. 15–23 weeks

C. 24–33 weeks

D. 29–36 weeks

54. In treating a pregnant woman with acute bacterial rhinosinusitis, the NP would likely *avoid* prescribing:

A. Amoxicillin

B. Cefuroxime

C. Azithromycin

D. Levofloxacin

55. According to the Infectious Disease Society of America recommendations, the duration of antimicrobial therapy for treatment of urinary tract infection in a pregnant woman is:

A. 3 days

B. 5 days

C. 7 days

D. 10 days

56. Selective serotonin reuptake inhibitor (SSRI) withdrawal syndrome is best characterized as:

A. Bothersome but not life-threatening

B. Potentially life-threatening

C. Most often seen with medications with a longer half-life (T½)

D. Associated with seizure risk

57. The placenta is best described as:

    A. Poorly permeable.
    B. An effective drug barrier.
    C. Best able to transport lipophilic substances.
    D. Capable of impeding substances with molecular weight (MW) <=300.

58. Preferred treatment options for a pregnant woman in the second trimester with migraine headache include:

    A. Sumatriptan
    B. Codeine
    C. Aspirin
    D. Ibuprofen

59. In counseling women about the use of an SSRI antidepressant during pregnancy, the NP considers that studies to date reveal:

    A. A teratogenic pattern has been identified.
    B. The drugs have a negative effect on intellectual development.
    C. No observable difference between children with intrauterine exposure and controls.
    D. Increased rate of seizure disorder in exposed offspring.

60. Which SSRI has the longest half-life?

    A. Paroxetine
    B. Fluoxetine
    C. Citalopram
    D. Sertraline

61. Among the most commonly used medications by women in the first trimester of pregnancy are:

    A. Antiepileptic drugs
    B. Antibiotics
    C. Antihypertensives
    D. Opioids

62. Benzodiazipine withdrawal syndrome is best characterized as:

    A. Bothersome but not life-threatening.
    B. Not observed during pregnancy.

    C. Most often seen with agents that have long half-lives.
    D. Associated with seizure risk.

63. The cornerstone controller therapy for chronic persistent asthma during pregnancy is the use of:

    A. Oral theophylline.
    B. Mast cell stabilizers.
    C. Short-acting beta agonists.
    D. Inhaled corticosteroids.

64. You examine a 24-year-old woman who is 24 weeks pregnant and has an acute asthma flare. Her medication regimen should be adjusted to include:

    A. Theophylline.
    B. Salmeterol (Servent).
    C. Prednisone.
    D. Montelukast (Singulair).

65. A drug that has shown to be harmful to the fetus in human and animal studies is assigned risk category:

    A. B.
    B. C.
    C. D.
    D. X.

66. Sertraline is pregnancy risk category:

    A. B.
    B. C.
    C. D.
    D. X.

67. Clonazepam is pregnancy risk category:

    A. B.
    B. C.
    C. D.
    D. X.

68. Bupropion is pregnancy risk category:

    A. B.
    B. C.
    C. D.
    D. X.

69. The tricyclic antidepressants are pregnancy risk category:

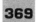

A. B.
B. C.
C. D.
D. X.

70. An example of an antimicrobial that is U.S. Food and Drug Administration (FDA) risk category B is:

    A. Clarithromycin.
    B. Doxycycline.
    C. Erythromycin.
    D. Ofloxacin.

71. An example of an antimicrobial that is pregnancy risk category D is:

    A. Amoxicillin.
    B. Levofloxacin.
    C. Tetracycline.
    D. Trimethoprim-sulfamethoxazole.

72. The penicillins are pregnancy risk category:

    A. B.
    B. C.
    C. D.
    D. X.

73. All of the following uropathogens are capable of reducing urinary nitrates to nitrites except:

    A. *Escherichia coli.*
    B. *Proteus spp.*
    C. *Klebsiella pneumoniae.*
    D. *Staphylococcus saprophyticus.*

74. Which of the following is FDA pregnancy risk category B until the 36th week of pregnancy?

    A. Gentamicin.
    B. Nitrofurantoin.
    C. Clarithromycin.
    D. Ciprofloxacin.

75. In the pregnant woman, asymptomatic bacteruria:

    A. Should be treated only if bladder instrumentation or surgery is planned.
    B. Needs to be treated to avoid complicated urinary tract infection (UTI).

C. Requires a 14-day course of antimicrobial therapy to eradicate.
D. Is a risk factor for hypertension.

76. Which of the following is the most common UTI organism in pregnant women?

    A. *Pseudomonas aeruginosa*
    B. *E. coli*
    C. *K. pneumoniae*
    D. *Proteus mirabilis*

77. Recommended length of antimicrobial therapy for a pregnant woman with asymptomatic bacteria is:

    A. 1–3 days.
    B. 2–5 days.
    C. 3–7 days.
    D. 10 days.

ANSWERS

45. B	**46.** A	**47.** D
48. B	**49.** C	**50.** D
51. B	**52.** C	**53.** D
54. D	**55.** C	**56.** A
57. C	**58.** D	**59.** C
60. B	**61.** B	**62.** D
63. D	**64.** C	**65.** D
66. C	**67.** C	**68.** A
69. C	**70.** C	**71.** C
72. A	**73.** D	**74.** B
75. B	**76.** B	**77.** C

DISCUSSION

Most women use more than three medications during the first trimester of pregnancy, but only about 40 percent of women report use of these drugs to their health care provider. Certain medications are potentially teratogenic, or capable of inducing birth defects, and should be avoided or used with great caution during pregnancy. By definition, a teratogenic drug is a substance that has the potential to create a characteristic set of malformations in the fetus. The classic teratogenic period occurs in a specific time of fetal development, usually between day 31 and day 81 following the last menstrual period, when organogenesis is taking place. For a teratogen to exert its effect, it must be taken at the point in the pregnancy when the affected organ system is developing. For example, lithium can cause a characteristic teratogenic cardiac defect when taken as the cardiac tube is forming; taken earlier or later in the organ development process, the drug has no effect on the heart. Fetal liver maturity also plays a role, because 40 to 60 percent of fetal blood circulation goes through the liver. With increasing maturity, the fetus's hepatic enzymes become more capable of metabolizing drugs. Prior to day 31 after the last menstrual period, the pregnancy exists as a group of poorly differentiated cells with no discrete organ systems to damage. Therefore, a teratogen could be taken at that point without causing damage because there are no organ systems to disrupt. After day 81 after the last menstrual period, the organs are formed but are still growing and developing. The likelihood of a substance exerting a teratogenic effect decreases.

Many factors influence drug transfer across the placenta, including the substance's MW, lipid solubility, and duration of exposure. Medications are usually passed by passive diffusion, in which the maternal drug level is greater than that of the fetus; more drug is passed when maternal levels are greatest. The degree of diffusion is influenced by a number of factors besides maternal drug levels, including the drug's MW and degree of lipophilicity. Drugs with low MWs (<500 g/mol) cross the placental barrier more easily than drugs with MWs greater than 500 g/mol, whereas drugs with a MW >1000 g/mol cross the placenta infrequently. The lower the MW, the greater the potential it has for passage through the placenta. Alcohol and cocaine have low MWs (<100 g/mol) and are easily passed, whereas insulin and heparin (MW >5000 g/mol) are examples of drugs that are poorly transported to the fetus and can be given with relative safety in pregnancy. Most oral over-the-counter and prescription medications have MWs of less than 500 g/mol and thus pass easily through the placenta, which preferentially allows highly lipophilic drugs to pass through. It is important to note that not all drugs with the same therapeutic endpoint have the same lipid solubility. Diphenhydramine (Benadryl) is a highly lipophilic antihistamine and penetrates the placenta and maternal central nervous system easily, causing sedation. In contrast, loratadine (Claritin) is more hydrophilic and thus has fewer fetal or maternal effects. Drugs with a long $T\frac{1}{2}$ or with extended-release formulations are usually held in maternal circulation for protracted periods of time and therefore have the potential to have a greater effect on the fetus than similar drugs with shorter half-lives or those metabolized more rapidly.

To help guide the health care provider choose the safest product possible for use during pregnancy, drug risk categories have been developed by the FDA to facilitate the quick recognition of drugs that may be harmful to take during pregnancy and lactation. Table 15–6 gives a description of the categories and examples for each. A quick way to remember the categories is as follows:

Category B for Best, as very few products are category A
Category C for Caution, as these products have demonstrated risk in animal models
Category D for Danger, as these products have demonstrated risk when used in human pregnancy but are used on occasion in life-threatening maternal disease
Category X for "Cross these drugs off the list," as these products have demonstrated teratogenic risk and have no therapeutic indication for use during human pregnancy.

Pregnant women have a similar incidence of acute and chronic illnesses as age-matched women who are not pregnant. An estimated 1 to 4 percent of all pregnancies are complicated by asthma, with documented increases in maternal morbidity and mortality during pregnancy for woman with the most severe asthma prior to conception. For the majority of pregnant asthmatics, symptoms will have no change or an improvement in symptoms may occur.

TABLE 15–6

FDA PREGNANCY RISK CATEGORIES

Category A	Category B	Category C	Category D	Category X
Well-controlled human study = No fetal risk in 1st trimester.	Animal studies do not demonstrate fetal risk but no controlled study in humans. OR	No controlled study in humans available. Animals reveal adverse fetal effects.	Positive evidence of human fetal risk. Use in pregnant woman occasionally acceptable despite risk.	Animal or human studies demonstrate fetal abnormality. Evidence of fetal risk based on human study.
No evidence of risk in 2nd and 3rd trimesters. Risk to fetus appears remote. Examples: insulin, thyroxine, vitamins in RDA doses	Animal studies show adverse effect but not demonstrated in human study. Examples: the penicillins, cephalosporins, acetaminophen	Examples: corticosteroids, fluoro-quinolones, SSRIs, TMP-SMX (1st and 3rd trimesters)	Examples: doxycycline, genta-micin, ARB and ACEI in 2nd and 3rd trimesters	No indication in pregnancy. Examples: Accutane, miso-prostol, thalido-mide

Braggs, G, Freeman, R, Yaffe, S. (2002). Drugs in Pregnancy and Lactation (6th ed.). Philadelphia: Lippincott, Williams and Wilkins.

Bronchospasm symptoms are usually worse between 29 and 36 weeks of gestation, due to esophageal irritation from gastroesophageal reflux disease. Symptoms usually improve late in gestation when gradual fetal descent occurs. Lifestyle changes that help improve gastroesophageal reflux disease symptoms will help with asthma management. In general, the risk of fetal hypoxia is greater than the risk of medication exposure, so standard asthma medications should be continued. Inhaled corticosteroids are FDA risk category C, a designation that is based on high oral or parenteral doses given to laboratory animals but appears to have little applicability in human use of inhaled medications that have low rates of systemic absorption. Oral corticosteroids have the same designation but should be used to treat an asthma flare. Beta$_2$-agonist bronchodilators are also category C, again based on studies on high oral doses in laboratory animals, and should be prescribed as a rescue drug for the pregnant woman with asthma. As these are newer medications, the leukotriene modifiers have not been as extensively studied in pregnant women and carry a risk category B or C.

Nausea and vomiting in pregnancy is often complicated by pre-existing conditions, such as gastritis. Although this has not yet been conclusively established, recent research indicated that women with hyperemesis gravidarum have a higher incidence of *Helicobacter pylori* infection. Preconceptual treatment of *H. pylori* should be considered for women with a history of a pregnancy complicated by severe nausea and vomiting or of recurrent gastrointestinal problems. Management is targeted toward relieving nausea by increasing rest and decreasing stress. Patients make their own ginger or lemon aromatherapy "kit." This is made by placing five ginger or lemon tea bags in an airtight plastic tub. The tub is opened and the vapors inhaled when nausea occurs. Treating the concomitant gastritis that often accompanies severe nausea and vomiting during pregnancy with a chewable calcium antacid tablet every 2 hours for 2 to 3 days can be helpful. Taking vitamin B$_6$, 25 mg, twice a day has been noted to prevent future nausea and vomiting. A 5HT$_3$-receptor antagonist, such as ondansetron (Zofran, pregnancy risk category B), can offer an effective therapeutic option for preventing severe morning sickness but is not effective in managing acute symptoms.

Among women with a migraine history, the majority will note fewer and less intense headaches during pregnancy. However, about 5 to 10 percent will have worsening headaches. Treatment options include acetaminophen and nonsteroidal anti-inflammatory drugs (except at term because of the potential risk of antiplatelet effect). The triptans are in the risk category, due in part to the C_M theoretical risk of vasoconstriction. However, no teratogenic effect in human pregnancy has been noted to date. Lidocaine 4 percent used as a nasal spray, applied to the nostril on the affected side of the head can help attenuate headache symptoms with minimal system drug absorption.

Women are twice as likely to experience a major depressive disorder. As a result, a significant number of women will either enter pregnancy in a depressed state or develop depression during the course of the pregnancy. Therapy for any mood disorder usually includes lifestyle changes, counseling, and drug therapy. Antidepressant therapy options include the serotonin and dopamine receptor modulators, the tricyclic antidepressants, and the benzodiazepines. Although the SSRIs drugs are all in risk category C, long-term observational study of the children born to women who took these medications during pregnancy has failed to note significant differences when compared with nonexposed matched controls. Bupropion is a dopamine receptor modulator that is in risk category B. Although at first glance, it would seem reasonable to switch a pregnant woman from a higher-risk category C SSRI to bupropion, this is not grounded in science because the medications work with different neurotransmittors; making this switch could actually cause depression to worsen. If the patient wishes to discontinue antidepressant therapy during pregnancy, she should be counseled about the risk of depression recurrence. A slow taper of approximately 25 percent of the total dose per week will be required in order to avoid SSRI withdrawal syndrome. The withdrawal syndrome is bothersome but not life-threatening and includes jitteriness, nausea, and sleep disturbance and is more severe with the SSRIs with a shorter $T\frac{1}{2}$, such as paroxetine ($T\frac{1}{2}$ = 26 hours), and less severe with the SSRIs with longer half-life, such as fluoxetine ($T\frac{1}{2}$ = 24 to 72 hours and metabolite $T\frac{1}{2}$ up to 26 hours). If SSRIs are used late in the third trimester, fetal withdrawal can also occur. Effects may last for as long as 30 days. Fetal effects are similar to maternal withdrawal and include irritability, protracted crying, and shivering.

The tricyclics antidepressants and benzodiazepines are risk category D and are therefore rarely prescribed during pregnancy. If an expectant mother has been on long-term benzydamine therapy, it is critical to taper doses gradually (25 percent per week) in order to avoid a withdrawal syndrome. Rapid withdrawal can lead to tremors, hallucinations, seizures, and a delirium tremens–like state and is most common with the use of products with a shorter $T\frac{1}{2}$. The onset of withdrawal symptoms occurs a few days after the last dose in a benzodiazepine with a shorter $T\frac{1}{2}$ (e.g., lorazepam) and to up to 3 weeks in products with a longer $T\frac{1}{2}$ (e.g., clonazepam).

Pregnancy-related anatomic changes in the urinary tract, such as pressure on the bladder from the enlarging uterus and increase in the size of the ureters, contribute to urinary reflux. UTI in the pregnant woman is a significant risk factor for low birth weight and prematurity.

Asymptomatic bacteriuria occurs in 5 to 9 percent of both nonpregnant and pregnant women. If this condition is left untreated in pregnancy, progression to symptomatic UTI, including acute cystitis and pyelonephritis, occur in 15 to 45 percent, or fourfold higher than in nonpregnant women. This is due largely to the lower interleukin-6 levels and serum antibody responses to *E. coli* antigens that occur during pregnancy, resulting in a less robust immune response.

Because asymptomatic bacteriuria, usually caused by aerobic gram-negative bacilli or *S. saprophyticus*, can lead to UTI, a urine culture should be obtained from all women early in pregnancy, even in the absence of UTI symptoms. Approximately 20 to 40 percent of women with bacteriuria will develop UTI during the course of the pregnancy; only 1 to 2 percent of those with a negative urine culture develop UTI. Bacteriuria should be treated with a 3- to 7-day course of antimicrobials, which reduces the risk of symptomatic UTI by 80 to 90 percent.

Therapeutic options for the treatment of asymptomatic bacteriuria and symptomatic UTI during pregnancy are guided by pathogen susceptibility, and preferred antimicrobials include those with FDA pregnancy risk category B. Table 15–7 identifies FDA pregnancy risk and Hale's lactation risk categories for commonly prescribed antimicrobials in UTI.

Antimicrobials in pregnancy risk category B include the beta-lactams (amoxicillin, cephalexin, cefpodoxime, cefixime, and amoxicillin/clavulanate) and nitrofurantoin. Nitrofurantoin has the advantage of sparing disruption of normal vaginal flora and consistent efficacy against *E. coli* and *S. saprophyticus*. Nitrofurantoin should be avoided after the 36th week of gestation due to the potential (although unlikely) risk for hemolysis if the fetus is G6PD-deficient and in infections caused by *P. mirabilis*. Beta-lactam use usually fails to erad-icate the offending pathogen from the periurethral and perivaginal areas, increasing the risk of reinfection.

Women with symptomatic UTI during pregnancy should be treated for 7 days. Once UTI is documented, monthly screening urine cultures should be obtained for the duration of the pregnancy. Daily antimicrobial prophylaxis with an appropriate agent should be considered with evidence of 2 days of a symptomatic UTI or persistent, unresolved bacteruria, in spite of effective antimicrobial therapy. Urologic evaluation should also be considered to rule out structural abnormality.

DISCUSSION SOURCES

Eisendrath, S., and Lichtmacher, J. (2003). Psychiatric disorders. In Tierney, L., McPhee, S., and Papadakis, M. (eds.). Current Diagnosis and Treatment (42nd ed.; pp. 1006–1066). New York: Lange Medical Books/McGraw-Hill.

Moore, K.L., and Peresaud, T.V.N. (1998). The Developing Human: Clinically Oriented Embryology (6th ed.). Philadelphia: W.B. Saunders.

Brown, K.P. (2004) Antenatal care. In: Management Guidelines for Nurse Practitioners Working with Women (2nd ed., pp 177–223). Philadelphia: F.A. Davis.

TABLE 15–7

HALE'S LACTATION RISK CATEGORIES

L1: Safest, controlled study = failed to demonstrate risk Examples: cromolyn, acetaminophen, Depo-Provera (=1 month postbirth)
L2: Safer, limited number of woman studied without risk Examples: nitrofurantoin, cephalosporins, 2nd-generation antihistamines, prednisone, SSRIs
L3: Moderately safe, no controlled study or controlled study shows minimal, non–life-threatening risk Examples: TMP-SMX, FQ antibiotics, 1st-generation antihistamines
L4: Hazardous, positive evidence of risk, may be used if maternal life-threatening situation exists Examples: lithium, ergot preparations
L5: Contraindicated, significant and documented risk Examples: radioactive isotopes, cocaine

Hale, T. (2004). Medications and Mothers' Milk (11th ed.) Amarillo, TX: Pharmasoft Medical Publishing.

78. Risk factors for preeclampsia include all of the following except:

    A. Low maternal weight.
    B. Age <16 years or >40 years.
    C. Collagen vascular disease.
    D. First pregnancy with a new partner.

79. Blood pressure changes in preeclampsia include increases of blood pressure over normotensive baseline of ___ mm Hg systolic and ___ mm Hg diastolic or more.

    A. 10, 5
    B. 20, 10
    C. 30, 15
    D. 40, 20

80. Preeclampsia presentation is noted after the ___ week of pregnancy.

    A. 10th
    B. 15th
    C. 20th
    D. 25th

81. The components of HELLP syndrome include all of the following except:

    A. Hepatic enzyme elevations.
    B. Thrombocytosis.
    C. Hemolysis.
    D. Eclampsia.

82. Which of the following is the most important part of care of the woman with preeclampsia?

    A. Antihypertensive therapy
    B. Anticonvulsant therapy
    C. Prompt recognition of the condition
    D. Referral to obstetric care

83. In neonatal group B streptococcus (GBS) disease, the NP considers that:

    A. This organism is harbored by about 50 to 70 percent of all pregnant women.
    B. There is no risk of disease with cesarean birth.
    C. The organism is most often acquired by vertical transmission in the second trimester of pregnancy.
    D. Intrapartum antimicrobials should be given to all women with evidence of GBS colonization.

84. From what location should GBS cultures be obtained?

    A. Cervix
    B. Urethra
    C. Urine
    D. Lower vagina and rectum

78. A	**79.** C	**80.** C
81. B	**82.** C	**83.** D
84. D		

Hypertensive disorders in pregnancy are usually divided into the following categories: chronic hypertension, that is, high blood pressure diagnosis that predates the pregnancy, and the hypertensive disorders acquired during pregnancy. Those acquired during pregnancy include gestational hypertension, preeclampsia, and eclampsia (Table 15–8). Preeclampsia risk factors include age (>40 years, <16 years), first pregnancy or first pregnancy with a new partner, pregestational diabetes mellitus, presence of collagen vascular disease, prepregnancy or primary hypertension, presence of renal disease, family history of pregnancy-induced hypertension, or multiple-gestation pregnancy. An early or milder case presentation of preeclampsia is usually characterized by an increase in systolic blood pressure (BP) of 30 mm Hg, an increase in diastolic BP of 15 mm Hg, or an absolute reading of 140 mm Hg/90 mm Hg in a pregnant patient with minimal proteinuria and pathologic edema, with presentation after the 20th week of gestation. Additional problems include right upper-quadrant abdominal pain,

TABLE 15–8

HYPERTENSIVE DISORDERS IN PREGNANCY

Category of Hypertensive Disorder During Pregnancy	Defining Characteristics of Disorder
Chronic HTN (CHTN)	High blood pressure diagnosed before pregnancy, present prior to the 20th week of pregnancy, and/or persisting more than 6 weeks postpartum
Gestational HTN (GHTN)	High blood pressure diagnosed after 20th week of pregnancy but resolving within 6 weeks postpartum but without significant proteinuria or other signs of preeclampsia
Preeclampsia	High blood pressure diagnosed after 20th week of pregnancy, accompanied by significant proteinuria (>300 mg protein in 24-hour urine collection) that cannot be attributed to another cause. Usually accompanied by increased edema.
Eclampsia	Presentation as in preeclampsia with tonic-clonic seizures or other alteration in mental status that cannot be attributed to another cause
HELLP syndrome	Preeclampsia accompanied by elevated hepatic enzyme levels and low platelet count.

Shubert, P., and Hackney, D. (2004). Hypertensive disorders in pregnancy. In: Rakel, R., Bope, E. (eds.) Conn's Current Therapy (pp. 1141–1145). Philadelphia: W.B. Saunders.

nausea, and vomiting. In more severe situations, a systolic BP greater than 160 mm Hg or a diastolic BP greater than 110 mm Hg with significant proteinuria (>5.0 g/d) and evidence of hepatic, renal, or central nervous system end-organ damage indicate severe preeclampsia. Preeclampsia can progress to the syndrome of hemolysis with resulting anemia, hepatocellular damage indicated by elevated liver enzyme levels, and low platelet count and eclampsia; this constellation is known as HELLP and is noted in 5 to 10 percent of patients with preeclamptic symptoms.

The most important intervention in preeclampsia is maintaining a high index of suspicion in women with considerable risk and prompt recognition of the condition. Once it is recognized, obstetric consultation should be obtained. Intervention includes rest, ongoing maternal and fetal monitoring, and antihypertensive and/or anticonvulsant medications; all of these measures have a small effect on outcome. Birth is the definitive intervention and is usually the treatment of choice in later pregnancy.

Prenatal care in later pregnancy should include screening for group B streptococcus (GBS). Neonatal infection with this organism remains one of the leading causes of newborn morbidity and mortality, resulting in an estimated 1600 early-onset cases and 80 deaths each year. Maternal lower genitourinary tract colonization with this organism is a major risk factor for early-onset, usually in the first week of life, GBS disease. The transmission of the organism from mother to fetus usually occurs after the onset of labor or membrane rupture. The lower gastrointestinal tract is the natural reservoir for this organism; this most likely contributed to GBS vaginal or rectal colonization in about 10 to 30 percent of pregnant women. GBS colonization is not considered to be a sexually transmitted infection and can be transient, chronic, or intermittent. Intrapartum antimicrobial chemoprophylaxis is currently the most effective intervention to help prevent infant GBS disease. As a result, GBS screening should be preformed in all women at 35 to 37 weeks of pregnancy, including women who will undergo cesarean birth, as the organism can cause infection across intact membranes. The culture should be obtained by swabbing the lower vagina and vaginal introitus, followed by the rectum, with insertion of the swab into the anal sphincter being needed for optimal results. The patient or health care provider can obtain the culture. No vaginal speculum is needed, and cervical cultures should not be obtained, as these can be negative in the presence of heavy lower vaginal GBS colonization.

DISCUSSION SOURCES

Brown, K.P. (2004) Antenatal care. In: Management Guidelines for Nurse Practitioners Working with Women (2nd ed., pp 177–223). Philadelphia: F.A. Davis.

Crombleholme., W. (2003). Obstetrics. In: Tierney, L., McPhee, S., and Papadakis, M. Current Medical Diagnosis and Treatment (42nd ed.; pp. 734–758). New York: Lange Medical Books/McGraw-Hill.

QUESTIONS

85. You note that a 28-year-old woman who is 4 months pregnant has bruises on her right shoulder. She states: "I fell up against the wall." The bruises appear finger-shaped. She denies that another person injured her. What is your best choice of statement in response to this?

    A. "Your bruises really look as if they were caused by someone grabbing you."
    B. "Was this really an accident?"
    C. "I notice the bruises are in the shape of a hand."
    D. "How did you fall?"

86. Which of the following is true concerning domestic violence during pregnancy?

    A. It is found largely among those of lower socioeconomic status.
    B. The woman in an abusive relationship usually seeks help.
    C. Routine screening is indicated during pregnancy.
    D. A predictable cycle of violent activity followed by a period of calm is the norm.

The following questions should be answered true or false:

87. Domestic abuse is uncommon in same-sex relationships.

88. Access to a firearm does not increase the rate of fatal episodes of domestic abuse.

89. Child abuse is present in about half of all homes where partner mistreatment occurs.

ANSWERS

85. C   86. C   87. False
88. False   89. True

DISCUSSION

Interpersonal violence among family members (i.e., domestic violence) is found in all socioeconomic and ethnic groups. However, because providers working with lower-income and select ethnic groups usually are more vigilant about domestic violence, there is often an appearance that the abuse is more of a problem in certain groups.

Domestic partner abuse can take a number of forms: psychological, financial, emotional, and physical. Acts of violence are typically thought to be against the victim but may include destruction of property, intimidation, and threats. A cycle of tension building, including criticism, yelling, and threats, followed by violence and then a quieter period of apologies and promises to change, is often seen. However, this cycle usually accelerates over time, with the violence being less predictable. Love for the perpetrator, hope that things will change, and fear of the consequences of leaving the relationship help to keep the victim in the relationship, particularly when the woman is pregnant with the perpetrator's baby and fears abandonment. As a result, the victim often does not come forth asking for help

As with counseling and screening for other health problems, using objective statements beginning with "I" is helpful. When a patient denies that finger-shaped bruises are caused by intentional injury by another person, an NP can simply state what is seen. This reinforces the assessment of abuse and allows the patient to offer more information. In a situation in which a patient is verbally abused in your presence, reinforce your role as patient advocate by stating that the behavior is unacceptable in your presence. Some may fear that this can possibly precipitate another episode of abuse. However, this is unlikely.

Applying the BATHE model is helpful in framing the problem and forming a therapeutic relationship and directing intervention. Developed by Stuart and Lieberman, this model provides a guide for gathering information while helping the patient reflect on the issues at hand. The components of the model are as follows:

BATHE

B—Background

- How are things at home? At work? Has anything changed? Good or bad? Anything you wish would change?

A—Affect, anxiety

- How do you feel about home life? Work? School? Life in general?

T—Trouble

- What worries you the most? How stressed are you about this problem?

H—Handling

- How are you handling the problems in your life? How much support do you get at home/work? Who gives you support in dealing with problems?

E—Empathy

- "That sounds difficult."

You may want to add SOAP to the BATHE.

S—Support

- Normalize problems, but do not minimize.
  - "Many people struggle with the same (similar) problem."
  - "What supports/resources can you use to help deal with this?"
- Some providers may use select self-disclosure for this. Self-disclosure usually works best in crises that are common and not of unusually tragic proportions, such as timely death or job change.

O—Objectivity

- Watch your reactions to the story. Maintain your professional composure without acting stonelike, but be mindful of "recoiling" gestures.
- Help client with objectivity.
  - What is the worst thing that can happen?
  - How likely is that?
  - Then what would happen?
- Present an accepting stance.
  - "That is an understandable way to feel."
  - "I think you have done well considering the stress."
- Coach the client to personal acceptance.
  - "I wonder if you are not being too hard on yourself."

Acknowledge client priorities.

- "It sounds like family is more important to you than your work."
- Acknowledge readiness/difficulty in making change.
  - "Change is hard and sometimes very scary."
  - "It sounds to me like you are (not) ready to make a change."

P—Present focus

- Assist client in focusing on the present, without minimizing concerns of the past and future.
  - "How could you cope better?"
  - "What could you do differently?"
  - What do you do after you have gathered this information?
- Negotiate a problem-focused contract for behavioral change.

- Repeat after me, "I promise not to harm myself or anyone else in any way between now and my next visit with_____."
- Homework assignment with "I" messages.
  - "I would like more help with the children."
  - "I feel really unimportant to you when _."
  - "I feel angry when_____."
- How do you keep this to 15 minutes?
  - Focus the client, using open- and close-ended questions. Tell client how much time you have, particularly with a revisit.
  - "We have 15 minutes to chat. What would you like to focus on?"
  - If the client cannot focus, ask, "If one problem in your life could just disappear, what would you choose?"

Interpersonal violence is likely as common in same-sex relationships as in opposite-sex relationships but not as well studied. Violent behavior by a woman against a male partner is unlikely to result in as serious an injury as in men's violence toward women. However, in all socioeconomic groups, access to a firearm by a male perpetrator is associated with increased risk of abuse toward women; indeed, this is also a risk for suicide. The nurse practitioner is in an ideal position to direct the couple to the appropriate resources for help in domestic violence but should not attempt to provide this counseling due to the complexity of this type of care. Individual treatment is the rule as long as the violent behavior continues. Child abuse is present in about half of all households where there is partner abuse.

DISCUSSION SOURCES

American Psychiatric Association. (1994). diagnostic and Statistical Manual of Mental Disorders (4th ed.) (DMS-IV). Arlington, VA: American Psychiatric Publishing, Inc.

Peace at Home, Inc. (1995). Domestic Violence: The Facts. Boston: Harvard Community Health Plan Foundation.

Stuart, M., and Lieberman, J. (2002). The 15-Minute Hour: Practical Therapeutic Intervention in Primary Care (3rd ed.). Philadelphia: W.B. Saunders

QUESTIONS

90. Approximately ___ percent of all clinically recognized pregnancies end in spontaneous abortion.

    A. 10
    B. 20
    C. 30
    D. 40

91. Approximately __ percent of spontaneous abortions result from chromosomal defects.

    A. 20 percent
    B. 40 percent
    C. 60 percent
    D. 80 percent

92. The classic clinical triad of ectopic pregnancy includes all of the following except:

    A. Abdominal pain.
    B. Vaginal bleeding.
    C. Large for gestational age uterus.
    D. Adnexal mass.

93. The classic clinical triad of ectopic pregnancy is found in no more than ___ percent of women presenting with this condition.

    A. 10
    B. 25
    C. 50
    D. 75

94. In the first weeks of a viable intrauterine pregnancy, serum quantitative hCG levels usually double every ___ hours.

    A. 24
    B. 48
    C. 72
    D. 96

95. In ectopic pregnancy, all of the following are true except:

    A. Serum progesterone level is usually less than 15 ng/mL.
    B. Sonographic evaluation fails to reveal abnormality in 20 to 30 percent of cases.

C. Location of the pregnancy is often on the ovary or cervix.

D. Risk factors include current pregnancy via assisted reproduction.

Match the clinical presentation of the following

_____96. Complete abortion

_____97. Inevitable abortion

_____98. Threatened abortion

_____99. Incomplete abortion

A. Uterine contents are in the process of being expelled.

B. Some portion of the products of conception remain in the uterus, although the pregnancy is no longer viable.

C. The products of conception have been completely expelled.

D. Ultrasound evaluation demonstrates a viable pregnancy, although vaginal bleeding is present.

ANSWERS

90. B	**91.** C	**92.** C
93. C	**94.** B	**95.** C
96. C	**97.** A	**98.** D
99. B		

DISCUSSION

Ectopic pregnancy is defined as any gestation that occurs outside of the uterus. Although reports of cervical, abdominal, and interstitial pregnancies exist, approximately 95 percent of all ectopic pregnancies are located in a fallopian tube. Because the physiologic and physical needs of the fetus cannot be met when pregnancy occurs outside the uterus, the pregnancy cannot progress beyond the earliest stages and will be lost. In fact, the majority of ectopic pregnancies resolve without intervention via miscarriage or involution of the gestation sac and reabsorption. However, those that do not resolve pose a significant risk to the mother.

Risk factors for ectopic pregnancy include factors that can influence normal tubal motility and patency, such as a history of pelvic inflammatory disease, prior ectopic pregnancy, current intrauterine device use, pregnancy achieved by means of in vitro fertilization or fertility drugs, prior tubal surgery (reconstruction or tubal ligation), and cigarette smoking. Increasing age is also an ectopic pregnancy risk factor.

The classic clinical triad of ectopic pregnancy—abdominal pain, vaginal bleeding, and an adnexal mass—is found in no more than 50 percent of women with the condition. As a result, careful clinical assessment to support or disprove the diagnosis is critically important. Diagnosis of ectopic pregnancy includes obtaining a beta-hCG level. Both urine and serum test results will usually be positive, and a negative result rules out the diagnosis. Usually, serum quantitative beta-hCG in ectopic pregnancy at gestational weeks 6 to 10, the most common weeks for clinical presentation, is in the range of 1000 to 6000 IU/m. This compares with =>40,000 IU/m for a viable intrauterine pregnancy. The normal rapid increase in serum quantitative beta-hCG level noted in a viable intrauterine pregnancy is missing, and the value tends to stall. With a positive beta-hCG level =>1000 IU/m, a gestational sac should be identifiable within the uterus on transvaginal sonogram with an intrauterine pregnancy; the presence of an intrauterine gestational sac effectively excludes the diagnosis of ectopic pregnancy. However, it is important to recall that 20 to 30 percent of women with ectopic pregnancies will have a nondiagnostic ultrasound; therefore, a normal ultrasound does not rule out the condition. The level of serum progesterone, a hormone produced by the developing chorion, should also be obtained if ectopic pregnancy is suspected. A level of less than 15 ng/mL is seen in only 11 percent of normal intrauterine pregnancies but will be noted in most ectopic pregnancies or inevitable abortions. On occasion, pelvic computed tomography or magnetic resonance imaging is indicated, with the recognition of the limitations of these studies in ectopic pregnancy but also their usefulness in identifying other reasons for abdominal pain.

Once the diagnosis of ectopic pregnancy is established, treatment is dependent on the patient's condition. If the patient is stable, evaluation for a concurrent (heterotopic) intrauterine pregnancy should be done as this condition can be found in up to 10 percent of women presenting with this condition. If the patient is hemodynamically unstable, immediate surgical intervention is warranted. If she is stable, surgical or medical intervention is warranted according to the availability of treatment options. Surgical treatments include salpingostomy, where the tube is opened and the pregnancy contents removed. The tube is then repaired. Salpingectomy is usually performed when the tubal rupture has occurred or tubal damage is severe and repair is not possible. Medical therapy with methotrexate, a medication that inhibits cell division and causes the pregnancy to regress and resolve, is an option when ectopic pregnancy is diagnosed early and the tube is intact. Close follow-up is critical with medical management of ectopic pregnancy to ensure pregnancy resolution, and surgical intervention is sometimes needed when this therapy fails. Considerable emotional support is also needed as the woman has faced a potentially life-threatening illness as well as the loss of a pregnancy. When compared with surgical therapy, tubal patency is usually better preserved with medical management.

Spontaneous abortion is defined as the natural ending of a pregnancy prior to 20 weeks' gestation. In about 60 percent of spontaneous abortions, chromosomal defects of maternal or paternal origin are responsible for the pregnancy loss. Maternal factors, such as trauma, illness, or infection, lead to the loss in about 15 percent of cases. In the remainder of the cases, no obvious cause can be found. With threatened pregnancy loss, intervention is aimed at maintaining a stable hemodynamic state and providing considerable emotional support.

About 25 to 30 percent of women experience some vaginal bleeding in the first trimester, with at least 50 percent of these women having pregnancy loss. Four terms are usually used to describe the condition of spontaneous abortion: threatened, inevitable, incomplete, and complete.

Threatened abortion presents as vaginal bleeding or brown spotting during early pregnancy that occurs with or without cramping but without cervical dilatation or change in cervical consistency. Ultrasound evaluation demonstrates a viable pregnancy, and serum quantitative hCG level is consistent with gestational age. Barring other complications, the pregnancy in threatened abortion progresses without problem. Intervention includes a few days of rest then resumption of normal activities, although even this common sense treatment likely makes little difference in the outcome. Less than half of the women who have vaginal bleeding during the first pregnancy trimester proceed to a complete abortion or miscarriage.

In an inevitable abortion, the cervix is open and the uterine contents are being expelled. The patient has cramping abdominal pain and usually brisk vaginal bleeding.

In an incomplete abortion, some portion of the products of conception remains in the uterus. The os is usually closed and minimal cramping is reported. Evacuation of the uterine contents by dilatation and aspiration is the usual intervention.

In a complete abortion, pregnancy-related uterine contents have been completely expelled. Quantitative hCG level is low for gestational age, and the ultrasound fails to identify a pregnancy. On examination, the patient has minimal cramping, the cervical os is likely still slightly open, and the uterine size is returning to normal.

DISCUSSION SOURCES

Bourgon, D. Emedicine: Ectopic Pregnancy. Available at http://www.emedicine.com/radio/topic231.htm, accessed 3/28/04.

Brown, K.P. (2004) Antenatal care. In: Management Guidelines for Nurse Practitioners Working with Women (2nd ed., pp 177–223). Philadelphia: F.A. Davis.

Crombleholme. W. (2003). Obstetrics. In: Tierney, L., McPhee, S., and Papadakis, M. (eds.). Current Medical Diagnosis and Treatment (42nd ed.; pp. 734–758). New York: Lange Medical Books/ McGraw-Hill.

QUESTIONS

100. First-time mothers usually have an average of __ hours of active first- and second-stage labor.

    A. 6
    B. 9
    C. 12
    D. 15

101. For women who have previously given birth, first- and second-stage labor usually lasts an average of __ hours.

    A. 4
    B. 6
    C. 8
    D. 10

ANSWERS

100. B   **101.** B

DISCUSSION

The NP must have knowledge of the normal process of labor in order to provide appropriate counseling. A number of theories exist as to why labor starts. These include factors related to placental aging and uterine distention. At the normal pregnancy term, a time between 38 and 42 weeks' gestation, the process of labor begins. Early labor, also called the latent phase of labor, is often the longest part, sometimes lasting 2 to 3 days, and is characterized by mild-to-moderate contractions that last about 30 to 45 seconds and are 5 to 20 minutes apart, often starting and stopping. The pregnant woman is usually able to be up and around during this period and may be frustrated by the apparent slow progress of labor. During this time, the cervix usually dilates to around 3 cm. The membranes are usually intact.

The first stage of active labor starts when the cervix is about 3 to 4 cm dilated and is complete when the cervix is fully dilated. Contractions become closer and more intense, culminating in transition when contractions occur every 2 to 3 minutes and last 50 to 70 seconds or more. The pregnant woman should be instructed to go to the hospital or birthing center when contractions are occurring every 5 minutes and lasting up to 1 minute. During active labor, the woman often feels restless and excited by the impending birth but is usually communicative between contractions. In transition, the woman is usually quite focused on getting through the birth process and may be distracted by the comments of others. However, the presence of a support person is important throughout the birth process.

The second stage of labor is the actual birth, a stage that can last a few minutes or a few hours. The mother often passes through this stage with a variety of emotions, from exhaustion to elation. The third stage of labor occurs when the placenta detaches and is expelled from the uterus.

First-time mothers usually have an average of 9 hours of first- and second-stage labor. For women who have previously given birth, first- and second-stage labor lasts an average of 6 hours.

The pregnant woman and her labor support should be encouraged to attend childbirth and infant care classes. Referral to these classes usually takes place during the second trimester of pregnancy.

DISCUSSION SOURCE

Labor and delivery. Available at http://www. marchofdimes.com/pnhec/240.asp, accessed 4/8/04.

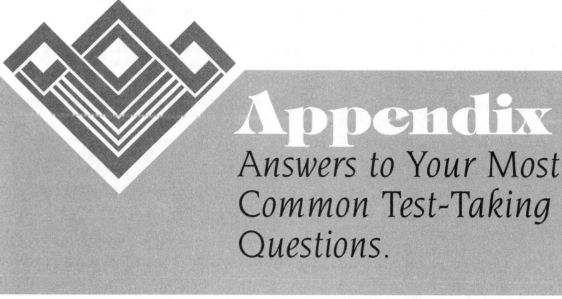

Appendix
Answers to Your Most Common Test-Taking Questions.

Are you getting ready to become a certified Nurse Practitioner (NP)? Are you confused about which organizations offer what kind of certification? Are you concerned about examination content or focus? Here are answers to frequently asked questions about the NP certification examinations.

What agencies offer NP certification examinations?

NP certification is offered by a variety of agencies, often affiliated with a professional organization. The American Nurses Credentialing Center (www.nursingworld.org/ancc) offers year-round computer-based testing for family, adult, acute care, geriatric and pediatric NP certification. The American Academy of Nurse Practitioners (www.aanp.org) offers family, adult, and NP certification, as well as computer-based testing offered during three testing seasons per year, while the National Certification Corporation (www.nccnet.com) offers paper-and-pencil testing as well as computer-based testing, year-round, for women's health NP and neonatal NP certifications. The National Certification Board of Pediatric Nurse Practitioners and Nurse, Inc. (www.pnpcert. org) offers year-round computer-based testing for pediatric NP certification.

What should I expect on the NP certification examination?

Each examination contains a set number of questions that contribute to your final score and likely a small number of additional sample items added for reliability and validity. The NP examinations contain sections that reflect the broad base of knowledge needed for entry-level NP practice. The largest sections of these examinations are typically dedicated to the evaluation of the certification candidate's ability to assess common health problems and develop an appropriate plan of intervention. The assessment section usually includes questions on obtaining an accurate, focused health history; identifying normal and abnormal findings in the physical examination; diagnostic studies and screening tests, and applying critical thinking skills vital to NP practice. Content in the intervention typically includes questions on both pharmacologic and nonpharmacologic therapies as well as principles of therapeutic communication. The remainder of the examination is usually devoted to areas such as health promotion, disease prevention, differential diagnosis skills, health care planning and education, epidemiology, pathophysiology, and evaluation, including response to treatment and quality assurance principles.

How do the NP examinations differ?

One obvious difference is the age or gender focus of many of the examinations. The adult nurse practitioner examination focuses on the care of the patient aged 13 years and older. The geriatric nurse practitioner examination focuses on health care issues for adults after age 50 years and contains a section on theories of aging. The pediatric nurse practitioner examinations focus on the care of children and young adults, usually up to age 22 years; a thorough knowledge of pediatric development and family systems is critical for success with this examination. The women's health NP examination's focus is on the primary care of women throughout the reproductive life span and beyond; about one quarter of the examination is on the care of the woman during pregnancy, and a similar amount is devoted to general primary care issues. The acute care NP examination focus is on the care of acutely or critically ill adults, but it also includes a section on health promotion and disease prevention as well as follow-up care. The family NP examination reflects a broad scope of knowledge needed to care for patients of all ages, with about one third of the examination devoted to pediatrics and care of the woman during pregnancy.

Should I expect questions on professional practice issues?

Each examination contains sections on issues such as scope of practice, health care ethics, and reimbursement. Generally, this section is about 5% to 6% of the total examination.

How can I find out the pass rates of the NP certification examinations?

Check the agency's Web site. Pass rates are often posted and are usually in the 70% to 85% range. Put another way, about one in four to one in five NP certification candidates does not pass the examination.

What kind of questions will I find on the NP certification examinations?

As mentioned, the NP certification examinations are composed of multiple-choice questions; there are no true/false, fill-in-the-blank, essay, or matching test items.

Are all of the examination questions at the same level of complexity or difficulty?

These examination questions are written on a number of levels of difficulty and depth, with the lowest level usually being the fact-oriented or knowledge questions. This type of question tests generalizations, principles, and widely recognized theories. When answering this question, you might read the question and instantly recognize the correct answer from a piece of information that was memorized long ago.

The following is an example of a fact-oriented question:

Pupillary constriction in reaction to light is in part a function of cranial nerve:

A. I
B. II
C. III
D. IV

Mnemonics or other memory aids may be helpful in answering a fact-oriented question. However, the certification examinations will likely contain many more complex types of questions that require application of clinical assessment and management skills. Examples of these include the comprehension question, where you must interpret the fact.

An example of a comprehension question is as follows:

The person with Bell palsy has paralysis of cranial nerve:

A. V
B. VI
C. VII
D. VIII

In order to respond correctly to this question, you must know that Bell palsy is a condition where the facial nerve (cranial nerve VII) is affected.

Likely the most common type of question found on the certification examinations is the application question. In this type, you analyze the information, then decide what is pertinent to the given situation. Look for key words in the stem (the question itself) that help set a priority. These include words such as first, initially, or most important action. If you are having difficulty ascertaining which action should be done first, particularly when the question poses many plausible actions, you should ask yourself, "What is the greatest risk in this situation?" Here is an example:

You are seeing Ms. Thomas, a 53-year-old woman who presents for a health examination. She smokes cigarettes and has a family history of premature heart disease. The most important part of her assessment is:

A. Chest x-ray study
B. Auscultation for S_3 and S_4 heart sounds
C. Blood pressure measurement
D. Cervical examination with Papanicolaou testing

When looking at this question, you may be struck with the fact that you would certainly perform a cardiac examination and Papanicolaou test. With the limited amount of information available on this patient, no indication for chest x-ray study is evident. So, how do you set the priority of the most important part of the assessment? Start with teasing out the facts and assumptions. Facts include two risk factors for cardiovascular disease: cigarette smoking and family history of premature heart disease. In addition, heart disease is the leading cause of death in American women. Assume that she is postmenopausal, because the average woman reaches this by age 50 years. This gives her an additional cardiovascular risk factor. Thus, the stage is set for her to be at high risk for cardiovascular disease. Another assumption is that the best evaluation is one that picks up early disease. Now, look at the answers given and think what you may expect for results.

In assessing Ms. Thomas, a chest x-ray study may reveal lung cancer or smoking-related lung disease. However, these changes will not be evident until these diseases are advanced. The presence of extra heart sounds would likely indicate systolic (S_3) and/or diastolic (S_4) cardiac dysfunction, again a marker of significant, usually advanced, cardiac problems. However, blood pressure measurement is critical, as it can detect hypertension in its asymptomatic, earliest state, and increases Ms. Thomas' risk of heart disease. Although screening for cervical neoplasia is important, intervening in hypertension would be more likely to improve this woman's shorter-term health.

How about some tips on answering multiple-choice questions?

A multiple-choice question has a number of components. Often, the first sentence is an introduction of a clinical scenario. Here is an example of a rather lengthy introduction, rich with information:

You see that 18-year-old Sam was seen yesterday at a local walk-in center for treatment of ear pain. He was diagnosed with left acute otitis media, and amoxicillin was prescribed. Today, Sam states that he has taken three amoxicillin doses but continues to have discomfort in the affected ear. The left tympanic membrane is red and immobile.

When responding to this question, remember that test questions are designed to have one best, although perhaps not perfect, answer. In clinical practice, you would likely gather more information than is given here. During the certification examination, you have to decide on the best response, simply given the information in front of you while applying sound clinical judgment. Here are the clinical points as these relate to this particular question. Consider the following:

As no chronic health problems are mentioned, assume that Sam is a young adult who is typically in good health. Acute otitis media (AOM) is a common episodic illness, usually caused by *Streptococcus pneumoniae, Haemophilus influenzae, Moraxella catarrhalis*, or respiratory virus.

One of the first-line antimicrobials for AOM treatment is amoxicillin, because when given in adequate amounts, it is effective against

S. pneumoniae, and non—beta-lactamase producing *H. influenzae* and *M. catarrhalis.* Nearly all *M. catarrhalis* and about 40% of *H. influenzae* produce beta-lactamase, rendering amoxicillin ineffective. Clavulanate is a beta-lactamase inhibitor and, when given in conjunction with amoxicillin, is an effective treatment option when AOM fails to respond to amoxicillin alone.

As inflammation and purulent exudate form in the middle ear, a small space rich with pain receptors, otalgia is an expected finding in AOM. This usually resolves after 2 to 3 days of antimicrobial therapy.

Tympanic membrane immobility is a cardinal sign of AOM that, in spite of antimicrobial therapy, does not resolve for a number of weeks.

The next part is the statement that poses the question to be answered.

Your next best action is to (this is an action-oriented question, directing you to consider Sam's care and chief complaint):

A. Advise Sam to discontinue the current antimicrobial and start a course of amoxicillin with clavulanate.

Choosing this response implies amoxicillin treatment failure. However, AOM antimicrobial treatment failure is usually defined as persistent otalgia with fever after 72 hours of therapy. Sam has taken less than 2 days of therapy, too short an interval to assign continued symptoms to ineffective antimicrobial therapy.

B. Perform tympanocentesis and send a sample of the exudate for culture and sensitivity.

AOM antimicrobial therapy is based on choosing an agent with activity against the most likely organisms, bearing in mind the most commonly resistant pathogens. Tympanocentesis is indicated only with treatment failure after 10 to 21 days of antimicrobial therapy with a second-line agent, with the goal of detecting a significantly resistant organism; at that point, culture and sensitivity of middle ear exudate would be appropriate. With less than 2 days of treatment, tympanocentesis is not indicated.

C. Have Sam return in 24 hours for reevaluation.

Certainly, if Sam's condition worsens in the next day, reevaluation is prudent. However, choosing this option ignores Sam's complaint of pain.

D. Recommend that Sam take ibuprofen for the next 2 to 3 days.

Choosing this response implies that treating Sam's pain is the most appropriate intervention. This is the best response and therefore the correct answer.

Now consider this question:

Which of the following best describes asthma?

No clinical scenario is presented, but the question simply asks for a definition of a pathologic state. When considering the options, the test taker must recall that asthma is a chronic inflammatory disease of the airways involving an increase in bronchial hyperresponsiveness. This leads to a potentially reversible decrease in forced expiratory volume in 1 second to vital capacity.

Consider these options:

A. Intermittent airway inflammation with occasional bronchospasm.
  • As asthma is a chronic, not intermittent, inflammatory airway disease, this option is incorrect.
B. A disease of bronchospasm leading to airway inflammation.
  As asthma is first a chronic inflammatory airway disease that leads to airway hyperresponsiveness, this option is incorrect.
C. Chronic airway inflammation with superimposed bronchospasm.
  This option most closely matches the definition of asthma and is the best option.
D. Relatively fixed airway obstruction.
  Because the airway obstruction in asthma is reversible, this option is incorrect.

What about test anxiety?

Everyone who sits for one of the certification examinations is anxious to some degree. This anxiety can be a helpful emotion, focusing the NP certification candidate on the task at hand, studying and successfully sitting for this important examination, a tangible end product of your graduate education. When excessive, however, anxiety can get in the way of your success.

So a little bit of anxiety is normal and helpful?

Yes. Stress yields anxiety, anxiety yields stress; one can be viewed as the product of the other. The stress of preparing for an important examination triggers the sympathetic nervous system to Seyle's three phases of the general adaptation syndrome: alarm, resistance, and exhaustion. In the alarm stage, perhaps triggered by contemplating the preparation needed to achieve certification success, the hypothalamus activates the autonomic nervous system, in turn triggering the pituitary and the body defenses, resulting in a heightened sense of awareness of surroundings, alertness, and focus. At this level of arousal, studying for and taking a test often yield great results. The well-prepared examination candidate is highly focused on what needs to be done to be successful on the examination. Distractions can be filtered out, extraneous information being discarded in favor of the essentials. During the examination, where anxiety and knowledge intersect, information retrieval is facilitated, and examination questions are fluidly processed. Difficult examination items are usually put in perspective, with the test taker recognizing that the majority of items were answered with relative ease. This NP certification candidate emerges from the test feeling challenged but confident.

Too much test anxiety is a problem?

Yes. Bringing together a sound knowledge base and a healthy dose of anxiety, most NP certification examination candidates proceed with confidence. However, a significant number do not move through the examinations in this manner. The process of completing a rigorous course of graduate education and study can result in a protracted period of stress. The formerly helpful stress leads to the second stage of the general adaptation syndrome, resistance, where epinephrine is released to help counteract or escape from the stressor. At that time, the feeling of milder anxiety present in the first stage gives way to a sense of greater nervousness, often accompanied by uncomfortable physical sensations, such as dry mouth, tachycardia, and tremor. Studying or taking an examination becomes difficult, and information retrieval is inhibited. This stage is mentally and physically taxing and, if left unchecked, can lead to exhaustion, complicating the challenging task of successful completion of the certification examination.

What exactly is test-taking anxiety?

Although often described as test-taking anxiety, the problem usually includes an excessive dose of anxiety while attempting to study for the examination, thus termed studying-testing anxiety. Although the reaction is most severe at the time of the test, most people who have severe test-taking anxiety have a similar, although milder, reaction with the deep study needed to prepare for a critical examination, such as NP certification. The following scenario describes the person with a problematic case of studying-testing anxiety:

The NP examination candidate is having a tough day, with a work shift that stretched for three unexpected hours and an unusually long commute, all following a poor night's sleep resulting from a noisy neighborhood party. To counteract this, the NP drank a few extra cups of strong coffee. However, studying was part of today's plan, so the NP sits down to prepare for the examination with great intentions of reviewing critical information. Surrounded by great stacks of study material, the examination candidate thinks about what might be on the examination and ponders the wide scope and knowledge base needed to be successful. Now the NP becomes aware of a dry mouth and a tight feeling in the throat. Determined, the NP sits down and decides to study about antimicrobial therapy. The words on the page seem to blur while the NP tries to read about an antibiotic's spectrum of activity; then, having difficulty keeping this information straight, the NP decides to skip that and focuses on memorizing a few antibiotic doses. Even with repeated tries, the NP cannot keep this information at hand and now feels even more anxious, with a feeling of tension in the back of the neck and a rapidly beating heart. The NP now shifts attentions, trying a few practice examination questions but answers three questions about the appropriate use of antimicrobial therapy in acute otitis media and gets all three items incorrect. Now, even the thought of sitting for the examination causes the NP to freeze.

How can this situation be altered?

Although developing a schedule of study is important, rescheduling the study time may be a good idea when a day has been particularly difficult. Trying to learn when exhausted and stressed by other influences is often counterproductive. Certain scents may be helpful for putting the NP in the right frame of mind to study, particularly under less-than-ideal conditions. These include basil, cinnamon, lemon, and peppermint for mental alertness and camomile, lavender, and orange for relaxation.

Learn a relaxation technique to use prior to studying or test taking. Start the session by reading or repeating a positive message about being successful on the examination. Avoid excessive amounts of caffeinated beverages that can add to anxious feelings.

The NP's anxiety started when pondering the wide range of possible of topics on the certification examination. Starting the session studying a narrowly focused topic with a specific outcome goal rather than simply studying might have averted this. Setting up a system of study can further enhance the success of a study session. One method is the SQ4R system, where the *s*tudy information is *S*urveyed to established goals; then, *Q*uestions about the information are formulated, then *R*ead to answer these questions, followed by *R*eciting the *R*esponses to the original questions, and *R*eviewing to see if the original goals were met. Study and test-taking anxiety can also be tamed with the help of a learning specialist who can work with the NP examination candidate to develop the needed skills. Learning specialists can usually be contacted through the academic support centers at universities.

What do NPs who have failed an NP certification examination offer as advice?

In the course of talking to candidates for certification, I often speak with NPs who do not pass the certification NP examination. I have learned from these conversations that this is a group of intelligent people who have completed a course of rigorous graduate study. In spite of this, they were unsuccessful at an examination that often dictates whether the NP can practice. This can be a devastating blow. However, in retrospect, most can say what it was that got in the way of success. Here is what they have shared:

"I expected to read a question and instantly recognize the answer."

Although this may happen with a low-level, fact-oriented question, such as one identifying an anatomic landmark, you should not expect this to be the case for most of the questions. Most items test your ability to assess or develop a plan of intervention for a clinical situation. Therefore, you should expect to apply clinical decision-making skills to the test question. Make sure you think through each question. In particular, bear in mind how the pathophysiology of the condition affects its presentation and treatment.

"I could not figure out what the question was asking."

Sometimes, identifying the verb in the question can help you determine the purpose of the question. In addition, look at the information presented, and then ask yourself, "Is this question a test of the ability to gather subjective or objective information? The ability to develop a diagnosis or to plan a course of intervention?" This will help focus your thought process as you choose the answer.

"More than one answer was applicable to the situation presented. I was not sure which response was correct."

Take another look at the question, and then choose the response most specific to the given situation. Also, sometimes questions that relate to presentation of disease have more than one applicable answer. However, the response with the most common presentation is likely to be correct. For example, an adult with bacterial meningitis can present with nuchal rigidity and papilledema. However, because nuchal rigidity is seen in most adults with this diagnosis and papilledema found far less often, nuchal rigidity is a better choice. In addition, childhood development questions often have more than one correct response. For example, a 4-month-old is expected to roll from stomach to back and smile. However, smiling is a developmental milestone achieved by age 2 months, whereas rolling is typically not seen until the baby is 4 months old. Therefore, rolling from stomach to back is most specific to that age.

"I work in an acute-care setting. The scenarios and treatment options presenting in the questions were quite different than what I am accustomed to seeing in my RN practice. I had a hard time choosing the best answer."

Many new NP graduates are seasoned RNs. It is important to remember that in the acute-care setting, you are typically seeing the "worst case scenario" of a disease state rather than how it would present in primary care, the practice setting of most NPs. Recall that the NP certification examination is a test of entry-level NP knowledge. The acute-care nurse is accustomed to seeing exceptions; the examination is likely to present situations that are more often the rule. For example, the chest pain associated with acute coronary syndrome or unstable angina can last for hours and is present at rest. Because the acute-care nurse likely has experience in caring for patients with unstable angina, this presentation may become the nurse's mindset of the typical presentation of angina pectoris. However, the chest pain episode of the community-dwelling elder with stable angina pectoris is usually infrequent and lasts less than 10 minutes. Relief of symptoms usually occurs promptly and is relieved with rest or cessation of the provoking activity. The test taker needs to apply primary, not acute-care, rules to the test.

How about some tips on approaching the certification examination?

Here are some certification examination "dos" and "don'ts."

Certification Examination Dos

Do read each question and the responses so that you mark your option choice only after you are sure you understand the concept being tested in the question. Answering a question may quickly lead to choosing a response that contains correct information about a given condition but might not be the correct response for that particular question.

Do be wary of options that include extreme words, such as "always," "never," "all," "best," "worst," or "none." Seldom is anything absolute in health care.

Do recall and jot down a few facts about the information if you are really stumped. Doing this may be enough to enable you to retrieve the information you need to more easily respond to the question.

Do remember that if the options cover a wide range of numerical values, a value at or near the middle is often correct.

Do make sure that the extra information usually found in a particularly long answer is pertinent to the question and not simply a distractor.

Do read the shortest answer with care before you reject it. Although the short option gives little detail, there still may be enough information in it to make it correct.

Do notice if two options look similar. Usually, one is the correct answer.

Do note when two options convey the same information or have the same meaning; usually, both are wrong.

Do read each option as if it were a true-false question, eliminating all the options that are false.

Do expect to answer about 60 to 70 or more multiple-choice questions per hour. This means that you may have less than minute, on average, to spend on each question. Some questions will take only a few seconds, whereas others will require more time for thought. Check yourself at 15- or 20-minute intervals to determine if you are progressing at an acceptable rate, setting a number of questions that you should have answered by a certain time.

Do expect that the topics you studied will be presented in random order. A question on diabetes mellitus may follow one on hypertension and can be preceded by a question on women's health.

Do recall that the certification examinations are geared to test the knowledge base of an entry-level NP knowledge. As a result, you may need to apply knowledge you have learned in a new or novel way in order to correctly answer a question.

Do use evidence- and consensus-based practice in the examination. Expect that advice on health screenings and interventions is based on nationally recognized standards of care from authorities such as the American Diabetes Association, the National Cholesterol Education Program, and the American Cancer Society, not simply what you have observed being done in clinical practice.

Certification Examination Don'ts

Don't forget that the computer-based test sites accommodate the needs of a number of different test candidates. Although these are generally quiet locations, people will be moving in and out of the test area. Bring along earplugs if you are easily distracted.

Don't be misled by the close-to-correct option that may precede the correct answer.

Don't assume that an answer is correct because this is what you have observed in your current nursing practice.

Don't dismiss an option because it seems too obvious and simple to be correct. If you are well prepared for the examination, some of the questions will appear very straightforward.

Don't select an option just because it contains factually correct information about the clinical situation. You have to make sure that it is the "correct" answer to the question.

Don't reject an answer just because you have answered three responses in a row with a given option, such as "B." If after careful consideration you deem a response correct, stick with that answer.

Don't answer every question that you are unsure about as a certain option, such as "C," or you will pick this one response too often. As a result of your NP studies and certification preparation, you should be able to draw on your knowledge base and be able to narrow choices to two options.

Don't pick an answer just because it seems to make sense. You are answering from your knowledge of the course content, not just from your general knowledge and logic.

Don't be taken in by the use of unfamiliar terms in the question. If you know you have studied the subject, few words should be unknown.

Don't get bogged down on one question part of the way through the examination if you are unsure or stumped about an answer. A better strategy is to move on and finish all of those questions that you can answer and then to come back later to process the problematic questions. The computer-based tests do have a mechanism to highlight questions you want to revisit.

Don't change an answer unless you first misinterpreted the question. If necessary, when looking over the questions again, change an answer only if you can logically justify the change.

Don't respond to self-defeating thoughts that may creep into your mind, such as, "I did not study enough," or "This test is too hard."

Recognize the time and energy you have put into your preparation.

When should I start studying for the NP certification examination?

I advise that you start at the beginning of your NP program! From your first day of NP study, think like an NP and work at developing the critical thinking and technical skills needed for success. The NP provides health care independently and as part of a health care team and assumes full accountability for clinical judgment. The content of the NP certification examinations reflect these fundamental components of NP practice.

How about some tips on how to prepare for NP practice as well as the certification examination?

Deep knowledge and appreciation of the pathophysiology and epidemiology of health problems inform NP practice. If you know what causes an illness, your job of figuring out how to help the person achieve health is greatly facilitated. Knowledge of disease epidemiology will help you recognize the most likely health problems in given patient groups.

Clinical practice and certification tip: Remember that common disease occurs commonly and that the uncommon presentation of a common disease is more common than the common presentation of an uncommon disease.

The fundamental tools of NP practice include the ability to comprehensively yet succinctly procure the information needed to develop an accurate diagnosis from subjective and objective information. Gathering the needed subjective and objective information for the care of the person with common acute, episodic, and chronic health problems is the most important skill the NP can develop. Develop the skill of taking the thorough yet concise health history that is pertinent to the patient's presenting complaint or health problem. As you proceed through the history, recall the rationale behind each question you ask and how a given response affects the possible etiology of the patient's health problem. Know

how to perform a thorough yet succinct symptom analysis—this is where the detective work of diagnosis starts. Use the physical examination to confirm the findings of the health history.

Clinical practice and certification tip: Remember that the physical examination is guided by the health history, not the other way around.

The advanced-practice NP role includes the responsibilities of arriving at a diagnosis, developing a treatment plan, and providing ongoing evaluation of response to treatment.

Clinical practice and certification tip: Learn to recognize the typical clinical presentation for the 10 most common health problems that present to your practice site, including chief complaint and physical examination findings and the needed diagnostics. Armed with this information, you can focus your study on a thorough knowledge of the assessment and the treatment of these conditions. Continue to evaluate the patient's response to therapy.

Ask your preceptor to save laboratory results, electrocardiograms, and other diagnostics for you to review for the next session. Do so with a clean eye, as if you were developing a plan of intervention/further diagnosis for the patient. This will help hone your skills. If you prescribed an intervention but will not have the opportunity to see the patient at a follow-up visit, ask your preceptor for an update.

Family, cultural, community, developmental, and environmental factors; lifestyle; and health behaviors influence patient health and NP–patient interaction. As an advanced-practice nurse, the NP provides holistic, wellness-oriented care on an ongoing or episodic basis.

Clinical practice and certification tip: Remember to address a patient's primary, secondary, and tertiary health care needs at every visit. Check for needed immunization, screening tests, and follow-up for previous health problems with every encounter. Think long term. Envision working with patients for years ahead, as well as the health problems you may help this person avoid by working together.

The health care provided by the NP is guided by health and wellness research. The NP is accountable for his or her ongoing learning and professional development and is a life-long learner. The NP is also knowledgeable in accessing resources to guide evidence-based care.

Clinical practice and certification tip: Ask preceptors and peers what references are most helpful for that particular practice. Armed with this information, develop your own reference library that you can use with ease. Your investment of time and money will pay off many times over as your knowledge base and clinical confidence grow.

REFERENCES

Nugent, P., and Vitale, B. (2004). Test-Taking Techniques for Beginning Nursing Students, 4th ed. Philadelphia: F.A. Davis.

Springhouse Corp. (2000). Studying and Test Taking Made Incredibly Easy. Springhouse, PA: Springhouse.

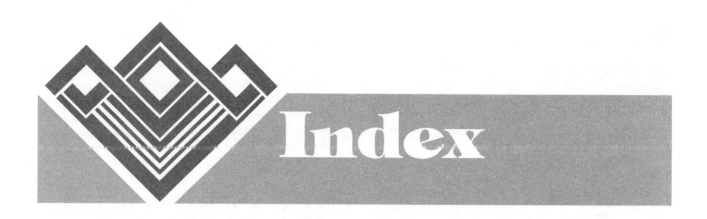

Index

Page numbers followed by "f" denote figures, "t" denote tables, and "b" denote boxes

A

Abducens nerve, 22
Abortion
  incomplete, 380
  inevitable, 380
  spontaneous, 378, 380
  threatened, 380
Absence seizure, 34
Abuse
  alcohol. *See* Alcohol abuse
  benzodiazepine, 265–266, 267t, 282, 284
  opiate, 265
  physical, 288
Acanthosis nigricans, 228
Accessory nerve, 22
Accolate. *See* Zafirlukast
Accutane. *See* Isotretinoin
Acetaminophen, 353
Achilles tendon reflex, 183
Acne neonatorum, 331
Acne vulgaris
  definition of, 45
  medications for, 45–47, 46t
Actinic keratoses, 58
Acute bacterial rhinosinusitis, 84, 85t
Acute cholecystitis, 129–131
Acute coronary syndrome
  pathophysiology of, 117
  questions about, 114–115
  signs and symptoms of, 116t
Acute epididymitis, 159
Acute febrile illness
  antipyretics for, 352–353
  description of, 352
  incidence of, 352–353
  questions about, 348, 351
Acute gastroenteritis, 345–346
Acute glomerulonephritis, 77, 146t
Acute gouty arthritis, 173
Acute interstitial nephritis, 146t
Acute limb ischemia, 212

Acute lumbosacral strain, 183–184
Acute myocardial infarction
  angiotensin-converting enzyme inhibitors for, 119
  chest pain associated with, 116t
  diagnostic tests for, 118
  fibrinolysis for, 118, 119t
  pathophysiology of, 117
  questions about, 114–115
  ST-segment elevated, 118, 119t
  treatment of, 118
Acute otitis media
  in children, 332–335
  definition of, 334
  description of, 66t, 74–75
  fever reduction in, 351
  Haemophilus influenzae and, 75, 333
  pathogens, 333
  questions about, 332–333
  recurrent, 332
  risk factors for, 333–334
  signs and symptoms of, 334
  Streptococcus pneumoniae and, 74–75, 333–334
  treatment of, 334–335
Acute prostatitis, 157t, 160–161
Acute pyelonephritis, 148
Acute renal failure, 145–146, 146t
Acute retroviral syndrome, 253t
Acute tubular necrosis, 146t
Acyclovir, 23
Adjustment disorder, 274–275
Adolescents, 319
Air trapping, 344
Airway inflammation, 89
Albuterol, 92t, 342, 343t
Alcohol abuse
  alkaline phosphatase and, 265
  aspartate aminotransferase levels in, 264
  during breast-feeding, 314, 316
  brief interventions for, 262, 263f
  CAGE questionnaire for, 262, 262b

Alcohol abuse *(Continued)*
  counseling for, 262–263
  detoxification, 263–264, 264b
  diagnosis of, 264
  during pregnancy, 361
  questions about, 261–262
  screening for, 3t, 262, 263f
  stages of change for, 263
Alcoholism, 262
Alcohol withdrawal
  benzodiazepines for, 264
  symptoms of, 263
Aldara. *See* Imiquimod
Alkaline phosphatase
  in acute cholecystitis, 129, 130t
  alcohol abuse and, 265
  in hepatitis, 143
Allergic conjunctivitis, 81t
Allergic rhinitis
  description of, 80–81, 81t–82t
  treatment of, 81t–82t, 82f–83f
Alpha-adrenergic agonists, 264
Alpha-fetoprotein, 364, 366
Alpha-glucosidase inhibitors, 216, 219t, 221
Alprazolam, 267t
Alzheimer disease, 38
Amantadine
  influenza treated with, 7
  Parkinson disease treated with, 33
American Cancer Society, 19t–20t
Amniocentesis, 364
Amoxicillin
  acute bacterial rhinosinusitis treated with, 85t
  peptic ulcer disease treated with, 136t
  pneumonia treated with, 103–104
  Streptococcus pneumoniae treated with, 103–104
Amoxicillin/clavulanate
  acute bacterial rhinosinusitis treated with, 85t
  acute otitis media treated with, 335
Amylase, 234, 234t
Anal fissures, 125–126
Anaphylaxis, 60, 241–242, 242t–243t
Androgens, 299–300
Anemia
  of chronic disease, 245, 250–251
  in chronic renal failure, 146
  clinical presentation of, 245
  definition of, 245
  etiology of, 245–246
  folate-deficiency
    causes of, 249
    overview of, 248–249
    questions about, 244
  hemograms, 246
  iron-deficiency
    causes of, 247
    iron therapy for, 247–248, 248t

  laboratory diagnosis of, 247
    questions about, 242–243
  pernicious, 244
  physical examination findings, 246
  during pregnancy, 360
  questions about, 242–245
Anergy testing, 99t
Angina pectoris
  grading of, 117t
  pathophysiology of, 115
  stable, 115
  treatment of, 115, 118
  unstable, 117t
Angiotensin-converting enzyme inhibitors
  acute myocardial infarction treated with, 119
  congestive heart failure treated with, 122–123
  hypertension treated with, 106–107
Angiotensin receptor blockers, 122–123
Angle-closure glaucoma, 68–69, 69f
Angular cheilitis, 64
Ankle sprain, 196
Annular, 40t
Anorexia nervosa, 269–271
Antacids, 138–139
Anterior epistaxis, 67
Anthralin, 56
Antidepressants
  depression treated with, 275–277, 276t–277t
  eating disorders treated with, 271
  during pregnancy, 372
  selective serotonin reuptake inhibitors, 276t–277t, 277, 279
  toxicity concerns, 277
  tricyclic
    depression treated with, 277, 279t, 280
    panic disorder treated with, 285
    pregnancy risk classification of, 368–369, 372
  types of, 276t–277t
Antiepileptic drugs, 34–35, 292–293
Antifungals
  Candida sp. treated with, 64
  onychomycosis treated with, 53
Antihistamines
  allergic rhinitis treated with, 80, 82t
  anaphylaxis treated with, 243t
  atopic dermatitis treated with, 51
  description of, 43–44
  Menière disease treated with, 72
Antimicrobial therapy
  acute bacterial rhinosinusitis treated with, 84
  microbe resistance to, 103
  pneumonia treated with, 103–104
Antinuclear antibodies, 179
Antipyretics, 348, 352–353
Antithrombin III, 203
Antithromboplastin III, 206
Anxiety disorders

benzodiazepines for, 284
depression and, 274, 283–284
description of, 283
generalized anxiety disorder, 283
herbal medications for, 286, 287t
questions about, 281–283
signs and symptoms of, 284
treatment of, 284
Aortic regurgitation, 110t, 190t
Aortic sclerosis, 110t
Aortic stenosis, 110t, 112, 188, 189t, 192, 350t
Appendicitis, 126–127
Arthritis
    gouty, 171–174
    osteoarthritis, 174–176
    Reiter syndrome, 185–186
    rheumatoid
        antinuclear antibodies associated with, 179
        definition of, 178
        diagnostic criteria for, 178, 178t
        disease-modifying antirheumatic drugs for, 179
        epidemiology of, 178
        erythrocyte sedimentation rate evaluations, 179
        nonsteroidal anti-inflammatory drugs for, 179–180
        questions about, 176–177
        tests for, 178–179
        treatment of, 179–180
Aspartate aminotransferase
    in acute cholecystitis, 130t
    alcohol abuse and, 264
    half-life of, 143, 264
    in hepatitis, 143
Asthma
    air trapping associated with, 344
    bronchospasm associated with, 89–90
    care guidelines for, 89–90
    in children, 91f
    chronic obstructive pulmonary disease treated with,
        96
    corticosteroids for, 90, 92t, 371
    definition of, 89
    diagnosis of, 89t, 340
    flare-ups, 90
    flaring of, 344
    in infants, 91f
    leukotriene receptor antagonists for, 90, 92t, 93
    maternal, during pregnancy, 367–368, 370–371
    questions about, 87–89, 338, 340–341
    treatment of, 89–93, 91f, 92t, 341–344, 343t–344t,
        371
Asymptomatic bacteriuria, 369, 372–373
Atarax. *See* Hydroxyzine
Ativan. *See* Lorazepam
Atopic dermatitis, 51, 332
Atopy, 242
Atrial septal defect, 111t, 191t, 193, 350t
Atrophic vaginitis, 300–301

Atrophy, 40t
Atrovent. *See* Ipratropium bromide
Attenuated influenza vaccine, 7, 323
Auditory nerve, 22
Azelaic acid (Azelex), 46t

B

Bacille Calmette-Guerin, 99t
Bacterial endocarditis, 113t
Bacterial meningitis, 30–31, 351
Bacterial pharyngitis, 77–78
Bacterial prostatitis, 157t–158t
Bacterial rhinosinusitis, acute, 84, 85t
Bacterial vaginosis, 302–303, 306t
Bacteriuria, asymptomatic, 369, 372–373
Bactroban. *See* Mupirocin
Bandemia, 127, 354
Barrett esophagus, 138
Basal cell carcinoma, 58
Bell palsy, 22–23
Benign prostatic hypertrophy, 153–154
Benign thyroid nodules, 236
Benzodiazepines
    abuse of, 265–266, 267t, 282, 284
    alcohol withdrawal managed using, 264
    anxiety managed using, 282, 284
    mechanism of action, 284
    physical dependence on, 268, 285
    psychological dependence on, 266, 268, 284–285
    toxicity associated with, 285
    withdrawal from, 368
Benzoyl peroxide, 46t
Beta-adrenergic agonists, 264
Beta-2 agonists, 90, 92t, 344t
Beta blockers
    acute myocardial infarction treated with, 118
    asthma treated with, 90
Beta-lactamases, 78
Beta-lactams, 102t
Betamethasone dipropionate, 43t
Beta$_1$ receptors, 90
Biguanides, 216–217, 219t
Bilirubin
    conjugated, 144
    unconjugated, 144
Binge eating disorder, 271
Bipolar disorder
    I, 281
    II, 281
    questions about, 272–273
    symptoms of, 280–281
    treatment of, 281
Bisphosphonates, 195
Bite wounds, 47, 48t
Black cohosh, 298
Bladder cancer, 128
Bladder outlet obstruction, 153

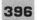

Blood coagulation, 203
Blood pressure
  elevated. *See* Hypertension
  measurement of, 106
  screening of, 3t
Blood urea nitrogen, 145–146
Borrelia burgdorferi, 257–258
Breakthrough bleeding, 289, 292
Breast cancer, 19t
Breast-feeding
  alcohol ingestion during, 314, 316
  guidelines for, 315b
  Hale's Lactation Risk Category, 367, 373t
  medication use during, 315–316
  nicotine use during, 316
  prevalence of, 314
  questions about, 313–314
  recommendations for, 3t
Breast milk
  benefits of, 314
  drug passage through, 314
Breast self-examination, 19t
Bronchiolitis, 330
Bronchospasm, 89–90, 371
Brudzinski sign, 30
Bulimia nervosa, 269–271
Bullae, 40t
Bupropion, 271, 278t, 368
Burns, 49
Bursitis, 169–171, 170t
Buspirone (BuSpar), 267t, 281

C

CAGE questionnaire, 262, 262b
Calcipotriene, 56
Calcitonin, 195
Calcium channel blockers, 107
Calcium intake
  osteoporosis prevention and, 194
  during pregnancy, 360–361
  recommendations for, 3t
Cancer
  American Cancer Society detection guidelines for,
    19t–20t
  bladder, 128
  breast, 19t
  cervical, 19t
  colorectal
    American Cancer Society detection guidelines for,
      19t
    description of, 131–132
    screening for, 3t
  endometrial, 20t
  oral, 72
  pancreatic, 234
  prostate, 161–162
Candida sp., 64

Candidiasis, 306t
Capillary hemangioma, 330–332
Carbamazepine, 35, 264
Cardiac rhythm disturbances, 188
Cardiovascular disease, 3t
Cardiovascular evaluation, before sports participation
  aortic regurgitation, 190t
  aortic stenosis, 188, 189t, 192
  atrial septal defect, 191t, 193
  cardiac rhythm disturbances, 188
  hypertension, 188
  hypertrophic cardiomyopathy, 191t, 193
  mitral regurgitation, 190t, 192
  mitral stenosis, 189t, 192
  mitral valve prolapse, 190t, 192
  murmurs, 188, 189t
  overview of, 187–188
  questions about, 186–187
  Still murmur, 191t
  ventricular septal defect, 191t, 193
Carpal tunnel syndrome, 181–182
Cat bite, 48t
Cefdinir, 85t
Cefpodoxime proxetil, 85t
Ceftriaxone, 354
Cefuroxime axetil, 85t
Celexa. *See* Citalopram
Cellulitis, 50, 70
Cephalosporins, 337
Certification examinations
  advice about, 388–389
  agencies that offer, 383
  anxiety before, 387–388
  differences among, 384
  guidelines for taking, 389–390
  multiple-choice questions on, 385–386
  pass rates for, 384
  questions on, 384–385
  recommendations for, 389–391
  structure of, 383
  studying for, 391
  tips for, 391–392
Certirizine, 51
Cervical disk lesion, 183–184
Cervix
  cancer of, 19t
  dilation of, 381
  pregnancy-related changes in, 363t
Chalazion, 70
Chancroid, 155, 156t, 306
Chemoprophylaxis, 2
Chest disorders
  asthma. *See* Asthma
  chronic obstructive pulmonary disease. *See* Chronic
    obstructive pulmonary disease
  congestive heart failure, 120–123
  heart murmurs. *See* Heart murmurs

hypertension, 104–107
pneumonia. *See* Pneumonia
tuberculosis, 97–100
Chickenpox, 14, 52. *See also* Varicella
Childbirth, 381
Children. *See also* Infants
  acute febrile illness in, 352–353
  acute otitis media in. *See* Acute otitis media
  aortic stenosis in, 112, 350t
  asthma in, 91f
  bacterial endocarditis prophylaxis in, 113t
  ear infections in. *See* Acute otitis media
  heart murmurs, 348
  Kawasaki disease in, 356–357
  lead poisoning in, 328–330
  pneumonia in, 355–356
  urinary tract infections in, 335–337
Chlamydial infection
  description of, 305
  screening for, 3t
Chlamydia trachomatis, 305
Cholecystectomy, 131
Cholecystitis, acute, 129–131
Cholelithiasis, 129
Cholesterol screening, 3t
Cholestyramine, 226t
Cholinesterase inhibitors, 38
Chondroitin, 176
Chronic bronchitis, 94
Chronic lymphocytic thyroiditis, 238
Chronic obstructive pulmonary disease
  chronic bronchitis associated with, 94
  clinical presentation of, 94–95
  corticosteroids for, 96, 97t
  definition of, 94
  emphysema associated with, 94
  exacerbations, 96, 97t
  management of, 95t–96t, 95–96
  questions about, 93–94
  stages of, 95t–96t
Chronic progressive multiple sclerosis, 32
Chronic prostatitis, 158t
Chronic renal failure
  description of, 146
  diabetes mellitus and, 221
Chronic venous insufficiency, 213
Cilostazol, 210
Cimetidine, 136
Circadian rhythms, 89, 342
Cirrhosis, 136
Citalopram, 276t
Claritin. *See* Loratadine
Clobetasol propionate, 43t
Clonazepam, 268t, 368
Clonidine, 269
Clostridium tetani, 14, 326
Clotting factors, 203

Cluster headache, 25t, 26
Coagulation, 203
Coagulation factors, 203
Coalescent, 40t
Coarctation of the aorta, 350t
Cocaine, 265, 269
Colchicine, 173
Colestipol, 226t
Colorectal cancer
  American Cancer Society detection guidelines for, 19t
  description of, 131–132
  screening for, 3t
Community-acquired cystitis, 150
Community-acquired pneumonia, 355–356
Complex partial seizure, 35t
Condyloma acuminatum, 157t, 166, 308t, 309–310
Confluent, 40t
Congestive heart failure
  clinical presentation of, 122
  laboratory testing in, 122
  pathophysiology of, 122
  questions about, 120–121
  treatment of, 122–123
Conjugated bilirubin, 144
Conjunctivitis
  allergic, 81t
  bacterial, 65, 66t
Contraception
  contraceptive patch, 291, 293
  diaphragm, 290, 294–295
  DMPA, 290, 293, 315
  emergency, 295–296, 296b
  estrogen-progestin injection, 293–294
  hormonal, 290
  intrauterine device, 290, 294, 296
  oral contraceptives. *See* Oral contraceptives
  postpartum, 315
  questions about, 289–291
Contrast venography, 204
COPD. *See* Chronic obstructive pulmonary disease
Coronary artery disease, 116, 116t
Corticosteroids
  allergic rhinitis treated with, 80, 82t
  anaphylaxis treated with, 243t
  asthma treated with, 90, 92t, 343t, 371
  atopic dermatitis treated with, 51
  Bell palsy treated with, 23
  chronic obstructive pulmonary disease treated with, 96, 97t
  definition of, 42
  giant cell arteritis treated with, 64
  gouty arthritis treated with, 173
  Menière disease treated with, 72
  psoriasis vulgaris treated with, 56
  types of, 43t
Cortisone, 97t
Corynebacterium diphtheriae, 15, 326

Counseling
   alcohol abuse, 262–263
   approach to, 18b
COX-1, 137, 177, 180
COX-2, 137, 177, 180
Cranial nerves, 21–22
C-reactive protein, 179
Creatine kinase-MB, 118
Creatine phosphokinase, 118
Creatinine, 145, 221
Cromolyn sodium, 92t, 343t
Cutaneous drug absorption, 42
Cyanocobalamin, 250
Cyclooxygenase-1, 137, 177, 180
Cyclooxygenase-2, 137, 177, 180
Cystitis
   community-acquired, 150
   hemorrhagic, 148
Cytochrome P-450, 35, 53

D

Dawn phenomenon, 220
Decongestants, 243t
Deep vein thrombophlebitis
   acute, 204
   chronic venous insufficiency secondary to, 213
   clinical presentation of, 204, 205t
   heparin for, 206–207
   pulmonary embolus caused by, 209
   questions about, 202
   treatment of, 206
   warfarin for, 207, 208t
Dehydration, 346, 346t
Delirium, 37–38
Dementia
   depression vs., 274
   description of, 38
Depo-Provera, 290, 293, 315
Depression
   antidepressants for, 275–277, 276t–277t
   anxiety associated with, 274, 283–284
   dementia vs., 274
   diagnostic criteria for, 273–274
   dysthymia, 272, 274
   herbal medications for, 286, 287t
   life stressors as cause of, 274–275
   prevalence of, 273
   questions about, 272–273
   relapse of, 275b
   signs and symptoms of, 273–274
   treatment of, 274
Dermatitis
   atopic, 51, 332
   seborrheic, 56–57
Dermatomal, 40t
Desoximetasone, 43t
Dexamethasone, 97t

Diabetes mellitus
   American Diabetes Association diagnosis of, 228–229
   chronic renal failure caused by, 221
   hyperglycemia in, 216, 218
   hypertension and, 216
   microalbuminuria
      questions about, 216–217
      screening for, 221–222
      treatment of, 217
   questions about, 215–218
   type 1
      characteristics of, 218
      clinical presentation of, 216
      dietary guidelines for, 219
      insulin for. *See* Insulin
   type 2
   alpha-glucosidase inhibitors for, 219t, 221
      diagnostic criteria for, 216
      dietary guidelines for, 219
      insulin resistance and, 218
      lifestyle changes for, 219
      meglitinides for, 219t, 221
      metformin for, 219t, 220–221
      obesity and, 218, 228
      risk factors for, 218–219
      screenings for, 219
      sulfonylureas for, 219t, 220
      testing for, 216
      thiazolidinediones for, 217, 219t, 221
      treatment of, 219t
Diabetic nephropathy, 221
Diaphragm, 290, 294–295
Diazepam, 264, 268t
Digoxin, 123
Dihydroergotamine, 27–28
Disease-modifying antirheumatic drugs, 179
Disk herniation, 183–184
Distance vision, 86
Diuretics
   congestive heart failure treated with, 123
   hypertension treated with, 106
Diverticulitis, 132–133
Diverticulosis, 132–133
Dix-Hallpike test, 72
DMPA, 290, 293, 315
Dog bite, 48t
Domestic violence
   description of, 286–288
   during pregnancy, 376–378
Down syndrome, 365–366
Doxycycline, 85t
Drithocreme. *See* Anthralin
Drospirenone, 293
Drusen, 86
Duodenal ulcer, 134–136, 135t
Duoderm. *See* Hydrocolloid gel
Dysthymia, 272, 274

E

Ear disorders
    acute otitis media, 66t, 74–75, 332–335
    Menière disease, 71–72
    otitis externa, 66t, 73
    presbycusis, 85–86
Ear infections. *See* Acute otitis media
Eating disorders, 269–271
Eclampsia, 375t
Ectopic pregnancy, 378–380
Eczema, 51, 331–332
Education, 18b
Edwards syndrome, 364–366
Effexor. *See* Venlafaxine
Egg allergy, 9
Elimite. *See* Permethrin
Emergency contraception, 295–296, 296b
Emphysema, 94
Endocarditis, 113t
Endometrial cancer, 20t
Epicondylitis
    lateral, 171, 172t
    medial, 172t
Epididymitis, acute, 159
Epididymoorchitis, 159
Epigastric pain, 129
Epinephrine, 243t
Epistaxis, 67
Epstein-Barr virus mononucleosis, 254, 257t, 340t
Erectile dysfunction, 166–167
Ergotamines, 28
Erosion, 40t
Erosive gastritis, 135t
Erythema toxicum neonatorum, 331
Erythrocyte sedimentation rate, 179
Erythromycin, 78
Erythropoietin, 146, 245, 251
Escherichia coli, 150
Escitalopram, 276t
Esophagus
    Barrett, 138
    gastroesophageal reflux disease-related injury to,
      138
Estrogen deficiency
    osteoporosis caused by, 194, 300
    vaginitis, 297, 300
Estrogen-progestin injection, 293–294
Estrogen receptors, 298–299
Euglycemia, 218
Eustachian tube dysfunction, 333
Eustachian tube obstruction, 333
Excedrin Migraine, 28
Excoriation, 40t
Exudative pharyngitis, 67t, 77, 338
Eye disorders
    chalazion, 70
    conjunctivitis, 65, 66t
    glaucoma, 68–69, 69f
    hordeolum, 70
    macular degeneration, 86
    open-angle glaucoma, 68–69, 69f
    ophthalmologic emergency, 68
    presbyopia, 86
Ezetimibe, 224, 226t

F

Facial nerve, 22
Febrile seizure, 352
Fecal occult blood test, 19t
Ferrous sulfate, 243, 361
Fetal alcohol syndrome, 361
Fever
    antipyretics for, 353
    causes of, 352–353
    description of, 352
    incidence of, 352–353
    in infants, 354t
    questions about, 348, 351
Fibrates, 224
Fibric acid derivatives, 226t
Fibrinolysis, 118, 119t
Fifth disease, 257t, 340t
Finasteride, 154
Fioricet, 28
First-degree burn, 49
First-generation antihistamines, 43
Fissure, 40t, 125–126
Flunitrazepam, 265–266, 269
Fluocinolone acetonide, 43t
Fluoroquinolones
    acute bacterial rhinosinusitis treated with, 85t
    bacterial pharyngitis treated with, 78
    otitis externa treated with, 73
Fluorouracil cream, 58
Fluoxetine, 272, 277t
Fluvoxamine, 276t
Folate-deficiency anemia
    causes of, 249
    overview of, 248–249
    questions about, 244
Folic acid
    deficiency of, 361
    description of, 248–249
    intake recommendations, 3t
    maternal deficiency of, 249
    during pregnancy, 249, 360–361
Follicle-stimulating hormone, 291, 299
Food allergies, 242
Foradil. *See* Formoterol
Forced expiratory volume in 1 second, 89
Forced vital capacity, 89
Formoterol, 92t, 344t
Formula-feeding, 313
Fukuda marching step test, 72

G

Gallstones, 129
Gamma-aminobutyric acid, 284
Gamma glutamyl transferase, 129, 130t
Gastric acid, 134
Gastric acid neutralization, 136
Gastric bypass, for obesity, 232–233
Gastric emptying, 138
Gastritis, 135t
Gastroenteritis, acute, 345–346
Gastroesophageal reflux disease, 138–139
Gastrointestinal irritation, 134
Gastropathy, 137, 176–177
Gemfibrozil, 226t
General adaptation syndrome, 387
Generalized anxiety disorder, 282, 283
Genital herpes, 156t
Genital warts, 157t, 166, 308t
Genitourinary infections
    bacterial vaginosis, 302–303, 306t
    candidiasis, 306t
    chancroid, 155, 156t, 306
    condyloma acuminatum, 157t, 166, 308t, 309–310
    genital warts, 157t, 166, 308t
    gonococcal urethritis, 157t, 307t
    human herpesvirus-2, 305, 306t
    lymphogranuloma venereum, 155, 156t, 158, 307
    nongonococcal urethritis, 156t, 307t
    pelvic inflammatory disease, 307t, 308–309
    syphilis, 164, 165t, 310–311
    trichomoniasis, 157t, 304, 307t
GERD. *See* Gastroesophageal reflux disease
Gestational hypertension, 375t
Giant cell arteritis, 63–64
Glaucoma, 68–69, 69f
Glomerulonephritis, 145, 146t
Glossopharyngeal nerve, 22
Glucosamine, 175–176
Glycated hemoglobin, 222
Gonococcal infection, 304–305
Gonococcal urethritis, 157t, 307t
Gonorrhea, 159–160, 305
Gout, 173
Gouty arthritis, 171–174
Graves disease, 235, 239
Group A beta-hemolytic streptococcus, 76
Group B streptococcus, 374–376

H

Haemophilus ducreyi, 155
Haemophilus influenzae
    otitis media caused by, 75, 333
    pneumonia caused by, 102, 104
    treatment for, 104
Hale's Lactation Risk Category, 367, 373t
Halobetasol propionate, 43t
Hand, foot, and mouth disease, 256t, 339t

Hashimoto thyroiditis, 238
Headache
    clinical presentation of, 25t
    cluster, 25t, 26
    description of, 24–25
    diagnosis of, 25t
    maternal, during pregnancy, 368, 372
    migraine
        abortive agents for, 26–27
        with aura, 25t, 26
        treatment of, 26–29
        without aura, 25t, 25–26
    neuroimaging evaluations, 25, 27t
    prophylactic therapy for, 29, 29t
    secondary, 29
    signs of, 26t
    tension-type
        characteristics of, 25t
        treatment of, 28
    treatment of
        goals for, 26–27
        lifestyle modifications, 29t
        medications for, 27–28, 29t
        prophylactic, 29, 29t
Hearing loss, 85–86
Hearing screening, 3t
Heart failure. *See* Congestive heart failure
Heart murmurs
    in children, 348, 349t–350t
    definition of, 109
    description of, 188, 189t, 246
    physiologic, 109, 110t
    types of, 110t–111t
Heart sounds, 115–116
Heat stroke, 222–223
Helicobacter pylori, 134, 135t
HELLP syndrome, 374–375, 375t
Hematuria, 128
Hemic murmur, 246, 349t
Hemoglobin A1C, 216, 222
Hemogram, 245–246
Hemorrhagic cystitis, 148
Hemorrhoids, 125–126
Heparin
    deep vein thrombophlebitis treated with, 206, 206t
    low-molecular-weight, 202, 206–207
    unfractionated, 202, 206–207
Hepatic enzymes
    in acute cholecystitis, 130t
    in hepatitis B, 142–143
Hepatitis A
    description of, 15–16, 141, 141t, 327
    treatment of, 144
    vaccination for, 4t, 5, 15–16, 17t, 322f, 327
Hepatitis B
    description of, 11, 141t, 142–143
    immune globulin, 11, 325

prevention of, 11
treatment of, 144
vaccination for, 4t, 5, 11, 11t, 17t, 322f, 324–325
viral structure of, 324
Hepatitis C, 142t, 143–144
Hepatitis D, 142t, 143
Hepatoiminodiacetic acid, 129
Herbal medications, 286, 287t
Hereditary nonpolyposis colon cancer, 20t
Herpes zoster, 52
High-density lipoprotein-cholesterol, 120t
Histamine 1 receptor, 43
Histamine 2 receptor antagonists, 248t
HIV
   acute retroviral syndrome, 253t
   clinical presentation of, 252
   counseling about, 253t, 253–254
   posttest counseling, 253t
   prejudice against, 252–253
   pretest counseling, 252t
   questions about, 251–252
   risk factors for, 252
   transmission of, 251–252
HMG-CoA reductase inhibitors, 224, 226t
Homan sign, 205t
Hordeolum, 70
Hormone therapy, postmenopausal, 297, 300
Hot flashes, 299, 301
H₂RA
   gastroesophageal reflux disease treated with, 139
   peptic ulcer disease treated with, 137
Human bite, 48t
Human herpesvirus-2, 305, 306t
Human herpesvirus-6, 256t, 339t
Human immunodeficiency virus. *See* HIV
Human papillomaviruses, 166–167, 309–310
Hydrocolloid gel, 59
Hydrocortisone, 43t, 97t
Hydrocortisone butyrate, 43t
Hydrocortisone valerate, 43t
Hydroxyzine, 51
Hyperbilirubinemia, 144
Hyperglycemia, 216, 218
Hyperinsulinemia, 227–228
Hyperlipidemia, 223–225, 226t–227t
Hypersensitivity reactions, 51, 55t, 60
Hypertension
   in African-Americans, 106–107
   angiotensin-converting enzyme inhibitors for, 106–107
   calcium channel blockers for, 107
   description of, 188
   diabetes mellitus and, 216
   gestational, 375t
   JNC-7 guidelines for, 106–107
   during pregnancy, 374–376
   pulmonary, 111t
   questions about, 104–106, 223–224
   stages of, 106
   treatment of, 188
Hyperthyroidism
   characteristics of, 237t
   questions about, 235
Hypertrophic cardiomyopathy, 113, 187–188, 191t, 193
Hypochondria, 274
Hypoglossal nerve, 22
Hypothyroidism
   characteristics of, 237t
   questions about, 235
   subclinical, 239
   treatment of, 239

I

Imiquimod, 61t
Immune globulin
   description of, 2
   hepatitis B, 11, 325
   tetanus, 15
   varicella, 14
Immunizations
   Haemophilus influenzae type B, 322f
   hepatitis A, 4t, 5, 15–16, 17t, 322f, 327
   hepatitis B, 4t, 5, 11, 11t, 17t, 322f, 324–325
   influenza, 3t–4t, 5, 7, 17t, 321–323, 322f
   measles, mumps, rubella, 3t–4t, 5–6, 8–9, 17t, 320–321, 322f
   meningococcal, 6, 17t
   pneumococcal, 3t–4t, 5, 9–10, 17t, 322f, 356
   poliovirus, 16, 322f, 328
   as primary prevention, 2
   recommendations for, 3t, 17t, 322f
   tetanus-diphtheria, 3t–4t, 5, 14–15, 17t, 322f, 326–327
   varicella, 3t–4t, 6, 12, 14, 17t, 322f, 325–326
Immunoglobulin E antibodies, 242
Immunoglobulin E-mediated hypersensitivity reaction, 55t, 60
Impetigo, 44
Impotency. *See* Erectile dysfunction
Inactivated poliovirus vaccine, 16, 322f, 328
Incomplete abortion, 380
Incontinence
   stress, 303t
   transient, 303t
   urge, 301–302, 303t
Inevitable abortion, 380
Infants. *See also* Children
   acute otitis media in. *See* Acute otitis media
   aortic stenosis in, 112, 350t
   asthma in, 91f
   breast-feeding of, 313–316
   bronchiolitis in, 330
   dermatologic conditions in, 330–332
   developmental milestones for, 316–317, 318t–319t

ear infections in. *See* Acute otitis media
fever in, 354t
hepatitis B in, 11
immunizations for. *See* Immunizations
lead poisoning in, 328–330
parental anticipatory guidance for, 317, 320
urinary tract infections in, 335–337
weight gain by, 314
Infectious diarrhea, 186
Infectious mononucleosis, 254–255, 257t, 338, 340t
Influenza
  attenuated influenza vaccine, 7, 323
  clinical features of, 7, 323
  treatment of, 7–8
  vaccination for, 3t–4t, 5, 7, 17t, 321–323, 322f
Insulin
  dawn phenomenon associated with, 220
  diabetes mellitus type 1 treated with, 219–220, 220t
  extended-acting, 220t
  intermediate-acting, 220t
  pharmacokinetics of, 220t
  pregnancy-related changes in, 363t
  short-acting, 220t
  Somogyi effect, 216, 220
  types of, 220t
  weight loss effects on, 229
Insulin G, 215
Insulin glargine, 220t
Insulin resistance
  acanthosis nigricans and, 228
  conditions associated with, 218, 228
  definition of, 218
  exercise and, 216, 219, 227, 229
  hypertension and, 229
  mechanism of action, 228
  metabolic syndrome and, 229
  obesity and, 218, 228
  prothrombotic and proatherogenic states associated
    with, 228
  treatment of, 229
Intal. *See* Cromolyn sodium
Interferon β-1a, 32
Interferon β-1b, 32
International normalized ratio, 207–208, 208t–209t
Interpersonal violence
  description of, 287–288
  during pregnancy, 376–378
Intrauterine device, 290, 294, 297
Intrinsic factor, 249
Ipratropium bromide
  asthma treated with, 93t, 344t
  chronic obstructive pulmonary disease treated with,
    95
Iron
  daily requirements, 247
  during pregnancy, 361
  supplements, 243

Iron-deficiency anemia
  causes of, 247
  iron therapy for, 247–248, 248t
  laboratory diagnosis of, 247
  questions about, 242–243
Isoniazid, 99
Isotretinoin, 46t, 47
Itching, 51
Itraconazole, 53

J

Joint replacement, for osteoarthritis, 176

K

Kava kava, 287t
Kawasaki disease, 356–357
Keratolytic agents, for warts, 61t
Kernig sign, 30–31
Klebsiella pneumoniae, 103
Klonopin. *See* Clonazepam
Kwell. *See* Lindane

L

Labor, 381
Lactic acidosis, 217
Lactobacilli, 150
Lamisil. *See* Terbinafine
Lansoprazole, 136
Laser therapy, 61t
Latent tuberculosis, 98
Lateral epicondylitis, 171, 172t
Latex allergy, 241
Lead poisoning, 328–330
Left bundle branch block, 118
Legionella sp., 102–103
Leukocyte esterase, 149t
Leukocytosis, 127, 354
Leukotriene antagonists, 343t
Leukotriene modifiers, 341, 343t, 344
Leukotriene receptor antagonists, 90, 92t, 93
Levalbuterol, 342
Levodopa, 33, 248t
Levonorgestrel intrauterine system, 291
Levothyroxine, 236, 238–239
Lichenification, 40t
Lindane, 54
Linear, 40t
Lipase, 234, 234t
Lipoproteins, 119, 120t
Liquid nitrogen, for warts, 61t
Lispro, 215
Liver enzymes
  in acute cholecystitis, 130t
  in hepatitis B, 142–143
Loratadine, 80
Lorazepam, 264, 267t
Low back pain, 183–185, 185t

Low-density lipoprotein-cholesterol, 120t
Lower extremity vascular disease
    acute limb ischemia caused by, 212
    aspirin therapy for, 212
    clinical presentation of, 211t
    diagnosis of, 211–212
    questions about, 209–210
    treatment of, 212
    venous stasis ulcers secondary to, 213
Low-molecular-weight heparin, 202, 206–207
Lumbar disk herniation, 183–184
Lumbar radiculopathy, 183
Lumbosacral strain, 183–184
Luteinizing hormone, 299
Luvox. See Fluvoxamine
Lyme disease, 257–259
Lymphadenopathy, 72, 255
Lymphogranuloma venereum, 155, 156t, 158, 307

M

Macular degeneration, 86
Macule, 40t
Magnetic resonance imaging
    meniscal tear evaluations, 181
    pancreatic cancer evaluations, 234
Malignant melanoma, 58
Malignant otitis externa, 66t
Mammography, 3t
Marijuana, 265, 269
Maxair. See Pirbuterol
McMurray test, 180–181
Mean corpuscular hemoglobin, 246
Measles, 256t, 339t
Measles, mumps, rubella
    questions about, 320
    vaccination against, 3t–4t, 5–6, 8–9, 17t, 320–321, 322f
Medial epicondylitis, 172t
Medroxyprogesterone acetate, 315
Meglitinides, 219t, 221
Ménière disease, 71–72
Ménière syndrome, 71
Meningitis
    description of, 30–31, 351
    treatment of, 354
Meningococcal vaccination, 6, 17t
Meniscal tear, 180–181
Menopause
    age of onset, 298
    androgen levels after, 299–300
    description of, 298
    estrogen deficiency associated with, 297, 300
    hot flashes associated with, 299, 301
    phytoestrogens for, 299
    postmenopausal hormone therapy, 297

questions about, 297–298
    vasomotor symptoms of, 299
Meridia. See Sibutramine
Metabolic syndrome
    definition of, 228
    insulin resistance and, 229
    questions about, 225–227
    terms for, 227–228
Metformin
    adverse effects of, 221
    description of, 229
    lactic acidosis associated with, 217
    questions about, 215, 227
    type 2 diabetes mellitus treated with, 219t, 220–221
Methicillin-sensitive Staphylococcus aureus, 44
Methylprednisolone, 97t
Metronidazole, 133, 309
Microalbuminuria
    description of, 106
    questions about, 216–217
    screening for, 221–222
    treatment of, 217
Midrin, 28
Migraine headache
    abortive agents for, 26–27
    with aura, 25t, 26
    treatment of
        goals for, 26–27
        medications, 27–29
    without aura, 25t, 25–26
Migrainous neuralgia, 26
Milia, 331
Mirtazapine, 278t
Mitral regurgitation, 111t, 112, 190t, 192
Mitral stenosis, 110t, 189t, 192
Mitral valve prolapse, 111t, 112–113, 190t, 192, 350t
Mongolian spots, 331
Monoamine oxidase inhibitors, 285–286
Mononucleosis, infectious, 254–255, 257t, 338, 340t
Montelukast, 92t
Moraxella catarrhalis, 75, 333–334
Multiple sclerosis, 32–33
Mupirocin, 44
Murmurs
    in children, 348, 349t–350t
    definition of, 109
    description of, 188, 189t, 246
    physiologic, 109, 110t
    types of, 110t–111t
Murphy's sign, 129
Mycobacterium tuberculosis, 98
Mycoplasma pneumoniae, 77
Myocardial infarction. See Acute myocardial infarction
Myoclonic seizure, 34

N

National Cholesterol Education Program, 228t
Nausea
    combined oral contraceptives and, 292
    during pregnancy, 371
Neck pain, 184–185
Nedocromil, 92t, 343t
Nefazodone, 278t
Neisseria gonorrhoeae, 157t, 160, 304
Neisseria meningitidis, 31
Neuralgia, 184
Neural tube defects, 244, 249, 360–361, 366
Neuroleptics, 28
Neurologic disorders
    headache. *See* Headache
    meningitis, 30–31
    multiple sclerosis, 32–33
    seizures, 34t, 34–35
    transient ischemic attack, 35–36
Neutrophilia, 127, 354
Newborns. *See* Infants
Niacin, 224, 226t
Nicotine, 316
Nitrates, 115
Nitrite test, 148, 149t
Nitrofurantoin, 152, 373
Nodule, 40t
Nonerosive gastritis, 135t
Nongonococcal urethritis, 156t, 307
Nonoxynol-9, 150, 291, 295
Nonsteroidal anti-inflammatory drugs
    carpal tunnel syndrome managed using, 182
    gastropathy induced by, 137, 176–177
    gouty arthritis treated with, 173
    headaches treated with, 28
    mechanism of action, 180
    osteoarthritis treated with, 175
    Reiter syndrome treated with, 186
    rheumatoid arthritis treated with, 179–180
    tendonitis treated with, 198
Nurse practitioner certification examinations. *See* Certification examinations

O

Obesity
    causes of, 230–231
    change strategies for, 232t
    classification of, 231t
    consequences of, 231
    gastric bypass for, 232–233
    incidence of, 230–231
    insulin resistance and, 218, 228
    pharmacotherapy for, 231–232
    questions about, 226–227, 230
    screening for, 3t
    sibutramine for, 231
    treatment of, 231

Obturator sign, 126
Oculomotor nerve, 21
Olecranon bursitis, 169, 170t
Olfactory nerve, 21
Omeprazole, 136
Ondansetron, 371
Onychomycosis, 53
Open-angle glaucoma, 68–69, 69f
Ophthalmologic emergency, 68
Opioids
    abuse of, 265
    migraine headaches treated with, 28–29
    withdrawal from, 268–269
Optic nerve, 21
Oral cancer, 72
Oral contraceptives
    combined
        breakthrough bleeding caused by, 289, 292
        discontinuation of, 291
        drug interactions, 292–293
        mechanism of action, 291
        missed, 292f
        nausea associated with, 292
        noncontraceptive benefits of, 292
        World Health Organization precautions for, 294t
    description of, 46t
    progestin-only pill, 289, 293, 315
    questions about, 289–290
    World Health Organization precautions for, 294t
Orlistat, 231
Oseltamivir, 7–8
Osteoarthritis, 174–176
Osteoporosis
    calcium intake to prevent, 194
    definition of, 194
    estrogen deficiency and, 194, 300
    questions about, 193–194
    risk factors for, 195t
    screening for, 3t, 193, 195t
    treatment of, 195, 195t
Otitis externa, 66t, 73
Otitis media
    acute
        in children, 332–335
        definition of, 334
        description of, 66t, 74–75
        fever reduction in, 351
        Haemophilus influenzae and, 75, 333
        pathogens, 333
        questions about, 332–333
        recurrent, 332
        risk factors for, 333–334
        signs and symptoms of, 334
        Streptococcus pneumoniae and, 74–75, 333–334
        treatment of, 334–335
    with effusion, 75, 333, 334t, 335

Oxazepam, 267t, 284
Oxybutynin, 302

P

Pain
    chest, 116t
    epigastric, 129
    low back, 183–185, 185t
    neck, 184–185
Pancreatic cancer, 234
Pancreatitis, 233–234
Panic attack, 285
Panic disorder, 282, 285
Papilledema, 69
Pap smear, 3t, 19t
Papule, 40t
Parental anticipatory guidance, 317, 320
Parietal cells, 134
Parkinson disease, 32–33
Paroxetine, 276t
Partial seizures, 35t
Parvovirus-B19, 257t, 340t
Patch, 40t
Patent ductus arteriosus, 350t
Patient education, 18b
Paxil. *See* Paroxetine
Pediatrics. *See* Children; Infants
Pelvic inflammatory disease, 307t, 308–309
Penicillin, 78
Peptic ulcer disease
    areas of, 134
    assessment of, 135t
    clinical presentation of, 134
    treatment of, 136–137
Perimenopause
    definition of, 298
    oral contraceptives for symptoms of, 299
    questions about, 297–298
Peripheral vascular disease
    aspirin therapy for, 212
    clinical presentation of, 211t
    definition of, 210
    questions about, 209–210
    risk factors for, 209–210
    treatment of, 212
    venous stasis ulcers secondary to, 213
Permethrin, 54
Pernicious anemia, 244
Persistent allergic conjunctivitis, 81t
Phalen sign, 181–182
Pharyngitis
    description of, 255
    exudative, 67t, 77, 338
    streptococcal, 337
Phenytoin
    acne caused by, 47
    seizures treated with, 35

Physiologic murmurs, 188, 189t
Phytoestrogens, 299
Pica, 360–362
Pilocarpine, 69
Pirbuterol, 92t, 342, 343t
Pityrosporum ovale, 57
Placental transfer of medications, 366–367, 370
Plaque, 40t
Plasminogen activator inhibitor, 226
Pleocytosis, 30–31, 354
Pletal. *See* Cilostazol
Plumbism, 328–329
Pneumatic otoscopy, 71–72
Pneumococcal disease
    description of, 10
    vaccination against, 3t–4t, 5, 9–10, 17t, 322f, 356
Pneumocystis carinii pneumonia, 150
Pneumonia
    in children, 355–356
    clinical features of, 102
    community-acquired, 355–356
    epidemiology of, 102
    Haemophilus influenzae, 102, 104
    mortality risks, 103
    pathogens associated with, 102–103, 355–356
    questions about, 100–101, 355
    signs and symptoms of, 355
    Streptococcus pneumoniae, 102–104
    treatment of, 102t, 103–104
Podophyllum resin, for warts, 61t
Polioviruses, 16, 322f, 328
Polycystic ovary syndrome, 228
Polymyalgia rheumatica, 64
Port-wine stain, 331
Posterior tibial reflex, 183
Post-herpetic neuralgia, 52
Postmenopausal hormone therapy, 297, 300
Postpartum contraception, 315
Postrenal azotemia, 145
Post-traumatic stress disorder, 282–283, 286
Pre-Achilles bursitis, 169, 170t
Precocious puberty, 346–348
Prednisolone, 97t
Prednisone, 97t
Preeclampsia, 374–375, 375t
Pregnancy
    anemia during, 360
    antidepressant use during, 372
    antimicrobials used during, 373
    asthma during, 367–368, 370–371
    asymptomatic bacteriuria during, 369, 372–373
    bronchospasms during, 371
    calcium intake during, 360–361
    cardiovascular system changes during, 363t
    contraception after, 315
    digestive system changes during, 363t
    domestic violence during, 376–378

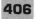

Pregnancy *(Continued)*
  ectopic, 378–380
  endocrine system changes during, 363t
  folic acid intake during, 249, 360–361
  headaches during, 368, 372
  hematologic system changes during, 363t
  hypertensive disorders during, 374–376
  influenza vaccination during, 7
  interpersonal violence during, 376–378
  iron requirements during, 360–361
  labor and delivery, 381
  medications during
    placental transfer of, 366–367, 370
    risk categories for, 370, 371t
    teratogenic, 369–370
  metabolic changes during, 363t
  migraine headaches during, 368, 372
  nausea and vomiting during, 371
  parental anticipatory guidance, 317, 320
  physiologic changes during, 362, 363t
  pica during, 360–362
  preeclampsia during, 374–375, 375t
  prenatal care, 362, 364t–365t
  prenatal screenings, 365–366
  questions about, 359–360
  renal changes during, 363t
  respiratory system changes during, 363t
  selective serotonin reuptake inhibitors during, 367–368, 372
  teratogenic periods during, 369–370
  urinary tract infections during, 367, 369, 372–373
  vaccinations during, 4t
  violence during, 376–378
  weight gain during, 360, 364t
Pregnancy-induced carpal tunnel syndrome, 182
Premature thelarche, 347
Prenatal care, 362, 364t–365t
Prerenal azotemia, 145
Presbycusis, 85–86
Presbyopia, 86
Preschoolers, 319
Prevacid. *See* Lansoprazole
Prevention
  primary, 2, 98–99
  secondary, 2
  tertiary, 2
Prilosec. *See* Omeprazole
Primary prevention, 2, 98–99
Progestin-only pill, 289, 293, 315
Propionibacterium acnes, 45
Prostate cancer, 20t, 161–162
Prostate gland
  alpha₁ receptor sites in, 153
  benign prostatic hypertrophy, 153–154
Prostate-specific antigen, 20t, 161–162
Prostatitis

  acute, 157t, 160–161
  chronic, 158t
Prosthetic heart valves, 113, 113t
Protein C, 203
Protein S, 203
Prothrombin time, 207–208
Proton pump inhibitors, 136–137
Proventil. *See* Albuterol
Prozac. *See* Fluoxetine
Pruritus, 51
Pseudomonas aeruginosa
  otitis externa caused by, 73
  pneumonia caused by, 103
Psoas sign, 126
Psoriasis vulgaris, 56
Pteroylglutamic acid. *See* Folic acid
Pulmonary embolus, 202, 205t, 209
Pulmonary hypertension, 111t
Pulmonary outflow ejection murmur, 349t
Pulmonary tuberculosis. *See* Tuberculosis
Pulmonic stenosis, 350t
Purpura, 40t
Pustule, 40t
Pyelonephritis, acute, 148

R

Rabies, 47, 48t
Raloxifene, 194, 301
Rat bite, 48t
Raynaud phenomenon, 199–200
Red blood cell(s), 149t, 246
Red blood cell distribution width, 246
Reflux esophagitis, 138
Reflux nephropathy, 337
Reiter syndrome, 185–186
Relapsing-remitting multiple sclerosis, 32
Remeron. *See* Mirtazapine
Renal failure
  description of, 145–146, 146t
  diabetes mellitus and, 221
Repaglinide, 221
Reperfusion, 118
Resins, 226t
Respiratory syncytial virus, 330
Reticular, 40t
Reticulocyte production index, 246–247, 247f
Reticulocytosis
  after folic acid therapy, 249
  after iron therapy, 248
Retinoic acid. *See* Tretinoin
Retrocalcaneal bursitis, 170t
Rheumatic fever, 77
Rheumatoid arthritis
  antinuclear antibodies associated with, 179
  definition of, 178
  diagnostic criteria for, 178, 178t

disease-modifying antirheumatic drugs for, 179
epidemiology of, 178
erythrocyte sedimentation rate evaluations, 179
nonsteroidal anti-inflammatory drugs for, 179–180
questions about, 176–177
tests for, 178–179
treatment of, 179–180
Rheumatoid factor, 179
Rhinitis, allergic
    description of, 80–81, 81t–82t
    treatment of, 81t–82t, 82f–83f
Rhinosinusitis, acute bacterial, 84, 85t
Rifampin, 85t
Rimantadine, 7
Rinne test, 71
Rohypnol. *See* Flunitrazepam
Romberg test, 72
Roseola, 256t, 339t
Rosiglitazone, 216
Rubella, 8–9, 256t, 321, 339t
Rubeola virus, 256t, 339t
Rule of nines, 49f

S

Salmeterol, 92t, 344t
Scabies, 54
Scale (skin lesion), 40t
Scarlet fever, 254, 256t, 339t
School-age children, 319
Sciatica, 184
Screenings, 3t
Seasonal allergic conjunctivitis, 81t
Seborrheic dermatitis, 56–57
Secondary prevention, 2
Second-degree burn, 49
Second-generation antihistamines, 43–44
Seizures, 34t, 34–35
Selective estrogen receptor modulator, 297, 301
Selective serotonin reuptake inhibitors
    eating disorders treated with, 271
    panic disorder treated with, 285
    during pregnancy, 367–368, 372
    sexual dysfunction caused by, 279
    side effects of, 277, 279
    tricyclic antidepressants vs., 280
    types of, 276t–277t
    withdrawal syndrome from, 273, 279–280, 367, 372
Sepsis
    evaluation for, 353–354
    laboratory findings in, 354
    questions about, 351
Serax. *See* Oxazepam
Serevent. *See* Salmeterol
Serotonin syndrome, 28
Sertraline, 272, 276t
Serzone. *See* Nefazodone

Sexually transmitted diseases
    chancroid, 155, 156t, 306
    condyloma acuminatum, 157t, 166, 308t, 309–310
    description of, 155
    genital herpes, 156t
    genital warts, 157t, 166, 308t
    gonorrhea, 159–160, 305
    lymphogranuloma venereum, 155, 156t, 158, 307
    syphilis, 164, 165t, 310–311
    trichomoniasis, 157t, 304, 307t
Shingles, 14, 52
Sibutramine, 231
Sildenafil, 167
Simple partial seizure, 35t
Singulair. *See* Montelukast
Sjögren syndrome, 180
Skin disorders
    antihistamines for, 43–44
    atopic dermatitis, 51
    bite wounds, 47, 48t
    burns, 49, 49f
    cellulitis, 50
    corticosteroids for, 42, 43t
    diagnosis of, 57–58
    herpes zoster, 52
    impetigo, 44
    onychomycosis, 53
    psoriasis vulgaris, 56
    scabies, 54
    seborrheic dermatitis, 56–57
    stasis ulcer, 59
    topical medications for, 41t, 41–42
    urticaria, 59–60
    verruca vulgaris, 60–61, 61t
Skin lesions, 40t
Smallpox, 12–13
Solar keratoses, 58
Somogyi effect, 216, 220
Sore throat, 76–78
Spermicides, 150, 295
Spider varicosities, 201
Spiriva. *See* Tiotropium bromide
Splenomegaly, 255
Spontaneous abortion, 378, 380
Sporanox. *See* Itraconazole
Sports participation, cardiovascular evaluation before
    aortic regurgitation, 190t
    aortic stenosis, 188, 189t, 192
    atrial septal defect, 191t, 193
    cardiac rhythm disturbances, 188
    hypertension, 188
    hypertrophic cardiomyopathy, 191t, 193
    mitral regurgitation, 190t, 192
    mitral stenosis, 189t, 192
    mitral valve prolapse, 190t, 192
    murmurs, 188, 189t

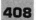

Sports participation *(Continued)*
 overview of, 187–188
 questions about, 186–187
 Still murmur, 191t
 ventricular septal defect, 191t, 193
Sprain, 196, 197t
St. John's wort, 287t
Staphylococcus aureus
 eye disorders caused by, 70
 methicillin-sensitive, 44
 pneumonia caused by, 103
Stasis ulcer, 59
Statin-induced myositis, 224
Still's murmur, 191t, 349t
Strain, lumbosacral, 183
Streptococcal pharyngitis, 337
Streptococcus pneumoniae
 acute bacterial rhinosinusitis caused by, 84
 acute otitis media caused by, 74–75, 333–334
 multidrug-resistant, 103, 334
 pneumococcal disease caused by, 10
 pneumonia caused by, 102–104, 356
Streptococcus pyogenes, 76–78
Stress incontinence, 303t
Stroke, acute, 36, 37t
Stroke output, 109
ST-segment elevated myocardial infarction, 118, 119t
Stye. *See* Hordeolum
Subscapular bursitis, 169, 170t
Substance abuse
 alcohol. *See* Alcohol abuse
 benzodiazepines, 266, 268
 definition of, 266
 diagnostic criteria for, 266
 gender prevalence of, 266
 marijuana, 265, 269
 questions about, 265–266
 in women, 266
Sucralfate, 139
Sulfonylureas, 216, 219t, 220
Sumatriptan, 27–28
Sun protection factor, 58
Superficial thrombophlebitis, 201–204
Suppurative conjunctivitis, 66t
Swine bite, 48t
Syphilis, 164, 165t, 310–311

T

Tamoxifen, 301
Temporal arteritis, 63–64
Tendonitis, 196–198
Tennis elbow. *See* Lateral epicondylitis
Tension-type headache
 characteristics of, 25t
 treatment of, 28
Teratogenic medications, 367, 369–370
Terbinafine, 53

Terodiline, 302
Tertiary prevention, 2
Testicular torsion, 162–163
Tetanus-diphtheria vaccination, 3t–4t, 5, 14–15, 17t, 322f, 326–327
Tetracycline, 248t
Thelarche, premature, 347
Theophylline, 90, 93t, 342, 344t
Thiazide diuretics, 106
Thiazolidinediones, 217, 219t, 221, 227, 229
third-degree burn, 49
Threatened abortion, 380
Thrombolytic therapy, 209
Thrombophlebitis
 deep vein
  acute, 204
  chronic venous insufficiency secondary to, 213
  clinical presentation of, 204, 205t
  heparin for, 206–207
  pulmonary embolus caused by, 209
  questions about, 202
  treatment of, 206
  warfarin for, 207, 208t
 questions about, 202
 risk factors for, 201–204
 superficial, 201–204
 treatment of, 204
Thyroid disease
 description of, 237–238
 Graves disease, 235, 239
 hyperthyroidism, 235, 237t
 hypothyroidism, 235, 237t, 239
Thyroiditis, 238–239
Thyroid nodule, 239
Thyroid-stimulating hormone, 238
Thyroxine, 238–239
Tilade. *See* Nedocromil
Tinel sign, 181–182
Tiotropium bromide
 asthma treated with, 93t, 344t
 chronic obstructive pulmonary disease treated with, 95
Tissue factor, 203
Tonic-clonic seizure, 35t
Topical medications
 amount needed, 41, 41t
 delivery vehicles for, 42
Total cholesterol, 120t
Total iron-binding capacity, 247
Transcobalamin I and II, 249
Transient ischemic attack, 35–36
Trazodone, 279t
Treponema pallidum, 164, 311
Tretinoin
 acne vulgaris treated with, 46t
 warts treated with, 61t
Triamcinolone acetonide, 43t, 97t

Trichomoniasis, 157t, 304, 307t
Tricyclic antidepressants
    depression treated with, 277, 279t, 280
    panic disorder treated with, 285
    pregnancy risk classification of, 368–369, 372
Trigeminal nerve, 22
Triglycerides, 120t
Triiodothyronine, 238–239
Trimethoprim-sulfamethoxazole, 150, 151t, 152
Triple screen test, 366
Triptans, 27–28
Trochanteric bursitis, 169, 170t
Trochlear nerve, 22
Troponins, 118
TST. *See* Tuberculin skin test
Tuberculin skin test, 98–99
Tuberculosis
    definition of, 98
    isoniazid for, 99
    latent, 98
    prevention of, 98–99
    questions about, 97–98
    testing for, 98–99, 99t
    treatment of, 99–100
Type 1 diabetes mellitus
    characteristics of, 218
    clinical presentation of, 216
    dietary guidelines for, 219
    insulin for. *See* Insulin
Type 2 diabetes mellitus
    alpha-glucosidase inhibitors for, 219t, 221
    diagnostic criteria for, 216
    dietary guidelines for, 219
    insulin resistance and, 218
    lifestyle changes for, 219
    meglitinides for, 219t, 221
    metformin for, 219t, 220–221
    obesity and, 218, 228
    risk factors for, 218–219
    screenings for, 219
    sulfonylureas for, 219t, 220
    testing for, 216
    thiazolidinediones for, 217, 219t, 221
    treatment of, 219t
Type I hypersensitivity, 60
Tzanck smear, 52

U

Ulcer
    characteristics of, 40t
    duodenal, 134–136, 135t
    gastric, 135t
    stasis, 59, 210, 213
    venous stasis, 210, 213
Unconjugated bilirubin, 144
Unfractionated heparin, 202, 206–207
Unstable angina pectoris, 117t

Urethral obstruction, 303t
Urethritis
    gonococcal, 157t, 307t
    nongonococcal, 156t, 307t
Urge incontinence, 301–302, 303t
Urinalysis, for urinary tract infection diagnosis, 148, 149t, 336
Urinary continence, 304t
Urinary tract infections
    bladder emptying to reduce risk of, 148, 150
    in children, 335–337
    complicated, 147
    culture testing for, 148
    description of, 147
    diagnosis of, 147–148, 336
    nonoxynol-9 and, 150
    nonpharmacologic treatment of, 152
    pathogens, 150
    during pregnancy, 367, 369, 372–373
    prophylaxis, 151
    questions about, 335–336
    recurrence of, 151–152
    risk factors, 148
    signs and symptoms of, 148
    spermicides and, 150
    treatment of, 150, 151t
    trimethoprim-sulfamethoxazole for, 150, 151t, 152
    urinalysis testing for, 148, 149t
    urinary tract abnormalities as cause of, 337
Urticaria, 59–60
Uterus, 363t

V

Vaccinations. *See* Immunizations
Vaccine-associated paralytic poliomyelitis, 16, 328
Vaginitis
    atrophic, 300–301
    estrogen deficiency, 297, 300
Vaginosis, bacterial, 302–303, 306t
Vagus nerve, 22
Valerian root, 287t
Valium. *See* Diazepam
Vardenafil, 167
Varicella
    description of, 325
    smallpox vs., 12
    vaccination against, 3t–4t, 6, 12, 14, 17t, 322f, 325–326
Varicella-zoster virus, 13–14, 52
Varicocele, 163–164
Varicose veins, 200–201
Venlafaxine, 278t
Venous hum, 349t
Venous stasis ulcers, 210
Venous thromboembolism, 202–203
Ventolin. *See* Albuterol
Ventricular septal defect, 191t, 193, 350t

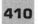

Verruca vulgaris, 60–61, 61t
Vesicle, 40t
Vesicoureteral reflux, 337
Vestibulocochlear nerve, 22
Violence
   description of, 286–288
   during pregnancy, 376–378
Virchow triad of venous stasis, 203–204
Vision screening, 3t
Vitamin B6, 299
Vitamin B$_{12}$, 249–250, 250t
Vitamin E, 299
Vitamin K, 207
Vomiting, during pregnancy, 371
Vulvovaginitis, 303

W

Warfarin
   deep vein thrombophlebitis treated with, 206t–208t
   drug interactions with, 207t
   food interactions with, 207t
   hemorrhage secondary to, 208–209
   indications for, 206t
   INR prolongation, 207–208, 208t–209t
   questions about, 202
Weber tuning test, 71
Wellbutrin. *See* Bupropion
Wheal, 40t
Withdrawal
   from alcohol
      benzodiazepines for, 264
      symptoms of, 263
   from benzodiazepines, 368
   from opioids, 268–269
   from selective serotonin reuptake inhibitors, 273, 279–280, 367, 372

X

Xanax. *See* Alprazolam

Z

Zafirlukast, 92t
Zanamivir, 7–8
Zetia. *See* Ezetimibe
Zoloft. *See* Sertraline
Zyrtec. *See* Certirizine